Adolescent Substance Abuse

Research and Clinical Advances

Adolescent drug abuse is one of the most challenging disorders to treat. It impacts on schools, community-based programs, mental health and medical facilities, and juvenile justice settings. This book provides practitioners, program developers, and policy makers with the most up-to-date and practical information for improving outcomes in adolescent substance abuse. The authors cover a range of issues, including empirically based treatment development protocols, how to incorporate innovative treatment models into diverse clinical settings, research advances, interventions with special populations, culturally based intervention guidelines, and recommendations for practice and policy.

Pre-publication comments on this book

There are some books that you wish you had the time to read and there are others that you simply make the time to read. This edited collection from Howard Liddle and Cynthia Rowe is of the "make-time-to-read" variety. Over the last few years many countries have witnessed a steady increase in adolescent drug abuse and are now looking to develop services that can meet the needs of these young people and their families. Liddle and Rowe have drawn on their own experience, over many years, to bring together some of the world's leading researchers and therapists in the field of adolescent drug abuse treatment. These authors were asked to set out the key achievements and future challenges in their field. The result is a book that will be an invaluable resource to all of those planning, researching and working in adolescent drug abuse treatment services for years to come.

Neil McKeganey
Professor of Drug Misuse Research
University of Glasgow

A hallmark of health services in the last decade has been the discovery that adolescence is different from adulthood, and that the methods to identify, treat, and prevent illness need to be different. Nowhere has this been more evident than in the substance abuse field. This book is evidence that this discovery has taken place and that the emergent field of adolescent substance abuse treatment is alive and well. It offers a comprehensive set of research-based summaries from the leaders in this area that needs to be read and thought about by anyone treating substance-abusing adolescents. It should also be extraordinarily useful for those involved in policy making.

Robert A. Zucker, Ph.D.
Professor of Psychology in Psychiatry and Psychology
Director, Substance Abuse Section, Department of Psychiatry,
Director, Addiction Research Center
University of Michigan

This monograph sits at the nexus of sophisticated research and statistical techniques, clinical practice and funding-policy addressing the challenging public health issues of adolescent substance use and sexual risk-taking. Many of the complex matters that make adolescent substance use an exemplar of the challenges and complexities that face those working with substance-use disorders in general, are taken up by the specialist researchers brought together in this book. It will be invaluable to all in the field as it not only offers scholarly literature reviews and discussions of developments in statistical and clinical practice and health service delivery, but the editors provide clear and reasonable suggestions in a call to action to promote the linkage of research and practice in adolescent substance use research, service delivery and policy development.

Dr. Jan Copeland
Senior Lecturer
National Drug and Alcohol Research Centre
School of Community Medicine and Public Health
University of South Wales

As substance misuse becomes increasingly prevalent in society, and particularly among the young, there is a need for authoritative evidence-based guidance on policy and treatment. Drs. Liddle and Rowe have provided the most comprehensive and timely review of the evidence base for treatment of adolescent substance abuse currently available. This will be of considerable value to clinicians, researchers and policy makers in this field as a state-of-the-art review of what is currently known, as well as identifying key gaps in knowledge and areas for future research. The assembled chapters will provide much needed impetus for the development of best practice in this field and stimulate rational service development internationally.

Professor Colin Drummond
St. George's Hospital Medical School
University of London

Adolescent Substance Abuse

Research and Clinical Advances

Edited by

Howard A. Liddle
University of Miami Miller School of Medicine Miami, USA

Cynthia L. Rowe
University of Miami Miller School of Medicine Miami, USA

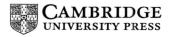

CAMBRIDGE
UNIVERSITY PRESS

CAMBRIDGE UNIVERSITY PRESS
Cambridge, New York, Melbourne, Madrid, Cape Town, Singapore,
São Paulo, Delhi, Dubai, Tokyo, Mexico City

Cambridge University Press
The Edinburgh Building, Cambridge CB2 8RU, UK

Published in the United States of America by Cambridge University Press, New York

www.cambridge.org
Information on this title: www.cambridge.org/9780521823586

© Cambridge University Press 2006

First published 2006
Reprinted 2007

A catalogue record for this publication is available from the British Library

ISBN 978-0-521-82358-6 Hardback
ISBN 978-0-521-53045-3 Paperback

Contents

Contributors

Dr. Marliyn Aguirre-Molina
Mailman School of Public Health,
Columbia University
60 Haven Avenue – B314,
New York, NY 10032, USA

Dr. Alison J. Boyd-Ball
Child and Family Center,
University of Oregon,
195 W. 12th Ave,
Eugene, OR 97403, USA

Dr. David W. Brook
New York University
School of Medicine,
215 Lexington Avenue, 15th Floor,
New York, NY 10016, USA

Dr. Judith S. Brook
New York University
School of Medicine,
215 Lexington Avenue, 15th Floor,
New York, NY 10016, USA

Dr. Sandra A. Brown
Department of Psychology,
University of California at San Diego,
9500 Gilman Drive, M/C 109
La Jolla, CA 92093-0109, USA

Dr. Oscar G. Bukstein
Child and Adolescent Psychiatry,
Western Psychiatric Institute and Clinic
of Presbyterian University Hospital,
3811 O'Hara St,
Pittsburgh, PA 15213, USA

Dr. Jack Cornelius
Child and Adolescent Psychiatry,
Western Psychiatric Institute and Clinic
of Presbyterian University Hospital,
3811 O'Hara St,
Pittsburgh, PA 15213, USA

Dr. Michael L. Dennis
Lighthouse Institute, Chestnut Health Systems,
720 West Chestnut,
Bloomington, IL 61701, USA

Dr. Jessy Dévieux
College of Health and Urban Affairs,
Florida International University,
AC1-260
Miami, FL 33199, USA

Dr. Thomas J. Dishion
Child and Family Center,
University of Oregon,
195 West 12th Avenue,
Eugene, OR 97401-3408, USA

Dr. Terry E. Duncan
Oregon Research Institute,
1715 Franklin Boulevard,
Eugene, OR 97403, USA

Dr. Susan C. Duncan
Oregon Research Institute,
1715 Franklin Boulevard,
Eugene, OR 97403, USA

Dr. Cecilia A. Essau
School of Human and Life Sciences,
Roehampton University,
Whitelands College, West Hill,
London SW15 3SN, UK

Dr. Jerry P. Flanzer
Division of Epidemiology Services and
Prevention Research,
National Institute on Drug Abuse,
6001 Exec Blvd, Room 4224,
Bethesda, MD 20892-9565, USA

Dr. Arlene Frank
Center for Treatment Research on
Adolescent Drug Abuse,
University of Miami Miller School
of Medicine,
PO Box 019132,
Miami, FL 33136, USA

Dr. Eilish Gilvarry
Centre for Alcohol and Drug Studies,
Northern Regional Drug and Alcohol
Services, Newcastle NHS Mental Health
Trust, Plummer Court,
Carliol Place,
Newcastle upon Tyne,
NE1 6UR, UK

Dr. Christine Grella
UCLA Drug Abuse Research Center,
1640 S Sepulveda Blvd, Suite 200,
Los Angeles, CA 90025, USA

Ms. Hollie Hix-Small
Oregon Research Institute,
1715 Franklin Boulevard,
Eugene, OR 97403, USA

Dr. Nancy Jainchill
National Development and Research
Institutes, 71 West 23rd St, 8th Floor,
New York, NY 10010, USA

Dr. Yifrah Kaminer
Department of Psychiatry and Alcohol
Research Center,
University of Connecticut
Health Center
263 Farmington Ave
Farmington, CT 06030-2103, USA

Dr. M. Katherine Kraft
19 Andrews Lane
Princeton, NJ 08540, USA

Dr. Howard A. Liddle
Center for Treatment Research on
Adolescent Drug Abuse,
University of Miami Miller School
of Medicine, PO Box 019132,
Miami, FL 33101, USA

Dr. Mark J. Macgowan
School of Social Work,
Florida International University,
University Park Campus, HIS-2 363B,
Miami, FL 33199, USA

Dr. Robert M. Malow
College of Health and Urban Affairs,
Florida International University,
3000 N.E. 151 St., AC1-260
Miami, FL 33181, USA

Dr. Paul McArdle
Fleming Nuffield Unit, Burdon Terrace,
Newcastle upon Tyne,
NE2 3AE, UK

Dr. Maite P. Mena
Center for Family Studies,
Department of Psychiatry and
Behavioral Sciences, University of
Miami Miller School of Medicine,
1425 NW 10th Avenue, Suite 301D,
Miami, FL 33136, USA

Dr. Hayrettin Okut
University of Yüzüncü Yyl,
65080 Van,
Turkey

Dr. Timothy J. Ozechowski
Oregon Research Institute,
1715 Franklin Boulevard,
Eugene, OR 97403, USA

Dr. Kerstin Pahl
New York University School
of Medicine,
215 Lexington Avenue,
New York, NY 10016, USA

Dr. Anna Pond
Anna Pond Consulting,
95 St. Marks Avenue,
Brooklyn, NY 11217, USA

Ms. Danielle E. Ramo
Department of Psychology,
University of California at San Diego,

9500 Gilman Drive, M/C 0109,
La Jolla, CA 92093-0109, USA

Dr. Paula D. Riggs
Department of Psychiatry,
University of Colorado School of Medicine,
4200 E. 9th Avenue C-268-35, Denver,
Colorado, CO 80262, USA

Dr. John M. Roll
Washington Institute for
Mental Illness Research and Training,
Washington State University
PO Box 1495, Spokane,
WA 99210-1495, USA

Dr. Rhonda Rosenberg
College of Health and Urban Affairs,
Florida International University,
3000 N.E. 151 St., AC1-260
Miami, FL 33199, USA

Dr. Cynthia L. Rowe
Center for Treatment Research on
Adolescent Drug Abuse,
University of Miami Miller School
of Medicine,
PO Box 019132,
Miami, FL 33101, USA

Dr. Daniel A. Santisteban
Center for Family Studies,
Department of Psychiatry and Behavioral
Sciences, University of Miami Miller
School of Medicine,
1425 N.W. 10th Avenue, Suite 301D,
Miami, FL 33136, USA

Ms. Kristin Schubert
Robert Wood Johnson Foundation,
PO Box 2316,
Princeton, NJ 08543, USA

Ms. Lisa Strycker
Oregon Research Institute,
1715 Franklin Boulevard,
Eugene, OR 97403, USA

Dr. Lourdes Suarez-Morales
University of Miami Miller
School of Medicine,
Department of Psychiatry
and Behavioral Sciences,
1425 N.W. 10th Avenue, Suite 301D,
Miami, FL 33136, USA

Dr. Janet C. Titus
Lighthouse Institute,
Chestnut Health Systems,
720 West Chestnut,
Bloomington, IL 61701, USA

Dr. Charles W. Turner
Oregon Research Institute,
1715 Franklin Boulevard,
Eugene, OR 97403, USA

Dr. Eric F. Wagner
College of Health and Urban Affairs,
Florida International University,
11200 SW 8th St, Marc Building 310
Miami, FL 33199, USA

Dr. Holly Barrett Waldron
Oregon Research Institute,
1715 Franklin Boulevard,
Eugene, OR 97403, USA

Dr. Donnie Watson
UCLA Integrated Substance Programs
and Friends Research Institute,
1001 W. Carson St, Suite S,
Torrance, CA 90502, USA

Dr. Elizabeth A. Whitmore
Department of Psychiatry,
University of Colorado School
of Medicine,
1611 S. Federal Blvd, 120 Denver,
Colorado 80219, USA

Dr. Kenneth C. Winters
Department of Psychiatry,
University of Minnesota
Medical School, F282/2A West,
2450 Riverside Avenue,
Minneapolis, MN 55454, USA

Forewords

Foreword 1

Alcohol and drug abuse continue to be perceived as extremely serious problems by all Americans. In volume alone, substance use disorders are daunting problems. For example, in 2001 (the latest data available in the US National Survey of Substance Abuse Treatment Services [2001]), 1.1 million US youth aged 12–17 were estimated to need substance abuse treatment. However, it seems clear from research in the UK and Europe that young people with substance abuse problems are not being identified accurately. Therefore, this very large prevalence figure may be a substantial underestimate. Finally, there is also indication that the situation may be getting worse. Surveys in the USA and a variety of other countries documented alarming increases in adolescent substance use throughout the 1990s and rates have remained steady and consistently high in the early years of this decade (see Ch. 6).

It is disturbing that of the 1.1 million identified adolescent abusers, fewer than 100 000 actually received treatment, leaving a significant "treatment gap" nationwide. Even worse, there is also concern regarding the effectiveness and worth of the treatment that is available. Indeed, a significant proportion of Americans – even those who work within healthcare settings – feel that "nothing works" for substance abuse. For instance, the Services Research Outcomes Study found in 1998 that while adult patients improved significantly in drug abuse programs, adolescents actually increased their alcohol and drug use in the years following treatment. In turn, research from the USA, the UK, and Europe suggests that the treatments being delivered to adolescents may not be developmentally appropriate, or based on research-derived approaches or interventions.

The poor public image of substance abuse treatment is made more disturbing because since the mid-1990s there have been significant advances in substance abuse treatment technology, such as the introduction of manual-driven, empirically validated treatment approaches (e.g. motivational enhancement therapy, 12-step facilitation therapy, etc.) and several new medications to assist in combating drug craving and withdrawal symptoms. Yet, much of this work remains isolated and disconnected from trends and developments that could enhance it. For instance, practitioners remain largely in the dark about the newer research findings and policy makers are unaware of the structural and regulatory changes that will be necessary to implement and support research-derived treatments and strategies. Legislatures, insurers, and the public at large have demanded more accountability and better performance from the specialty treatment programs in their states. Consequently, despite substantial research progress there remains uncertainty and even doubt about the effectiveness of treatments for alcohol and drug dependence in the real world.

Adolescent Substance Abuse: Research and Clinical Advances is a volume of interesting, timely, practical, and scientifically rigorous papers that is placed squarely at the intersection of three significant forces affecting our field:
- increases in the prevalence and severity of adolescent substance use
- public concern regarding the availability and quality of substance abuse treatment for adolescents
- scientific advances in our understanding about the prevention and treatment of adolescent substance abuse.

The book includes chapters addressing all three of these forces and is designed to address the gap between what we could provide to substance-abusing adolescents and what is currently available. In the five sections of this volume, readers will find the latest treatment research advances, presented in clinically relevant ways and offering practical steps for policy makers and practitioners to advance the field into the next developmental stage of adolescent substance abuse treatment research. The work presented comes from the very best researchers and clinicians in our field. Therefore, this volume should be relevant for and appeal to a wide audience from the many groups of providers, researchers, and policy makers that work with adolescent drug abuse. Though the findings from these papers may provoke serious concerns regarding the current effectiveness of adolescent substance abuse treatment, the suggestions to improve that treatment are sensible, timely, objective, and practical – but not too simple. Adolescent substance abuse treatment is at a serious crossroads and there are no simple fixes that will assure more availability and better quality. Adolescent addiction treatment needs political commitment to address the many problems as well as practical science working with committed clinicians to engineer new solutions supported by financial and technical investment and incentives to raise quality and to attract the best personnel. Achieving the public expectations for adolescent substance abuse treatment will not be quick or easy, but with guidance from the science-based findings, principles, and recommendations within this volume, there is reason for optimism that better days lie ahead.

A. Thomas McLellan
Director, Treatment Research Institute
Professor, University of Pennsylvania School of Medicine

Foreword 2

Compliments from Europe!

That was the first phrase that came to mind after I had finished reading this informative and remarkable book. A few years ago, when the University of Miami sponsored a meeting that ultimately resulted in this book, many considered adolescent substance abuse science to be in the toddler stage. Yet, behold, it is now rapidly evolving into a new developmental period. In the past decades, but with accelerated speed in the past few years, sizable advances have been made in:

- understanding the determinants of substance use disorders in youth from a longitudinal perspective
- accepting co-morbidity and "multidimensionality" as real issues in the causation, perseverance, and exacerbation of these disorders
- developing tools and methods to measure problems, to target actions, and to evaluate intervention outcomes
- designing and implementing efficacious and perhaps even effective treatments.

One would hope that the next stride forward in this relatively young field of science and practice would be as big as the one made in this book. Europeans should be grateful to our American colleagues for paving the way. The next book should contain not only descriptions but also data from trials in Europe. There are presently efforts underway to transport interventions developed in the USA to European contexts. There is a fair amount of competition here, with "American" treatments outbidding each other. I sincerely hope that science will prevail here, in the tradition established by this book.

I also hope that policy generation by policy makers and politicians will start to acknowledge that substance use disorder in "multiproblem kids" is something far more serious and worthy of preventive and therapeutic intervention than has been, until recently, accepted in debates dominated by ideology. Researchers cannot take over the tasks of policy makers, but they can be helpful. Improve the world, but start with sound research.

In sum, this volume characterizes the specialty's current state and offers ideas about directions needed. Any researcher or therapist with interest in the exciting area of youth substance use and misuse should read this book.

Henk Rigter
Professor of Public Health
Erasmus University Rotterdam, The Netherlands

Acknowledgements

Numerous people contributed to the development of this comprehensive volume, which was inspired by the October 2001 conference held in Coral Gables, Florida, *Treating Adolescent Substance Abuse: State of the Science*. The conference was made possible through a grant from the National Institute on Drug Abuse (grant no. 1 R13 DA13395-01A1, H. Liddle, PI). We acknowledge our original conference presenters, Dr. Michael Dennis, Dr. James Alexander, Dr. Sandra Brown, Dr. Richard Catalano, Dr. Nancy Jainchill, Dr. Ken Winters, Dr. Oscar Bukstein, Dr. Gayle Dakof, Dr. Paula Riggs, Dr. Daniel Santisteban, Dr. Duncan Stanton, Dr. Peter Monti, Dr. Eric Wagner, Dr. Holly Waldron, and Dr. Yifrah Kaminer for helping to develop many of the themes and questions that are addressed in the volume. We thank each author for their unique contribution to the volume. We also owe a debt of gratitude to many others who helped in the review and editing process, including Dr. Arlene Frank, Dr. Paul Greenbaum, Dr. Craig Henderson, and Dr. Gayle Dakof. Ligia Gómez worked tirelessly to coordinate with contributors and with the team at Cambridge in the final stage of the volume's production. Finally, we offer many thanks to Pauline Graham and the production team at Cambridge University Press for making this book a reality.

Abbreviations

ASAM	American Society of Addiction Medicine
CJ-DATS	Criminal Justice Drug Abuse Treatment Studies
CSAT	Center for Substance Abuse Treatment
CTN	Clinical Trials Network
DARP	Drug Abuse Reporting Program
DATOS-A	Drug Abuse Treatment Outcome Studies in Adolescents
DSM	Diagnostic and Statistical Manual
EMCDDA	European Monitoring Centre for Drugs and Drug Addiction
ESPAD	European Schools Project on Alcohol and Other Drugs
HBSC	Health Behaviour in School-aged Children
MTF	Monitoring the Future [project]
NCADI	National Clearing House on Alcohol and Drug Information
NHSDA	National Health Survey of Drug Abuse
NIAAA	National Institute on Alcohol Abuse and Alcoholism
NIDA	National Institute on Drug Abuse
NIH	National Institutes of Health
NIMH	National Institute of Mental Health
NITIES	US National Treatment Improvement Evaluation Study
SAMHSA	Substance Abuse and Mental Health Services Administration
SASATE	Society for Adolescent Substance Abuse Treatment Effectiveness
TOPS	Treatment Outcome Perspectives Study

Treating adolescent substance abuse: state of the science

Cynthia L. Rowe and Howard A. Liddle

University of Miami Miller School of Medicine, Miami, FL, USA

In October, 2001, just a month after the World Trade Center tragedy, a 2-day conference was scheduled to be held in Coral Gables, Florida entitled *Treating Adolescent Substance Abuse: State of the Science* funded by the National Institute on Drug Abuse (grant 1 R13 DA13395-01A1, H. Liddle, PI). It was hosted by the University of Miami Center for Treatment Research on Adolescent Drug Abuse. The conference objective was to characterize and articulate the developmental status of the research specialty in adolescent drug abuse treatment. Specifically, we aimed to explore the specialty's readiness to adopt or adapt existing treatment development models, and to develop new empirical and clinical frameworks. A broader function of the conference was to disseminate the latest research-based work on a range of core topics in adolescent substance abuse treatment to a diverse audience. With a diversity of research and clinical interests, viewpoints, and settings represented, we hoped that the conference would facilitate dialogue and specify unanswered empirical questions and points of controversy. In addition, if issues of this kind could be addressed successfully, additional advances in the adolescent substance abuse treatment research specialty could occur.

In the weeks after the terrorist attacks, amidst threats of continued violence, fears of flying, and the anthrax outbreak only miles from the conference venue, serious questions emerged: could the conference proceed at all, and if it did, would more than a handful of participants attend? We held the meeting and the participants turned up. We were relieved and amazed to see that there was standing room only throughout the 2-day event, and that participants and presenters came from across the USA to attend. The conference exceeded all expectations. The capacity turnout and enthusiastic discussions following the presentations testified to the fact that research on adolescent substance abuse treatment had come of age and had taken its place in the substance abuse field. There was a sense of looking back, reviewing progress, and taking stock of where we had come as a field in our short history. But more pronounced was the excitement about where we could go together if we focused less on our theoretical and clinical differences and more on the cross-cutting themes of our work. The Roman mythical god Janus was the god of both beginnings and endings. Like Janus, the conference looked to the past but also faced the future. Consensus was that we were turning a page as well as trying to specify what needs to come next in the field.

The conference turned out to be more than just a 2-day event. New collaborations were formed among researchers who had never met before. Partnerships also were forged among providers, research teams, and representatives of state and federal funding agencies and policy makers. The first adolescent-focused substance abuse treatment association, the Society for Adolescent Substance Abuse Treatment Effectiveness (SASATE), was created. SASATE now holds a full-day meeting in conjunction with the annual conference of the College on Problems of Drug Dependence (CPDD). With funding from the Center for Substance Abuse Treatment (CSAT), SASATE also maintains a list-serve to promote regular dialogue among clinicians, researchers, program directors, funders, and policy makers.

The conference also created the foundation for this book. While the scope of the volume far exceeds what we were able to cover in the 2 days of the event, the overall objective and the themes of the book grew from the seeds planted in the conference presentations and discussions. Like the conference, the book covers a range of issues. It includes theoretical models that provide a foundation for adolescent substance abuse interventions, research innovations, specific empirical findings supporting assessment and treatment techniques and interventions with special populations, as well as research funding trends and practice and policy guidelines. We aim to reach a wide audience that includes researchers in adolescent substance abuse, researchers and therapists who are training, clinical program administrators, funders, and practitioners interested in the latest scientific issues and advances in treating adolescent drug abuse.

Like the guiding objectives and themes for the conference, the book's primary purpose is to organize state-of-the-science treatment research findings in conceptually coherent and clinically meaningful ways, and to show how advances across our specialty can be brought to bear in improving research, clinical work, and the connection between these realms. Five major sections organize the volume: Theoretical, empirical, and methodological foundations for research into treatment of adolescent substance abuse; Practice and policy trends in treatment for adolescent substance abuse; Comprehensive assessment and integrative treatment planning with adolescent substance abusers; Empirically based interventions for adolescent substance abuse: research and practice implications; and Culturally based treatment development for adolescent substance abusers. Contributors were asked to address the following points and questions in summarizing progress and new directions in their subspecialty area.

- Define the relevant background and history of your subspecialty relative to the broader adolescent substance abuse specialty.
- Why is this focal area and content important in the field?
- What research has been done in this area, and what are the most important findings?
- Explain the clinical relevance of these findings.
- What are the limitations of this particular specialty area?
- What is needed to advance the research and/or clinical work in this area?

In expanding the volume beyond the scope of the conference, we sought a diverse collection of experienced scholars with expertise in a variety of subspecialties within the adolescent substance abuse treatment field and experience with a variety of client groups and treatment and research settings. The following sections offer a brief history and status report on the field's progress and introduce the themes and content areas to be covered in the chapters that follow.

A brief history of adolescent substance abuse treatment research

Adolescent substance abuse treatment has evolved into a robust, well-defined specialty since the mid-1990s. Indeed, the proliferation of studies on adolescent substance abuse treatment in recent years can be characterized as nothing short of a "research renaissance" (Liddle, 2002a). Since the National Institute on Drug Abuse (NIDA) released its first solicitation for adolescent-specific drug abuse research nearly 20 years ago, the specialty has matured a great deal. Emerging from the shadows of adult studies, adolescent-focused research has firmly established its own identity distinct from both adult drug abuse treatment and substance abuse prevention (Liddle, 2004). One developmental marker is the increase in the number of published and funded studies. Between 1997 and 2001 alone, studies on adolescent substance abuse treatment doubled, and taking into account funded, in-process research, an even larger increase is forecasted in this decade (Dennis, 2002).

Several interacting factors account for this research bonanza. First, there was the rapidly changing epidemiology of teen drug use. Surveys in the USA and a variety of other countries documented alarming increases in adolescent substance use throughout the 1990s, and rates have remained steady and consistently high in the early years of this century (Johnston, O'Malley, & Bachman, 2003; Gilvarry, 2000; see Ch. 6). The high prevalence of adolescent substance abuse was evident across all sectors of care – not only in the substance abuse treatment system but in mental health, juvenile justice, child welfare, and the schools (Aarons *et al.*, 2001). At the same time, data from large-scale evaluation studies revealed that standard, community-based substance abuse programs that were available in the 1990's were not effective with adolescents nor were they meeting the needs of most adolescents with substance abuse and related problems (Dennis et al., 2003; Etheridge et al., 2001). For instance, the Services Research Outcomes Study (SROS) of the Substance Abuse and Mental Health Services Administration (SAMHSA) found that while adult patients improved significantly in drug abuse programs, adolescents actually increased their alcohol and drug use in the years following treatment (SAMHSA, 1998a). Other basic and applied research began to delineate more clearly the unique developmental and treatment needs of referred adolescents (e.g., Winters, Latimer, & Stinchfield, 1999), and the complexity of adolescent substance abuse and its corresponding impairments (Bukstein, Glancy, & Kaminer, 1992). Consequently, it became increasingly clear that treatment models borrowed from adult addiction programs were inappropriate for teenagers (Deas et al., 2000). But this insight could not solve a troubling conundrum. The need for effective, developmentally tailored adolescent substance abuse treatment continued to grow (Kaminer, 2001), while funding, capacity, and resources in standard treatment practice dwindled (Muck et al., 2001). These circumstances created fertile soil for major advances in research on adolescent substance abuse treatment.

In response to these multiple interacting forces, funding for research into adolescent-focused substance abuse treatment increased steadily, and major initiatives were launched in the USA and in Europe. In 1993, NIDA identified adolescent drug treatment as a high priority area in its *Behavioral Therapies Development* program (NIDA, 1993). Five years later, the National Institute on Alcohol Abuse and Alcoholism (NIAAA) launched its own adolescent treatment research program in partnership with the Center for Substance Abuse Treatment CSAT (NIAAA, 1998). That initiative called for clinical trials to establish the efficacy of well-defined, developmentally appropriate treatment models, as well as scientifically rigorous studies to examine the effectiveness of standard practice for adolescents with primary alcohol abuse. NIAAA subsequently released another solicitation for adolescent-focused treatment studies in 2003, calling for research to build on its developing program and fill in gaps in identified areas, such as diminishing the substance abuse potential of high-risk groups including children of alcoholics (NIAAA, 2003). Also in 2003, NIDA funded several new adolescent treatment studies through its initiative designed to stimulate research that would improve behavioral health services and treatment for adolescent drug abuse (NIDA, 2002a). At around the same time, CSAT was developing its own adolescent substance abuse treatment portfolio. In 1998, CSAT launched its multisite Cannabis Youth Treatment study (Ch. 5) and the Adolescent Treatment Models program announcement was released that same year and again in 1999 (SAMHSA, 1998b, 1999). These multisite initiatives represented major advances in identifying and disseminating effective treatment models for adolescent substance abusers in the USA (Dennis *et al.*, 2003, 2004).

Interest in youth substance misuse and funding for new research initiatives has also increased substantially in the UK and Europe (EMCDDA, 2003a; EORG, 2002; Rigter *et al.*, 2004; UK Department of Health, 2002). Government-funded reports across the UK and European nations reveal disturbing trends in recent years, including exposure to and access to a wide range of drugs by young people, increases in the number of young teens who have used drugs, higher rates of youth presenting for treatment, and increases in drug misuse among younger adolescents (EMCDDA, 2003b; McKeganey *et al.*, 2003; UK Drug Strategy Directorate, 2002). Consistent with research on adolescent drug abuse in the USA (e.g., Hawkins, Catalano, & Miller, 1992), drug use among young people in the UK and Europe is associated with a challenging set of problems, including delinquent behavior; peer drug use; school exclusion; and family dysfunction such as marital discord, poor parental supervision and management, and family substance abuse and disruption (EMCDDA, 2003b; Scottish Executive, 2003). Further, research reveals that young people with substance misuse problems in the UK and Europe are not being identified accurately or treated with integrative, developmentally appropriate, research-supported interventions (Burniston, *et al.*, 2002; DrugScope, 2003; Scottish Executive, 1999; Strijker *et al.*, 2001). With growing recognition and concern about the multifaceted nature of the clinical problem, the increase in the numbers of substance involved youth, and the lack of services for substance-abusing teens, many nations have given a high priority to the problem of youth substance misuse in their recently released national strategies for addressing substance misuse (Ketelaars *et al.*, 2002; Scottish Executive, 2003; UK Anti-Drugs Co-Ordinator, 2000). In one current study, for instance, scientists from five European countries are working together with funding from their Health Ministers to embark on new research to examine treatment approaches for adolescent cannabis misuse. This collaborative will attempt to replicate the impressive effects of a multisystem-oriented, family-based intervention established in the USA (Rigter, 2003).

Beyond the obvious commitment of federal funding bodies to improving adolescent substance abuse treatment and increasing the research base for effective interventions, evidence of the specialty's maturation is apparent in several areas. One is in the proliferation of specialized adolescent-focused methods of assessment (Ch. 11) and intervention (Liddle *et al.*, 2000; Wagner & Waldron, 2001) based largely on developmental research and studies of risk factors for adolescent substance abuse (Ch. 2). Many treatments are now available as studies have shown that even complex adolescent treatment models can be translated into practical manuals, and that these are not only acceptable to and feasible for training community-based providers (Godley *et al.*, 2001; Liddle *et al.*, 2002) but also, critically, are efficacious in curtailing drug use and improving functioning among drug-abusing adolescents (e.g., Liddle *et al.*, 2001, 2004). The literature has expanded accordingly. Since 2000, three comprehensive volumes on treatment of adolescent substance abuse have been published (Monti, Colby, & O'Leary, 2001; Stevens and Morral, 2003; Wagner & Waldron, 2001). Special issue publications have been compiled on timely and clinically important topics in adolescent substance abuse treatment, such as national trends in drug treatment evaluation for adolescents (the Drug Abuse Treatment Outcome Studies in Adolescents [DATOS-A]; Fletcher & Grella, 2001; Ch. 7), qualitative methods for evaluating adolescent substance abuse treatment (Currie, Duroy, & Lewis, 2003), the prevalence and clinical implications of child abuse among adolescent substance abusers (Dennis & Stevens, 2003), empirically supported treatment approaches for adolescent substance abusers (Cavanaugh & Muck, 2004; Fromme & Brown, 2000), and a report on the first multisite field trial of several manual-guided interventions for teenage cannabis abuse (Dennis *et al.*, 2002). The adolescent specialty also is now regularly represented in special journal issues and featured articles on important cross-disciplinary topics such as bridging the research–practice gap and conducting state-of-the-art economic evaluations of adolescent drug treatment (Liddle *et al.*, 2002; Roebuck, French, & McLellan, 2003).

Dennis (2002, p. 2) summarized the specialty's growth in the following way: "We've seen major methodological advances in screening and assessment, placement, manual-guided approaches for targeted interventions and for more comprehensive program management that can be easily disseminated, treatment engagement and retention, recovery management, follow-up and outcome assessment, and economic analysis, as well as organizational changes in treatment delivery and financing systems."

These numerous and diverse signs of progress place this specialty at an interesting crossroad. On the one hand, a solid foundation of research on adolescent substance abuse treatment has been constructed and enormous excitement has been generated by the development of more and more sophisticated, empirically supported treatments. On the other hand, much of this work remains isolated and disconnected from trends and developments that could enhance it. For instance, practitioners remain largely unaware of the important empirical advances that have been made and are necessary to implement effective strategies with this difficult-to-treat population. This volume is designed to address some of these limitations by presenting the latest treatment research advances in clinically relevant ways, by inspiring thoughtful reflection, and by offering practical steps that can be taken to advance the field into the next developmental stage.

Theoretical, empirical, and methodological foundations for research

Part I contains four chapters highlighting some of the advances in theory and science that have provided a foundation for the field; at the same time, they address potential paths that might be followed. Brook *et al.* (Ch. 2) present the developmentally oriented framework of risk and protective factors that has guided and served as the basis for much of the current treatment development work and research. Research methodologies have improved since the first studies of treatment for adolescent substance abuse were carried out, with features such as intervention manuals (e.g., Liddle, 2002b) and adherence evaluations (Hogue *et al.*, 1998), now being considered necessary standards: a feature of treatment and prevention science generally. Statistical methods for analyzing data both during and following treatment are more sophisticated; they enable investigators to answer more nuanced questions about the effects of interventions on youth and their families (Ch. 3). The use of more rigorous methods for following teens post-treatment (Meyers *et al.*, 2003) has provided a knowledge base about the longer-term impact of adolescent substance abuse treatment (Ch. 3). A major development in the field's history, CSAT's Cannabis Youth Treatment Initiative, (Ch. 4), describes the first multisite study of adolescent substance abuse treatment, the methods that led to its successful implementation, and its key findings. Building on these theoretical and scientific advances and following the recommendations of these and other investigators for new research directions, the field's promise for continued growth is considerable.

Practice and policy trends in treatment for adolescent substance abuse

The potential for this specialty to improve the quality of care for adolescent substance abusers will depend in large part on the field's examining and making critical changes in the context of service delivery. The gulf between science and practice has been criticized by researchers and clinicians alike (Brown & Flynn, 2002), and this disconnection impacts the work of all stakeholders involved in efforts to improve treatment for substance abusers (Institute of Medicine, 1998). Empirical studies are now showing that research-based adolescent substance abuse interventions can influence the day-to-day practice of community providers (Liddle *et al.*, 2002), and more empirical support exists for a range of models (Stevens & Morral, 2003). However, changes in the service delivery systems themselves will be necessary before widespread dissemination of evidence-based practices will be possible. Even though providers may be motivated to adopt effective models and may be supportive of change, implementation capacity in most programs remains limited (Burke & Early, 2003).

Systems-level organizational factors impede technology-transfer efforts (Simpson, 2002). Adolescent substance abusers are involved in multiple social systems, yet the coordination of care among systems – substance abuse treatment, juvenile justice programs, mental health treatment, and the schools – is notoriously poor (CSAT, 1999). Fragmentation of services has been identified as a major obstacle in treating youth effectively (Aarons *et al.*, 2001; Garland *et al.*, 2001). Recommendations from expert panels suggest that new linkages and partnerships among juvenile justice officials, substance abuse treatment providers, community health agencies, and social service agencies, as well as between these and researchers, must be made in order to create effective treatment systems and promote the use of evidence-based practices (CSAP, 2000; CSAT, 1995 NIDA, 2002a; Robert Wood Johnson Foundation, 2001).

Part II provides a briefing on some important practice and policy trends and on existing barriers to improving services for adolescent substance abusers. For instance, our understanding of the evolution of substance abuse services for adolescents can be enhanced by first understanding epidemiological trends in youth substance use. Essau (Ch. 6) discusses the trends seen in Europe and their treatment implications, while Grella (Ch. 7) describes parallel findings from national drug treatment evaluation studies done in the USA and their influence on practice patterns. Some of the more specific challenges of service implementation are presented in chapters discussing the systems of care for adolescent substance misusers in the USA (Ch. 8) and the UK (Ch. 9). Finally, Flanzer (Ch. 10) identifies a broad range of research issues in health services that will be important to address successfully if we are to make progress in bridging the research–practice divide in adolescent substance abuse treatment.

Comprehensive assessment and integrative treatment planning with adolescent substance abusers

Among the most consistent and clinically pertinent findings to emerge from basic and applied research with this population since the mid-1980s is the complexity, heterogeneity, and multiplicity of problems associated with adolescent substance abuse (Grella *et al.*, 2001; Rowe *et al.*, 2004). Adolescent substance abuse is no longer considered as an isolated clinical problem since these youth almost without exception suffer multiple interrelated deficits that together form what has been called a "problem behavior syndrome" (Jessor & Jessor, 1977). Contemporary assessment and treatment development efforts are, therefore, organized around the constellation of problems that typically co-occur with adolescent substance abuse: psychiatric disorders and symptoms, school problems, delinquency, and high-risk sexual behavior (Dennis *et al.*, 2003). Unfortunately, although strong statements have been made about the need for changes in this area (Drug Strategies, 2003), most adolescent substance abusers in community-based treatment programs do not receive comprehensive interventions to address their multiple needs (Jaycox, Morral, & Juvonen, 2003), and there is a well-documented mismatch between the services that are offered and the service needs of the clients (Grella *et al.*, 2001). In the absence of coordinated and targeted interventions, youth with comorbid conduct problems are at especially high risk to drop out of treatment (Kaminer *et al.*, 1992), have poor long-term outcomes (Crowley *et al.*, 1998), and are likely to reoffend following treatment (Farabee *et al.*, 2001).

In part III, the contributors address ways in which effective assessment and treatment can be achieved with adolescents with multiple problems. Chapter 11 reviews and discusses assessment issues and challenges, as well as the latest assessment methods and their application in practice. Two chapters address in different ways some of the challenges and effective approaches for treating adolescent substance abusers with comorbid psychiatric problems: Ch. 12 discussing integrative psychopharmacological interventions and Ch. 13 presenting a broad-based review and discussion of treatment and research issues pertaining to comorbidity. Finally, Ch. 14 is a summary of the latest in human immuno-deficiency virus (HIV)/acquired immunodeficiency disease (AIDS) prevention for this population, discussing approaches that have the potential for integration within adolescent substance abuse programs. These topics represent some of the most perplexing and important issues in the field today.

Empirically based interventions for adolescent substance abuse: research and practice implications

Remarkable advances have been made since the mid-1990s in the development and testing of promising interventions for adolescent substance abuse and its associated problems (Weinberg *et al.*, 1998). Much of this progress has been based on the considerable knowledge gained from developmental psychopathology research (e.g., Dishion & Kavanagh, 2003). Interventionists have used basic research about normative and atypical development to design interventions that address the multiple interacting risk and protective factors contributing to adolescent substance abuse (Liddle *et al.*, 2000). A second important theme of treatment development efforts has been a focus on integration: not only in terms of incorporating traditional drug counseling techniques (Liddle, 2002b; Randall *et al.*, 2001; Rowe *et al.*, 2002) but also in blending therapeutic models to have maximum impact (Latimer *et al.*, 2003; Ch. 17). Many of the most promising empirically supported models are based on systemic sensibilities that represent a break with traditional disease models of addiction or with reductionistic thinking that locates the problem within the individual adolescent (Liddle, 1999). In fact, family-based interventions with an ecological and developmental orientation are widely recognized as the most effective approaches for adolescent substance abuse (NIDA, 2002a; Rowe & Liddle, 2003; Weinberg *et al.*, 1998; Williams & Chang, 2000).

A greater number of adolescent substance abuse interventions are available than ever before, with roots in a range of theoretical orientations including family therapy, cognitive–behavioral treatment, behavioral therapy, psychopharmacology, and the 12-step approaches (Deas & Thomas, 2001). Since 1998 alone, NIAAA (2003) has identified 10 effective interventions for adolescent alcohol abusers, with several more being studied in new projects. The CSAT multisite study identified five Cannabis Youth Treatment interventions that were effective in adolescents for reducing marijuana use and maintaining gains following treatment (Ch. 5); the CSAT Adolescent Treatment Models initiative identified 10 promising interventions and evaluated them up to 12 months after intake (see Cavanaugh & Muck, 2004). Three promising approaches specific for adolescents were also profiled by NIDA (1999a) in a publication outlining the principles of effective interventions for drug abuse. With sufficient empirical support and replication in rigorously controlled trials, some of these models have reached "best practice" status on sites such as the USA Department of Health and Human Services Best Practice Initiative (http://phs.os.dhhs.gov/ophs/BestPractice).

While the treatment models are diverse and represent a range of theoretical frameworks, their essential elements are generally consistent across different disciplines and sources. For instance, the practice parameters for treating adolescent substance abuse published by the *Journal of the American Academy of Child and Adolescent Psychiatry* (Bukstein, 2004) state that interventions need to be focused on achieving and maintaining abstinence from substances, as well as targeting associated problems across domains of functioning (e.g., coexisting psychiatric and behavioral problems, family functioning, interpersonal relationships, and academic factors). According to these guidelines, treatment for adolescent substance abuse must be of sufficient duration and intensiveness; should be comprehensive and provide after-care or follow-up sessions; be sensitive to cultural, racial, and socioeconomic factors; include families; facilitate collaboration with social services agencies; promote prosocial activities and a drug-free lifestyle (including involvement in self-help groups); and should be provided in the least-restrictive setting that is safe and effective. Similarly, in a recent publication focusing exclusively on adolescent substance abuse treatment, Drug Strategies (2003) presented nine principles illustrating practices common to the most effective programs (see Box 1.1).

> ## Box 1.1 Principles of effective drug treatment
>
> 1. **Assessment and treatment matching.** Programs should use standard screening instruments and comprehensive assessment throughout the course of treatment to provide further guidance based on the adolescent's progress.
> 2. **Comprehensive, integrated treatment approach.** Provision of an integrated treatment approach maximizes the chances that the adolescent will be able to reduce both his/her substance use and other problem behaviors.
> 3. **Family involvement.** Engaging parents/caregivers in the treatment process increases the probability that the adolescent will remain in treatment and that the treatment gains will be maintained after treatment has ended.
> 4. **Developmentally appropriate program.** Treatment approaches for adolescents must take into consideration the biological, behavioral, and cognitive changes that characterize this stage and must also incorporate the different contexts that are meaningful to this age group.
> 5. **Engage and retain adolescents in treatment.** In order for the adolescent to become fully engaged in treatment, the therapist must elicit a commitment on his/her part to change and facilitate his/her realization that a productive life is possible without the use of substances.
> 6. **Qualified staff.** Staff should have training and experience in diverse areas related to co-occurring problems of adolescents. Staff should also have a strong understanding of adolescent development and have experience of working with adolescents and families.
> 7. **Gender and cultural competence.** A thorough understanding of gender and cultural issues is essential to the development of a strong therapeutic alliance.
> 8. **Continuing care.** Examples of continuing care services include relapse-prevention training, follow-up plans and referrals to community agencies, and check-ups.
> 9. **Treatment outcomes.** Routine measures of client progress, such as clean urine tests, improved school performance, and enhanced family communication, should be carried out during and up to 1 year after treatment.
>
> *Note:* From Drug Strategies. (2003).

The purpose of Part IV is to present the most up-to-date empirical findings supporting the use of specific intervention modalities with adolescent substance abusers. Individual chapters focus on therapeutic community treatment (Ch. 15), school-based interventions (Ch. 16), integrative family and behavioral interventions (Ch. 17), behavioral management approaches (Ch. 18), and cognitive–behavioral therapy (Ch. 19). This is only a sampling of the range of models that are accumulating empirical support. A sturdy foundation of empirical knowledge about effective interventions for adolescent substance abuse has been built; however, new studies that extend and test the limits of these scientific developments are still required.

Culturally based treatment development for adolescent substance abusers

Despite the progress that has been made in developing effective interventions for substance-abusing youth, much remains to be done in order to ensure that all affected adolescents receive and benefit from these services. This is especially true for minority teens and their families (NIAAA, 2001). Minority youth are at particular risk for developing substance-related problems (Kumpfer & Alvarado, 1995), and as adults they suffer disproportionately from the detrimental effects of heavy substance use (Wallace, 1999; Zucker et al., 1996). Minorities have less access to services for substance abuse (Wells, Koike, & Sherbourne, 2001) and have been historically underrepresented in substance abuse intervention studies (Monti et al., 2001). Minority youth and families tend to underutilize the services that are available (Garland et al., 2000; Wallace, 1999), and when they do enter substance abuse treatment, they drop out at disproportionately high rates (Agosti, Nunes, & Ocepeck-Welikson, 1996). To date, however, very little is known about cultural factors related to treatment success and failure among adolescent substance abusers and those therapeutic interventions and processes that might be used to counteract existing health disparities.

Initial efforts in this regard are underway. For example, process research with African-American substance abusing youth in Multidimensional Family Therapy (Liddle, 2002b) has shown that articulation of culturally meaningful themes in therapy (such as those involving the exploration of anger, alienation, and the journey from boyhood to manhood) are directly linked to adolescent investment in the treatment process (Dakof, 2003; Jackson-Gilfort et al., 2001). Treatment developers have used such process research findings to design more appropriate interventions for minority youth. In addition, intervention researchers have begun to apply the results of empirical studies suggesting that specific factors may be particularly critical in determining substance abuse risk among minority youth (Bradizza, Reifman, & Barnes, 1999) and in guiding the selection of intervention targets. For instance, positive self-esteem (Alva & Jones, 1994; Rodney, Mupier, & Crafter, 1996) and positive ethnic identity (Brook et al., 1998; Scheier et al., 1997) appear to play an important protective function against substance use for minority teens. Level of acculturation appears to be a particularly important risk factor for substance use among minority youth (Bettes *et al.*, 1990; de la Rosa, Vega, & Radisch, 2000). Yet the impact of acculturation on substance abuse risk can only be understood in the context of familial processes such as parental support, communication, and family disruption (Gil, Vega, & Biafora, 1998). The contributors in Part V have described how research findings such as these have helped to guide treatment development efforts with American Indian (Ch. 20) and Hispanic (Ch. 21) youth and families. These chapters, which outline steps in treatment development that can be applied to other special populations, represent the latest advances in treatment research with understudied groups of adolescent drug abusers.

Next steps in adolescent substance abuse treatment research

In the final chapter, Liddle and Frank have summarized the themes presented by the contributors and the key conclusions, and then outlined priorities for the next generation of studies in this specialty.

In a recent request for applications for treatment and services research with adolescent drug abusers, NIDA (2002a, p. 3) concluded:

Despite these exciting successes, rates of engagement, retention, and long-term positive outcomes are far from perfect, suggesting that more work is needed to produce maximally effective treatments. This work includes all stages of treatment development (i.e., developing and testing new treatments, adapting existing treatments, examining moderators and mediators of treatment efficacy, and testing strategies for training and supervising community providers in efficacious treatments).

Some of this work has already been launched. For instance, evidence-based adolescent substance abuse interventions are being tested in major multisite NIDA-funded initiatives including the Criminal Justice–Drug Abuse Treatment Studies (CJ–DATS; NIDA, 2002b) and the Clinical Trials Network (CTN; NIDA, 1999b). NIDA is also funding innovative studies investigating empirically supported adolescent substance abuse interventions in community and practice settings such as juvenile drug courts (Dakof, 2003). NIAAA has likewise funded a new cohort of studies with adolescent alcohol abusers testing a range of interventions, including brief motivational interviewing, after-care models, school-based approaches, and pharmacological trials for youth with comorbid alcohol abuse and mental health problems (NIAAA, 2003).

Priority areas for the next wave of studies in this field have been outlined (NIDA, 2002a; NIAAA, 2003). The following 10 areas have been identified and discussed frequently: (1) developing better methods for assessing the unique treatment needs of adolescent substance abusers; (2) developing more effective interventions to meet those needs and for youth with comorbid substance abuse and psychiatric problems; (3) investigating mediators and moderators of change; (4) exploring predictors of long-term, post-treatment outcomes; (5) examining assessment and intervention approaches for different cultural, gender, and age groups; (6) investigating workforce issues and other barriers to implementing evidence-based practices in the community; (7) studying availability, accessibility, organization, and financing of services; (8) developing and testing continuing care models for youth with multiple problems in different service delivery systems and settings; (9) integrating HIV prevention with adolescent substance abuse treatment; and (10) translating evidence-based interventions to practice settings, and training community-based providers in their use.

Recent work by Tom McLellan has challenged the drug abuse research and practitioner establishments to think through the inconsistencies between the particular characteristics and features of the clinical drug problems that we treat and the treatment and research models we use to intervene and evaluate our work (McLellan, 2004). We hope this book offers a window into the state of the science of adolescent drug abuse treatment research, and that the work represented here provides a basis for necessary and potentially productive challenges to our specialty in the way that McLellan's work has challenged the field at large.

REFERENCES

Aarons, G. A., Brown, S. A., Hough, R. L., Garland, A. F., & Wood, P. A. (2001). Prevalence of adolescent substance abuse disorders across five sectors of care. *Journal of the American Academy of Child and Adolescent Psychiatry*, **40**, 419–426.

Agosti, V., Nunes, E., & Ocepeck-Welikson, K. (1996). Patient factors related to early attrition from an outpatient cocaine research clinic. *American Journal of Drug and Alcohol Abuse*, **22**, 29–39.

Alva, S. A. & Jones, M. (1994). Psychosocial adjustment and self-reported patterns of alcohol use among Hispanic adolescents. *Journal of Early Adolescence*, **14**, 432–448.

Bettes, B. A., Dusenbury, L., Kerner, J., James-Orvitz, S., & Botvin, G. J. (1990). Ethnicity and psychosocial factors in alcohol and tobacco use in adolescence. *Child Development*, **61**, 557–565.

Bradizza, C. M., Reifman, A., & Barnes, G. M. (1999). Social and coping reasons for drinking: predicting alcohol misuse in adolescents. *Journal of Studies on Alcohol*, **60**, 491–499.

Brook, J. S., Balka, E. B., Brook, D. W., Win, P. T., & Gursen, M. D. (1998). Drug use among African-Americans: ethnic identity as a protective factor. *Psychological Reports*, **83**, 1427–1446.

Brown, B. S. & Flynn, P. M. (2002). The federal role in drug abuse technology transfer: a history and perspective. *Journal of Substance Abuse Treatment*, **22**, 245–257.

Bukstein, O. G. For the Work Group on Quality Issues (2004). *The practice parameters for the assessment and treatment of children and adolescents with substance use disorders.* www.aacap.org/clinical/parameters/fulltext/SubstanceUseDisorder.pdf. Retrieved July 5, 2004.

Bukstein, O. G., Glancy, L. J., & Kaminer, Y. (1992). Patterns of affective comorbity in a clinical population of dually diagnosed adolescent substance abusers. *Journal of the American Academy of Child and Adolescent Psychiatry*, **31**, 1041–1045.

Burke, A. & Early, T. J. (2003). Readiness to adopt best practices among adolescents' AOD treatment providers. *Health and Social Work*, **28**, 99–105.

Burniston, S., Dodd, M., Elliott, L., Orr, L., & Watson, L. (2002). *Drug Treatment Services for Young People: A Research Review.* Edinburgh: Scottish Executive Effective Interventions Unit, Substance Misuse Division.

Cavanaugh, D. A. & Muck, R. D. (2004). Using research to improve treatment for adolescents: findings from two CSAT demonstrations. *Journal of Psychoactive Drugs*, **36**, 1–3.

CSAP (Center for Substance Abuse Prevention) (2000). *Strengthening America's Families: Model Family Programs for Substance Abuse and Delinquency Prevention.* Salt Lake City, UT: University of Utah.

CSAT (Center for Substance Abuse Treatment) (1995). *Planning for Alcohol and other Drug Abuse Treatment for Adults in the Criminal Justice System. [Treatment Improvement Protocol Series, No. 17.]* Washington, DC: Substance Abuse and Mental Health Services Administration, Department of Health and Human Services.

(1999). *Treatment of Adolescents with Substance Use Disorders. [Treatment Improvement Protocol Series, No. 32.]* Washington, DC: Government Printing Office.

Crowley, T. J., Mikulich, S. K., MacDonald, M., Young, S. E., & Zerbe, G. O. (1998). Substance-dependent, conduct-disordered adolescent males: severity of diagnosis predicts 2-year outcome. *Drug and Alcohol Dependence*, **49**, 225–237.

Currie, E., Duroy, T. H., & Lewis, L. (2003). Introduction to the special section: qualitative explorations of adolescents in treatment. *Journal of Drug Issues*, **33**, 769–776.

Dakof, G. A. (2003). *Family-based Juvenile Drug Court Services.* [Grant 1R01 DA17478] Rockville, MD: National Institutes of Health.

de la Rosa, M., Vega, R., & Radisch, M. A. (2000). The role of acculturation in the substance abuse behavior of African-American and Latino adolescents: advances, issues, and recommendations. *Journal of Psychoactive Drugs*, **32**, 33–42.

Deas, D. & Thomas, S. E. (2001). An overview of controlled studies of adolescent substance abuse treatment. *American Journal on Addictions*, **10**, 178–189.

Deas, D., Riggs, P., Langenbucher, J., Godman, M., & Brown, S. (2000). Adolescents are not adults: developmental considerations in alcohol users. *Alcoholism: Clinical and Experimental Research*, **24**, 232–237.

Dennis, M. L. (2002). *Treatment Research on Adolescent Drug and Alcohol Abuse: Despite Progress, Many Challenges Remain.* Washington, DC: Academy for Health Services Research and Health Policy.

Dennis, M. L. & Stevens, S. J. (2003). Maltreatment issues and outcomes of adolescents enrolled in substance abuse treatment. *Child Maltreatment: Journal of the American Professional Society on the Abuse of Children*, **8**, 3–6.

Dennis, M. L., Titus, J. C., Diamond, G., *et al.* & the CYT Steering Committee. (2002). The Cannabis Youth Treatment (CYT) experiment: rationale, study design, and analysis plan. *Addiction*, **97**(Suppl. 1), 16–34.

Dennis, M. L., Dawud-Noursi, S., Muck, R. D., & McDermeit, M. (2003). The need for developing and evaluating adolescent treatment models. In S. J. Stevens & A. R. Morral (eds.), *Adolescent Substance Abuse Treatment in the United States: Exemplary Models from a National Evaluation Study* (pp. 3–34). New York: Haworth Press.

Dennis, M. L., Godley, S. H., Diamond, G., *et al.* (2004). The Cannabis Youth Treatment (CYT) study: main findings from two randomized trials. *Journal of Substance Abuse Treatment*, **27**, 197–213.

Dishion, T. J. & Kavanagh, K. (2003). *Intervening in Adolescent Problem Behavior: A Family-centered Approach.* New York: Guilford Press.

DrugScope (2003). Linking practice to research/research to practice: what works, what doesn't, what could be done better. *Drug and Alcohol Findings* **7**, 13.

Drug Strategies (2003). *Treating Teens: A Guide to Adolescent Drug Problems.* Washington, DC: Drug Strategies.

EMCDDA (European Monitoring Centre for Drugs and Drug Addiction) (2003a). *2003 Annual Report on the Drug Situation in the EU and Norway: Some 'Cautious Optimism' but Beware of Complacency, Warns Agency.* Lisbon: EMCDDA. Retrieved June 21, 2004 from http://annualreport.emcdda.eu.int/download/mainreport-en.pdf.

    (2003b). Drug use amongst vulnerable young people. *Drugs In Focus, 10.* Lisbon: EMCDDA. Retrieved June 21, 2004, from http://www.emcdda.eu.int/multimedia/publications/Policy_briefings/10_12/pb_10_en.pdf.

EORG (European Opinion Research Group) (2002, October). *Attitudes and Opinions of Young People in the European Union on Drugs* (Eurobarometer 51.2/Special Eurobarometer 172). Brussels: EORG. Retrieved June 21, 2004 from http://europa.eu.int/comm/public_opinion/archives/eb/ebs_172_en.pdf.

Etheridge, R. M., Smith, J. C., Rounds-Bryant, J. L., & Hubbard, R. L. (2001). Drug abuse treatment and comprehensive services for adolescents. *Journal of Adolescent Research*, **16**, 563–589.

Farabee, D., Shen, H., Hser, Y., Grella, C. E., & Anglin, M. D. (2001). The effect of drug treatment on criminal behavior among adolescents in DATOS-A. *Journal of Adolescent Research*, **16**, 679–696.

Fletcher, B. W. & Grella, C. E. (2001). The Drug Abuse Treatment Outcome Studies for Adolescents. [Preface to the *JAR* Special Issue.] *Journal of Adolescent Research*, **16**, 537–544.

Fromme, K. & Brown, S. A. (2000). Empirically based prevention and treatment approaches for adolescent and young adult substance. *Cognitive and Behavioral Practice*, **7**, 61–64.

Garland, A. F., Aarons, G. A., Saltzman, M. D., & Kruse, M. I. (2000). Correlates of adolescents' satisfaction with mental health services. *Mental Health Services Research*, **2**, 127–139.

Garland, A. F., Hough, R. L., Landsverk, J. A., & Brown, S. A. (2001). Multi-sectors of systems of care for youth with mental health needs. *Children's Services: Social Policy, Research, and Practice*, **4**, 123–140.

Gil, A. G., Vega, W. A., & Biafora, F. (1998). Temporal influences of family structure and family risk factors on drug use initiation in a multiethnic sample of adolescent boys. *Journal of Youth and Adolescence*, **27**, 373–393.

Gilvarry, E. (2000). Substance abuse in young people. *Journal of Child Psychology and Psychiatry and Allied Disciplines*, **41**, 55–80.

Godley, S. H., White, W. L., Diamond, G., Passetti, L., & Titus, J. C. (2001). Therapist reactions to manual-guided therapies for the treatment of adolescent marijuana users. *Clinical Psychology: Science and Practice*, **8**, 405–417.

Grella, C. E., Hser, Y. I., Joshi, V., & Rounds-Bryant, J. (2001). Drug treatment outcomes for adolescents with comorbid mental and substance use disorders. *Journal of Nervous and Mental Diseases*, **189**, 384–392.

Hawkins, J. D., Catalano, R. F., & Miller, J. Y. (1992). Risk and protective factors for alcohol and other drug problems in adolescence and early adulthood: implications for substance abuse prevention. *Psychological Bulletin*, **112**, 64–105.

Hogue, A., Liddle, H. A., Rowe, C., Turner, R. M., Dakof, G. A., & LaPann, K. (1998). Treatment adherence and differentiation in individual versus family therapy for adolescent substance abuse. *Journal of Counseling Psychology*, **45**, 104–114.

Institute of Medicine (1998). *Bridging the Gap between Practice and Research: Forging Partnerships with Community-based Drugs and Alcohol Treatment*. Washington, DC: National Academy Press.

Jackson-Gilfort, A., Liddle, H. A., Tejeda, M. J., & Dakof, G. A. (2001). Facilitating engagement of African-American male adolescents in family therapy: a cultural theme process study. *Journal of Black Psychology*, **27**, 321–340.

Jaycox, L. H., Morral, A. R., & Juvonen, J. (2003). Mental health and medical problems and service use among adolescent substance abusers. *Journal of the American Academy of Child and Adolescent Psychiatry*, **42**, 701–709.

Jessor, R. & Jessor, S. L. (1977). *Problem Behavior and Psychosocial Development: A Longitudinal Study in Youth*. New York: Academic Press.

Johnston, L. D., O'Malley, P. M., & Bachman, J. G. (2003). *Monitoring the Future National Survey Results on Adolescent Drug Use: Overview of Key Findings, 2002*. [Report 03-5374] Bethesda, MD: National Institute on Drug Abuse.

Kaminer, Y. (2001). Adolescent substance abuse treatment: where do we go from here. *Alcohol and Drug Abuse*, **52**, 147–149.

Kaminer, Y., Tarter, R. E., Bukstein, O. G., & Kabene, M. (1992). Comparison between treatment completers and noncompleters among dually diagnosed substance-abusing adolescents. *Journal of the American Academy of Child and Adolescent Psychiatry*, **31**, 1046–1049.

Ketelaars, T., van Laar, M. W., van Gageldonk, A., & Cruts, A. A. N. (2002). *Report to the EMCDDA by the Retoix National Focal Point: The Netherlands Drug Situation 2001*. Lisbon: EMCDDA. Retrieved June 21, 2004, from http://www.emcdda.eu.int/multimedia/ publications/national_reports/2002/Netherlands/NR2002_Netherlands.pdf.

Kumpfer, K. L. & Alvarado, R. (1995). Strengthening families to prevent drug use in multiethnic youth. In G. J. Botvin, S. Schinke, & M. A. Orlandi (eds.), *Preventing Childhood Disorders, Substance Abuse, and Delinquency* (pp. 241–267). Thousand Oaks, CA: Sage.

Latimer, W. W., Winters, K. C., D'Zurilla, T., & Nichols, M. (2003). Integrated family and cognitive–behavioral therapy for adolescent substance abusers: a stage I efficacy study. *Drug and Alcohol Dependence*, **71**, 303–317.

Liddle, H. A. (1999). Theory development in a family-based therapy for adolescent drug abuse. *Journal of Clinical Child Psychology*, **28**, 521–532.

(2002a). *Cannabis Youth Treatment (CYT) Series, Vol. 5: Multidimensional Family Therapy for Adolescent Cannabis users*. Rockville, MD: Center for Substance Abuse Treatment, Substance Abuse and Mental Health Services Administration.

(2002b). Advances in family-based therapy for adolescent substance abuse: findings from the Multidimensional Family Therapy research program. In L. S. Harris (ed.), *Problems of Drug Dependence 2001: Proceedings of the 63rd Annual Scientific Meeting*. [*NIDA Research Monograph* No. 182, pp. 113–115.] Bethesda, MD: National Institute on Drug Abuse.

(2004). Family-based therapies for adolescent alcohol and drug abuse: research contributions and future research needs. *Addiction* **99**, (Suppl. 2): 76–92.

Liddle, H. A., Rowe, C. L., Diamond, G. M., *et al.* (2000). Towards a developmental family therapy: the clinical utility of adolescent development research. *Journal of Marital and Family Therapy*, **26**, 491–506.

Liddle, H. A., Dakof, G. A., Parker, K., *et al.* (2001). Multidimensional Family Therapy for adolescent drug abuse: results of a randomized clinical trial. *American Journal of Drug and Alcohol Abuse*, **27**, 651–687.

Liddle, H. A., Rowe, C. L., Quille, T., *et al.* (2002). Transporting a research-based adolescent drug treatment into practice. *Journal of Substance Abuse Treatment*, **22**, 1–13.

Liddle, H. A., Rowe, C. L., Ungaro, R. A., Dakof, G. A., & Henderson, C. E. (2004). Early intervention for adolescent substance abuse: pretreatment to post-treatment outcomes of a randomized controlled trial comparing multidimensional family therapy and peer group treatment. *Journal of Psychoactive Drugs*, **36**, 2–37.

McKeganey, N., McIntosh, J., MacDonald, F., *et al.* (2003). *Preteens and Illegal Drug Use: Use, Offers, Exposure and Prevention*. Glasgow: Department of Health Policy Research Program.

McLellan, A. T. (2004). Have we evaluated addiction treatment correctly? Implications from a chronic care perspective. *Addiction*, **97**, 249–252.

Meyers, K., Webb, A., Frantz, J., & Randall, M. (2003). What does it take to retain substance-abusing adolescents in research protocols? Delineation of effort required, strategies undertaken, costs incurred, and 6-month post-treatment differences by retention difficulty. *Drug and Alcohol Dependence*, **69**, 73–85.

Monti, P. M., Colby, S. M., & O'Leary, T. A. (2001). Introduction. In P. M. Monti, S. M. Colby, & T. A. O'Leary (eds.), *Adolescents, Alcohol, and Substance Abuse: Reaching Teens through Brief Interventions* (pp. 1–16). New York: Guilford Press.

Muck, R., Zempolich, K. A., Titus, J. C., *et al.* (2001). An overview of the effectiveness of adolescent substance abuse treatment models. *Youth and Society*, **33**, 143–168.

NIAAA (National Institute on Alcohol Abuse and Alcoholism) (1998). *Treatment for Adolescent Alcohol Abuse and Alcoholism*. [RFA-AA-98-003] Bethesda, MD: NIAAA. Retrieved May 15, 2004, from http://grants2.nih.gov/grants/guide/rfa-files/RFA-AA-98-003.html.

(2001). *Strategic Plan to Address Health Disparities.* Bethesda, MD: NIAAA. Retrieved May 15, 2004, from http://www.niaaa.nih.gov/about/health.PDF.

(2003). *Treatment of Adolescents with Alcohol Use Disorders.* [PA-03-088] Bethesda, MD: NIAAA. Retrieved May 15, 2004, from http://grants2.nih.gov/grants/guide/pa-files/PA-03-088.html.

NIDA (National Institute on Drug Abuse) (1993). *Behavioral Therapies Development Program.* Rockville, MD: National Institutes of Health. Retrieved May 15, 2004 from http://grants.nih.gov/grants/guide/rfa-files/RFA-DA-94-002.html.

(1999a). *Principles of Drug Addiction Treatment: A Research-based Guide.* [Report No. 99–4180] Rockville, MD: National Institute of Health.

(1999b). *National Drug Abuse Treatment Clinical Trials Network.* [RFA-DA-99-004]. Rockville, MD: National Institute on Drug Abuse. Retrieved May 5, 2005, from http://grants1.nih.gov/grants/guide/rfa-files/RFA-DA-99-004.html.

(2002a). *Improving Behavioral Health Services and Treatment for Adolescent Drug Abuse.* [Report RFA-DA-03-003] Rockville, MD: National Institutes of Health. Retrieved May 15, 2004 from http://grants1.nih.gov/grants/guide/rfa-files/RFA-DA-03-003.html.

(2002b). *National Criminal Justice Drug Abuse Treatment Services Research System.* [Report RFA-DA-02-011] Rockville, MD: National Institutes of Health. Retrieved May 15, 2004 from http://grants2.nih.gov/grants/guide/rfa-files/RFA-DA-02-011.html.

Randall, J., Henggeler, S. W., Cunnigham, P. B., Rowland, M. D., & Swenson, C. C. (2001). Adapting multisystemic therapy to treat adolescent substance abuse more effectively. *Cognitive and Behavioral Practice,* **8**, 359–366.

Rigter, H. (2003). *Action Plan on Cannabis Research 2003–2006: Belgium, Germany, France, the Netherlands, Switzerland.* The Hague: National Drug Monitor/Trimbos Institute.

Rigter, H., van Gageldonk, A., Ketelaars, T., & van Laar, M. (2004). *Helping Problem Users of Drugs. The Science Base for Treatments and Other Interventions.* Utrecht: National Drug Monitor/Trimbos Institute.

Robert Wood Johnson Foundation. (2001). *Reclaiming Futures: Building Community Solutions to Substance Abuse and Delinquency.* Princeton, NJ: Robert Wood Johnson Foundation. Retrieved July 15, 2004 from http://www.reclaimingfutures.org/.

Rodney, H. E., Mupier, R., & Crafter, B. (1996). Predictors of alcohol drinking among African-American adolescents: implication for violence prevention. *Journal of Negro Education,* **65**, 434–444.

Roebuck, M. C., French, M. T., & McLellan, A. T. (2003). DATStats: Summary results from 85 completed drug abuse treatment cost analysis programs (DATCAPs). *Journal of Substance Abuse Treatment,* **25**, 51–57.

Rowe, C. L. & Liddle, H. A. (2003). Substance abuse. *Journal of Marital and Family Therapy,* **29**, 97–120.

Rowe, C. L., Liddle, H. A., McClintic, K., & Quille, T. J. (2002). Integrative treatment development: multidimensional family therapy for adolescent substance abuse. In J. Lebow & F. W. Kaslow (eds.), *Comprehensive Handbook of Psychotherapy Integrative/Eclectic* 4th edn, Vol. 4 (pp. 133–161). New York: John Wiley.

Rowe, C. L., Liddle, H. A., Greenbaum, P. E., & Henderson, C. (2004). Impact of psychiatric comorbidity on treatment outcomes of adolescent drug abusers. *Journal of Substance Abuse Treatment*, **26**, 1–12.

SAMHSA (Substance Abuse and Mental Health Services Administration) (1998a). *Services Research Outcomes Study (SROS)*. Rockville, MD: Department of Health and Human Services, Substance Abuse and Mental Health Services Administration, Office of Applied Studies.

(1998b). *Grants for the Identification of Exemplary Treatment Models for Adolescents*. [GFA No. TI-98-007] Rockville, MD: Department of Health and Human Services, Substance Abuse and Mental Health Service Administration.

(1999). *Grants for the Evaluation of Treatment Models for Adolescents*. [GFA No. TI-99-001] Rockville, MD: Department of Health and Human Services, Substance Abuse and Mental Health Service Administration.

Scheier, L. M., Botvin, G. J., Diaz, T., & Ifill-Williams, M. (1997). Ethnic identity as a moderator of psychosocial risk and adolescent alcohol and marijuana use: Concurrent and longitudinal analyses. *Journal of Child and Adolescent Substance Abuse*, **6**, 21–47.

Scottish Executive (1999). *Tackling Drugs in Scotland: Action in Partnership*. Edinburgh: The Scottish Office.

(2003). *A Guide to Working in Partnership: Employability Provision for Drug Users*. Edinburgh: Scottish Executive Effective Interventions Unit.

Simpson, D. D. (2002). A conceptual framework for transferring research to practice. *Journal of Substance Abuse Treatment*, **22**, 171–182.

Stevens, S. & Morral, A. R. (2003). *Substance Abuse Treatment in the United States*. New York: Haworth Press.

Strijker, J., Boersma, C. J., Zandberg, T. J., & Rink, J. E. (2001). *Jong en verslaafd. Onderzoek naar nut en noodzaak van intersectorale behandeling voor verslaafde jongeren in het Bauhuus*. Groningen: Rijk university.

UK Anti-Drugs Co-Ordinator (2000). *UKADC Second National plan 2000/2001: Tackling Drugs to Build a Better Britain*. London: Cabinet Office.

UK Department of Health (2002). *Statistics on Young People and Drug Misuse: England, 2000 and 2001*. [*Statistical Bulletin 2002/15*] London: Department of Health.

UK Drug Strategy Directorate (2002). *Updated Drug Strategy 2002*. London: Home Office Research.

Wagner, E. F., & Waldron, H. B. (2001). *Innovations in Adolescent Substance Abuse Interventions*. Amsterdam, Pergamon.

Wallace, J. M. J. (1999). The sociology ecology of addiction: race, risk, and resilience. *Pediatrics*, 1122–1127.

Weinberg, N. Z., Rahdert, E., Colliver, J. D., & Glantz, M. D. (1998). Adolescent substance abuse: a review of the past 10 years. *Journal of the American Academy of Child and Adolescent Psychiatry*, **37**, 252–261.

Wells, K., Koike, A., & Sherbourne, C. (2001). Ethnic disparities in unmet need for alcoholism, drug abuse, and mental health care. *American Journal of Psychiatry*, **58**, 2027–2032.

Williams, R. J. & Chang, S. Y. (2000). A comprehensive and comparative review of adolescent substance abuse treatment outcome. *Clinical Psychology: Science and Practice*, **7**, 138–166.

Winters, K. C., Latimer, W. L., & Stinchfield, R. D. (1999). Adolescent treatment. In P. J. Ott, R. E. Tarter, & R. T. Ammerman (eds.), *Sourcebook on Substance Abuse: Etiology, Epidemiology, Assessment, and Treatment* (pp. 350–361). Boston, MA: Allyn and Bacon.

Zucker, R. A., Ellis, D. A., Bingham, C. R., & Fitzgerald, H. E. (1996). The development of alcoholic subtypes: risk variation among alcoholic families during the early childhood. *Alcohol Health and Research World*, **20**, 46–54.

Part I

Theoretical, empirical, and methodological foundations for research into treatment of adolescent substance abuse

The developmental context for adolescent substance abuse intervention

Judith S. Brook, David W. Brook, and Kerstin Pahl

New York University School of Medicine, New York, USA

The first purpose of this chapter is to identify the risk and protective factors related to adolescent drug use, emphasizing the importance of the parent–child relationship. The framework is derived from family interactional theory. Operating within a developmental perspective, we explore the interrelations of risk and protective factors related to drug use. A second goal of the chapter is to elucidate the protective factors that mitigate adolescents' vulnerability to drug use, as well as enhance other protective factors. Finally, we consider the implications of etiological research on the risk and protective factors and their interactions for prevention and treatment based on a number of major studies undertaken since the mid-1990s.

Drug use and abuse are costly problems that affect the health and well-being of individuals and families. Despite a decline in drug use during the early 1990s, there has since been a subsequent increase (Bachman *et al.*, 1997). The personal, social, medical, and legal costs of adolescent drug use and abuse are considerable (Hawkins, Catalano, & Miller, 1992; Wallace & Muroff, 2002).

This chapter integrates findings from several cross-sectional and longitudinal studies conducted since the late 1980s on the psychosocial risk and protective factors for drug use and abuse. Risk factors precede drug use, increasing the probability of later drug use and abuse. Protective factors ameliorate the effect of these risk factors or enhance those of other protective factors leading to less drug use. Numerous studies conducted since the 1970s have contributed to an understanding of the etiology of drug use (Brook *et al.*, 1990; Hawkins *et al.*, 1992; Oetting & Donnermeyer, 1998).

The main goals of our own research have been to understand the underlying causes of adolescent drug use and abuse within a developmental framework, and to test hypothetical relationships among developmental, familial, personality, peer, and contextual factors. The data from these studies (Brook *et al.*, 1990, 1997a,b; Brook,

Adolescent Substance Abuse: Research and Clinical Advances, ed. Howard A. Liddle and Cynthia L. Rowe.
Published by Cambridge University Press. © Cambridge University Press 2006.

Cohen, & Brook, 1998a; Brook *et al.*, 1998b) are generally consistent with the findings of other researchers in the field. While our research complements that of others, it is also unique in several important ways. First, some of our longitudinal studies began when the participants were in early childhood. This developmental approach to studying adolescent drug use and abuse allows us to include in our research the childhood factors that are antecedent to and underlie later determinants of drug use and abuse in adolescence. While the pathways leading to adolescent drug use begin early in childhood, they may be influenced later by many different events and circumstances. In addition, we have assessed the risk and protective factors involved in adolescent substance use and abuse and integrated our findings regarding these issues into a further understanding of etiology. The result is a family interactional theory of adolescent substance use (Brook *et al.*, 1990), which provides a developmental framework to assess some of the determinants of drug use and abuse.

The developmental model

Operating within the framework of family interactional theory, the developmental model that forms the basis for our research on adolescent drug use has been tested and supported in a number of cross-sectional and longitudinal studies (Fig. 2.1).

This theoretical framework posits that adolescent drug use is determined by the interrelationships between factors in several psychosocial domains, including the adolescent's personality characteristics (e.g., ego integration), previous drug use, parental characteristics (e.g., parental depression and drug use), the adolescent's relationships with family members (e.g., mutual attachment), and features of the environment (e.g., neighborhood characteristics).

Of central importance to this model is the parent–child relationship, in particular the presence of a close affectional bond, non-conflictual relations between child and parents, and the adolescent's identification with the parent. Our research has shown that a positive mutual attachment in the parent–child relationship is critical in preventing drug use (Brook *et al.*, 1990, 1998c, 2001).

The basic pathways to adolescent drug use and abuse are summarized below.

1. Internalization of societal values by the parent and the absence of parental drug use and psychopathology create a warm, conflict-free parent–child relationship, which leads to the adolescent's identification with the parent. The result is a firm mutual attachment relationship between parent and child.

2. As a consequence of this attachment and the child's identification with the parent, the child internalizes the conventional parts of the parent's personality, attitudes, and behaviors, which, in turn, leads to the formation of a psychologically healthy and conventional personality in adolescence.

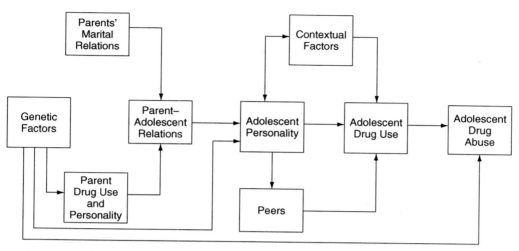

Fig. 2.1   Family interactional theory: the developmental model.

3. Healthy adolescent personality characteristics (e.g., conventionality, control of emotions) are then expressed in attitudes and behaviors that discourage affiliations with peers who use drugs, supporting the adolescent's own abstinence from drug use and, ultimately, from substance abuse. Drug use is always a mediating step between various psychosocial domains and the development of substance abuse (Brook, Rosen, & Zhang, 2002a; Glantz et al., 1999).

In addition, family interactional theory also emphasizes the importance of the adolescent's context for determining his/her drug use. For example, being exposed to environments in which drugs are readily available heightens the chances of getting involved in substance use. Relationships among psychosocial domains may also be culture specific, and so particular pathways may differ from one cultural context to another. For example, an important finding of our research in Colombia, South America, is that contextual violence moderates the relationship between adolescents' illegal drug use and risky sexual behaviors (Brook et al., 2002b).

A basic feature of our developmental model is the assumption that pathways to adolescent drug use and abuse have their origins in childhood. In one of our longitudinal studies (Brook et al., 1997b), we tested the linkages between a set of child personality, family, and ecological factors and domains of adolescent personality and parent–adolescent relations and found several continuities between childhood and adolescence (see below).

The influence of each domain

The childhood domain

There are important continuities from childhood to adolescence. Early temperamental dispositions, family experiences, and interactions with the environment influence whether the adolescent will develop a conventional or an unconventional (i.e., drug-use prone) personality. Several investigators have found childhood aggression to be a powerful predictor of adolescent and adult drug use (Brook *et al.*, 1998c; Brook & Newcomb, 1995; Kaplan, 1995; McCord, 1988). Certain personality predispositions that are related to later drug use and abuse, such as antisocial behavior and aggression, appear to be moderately stable from childhood through adolescence (Cohen & Brook, 1987; Moffitt, 1993). A review of the literature (Windle & Windle, 1993) has shown that externalizing behaviors are not only stable over time but also predictive of substance abuse.

Childhood psychopathology is a great risk factor for problem behaviors, including substance abuse, later in life. Two of the most common psychiatric disorders that have been identified as risk factors for substance abuse are major depressive disorder and antisocial personality disorder (Capaldi & Stoolmiller, 1999). Studies of clinical and epidemiological samples have also suggested that drug abuse and psychopathology are often linked (Kessler *et al.*, 1996). Survey research has shown that psychiatric disorders, including conduct and oppositional disorder, attention deficit disorder, anxiety disorders, particularly phobic disorders, and major depressive disorder are related to an increased risk of alcoholism and drug abuse (Fergusson, Horwood, & Lynskey, 1994; Glantz *et al.*, 1999; Kessler *et al.*, 1996).

Together, our findings show that the effects of a pattern of childhood personality, familial, and ecological risk factors for adolescent drug use are mediated by adolescent personality traits and the parent–adolescent attachment. Further, our longitudinal research also supports the view that childhood factors may interact with adolescent factors to affect the adolescent's use of drugs (Brook *et al.*, 1990). Our findings indicated that an early risk factor can be moderated by the presence or absence of a protective factor at a later point in time, reducing or increasing the risk of adolescent drug use.

The adolescent personality domain

The domain of adolescent personality characteristics has a powerful impact on the adolescent's drug use (Bachman *et al.*, 1997; Brook *et al.*, 1990; Kaplan, 1995). In our research, we have studied four distinct aspects of the personality domain: conventionality/unconventionality, emotional control, intrapersonal functioning, and interpersonal relatedness. Of these, the most powerful predictors of more frequent drug use are the variables reflecting unconventionality: namely sensation seeking, rebelliousness, tolerance of deviance, and low school achievement.

In our research, dimensions of unconventionality affected drug use independently of family or peers; that is, despite benign family and peer conditions, drug-prone personality traits contributed to involvement in drug use. However, we found the personality domain to be related to substance use disorders indirectly, via prior drug use (Brook *et al.*, 2002a).

As noted above, psychopathology is another important risk factor for adolescents' drug use and abuse (Glantz *et al.*, 1999). In particular, substance use disorders tend to be comorbid with other psychiatric diagnoses such as bipolar disorder (Kessler *et al.*, 1996), schizophrenia, and eating disorders (Holderness, Brooks-Gunn, & Warren, 1994).

The family relations domain
Parent–adolescent mutual attachment

The parent–child mutual attachment relationship is important both directly and indirectly in terms of its effect on adolescent drug use (Wills *et al.*, 2001). A mutually affectionate, conflict-free attachment promotes the adolescent's identification with the parent and ultimately leads to the adolescent's introjection of the parents' values and behaviors (Brook *et al.*, 1998c). Thus mutual attachment and identification with parents who are traditional promotes the development of conventional and well-adjusted adolescents. Parents of non-users, in comparison with parents of users, tend to report greater warmth (more child-centeredness, affection, and communication) and less conflict in the relationship with their children (Brook *et al.*, 1998c, 1999).

In one of our recent studies, we found that low family bonding, including low marital harmony, parent–adolescent conflict, and less maternal satisfaction with the adolescent, predicted early substance use disorders directly in a sample of young adults (Brook *et al.*, 2002a). Together, these findings suggest that an affectionate and non-conflictual parent–adolescent attachment relationship helps adolescents to abstain from drug use and abuse.

Parental discipline

Another way in which parents help to shape the behavior of the adolescent is through control (disciplinary techniques). This includes physical and psychological forms of discipline. In our research, parental control patterns that involve setting clear requirements for mature and responsible behavior, in contrast to power-assertive (authoritarian) techniques of discipline, resulted in less drug use. Formulating clear behavioral expectations on the one hand while maintaining high levels of involvement on the other (two aspects of authoritative parenting) have been linked with adolescents' psychological well-being (Brook *et al.*, 1990; Kosterman *et al.*, 2000).

Furthermore, appropriate parental monitoring, another aspect of authoritative parenting, has been found to be effective in reducing delinquency and substance use and abuse (Dishion & McMahon, 1998; Fletcher, Darling, & Steinberg, 1995; LeDoux *et al.*, 2002).

The parental drug use and personality domain

Parental drug use has been found by many investigators to be related to the adolescent's own drug use (Peterson *et al.*, 1995). Further, having had family members with alcohol or drug use problems increases adolescents' risk for drug abuse/dependence (Brook *et al.*, 2002a; Kilpatrick *et al.*, 2000), and substance use disorders in young adulthood are directly affected by parental drug use, including illegal drugs and alcohol (Brook *et al.*, 2002a). Intergenerational transmission may be influenced by genetic factors and/or reflect parental modeling of drug use.

There are also indirect effects of parental drug use on the adolescent's own use of drugs (Hansen *et al.*, 1987). Specifically, parental drug use is associated with the adolescent's selection of friends who use drugs, which, in turn, is related to the adolescent's own drug use.

We also found that parental personality factors and attitudes towards the child's drug use played a significant role in the adolescent's drug use and abuse, with most of their effects mediated by other domains, especially the parent–adolescent attachment relationship (Brook *et al.*, 1990). The parental personality variables that play a protective role in the adolescent's drug use and abuse include the parents' endorsement and modeling of traditional values and behaviors (e.g., conventional attitudes and impulse control).

The marital relationship domain

The relationship between the adolescent's parents needs to be considered when trying to understand the adolescent's development. Family conflict and having parents who are not emotionally supportive are associated with a higher risk for delinquency and drug use. Marital conflict is likely to interfere with the development of mutual attachment between the parent and the child, reducing the opportunity for the parent to influence the child and for the child to internalize conventional rules. Marital discord has also been found to affect the quality of parenting (Finchmam, Grych, & Osborne, 1994) and may result in an increased risk of drug use. Indeed, parental conflict may be a greater risk factor for adolescent drug use than parental absence (Farrington, 1991).

The peer domain

The percentage of variance in drug use contributed by the peer domain exceeds that of all other intrapersonal or interpersonal domains (Kandel, 1996). Peers have been found to have a greater effect than parents on adolescent drug use among Whites, African-Americans, Asians, and Latinos (Newcomb & Bentler, 1986). In general, the importance of the peer group is consistent across a variety of studies and cultures (Donovan, 1996; Swaim, Bates, & Chavez, 1998).

Unconventional adolescents are likely to have friends who use drugs. This may be explained in part by assortative peer selection, which refers to the process of selecting friends who are similar to oneself (Kandel, 1996). If an adolescent is using drugs, he or she is more likely to associate with drug-using peers, which, in turn, increases the chance of the adolescent's maintaining or increasing his or her own drug involvement. Unconventional (i.e., drug-prone) adolescents tend to select deviant peers who share characteristics similar to their own personality attributes (Brook *et al.*, 1990). Deviant peers, in turn, influence deviant attitudes and behavior via role modeling, which further increases the probability of adolescent drug use.

In summary, peers are most important in the initiation and maintenance of drug use, but not drug abuse. While drug-abusing individuals tend to socialize with other drug abusers, peer drug use does not seem to lead directly to drug abuse as much as do other factors (e.g., self-drug use, biological vulnerabilities, parental drug use). One of our recent studies found that peer drug use was directly related to self-drug use but indirectly related to substance abuse disorders (Brook *et al.*, 2002c).

The larger context

In this domain, environmental factors, such as drug availability, adverse economic conditions, a high crime rate, and neighborhood disorganization, have all been found to be related to drug use (Ryan *et al.*, 1999; Sampson, Raudenbush, & Earls 1997). In addition, the macro environment, including the effects of media, advertising, and social and legal policies, has important effects on adolescent drug use. The influence of cultural and ecological factors on drug use and abuse is mediated by their effects on family relations, personality, and peer factors.

For example, among other factors, having been a victim of violence or having witnessed violent acts puts adolescents at higher risk for drug abuse (Kilpatrick *et al.*, 2000). Our research in Colombia, South America, a country in which levels of drug availability and violence exceed that in the USA, has found that such factors are highly related to adolescent drug use. However, several cultural characteristics also serve as protective factors to buffer the effects of the numerous psychosocial and environmental risk factors (Brook *et al.*, 1998d). For example, religion, familism (a system of values that places the needs and rights of the family and community over individual needs and rights), and a respect for one's elders and authority all serve as protective or mitigating factors for drug use among Colombian youth. Family interactional theory, in which the personality and peer domains play a prominent role, best explains the pathways to adolescent marijuana use among Colombian youth.

Ethnicity

Ethnic and socioeconomic factors have main and moderator effects on drug use and abuse (Brook *et al.*, 1998b; Félix-Ortiz & Newcomb, 1999). Ethnic minority group membership can pose both risk and protective factors for drug use and abuse, as adolescents of different ethnic groups may be either differentially exposed and/or vulnerable to certain risk factors (Nurco *et al.*, 1997).

One way in which belonging to an ethnic/racial minority group may act as a risk factor for drug use and abuse is via its association with being marginalized. For example, in many urban ethnic and racial minority communities in the USA (e.g., African-American, Latino), individuals have little access to resources and opportunities, which can lead to indifference or even opposition to dominant social norms. This detachment from social norms may ultimately be expressed in high levels of substance use and abuse. Further, drug use may function as self-medication in the face of lack of opportunity and discrimination.

Among young Native Americans, many of whom are isolated on reservations, the most proximal risk factors for alcohol and illicit drug use and abuse are family problems and family dysfunction. This may be caused by the marginalized status of this group. Because of limited access to employment and educational opportunities, school drop-out rates and unemployment rates in Native American communities are often high (Chavers, 1991). Further, high levels of exposure to poverty and violence contribute to the production of conditions in which drug use and abuse can flourish (Fisher, Storck, & Bacon, 1999). However, there are also a number of protective factors to be found within Native American communities, including the adherence to traditional practices and values (Fisher *et al.*, 1999).

Among Latino adolescents, acculturative stress has been identified as a risk factor for drug use and abuse (Félix-Ortiz & Newcomb, 1999). Similarly, perceived discrimination has been found to be associated with elevated drug use among Latinos (Vega *et al.*, 1993). Further, gender differences in substance use in this ethnic group are pronounced. While many males tend to be heavy users of alcohol, women are likely to abstain (Canino, Burnam, & Caetano, 1992). This seems to be related to women's roles in traditional Latino culture. Church attendance and religiosity are correlated with lower levels of drug use, particularly among Latinos (Félix-Ortiz & Newcomb, 1999). Ethnic identity, familism, and religiosity serve as protective factors against adolescent drug use among Puerto Rican adolescents (Brook *et al.*, 1998b).

Research on drug use among African-American adolescents has shown that adolescents from this ethnic/racial group tend to use drugs less than White (Catalano *et al.*, 1993; Maddahian, Newcomb, & Bentler, 1988) and Puerto Rican (Brook *et al.*, 1997b) adolescents. This is the case despite that fact that African-American youth tend to be more exposed to a number of important contextual risk factors associated with adolescent substance use and abuse, including drug availability (LaVeist & Wallace, 2000), drug offers (Wallace & Muroff, 2002), and economic deprivation (Wallace & Muroff, 2002). African-American adolescents also seem to have a number of intra- and interpersonal protective factors that help them to abstain from drug use and may account for their lower levels of drug use compared with Whites, such as high levels of family bonding, religiosity, and less sensation seeking (Wallace & Muroff, 2002). Researchers concluded that, when other factors were controlled, African-American youth were at one third of the risk for substance abuse than their White counterparts (Kilpatrick *et al.*, 2000). As with Latinos, our own research showed that ethnic identity in African-American youth served as a protective factor against drug use (Brook *et al.*, 1998e).

Similarly, the cultural and ecological factors unique to Colombian youth provide differences in specific risk factors for marijuana use. Our study found that intrapersonal distress (depression, anxiety, and interpersonal difficulty), peer drug use, violence, and drug availability all had a greater impact on drug use in Colombia than in the USA (Nurco *et al.*, 1997). Furthermore, two important cultural factors, religion and familism, were more likely to protect adolescents from drug use in Colombia than in the USA.

The biological domain

Since the late 1980s, much progress has been made toward understanding the biological and genetic risk factors for drug use and drug abuse. Family studies have been undertaken to identify genetic vulnerability for drug abuse; for example, one line of research suggests that sons and daughters of alcoholics have a three- to fourfold risk for developing alcoholism (Institute of Medicine, 1996). While family studies identify genetic vulnerability, they cannot definitively determine the effects of genes compared with those of environmental factors on the development of alcoholism or drug abuse.

Another approach to the study of genetic vulnerability is the twin study paradigm, used to identify the role of genetic factors in the etiology of substance abuse in twins (Tsuang *et al.*, 2001). Overall, the results of these studies indicate that genetic factors do explain a proportion of the variance in the development of drug abuse. Furthermore, a proportion of the heritability of drug abuse in adulthood may be attributed to the same genetic factors as those that underlie the development of behavior problems in childhood. In addition to twin studies, adoption studies have been used with some success to examine the respective roles of genetic and environmental factors in problem behavior, alcoholism, and drug abuse (Tsuang *et al.*, 2001). Children of alcoholics who are raised by non-alcoholic parents have been shown to have a three- to fourfold increased risk for alcohol abuse compared with adoptees whose biological parents were not alcoholics.

Physiological factors may enhance the individual's vulnerability to drug and alcohol abuse (Tabakoff *et al.*, 1988). Such physiological influences include neurochemical impairment and metabolic variations in susceptibility to drugs (Cloninger, 1987). Indeed, there are large variations between individuals and ethnic groups in the physiological susceptibility to drugs and alcohol. The decreased ability to metabolize alcohol may be a protective factor in some Asians in preventing continued exposure. In contrast, efficient metabolism may permit higher levels of exposure, which is more conducive to the development of abuse and dependence.

Interactions of individual, family, peer, and environmental factors

Earlier in this chapter, we identified numerous risk and protective factors for adolescent drug use and abuse. Certainly, the goal of many prevention programs should be toward early risk reduction. Another approach is to enhance protective factors that serve to buffer such risks, ultimately leading to less drug use (Jessor *et al.*, 1995). In our view, risk and protective factors are not always simply the two ends of a continuum of risk (a linear relationship); in other words, the absence of a particular risk does not automatically qualify as a protective factor. Equally, the absence of a particular protective factor does not necessarily pose a risk for a particular problem behavior such as drug use and abuse (Fisher *et al.*, 1999). Rather, some risk and protective factors have interactive relationships with one another in their effects on adolescent drug abuse (Hawkins *et al.*, 1992). In our research (Brook *et al.*, 1990, 1998b), we have focused on two types of interactive process that can either offset risk factors or enhance protective factors. We have considered the interactive relationships between a number of variables from the domains of personality, family, peers, and the adolescents' environment, reflecting risk or protection against risk. In the first type of interaction (risk/protective), risk factors are attenuated by protective factors. The buffering model posits that certain factors buffer (protect) individuals from the potentially pathogenic influences of risk factors. Evidence has shown that adolescents may be resilient even under the most damaging circumstances (Wallace & Muroff, 2002).

The second type of interaction (protective/protective) is a synergistic process, in which one protective factor potentiates another protective factor, so that the multiplicative effect of both protective factors is greater than their sum. In the following paragraphs, we will review our own findings as well as those of other researchers, dividing them into risk/protective interactions and protective/protective interactions, as well as by domains of psychosocial influences.

Risk/protective interactions
Individual characteristics as buffers

Our research has shown that aspects of the adolescent or young adult's personality can buffer against the risks for drug use and abuse stemming from a variety of domains, including peers and family (Brook, 1993; Brook et al., 1990, 1992a, 1997b, 2000, 2001). Adolescent conventionality, in particular, serves a strong protective function, particularly for girls, in offsetting risks for drug use (Brook et al., 1990, 1997c, 2000, 2001). For example, we found that adolescent church attendance buffered against the risks posed by paternal marijuana use (Brook et al., 2001), and being oriented towards one's parents protected against peer marijuana use and associating with deviant peers (Brook et al., 1992a; Brook, 1993). Kendler, Gardner, and Prescott (1997) also identified personal devotion (religiosity) as a buffer against the risks posed by negative life events. We also found that low levels of depressive mood and social isolation acted as buffers against the risk posed by peer deviance (Brook et al., 1997c).

Hussong and Chassin (1997) further found that perceived control over external events as well as cognitive coping offset the risk of having an alcoholic parent for the onset of adolescent substance use. Similarly, emotional self-control can protect adolescents from the risks for drug abuse posed by peers, family, and the environment. Wills, Sandy, and Yaeger (2002) found that self-regulation acted as a moderator of the level of substance use and problems associated with it.

Other researchers have found that adolescent values and attitudes may act as protective factors against drug risks. For example, Reifman et al. (2002) found that health values buffered against an index of risks for alcohol misuse, including peer deviance, parental alcohol abuse, and low parental monitoring. Furthermore, Tiet et al. (1998) found that the intelligence quotient (IQ) buffered against the risk of negative life events. Those high-risk adolescents (i.e., those who had experienced more negative life events) with higher IQs evidenced higher levels of adjustment (including the absence of substance use disorder) than those with lower IQ levels.

Ethnic identity as a protective factor

Some of our recent research with African-American and Puerto Rican teenagers has shown that a firm sense of belonging to one's ethnic group, ethnic pride, and knowledge about one's ethnic group were able to offset a variety of risk factors for adolescent drug use including perceived low drug risk, parental drug use, drug availability, and peer drug use and pro-drug attitudes (Brook *et al.*, 1998e,f; Brook & Pahl, 2005). Scheier *et al.* (1997) also investigated ethnic identity as a moderator of risk factors for drug use among adolescents from an ethnic minority. However, their findings were mixed: while some interactions were risk/protective in nature, there were two instances in which high levels of ethnic identity potentiated risks for drug use. We are not aware of other research investigating ethnic identity and related constructs within an interactive risk/protective paradigm. More research is needed to illuminate further the role of ethnic identity as a buffer against drug risks.

Familial factors as buffers

Among familial factors that serve as buffers against peer drug risks, we have identified parental conventionality and a strong parent–adolescent mutual attachment relationship (Brook *et al.*, 1990, 1992a, 2001; Brook, 1993; Morojele & Brook, 2001). Parental models of low drug use, conventionality, and adjustment may counteract the effects of drug-using models presented by the peer group. A strong mutual attachment between parent and child may offset such peer risk factors because parental attachment provides adolescents with a feeling of being worthy, a sense of predictability in their lives, and a general expectation of support, all of which help to mitigate the influences of peer drug use. Wills and Cleary (1996) found that the relationship between an index of negative life events and substance use was attenuated by parental support in a sample of adolescents. Furthermore, they found that the effects of peer affiliations and tolerance of deviance were buffered by parental support. In accord with social learning theory, it is likely that close relationships with parents decrease the need for adolescents to depend on peers for approval, which, in turn, reduces adolescent vulnerability to peer pressure for conformity to peer norms. A lower level of substance use by African-American youths may be related to the fact that they are less peer oriented and more parent oriented than their White counterparts (Wallace & Muroff, 2002).

Parental behaviors, such as high levels of parental monitoring, also buffer against peer (e.g., peer drug use) and personality (e.g., sensation seeking) risks (Morojele & Brook, 2001). In addition, Mounts (2002) found that parenting styles moderated the effect of parenting behaviors, such as monitoring, on their children's drug use and association with drug-using friends. For example, for adolescents whose parents were authoritarian (a parenting style often associated with negative outcomes), parental neutrality vis-à-vis their children's choices of friends was associated with choosing friends with lower levels of drug use. Furthermore, for adolescents with uninvolved parents, high levels of guiding children in their choice of friends were associated with lower levels of self-drug use.

To our knowledge, there has been no systematic study of the differential impact of one parent on risk factors associated with the other parent. We have found that risks stemming from the father–child relationship and from paternal drug use can be offset by the mother's conventionality and psychological adjustment and by a close mother–child attachment (Brook *et al.*, 1990).

Environmental factors as buffers

Environmental or contextual variables, such as neighborhood factors or a person's socioeconomic status, can further moderate the relationship between individual, peer, or family risks and adolescent drug use and abuse. For example, Wills *et al.* (1995) found that socioeconomic status moderated the relationship between certain risk factors (e.g., negative life events, peer drinking) and drug use. The relationship between the risk factors and substance use was greater for adolescents with lower socioeconomic status. Thus higher socioeconomic status acted as a protective factor. Furthermore, Legrand, McGue, and Iacono (1999) found that low levels of environmental risks buffered against a familial (genetic) risk of drug use.

Protective/protective interactions

Individual characteristics as enhancers of protective factors

In our research about the extent to which protective factors are further enhanced by other protective or resource factors in reducing the likelihood of adolescent drug use, we have again found that adolescent conventionality is an important target for intervention (Brook *et al.*, 1990, 1997c). Conventionality enhanced the effects of low peer drug use and low deviance. Furthermore, dimensions of emotional control, including ego integration and low levels of interpersonal aggression, enhanced the effect of these resource factors.

Ethnic identity as an enhancer of protective factors

Similarly, in our research, ethnic identity and other culture-specific variables acted to strengthen protective factors from various domains, including having achieving friends, non-conflictual relations with one's mother, low levels of family drug use, and high levels of ego integration. In particular, we found that, for Puerto Rican adolescents, affiliating with other Puerto Ricans and high levels of familism enhanced the protective effect of low levels of family drug use (Brook *et al.*, 1998f). For African-American youths, African-American awareness, ethnic identity, pride, and familism enhanced the protective effects of high ego integration, low rebelliousness, low depression, low family and peer drug use, non-conflictual relations with parents, associating with achieving peers, and low drug availability (Brook *et al.*, 1998e).

Familial factors as enhancers of protective factors

In our work, we have identified numerous protective factors from the family that enhance the effect of resource factors. In particular, parental warmth, child-centeredness, and communication have emerged as enhancers of adolescent conventionality, such as school achievement, intolerance of deviance, non-deviance, and non-rebelliousness (Brook *et al.*, 1997b).

Our most outstanding finding is the crucial role of the father in protective/protective interactions. Protective characteristics of the father (i.e., his general emotional stability, a strong father–adolescent bond, conventionality) enhance other protective factors, such as adolescent conventionality, positive maternal characteristics (non-use of drugs, positive child-rearing practices), and marital harmony (Brook *et al.*, 1990, 1997c).

In her study of the interactions of parenting styles and behaviors, Mounts (2002) identified the following protective/protective interactions: for adolescents from authoritative (a parenting style associated with positive adolescent outcomes) homes, high levels of guiding teens in their friendship choices was associated with low levels of drug use. Similarly, for adolescents with authoritative parents, higher levels of monitoring were associated with lower levels of peer drug use.

Peer factors as enhancers of protective factors

In two of our studies (Brook *et al.*, 1992b, 1997c) we also found that positive peer factors interacted with another protective factor to lower the likelihood of substance use. In particular, low levels of peer drug use and deviance enhanced the protective effects of intolerance of deviance, paternal affection, and low levels of the adolescent's interpersonal aggression. We are not aware of any other research identifying peer factors as interacting with other protective variables.

In sum, our findings suggest that in designing intervention programs, it is necessary not only to reduce risk factors but also to enhance protective factors for adolescent drug use and abuse. Furthermore, because risk and protective factors can occur across a variety of contexts of the adolescent's social environment, a broad-based, multidisciplinary approach to drug prevention and treatment should be pursued. Finally, with recent advances in the study of the genetics of drug abuse, research should focus on the interactions between psychosocial variables and genetic risk and protective factors for drug abuse.

Implications for prevention and treatment

Substance abuse is a chronic relapsing disease of the brain with biopsychosocial and cultural antecedents, concomitants, and consequences. The psychosocial roots of substance abuse in adolescence often are found in the interactions in the family and in the many groups in which the individual participates in the course of growth and development. For this reason, the treatment of adolescent substance abuse can involve many different methods, depending on the circumstances. Substance abuse is the phenotypic expression of the interaction of a genetic predisposition(s) (genotype) to substance abuse, certain personal or environmental risk factors, and the psychopharmacological effects of the drugs themselves. Certain medications are used to treat the underlying pathophysiological predisposition, as well as any comorbid psychiatric disorders (occurring in a large number of adolescent substance abusers). Environmental factors are treated by intervening to change the risk and protective factors for substance abuse, which are discussed elsewhere in this chapter. Group and family interventions also try to treat the behavioral effects of the drugs themselves, particularly focusing on craving, relapse prevention, and rehabilitation. Treatment programs that combine different kinds of psychosocial therapies and other elements of treatment are often most effective.

Although a detailed discussion of the medications useful in treating substance abuse is beyond the scope of this chapter, a number of medications are available to treat substance abuse/dependence in combination with the use of psychosocial treatments (including methadone, naltrexone, buprenorphine, disulfiram, and a few others). Although addiction to illegal substances of abuse is less common in adolescence than in adulthood, addictions to the legal substances of abuse (alcohol and tobacco) are common and most often begin during adolescence. Medications are most effective, and often only effective, when used in conjunction with psychosocial treatments.

The treatment of adolescent substance abusers can take place in a number of different settings. These can include outpatient treatment, inpatient treatment, residential long-term treatment, specialized therapeutic communities, and self-help treatments. For many adolescents, treatment may require many attempts at helping the adolescent over a prolonged period of time. Generally speaking, the longer the adolescent stays in treatment, the more effective the treatment. Sometimes beneficial therapeutic effects may continue to occur even after the adolescent stops treatment (Carroll *et al.*, 1994).

As a general principle, we would like to emphasize the importance of adapting treatment to the needs of the individual adolescent and his/her specific context (e.g., family situation, neighborhood setting, peer group). Because research, including our own, has demonstrated the complex interactions between psycho-social domains of influence, treatment should try at least to address, if not include, risk and protective factors at the different levels of the adolescent's development and environment. Interventions can take place, simultaneously or sequentially, at all levels, depending on the individual adolescent's situation. For example, if the adolescent's family is not willing or able to participate in treatment, therapists should try to focus on other important areas of the adolescent's environment (e.g., the peer group).

Another important principle in treating adolescent substance abuse is that interventions should be developmentally appropriate. The timing of the specific intervention should be synchronized not only with the adolescent's specific psychosocial context but also with his/her developmental level. For example, intervention with the parents and the child to improve their relationship is appropriate for early adolescence, while in later adolescence intervention with the parents alone or with the adolescent in adolescent group therapy might be more effective.

Finally, we would like to emphasize the importance of the cultural appropriate-ness of any kind of treatment for adolescent substance abuse. It is important to take into consideration the cultural variations that exist within the psychosocial domains that make up the adolescent's psychosocial context. Differences in certain constructs (e.g., family relationships) and in their meanings, exist across different ethnic and racial groups. These differences should be respected and included into any kind of treatment modality in a sensitive manner. For example, in a therapeutic setting, the therapist should be familiar with important constructs that are specific to the adolescent's culture. Cultural awareness and culturally competent interventions are necessary for effective treatment.

Individual treatment

Individual therapy for the treatment of drug abuse includes a number of approaches that have been used successfully. This form of therapy seems to be most effective in strengthening the protective factors from the personality domain, which have been found to interact with risks from other psychosocial domains (see above). In particular, individual treatments should focus on fostering the adolescent's conventionality, commitment to traditional values and academic achievement, responsibility, self-esteem, dimensions of emotional control, and his/her overall mental health.

Individualized drug counseling uses short-term goals, which aim to change behavior and assist the patient in developing more effective methods of coping and refraining from drug use. Supportive–expressive psychotherapy focuses on helping patients to talk about their own use of drugs, and to express their feelings and difficulties experienced in interpersonal relationships. The therapist may focus on the relationship of drug use to difficulties in feelings and behavior, and on enhancing the person's ability to deal with problems without using drugs. This approach may be particularly effective in improving the adolescent's emotional control, which has been shown to buffer drug risks from the family, peer, and environmental domains (Wills *et al.*, 2002). Moreover, learning to express one's feelings in a constructive and socially acceptable fashion can improve difficult family relationships, another risk factor for adolescent drug abuse.

Another form of individual therapy with longer-term treatment and goals is behavioral treatment, which often involves a cognitive–behavioral approach. This approach focuses on delineating the pathways to changing harmful behaviors. Changing behavior and changing thinking that supports adverse or self-destructive behavior, for example, through cognitive restructuring can result in a decrease in such harmful behavior and an increase in a healthful lifestyle. Cognitive restructuring can also aid in raising the adolescent's sense of control over his/her environment, which has been shown to buffer family risks for drug use (Hussong & Chassin, 1997). Behavioral treatments teach coping skills to help adolescents to avoid aspects of their lives previously associated with drug use (people, places, and things) and encourage prosocial, non-drug-related activities. Behavioral treatments often make use of the involvement of significant people in the adolescent's environment, including family members, friends, social workers, and sometimes teachers. These significant others may be asked to help the adolescent to achieve healthful goals and behaviors in a number of life areas, including school, family, psychiatric symptoms, legal issues, and peer relationships. This approach directly incorporates the interactions of protective factors from these multiple domains of influence.

Family treatment

Family therapeutic approaches are often effective ways to achieve abstinence and focus on decreasing risk factors and enhancing protective factors. Because of the importance of close family bonding in reducing adolescent drug use, both as a main effect and as a moderator of other risk and protective factors, family therapy approaches seem particularly suited for the treatment of adolescent drug abuse. One of the important dimensions of family functioning to be addressed in family therapy is the development of a close parent–child mutual attachment relationship, which has been shown to buffer against risks from other domains (Brook *et al.*, 1990, 1997b,c; Brook, 1993). This facet of the family relationship can be addressed in an age-appropriate fashion. Furthermore, parental modeling of conventional behaviors and parental monitoring are important parenting skills that should be stressed in interventions that include parental figures (Brook *et al.*, 1997a,b; Mounts, 2002).

One family therapy approach, which has been extensively studied, is multi-dimensional family therapy, as developed and applied by Liddle and colleagues (Liddle *et al.*, 2001). In general, this approach focuses on changing family functioning, as well as addressing systemic issues such as school performance, peer relationships, antisocial behavior and legal issues, and community-related factors. Positive changes in the family become the vehicle for changes in the adolescent's life and interactions with others. This approach is particularly promising in addressing the interactions between multiple psychosocial domains of influence. Research studies have demonstrated the effectiveness of such treatment in decreasing adolescent drug use, antisocial behavior, and family conflict (Liddle & Rowe, 2002).

Other forms of family therapy include multisystemic therapy, developed by Henggeler *et al.* (2002), in which the family members and the adolescent are helped to monitor at-risk behavior, and to provide positive reinforcements for responsible behavior and a more functional family structure. Szapocznik and Kurtines (1989) have developed brief strategic family therapy, which uses a structural strategic systems approach and attempts to have an impact on intergenerational and cultural differences in the family. This therapeutic context would lend itself to fostering attachment to family and one's culture, which, with ethnic identification, have been found to buffer other risk factors for drug use (Brook *et al.*, 1998e,f). Other family therapy approaches include functional family therapy and cognitive–behavioral therapy. Space limitations prevent further discussion of these approaches in this chapter.

Group treatments

Group treatments are among the most widespread forms of psychosocial interventions used in the treatment of substance-abusing adolescents. There are a number of different group approaches, some of which will be described below, but they often involve adolescents meeting together in a group with a therapist, and sometimes a co-therapist as well. Group therapy with substance-abusing adolescents can be very difficult to conduct, as many such adolescents have comorbid psychiatric disorders in addition to common adolescent developmental issues, such as rebelliousness, separation issues, and an increase in the influence of the peer group.

As will be noted below, many kinds of group therapy allow the group to focus on the risk and protective factors for substance abuse more readily than in individual therapy. This can occur through the use of peer pressure, which can make it difficult for the adolescent to avoid confronting her/his self-destructive and risky drug-abusing and related behaviors. As mentioned above, our research has found that interacting with prosocial peers (who do not use drugs) can heighten the effect of other protective factors, such as paternal affection. In group therapy, social skills necessary to befriend prosocial peers can be learned and practised. Family issues can also be more readily addressed in group settings through the fostering of group discussion and through the group's support, thus beneficially interweaving the psychosocial domains of family and peers.

As with other forms of treatment, group treatments can take place in a wide variety of settings. For example, cognitive–behavioral group therapy can occur on an outpatient basis, in a residential treatment setting, or in a therapeutic community. Cognitive–behavioral therapy utilizes the group to help adolescents to modify their thinking about risk-taking behavior, including drug use and abuse. Through changes in thinking, adolescents can focus on reevaluating and changing their behaviors, including such risk-taking behaviors as risky sexual behavior, associating with drug-using peers, dropping out of school, and involvement in antisocial or criminal behavior.

Psychodynamic approaches can be helpful in treating adolescent substance abusers. The risk with such approaches is that, despite talking about seemingly relevant important dynamic issues, adolescents may continue to use or abuse drugs. However, sometimes approaches such as modified dynamic group therapy or interpersonal group psychotherapy can enable adolescents to observe their own behaviors with constructive results. The former involves focusing on disorders of self-regulation, including affective dysregulation, poor self-care, disturbed peer relationships, and the use of drugs in attempts at regulation of self-esteem (Albanese & Khantzian, 2002). As mentioned above, emotional control, an aspect of self-regulation, has been identified as a protective factor that can enhance the positive effects of other protective factors from the peer group (Brook et al., 1997b). The group process can help group members to focus on such disturbances as risk factors for drug use and can offer group members a safe environment in which to address more constructive and healthier methods of self-regulation. Interpersonal group therapy uses the group process to address individual self-regulatory processes, which affect both neurobiological and interpersonal functioning. Changing interpersonal relationships and interactions in the group can result in improved self-regulation and biopsychosocial functioning, which, in turn, can lead to decreased drug use and other problem behaviors, and improved self-esteem, interpersonal relationships, and academic and vocational productivity – and perhaps an improvement in aspects of health (Flores, 2002; Brook et al., 2002d).

Another form of group treatment for substance-abusing adolescents is network therapy (Galanter, 1993). This uses all the significant others in the adolescent's life as members of a group, including the adolescent, to help the adolescent to achieve freedom from substance abuse. All the members of this "extended family" are regarded as responsible for the adolescent's behavior. Through the interactions with these group members, who care about the adolescent, progress can be made in helping the adolescent to deal with her/his substance abuse. This approach is particularly promising in addressing the multiple psychosocial domains of influence in the adolescent's life and their complex interactions.

Large group/community approaches

Self-help groups can be quite useful for selected adolescents. Alcoholics Anonymous has groups for adolescents, as well as groups for members of the adolescent's family in Al-Anon. These large self-help groups can be as effective for adolescents as they are for adults.

Furthermore, group interventions in community settings lend themselves to fostering protective factors against drug use in an effort toward enhancing prevention. Importantly, interventions aimed at the development of a strong cultural attachment and ethnic identification are promising in preventing and reducing drug use among adolescents from ethnic minorities (Belgrave, 2002; Townsend & Belgrave, 2000).

Residential therapeutic community programs can also be useful for adolescents. These often involve a structured program, including group therapy, and try to help the adolescent to focus on adapting to life in a structured residential setting without the expression of self-destructive behavior. Managing adolescent rebelliousness and aggression is often a focus of groups in such a setting, but many other kinds of group can be utilized at the same time. Adolescents in such a setting are often given jobs that they are expected to carry out, and responsibility to the community is an important focus.

Conclusions

This chapter has presented a summary of findings from a number of recent studies exploring the psychosocial risk and protective factors for drug use and abuse using a developmental approach. This approach emphasizes the centrality of the parent–child relationship, especially the non-conflictual mutual attachment between parents and child. Family interactional theory posits that such an attachment is of great importance in preventing the development of risk factors for drug use. Risk and protective factors in a number of psychosocial domains are discussed, focusing on the developmental pathways of risk and protective factors to drug use, beginning in childhood. The chapter has also presented research on the risk/protective and protective/protective interactions between psychosocial factors related to drug use/abuse. In designing interventions, it is, therefore, of particular importance to keep the adolescent's entire psychosocial environment in perspective. Because of the complex interactions between the different psycho-social domains, it is essential to strengthen protective factors (e.g., enhance family functioning) in those areas that will be the most promising in offsetting risk factors, in addition to having a direct effect on the adolescent's substance use. Furthermore, it is important that these interventions be developmentally, as well as culturally, appropriate. Together, these principles suggest that the course of adolescent substance abuse treatment be tailored to the individual adolescent, taking into consideration his/her psychosocial and cultural environment, as well as his/her developmental level.

While research has definitively identified certain psychosocial risk and protect-ive factors with regard to adolescent substance use and abuse, many unanswered questions remain to be explored by future research in this area. The first step is to expand our limited knowledge of the genetic bases for substance abuse. Research needs to identify variations in specific genes that affect risk or protective factors for substance use/abuse. A second step is to examine the interactions between these genetic vulnerabilities and the environment to which the individual is exposed. Assessments of both gene–environment and gene–gene interactions are needed. In order to do these assessments, we also need to improve our ability to capture and accurately measure the different facets of the individual's environ-ment by developing innovative and creative research designs. By meeting these challenges, we can develop a truly biopsychosocial perspective of the development of adolescent substance abuse.

ACKNOWLEDGEMENTS

This research was supported by Research Scientist Award 1 K05 DA 00244 and grants DA 03188, DA 05702, DA 10348, and DA 12637, awarded by the National Institute on Drug Abuse, and grant CA 84063, awarded by the National Cancer Institute, to Dr Judith S. Brook, and grants DA 09950 and DA 11116, awarded by the National Institute on Drug Abuse to Dr David W. Brook. We wish to thank Jacques Normand Ph.D. for his support and encouragement. We gratefully acknowledge the assistance of Linda Capobianco for her help in the preparation of the manuscript.

REFERENCES

Albanese, M. J. & Khantzian, E. J. (2002). Self-medication theory and modified dynamic group therapy. In D. W. Brook & H. I. Spitz (eds.), *The Group Therapy of Substance Abuse* (pp. 79–96). New York: Haworth Press.

Bachman, J. G., Wadsworth, K. N., O'Malley, P. M., Johnston, L. D., & Schulenberg, J. E. (1997). *Smoking, Drinking, and Drug Use in Young Adulthood: The Impacts of New Freedoms and New Responsibilities*. Hillsdale, NJ: Lawrence Erlbaum.

Belgrave, F. Z. (2002). Relational theory and cultural enhancement interventions for African-American girls. *Public Health Reports*, **117**, S76–S81.

Brook, D. W., Brook, J. S., Whiteman, M., *et al.* (1997a). Psychosocial risk factors for HIV transmission in female drug abusers. *American Journal on Addictions*, **6**, 124–134.

Brook, D. W., Brook, J. S., Pahl, T., & Montoya, I. (2002b). The longitudinal relationship between drug use and risky sexual behaviors among Colombian adolescents. *Archives of Pediatrics and Adolescent Medicine*, **156**, 1101–1107.

Brook, D. W., Brook, J. S., Zhang, C., Cohen, P., & Whiteman, M. (2002c). Drug use and risk of major depressive disorder, alcohol dependence, and substance use disorders. *Archives of General Psychiatry*, **59**, 1039–1044.

Brook, J. S. (1993). Interactional theory: Its utility in explaining drug use behavior among African-American and Puerto Rican youth. In M. R. de la Rosa & J. R. Adrados (eds.), *Drug Abuse Among Minority Youth: Methodological Issues and Recent Research Advances*. [*NIDA Research Monograph Series* No. 130, pp. 79–101.] Rockville, MD: National Institute on Drug Abuse.

Brook, J. S. & Newcomb, M. D. (1995). Childhood aggression and unconventionality: impact on later academic achievement, drug use, and workforce involvement. *Journal of Genetic Psychology*, **4**, 393–410.

Brook, J. S. & Pahl, K. (2005). The protective role of ethnic and racial identity and aspects of an Africentric orientation against drug use among African American young adults. *Journal of Genetic Psychology*, **166**, 329–345.

Brook, J. S., Brook, D. W., Whiteman, M., Gordon, A. S., & Cohen, P. (1990). The psychosocial etiology of adolescent drug use and abuse. *Genetic, Social and General Psychology Monographs*, **116**, 111–267.

Brook, J. S., Whiteman, M., Balka, E. B., & Hamburg, B. A. (1992a). African-American and Puerto Rican drug use: personality, familial, and other environmental risk factors. *Genetic, Social, and General Psychology Monographs*, **118**, 417–438.

Brook, J. S., Cohen, P., Whiteman, M., & Gordon, A. (1992b). Psychosocial risk factors in the transition from moderate to heavy use/abuse of drugs. In M. Glantz & R. Pickens (eds.), *Vulnerability to Drug Abuse* (pp. 359–388). Washington, DC: American Psychological Association.

Brook, J. S., Whiteman, M., Balka, E. B., Win, P. T., & Gursen, M. D. (1997b). African-American and Puerto Rican drug use: a longitudinal study. *Journal of the American Academy of Child and Adolescent Psychiatry*, **36**, 1260–1268.

Brook, J. S., Balka, E. B., Gursen, M. D., *et al.* (1997c). Young adults' drug use: a 17-year longitudinal inquiry of antecedents. *Psychological Reports*, **80**, 1235–1251.

Brook, J. S., Cohen, P., & Brook, D. W. (1998a). Longitudinal study of co-occurring psychiatric disorders and substance use. *Journal of the American Academy of Child and Adolescent Psychiatry*, **37**, 322–330.

Brook, J. S., Whiteman, M., Balka, E. B., Win, P. T., & Gursen, M. D. (1998b). Similar and different precursors to drug use and delinquency among African-Americans and Puerto Ricans. *Journal of Genetic Psychology*, **159**, 13–29.

Brook, J. S., Whiteman, M., Finch, S., & Cohen, P. (1998c). Mutual attachment, personality, and drug use: pathways from childhood to young adulthood. *Genetic, Social, and General Psychology Monographs*, **124**, 492–510.

Brook, J. S., Brook, D. W., de la Rosa, M., *et al.* (1998d). Pathways to marijuana use among adolescents: cultural/ecological family, peer, and personality influences. *Journal of the American Academy of Child and Adolescent Psychiatry*, **37**, 759–766.

Brook, J. S., Balka, E. B., Brook, D. W., *et al.* (1998e). Drug use among African-Americans: ethnic identity as a protective factor. *Psychological Reports*, **83**, 1427–1446.

Brook, J. S., Whiteman, M., Balka, E. B., Win, P. T., & Gursen, M. D. (1998f). Drug use among Puerto Ricans: ethnic identity as a protective factor. *Hispanic Journal of Behavioral Science*, **20**, 241–254.

Brook, J. S., Brook, D. W., de la Rosa, M., Whiteman, M., & Montoya, I. D. (1999). The role of parents in protecting Colombian adolescents from delinquency and marijuana use. *Archives of Pediatrics and Adolescent Medicine*, **153**, 457–464.

Brook, J. S., Whiteman, M., Finch, S., & Cohen, P. (2000). Longitudinally foretelling drug use in the late twenties: adolescent personality and social-environmental antecedents. *Journal of Genetic Psychology*, **161**, 37–51.

Brook, J. S., Brook, D. W., de la Rosa, M., *et al.* (2001). Adolescent illegal drug use: the impact of personality, family, and environmental factors. *Journal of Behavioral Medicine*, **24**, 183–203.

Brook, J. S., Rosen, Z., & Zhang, C. (2002a). Universal risk factors for substance use and the transition from substance use to substance abuse. In *Proceedings of the XIII Medical Symposium of the Yrjö Jahnsson Foundation: Youth and Substance Use*, Porvoo, Finland.

Brook, J. S., Finch, S., Whiteman, M., & Brook. D. W. (2002d). Drug use and neurobehavioral, respiratory, and cognitive problems: precursors and mediators. *Journal of Adolescent Health*, **30**, 433–441.

Canino, G., Burnam, A., & Caetano, R. (1992). The prevalence of alcohol abuse and/or dependence in two Hispanic communities. In J. Helzer and G. Canino (eds.), *Alcoholism in North America, Europe, and Asia* (pp. 131–154). New York: Oxford University Press.

Capaldi, D. M. & Stoolmiller, M. (1999). Co-occurrence of conduct problems and depressive symptoms in early adolescent boys: III. Prediction to young-adult adjustment. *Development and Psychopathology*, **11**, 59–84.

Carroll, K. M., Rounsaville, B. J., Nich, C., *et al.* (1994). One-year follow-up of psychotherapy and pharmacotherapy for cocaine dependence. Delayed emergence of psychotherapy effects. *Archives of General Psychiatry*, **51**, 989–997.

Catalano, R. F., Hawkins, J. D., Krenz, C., *et al.* (1993). Using research to guide culturally appropriate drug abuse prevention. *Journal of Consulting and Clinical Psychology*, **61**, 804–811.

Chavers, D. (1991). Indian education: dealing with disaster. *Principal*, **70**, 28–29.

Cloninger, C. R. (1987). Neurogenetic adaptive mechanisms in alcoholism. *Science*, **236**, 410–416.

Cohen, P. & Brook, J. S. (1987). Family factors related to the persistence of psychopathology in childhood and adolescence. *Psychiatry*, **50**, 332–345.

Dishion, T. J. & McMahon, R. J. (1998). Parental monitoring and the prevention of child and adolescent problem behavior: a conceptual and empirical formulation. *Clinical, Child, and Family Psychology Review*, **1**, 61–75.

Donovan, J. E. (1996). Problem-behavior theory and the explanation of adolescent marijuana use. *Journal of Drug Issues*, **26**, 379–404.

Farrington, D. P. (1991). Childhood aggression and adult violence: early precursors and later life outcomes. In D. J. Pepler and K. H. Rubin (eds.), *The Development and Treatment of Childhood Aggression* (pp. 5–29). Hillsdale, NJ: Lawrence Erlbaum.

Félix-Ortiz, M. & Newcomb, M. D. (1999). Vulnerability for drug use among Latino adolescents. *Journal of Community Psychology*, **27**, 257–280.

Fergusson, D. M., Horwood, L. J., & Lynskey, M. (1994). The childhood of multiple problem adolescents: a 15-year longitudinal study. *Journal of Child Psychology and Psychiatry*, **35**, 1123–1140.

Finchham, F. D., Grych, J. H., & Osborne (1994). Does marital conflict cause child maladjustment? Directions and challenges for longitudinal research. *Journal of Family Psychology*, **8**, 128–140.

Fisher, P. A., Storck, M., & Bacon, J. G. (1999). In the eye of the beholder: risk and protective factors in rural American Indian and Caucasian adolescents. *American Journal of Orthopsychiatry*, **69**, 294–304.

Fletcher, A. C., Darling, N. E., & Steinberg, L. (1995). The company they keep: relation of adolescents' adjustment and behavior to their friends' perceptions of authoritative parenting in the social network. *Developmental Psychology*, **31**, 300–310.

Flores, P. J. (2002). The interpersonal approach. In D. W. Brook & H. I. Spitz (eds.), *The Group Therapy of Substance Abuse* (pp. 19–36). New York: Haworth Press.

Galanter, M. (1993). Network therapy for addiction: a model for office practice. *American Journal of Psychiatry*, **150**, 28–36.

Glantz, M. D., Weinberg, N. Z., Miner, L. L., & Colliver, J. D. (1999). The etiology of drug abuse: mapping the paths. In M. D. Glantz & C. R. Hartel (eds.), *Drug Abuse, Origins, and Interventions* (pp. 3–45). Washington, DC: American Psychological Association.

Hansen, W. B., Graham, J. W., Sobel, J. L., *et al.* (1987). The consistency of peer and parent influences on tobacco, alcohol, and marijuana use among young adolescents. *Journal of Behavioral Medicine*, **10**, 559–579.

Hawkins, J. D., Catalano, R. F., & Miller, J. Y. (1992). Risk and protective factors for alcohol and other drug problems in adolescence and early adulthood: implications for substance abuse prevention. *Psychological Bulletin*, **112**, 64–105.

Henggeler, S. W., Clingempeel, W. G., Brondino, M. J., & Pickrel, S. G. (2002). Four-year follow-up of multisystemic therapy with substance-abusing and substance-dependent juvenile offenders. *Journal of the American Academy of Child and Adolescent Psychiatry*, **41**, 868–874.

Holderness, C. C., Brooks-Gunn, J., & Warren, M. P. (1994). Comorbidity of eating disorders and substance abuse: review of the literature. *International Journal of Eating Disorders*, **16**, 1–34.

Hussong, A. M. & Chassin, L. (1997). Substance use initiation among adolescent children of alcoholics: testing protective factors. *Journal of Studies on Alcohol*, **58**, 272–279.

Institute of Medicine (1996). *Pathways of Addiction: Opportunities in Drug Abuse Research*. Washington, DC: National Academy Press.

Jessor, R., van den Bos, J., Vanderryn, J., Costa, F. M., & Turbin, M. S. (1995). Protective factors in adolescent problem behavior: moderator effects and developmental change. *Developmental Psychology*, **31**, 923–933.

Kandel, D. B. (1996). The parental and peer contexts of adolescent deviance: an algebra of interpersonal influences. *Journal of Drug Issues*, **26**, 289–315.

Kaplan, H. B. (1995). Drugs, crime, and other deviant adaptations. In H. B. Kaplan (ed.), *Drugs, Crime, and Other Deviant Adaptations* (pp. 3–46). New York: Plenum Press.

Kendler, K. S., Gardner, C. O., & Prescott, C. A. (1997). Religion, psychopathology, and substance use and abuse: a multimeasure, genetic-epidemiologic study. *American Journal of Psychiatry*, **154**, 322–329.

Kessler, R. C., Nelson, C. B., McGonagle, K. A., *et al.* (1996). The epidemiology of co-occurring addictive and mental disorders: implications for prevention and service utilization. *American Journal of Orthopsychiatry*, **66**, 17–30.

Kilpatrick, D. G., Acierno, R., Saunders, B., *et al.* (2000). Risk factors for adolescent substance abuse and dependence: data from a national sample. *Journal of Consulting and Clinical Psychology*, **68**, 19–30.

Kosterman, R., Hawkins, J. D., Guo, J., Catalano, R. F., & Abbott, R. D. (2000). The dynamics of alcohol and marijuana initiation: patterns and predictors of first use in adolescence. *American Journal of Public Health*, **90**, 360–366.

LaVeist, T. L. & Wallace, J. M. Jr. (2000). Health risks and the inequitable distribution of liquor stores in African-American communities. *Social Science and Medicine*, **51**, 613–617.

LeDoux, S., Miller, P., Choquet, M., & Plant, M. (2002). Family structure, parent–child relationships, and alcohol and other drug use among teenagers from France and the United Kingdom. *Alcohol and Alcoholism*, **37**, 52–60.

Legrand, L. N., McGue, M., & Iacono, W. G. (1999). Searching for interactive effects in the etiology of early-onset substance use. *Behavior Genetics*, **29**, 433–444.

Liddle, H. A. & Rowe, C. L. (2002). Multidimensional Family Therapy for adolescent drug abuse: making the case for a developmental, contextual, family-based intervention. In D. W. Brook & H. I. Spitz (eds.), *The Group Therapy of Substance Abuse* (pp. 275–291). New York: Haworth Press.

Liddle, H. A., Dakof, G. A., Parker, K., *et al.* (2001). Multidimensional Family Therapy for adolescent drug abuse: results of a randomized, clinical trial. *American Journal of Drug and Alcohol Abuse*, **27**, 651–688.

Maddahian, E., Newcomb, M. D., & Bentler, P. M. (1988). Risk factors for substance use: ethnic differences among adolescents. *Journal of Substance Abuse*, **1**, 11–23.

McCord, J. (1988). Identifying developmental paradigms leading to alcoholism. *Journal of Studies on Alcohol*, **49**, 357–362.

Moffitt, T. E. (1993). Adolescence-limited and life-course persistent antisocial behavior: a developmental taxonomy. *Psychological Review*, **100**, 674–701.

Morojele, N. D. & Brook, J. S. (2001). Adolescent precursors of intensity of marijuana and other illicit drug use among adult initiators. *Journal of Genetic Psychology*, **162**, 430–450.

Mounts, N. (2002). Parental management of adolescent peer relationships in context: the role of parenting style. *Journal of Family Psychology*, **16**, 58–69.

Newcomb, M. D. & Bentler, P. M. (1986). Substance use and ethnicity: differential impact of peer and adult models. *Journal of Psychology*, **120**, 83–95.

Nurco, D. N., Hanlon, T. E., O'Grady, K. E., & Kinlock, T. W. (1997). The early emergence of narcotic addict types. *American Journal of Drug and Alcohol Abuse*, **23**, 523–542.

Oetting, E. R. & Donnermeyer, J. F. (1998). Primary socialization theory: the etiology of drug use and deviance. Part I. *Substance Use and Misuse*, **33**, 995–1026.

Peterson, P. L., Hawkins, J. D., Abbott, R. D., & Catalano, R. F. (1995). Disentangling the effects of parental drinking, family management, and parental alcohol norms on current drinking by black and white adolescents. In G. M. Boyd, J. Howard, *et al.* (eds.), *Alcohol Problems among Adolescents: Current Directions in Prevention Research* (pp. 33–57). Hillsdale, NJ: Lawrence Erlbaum.

Reifman, A., Barnes, G. M., Dintcheff, B. A., Uhteg, L., & Farrell, M. P. (2002). Health values buffer social-environmental risks for adolescent alcohol misuse. *Psychology of Addictive Behaviors*, **15**, 249–251.

Ryan, J. A., Abdelrahman, A. I., French, J. F., & Rodriguez, G. (1999). Social indicators of substance abuse prevention: a need-based assessment. *Social Indicators Research*, **46**, 23–60.

Sampson, R. J., Raudenbush, S. W., & Earls, F. (1997). Neighborhoods and violent crime: a multilevel study of collective efficacy. *Science*, **277**, 918–924.

Scheier, L. M., Botvin, G. J., Diaz, T., & Ifill-Williams, M. (1997). Ethnic identity as a moderator of psychosocial risk and adolescent alcohol and marijuana use: concurrent and longitudinal analyses. *Journal of Child and Adolescent Substance Abuse*, **6**, 21–47.

Swaim, R. C., Bates, S. C., & Chavez, E. L. (1998). Structural equation socialization model of substance use among Mexican-American and white non-Hispanice school drop-outs. *Journal of Adolescent Health*, **23**, 128–138.

Szapocznik, J. & Kurtines, W. N. (1989). *Breakthroughs in Family Therapy with Drug-abusing Problem Youth*. New York: Springer.

Tabakoff, B., Hoffman, P. L., Lee, J. M., *et al.* (1988). Differences in platelet enzyme activity between alcoholics and nonalcoholics. *New England Journal of Medicine*, **318**, 134–139.

Tiet, Q. Q., Bird, H. R., Davies, M., *et al.* (1998). Adverse life events and resilience. *Journal of the American Academy of Child and Adolescent Psychiatry*, **37**, 1191–1200.

Townsend, T. G. & Belgrave, F. Z. (2000). The impact of personal identity and racial identity on drug attitudes and use among African-American children. *Journal of Black Psychology*, **26**, 421–436.

Tsuang, M. T., Bar, J. L., Harley, R. M., & Lyons, M. J. (2001). The Harvard twin study of substance abuse: What we have learned. *Harvard Review of Psychiatry*, **9**, 267–279.

Vega, W. A., Gil, A., Warheit, G. J., Zimmerman, R., & Apospori, E. (1993). Acculturation and delinquent behavior among Cuban-American adolescents: toward an empirical model. *American Journal of Community Psychology*, **21**, 113–125.

Wallace, J. M. & Muroff, J. R. (2002). Preventing substance abuse among African-American children and youth: race differences in risk factor exposure and vulnerability. *Journal of Primary Prevention*, **3**, 235–261.

Wills, T. A. & Cleary, S. D. (1996). How are social support effects mediated? A test with parental support and adolescent substance use. *Journal of Personality and Social Psychology*, **5**, 937–952.

Wills, T. A., McNamara, G., & Vaccaro, D. (1995). Parental education related to adolescent stress-coping and substance use: development of a mediational model. *Health Psychology*, **14**, 464–478.

Wills, T. A., Sandy, J. M., Yaeger, A., & Shinari, O. (2001). Family risk factors and adolescent substance use: moderation effects for temperament dimensions. *Developmental Psychology*, **37**, 283–297.

Wills, T. A., Sandy, J. M., & Yaeger, A. M. (2002). Moderators of the relation between substance use level and problems: test of a self-regulation model in middle adolescence. *Journal of Abnormal Psychology*, **111**, 3–21.

Windle, M. & Windle, R. C. (1993). The continuity of behavioral expression among disinhibited and inhibited childhood subtypes. *Clinical Psychology Review*, **13**, 741–761.

3

Recent methodological and statistical advances: a latent variable growth modeling framework

Terry E. Duncan, Susan C. Duncan, Lisa A. Strycker, Hayrettin Okut, and Hollie Hix-Small

Oregon Research Institute, Eugene, OR, USA

Since the late 1970s, we have witnessed a gradual increase in the complexity of theoretical models that attempt to explain development in substance use and related problem behaviors (e.g., Akers & Cochran, 1985; Patterson *et al.*, 1992; Sampson, 1988, 1992; Sampson & Laub, 1990). The field has moved away from an emphasis on cross-sectional person-centered data toward a wider examination of the developmental nature of behavior over time, person–environment interactions, and the social context as an interactive, interdependent network that exerts influence on all its members (e.g., Conger, 1997). This social–contextual framework for studying change necessitates a broad conceptual approach that is not subsumed by any single theory. The conceptual movement to examine substance use behavior from both a developmental and contextual perspective parallels recent methodological and statistical advances in the analysis of change. The search for the best methods to address complex issues in behavior change has been a persistent theme of recent developmental research (e.g., Collins & Horn, 1991; Collins & Sayer, 2001; Duncan *et al.*, 1999; Gottman, 1995) and has prompted a shift in analytic strategies. Rather than focusing on homogeneous populations and inter-individual variability, analysts are turning to new methods to explore both inter- and intra-individual variability and heterogeneity in growth trajectories of substance use.

Historically, research into prevention intervention has included efficacy and effectiveness studies, both of which generally incorporate a longitudinal design to examine mediators and long-term effects. Research has focused on factors and patterns associated with the longitudinal nature (e.g., initiation, escalation, continuation, and cessation) of drug use and associated antisocial, health-threatening, and other problem behaviors. Researchers have also identified specific areas in

Adolescent Substance Abuse: Research and Clinical Advances, ed. Howard A. Liddle and Cynthia L. Rowe.
Published by Cambridge University Press. © Cambridge University Press 2006.

need of development, including: (a) more powerful designs for detecting differences in program effectiveness by attributes such as subgroup membership, content delivered, and content exposure; (b) methodologies reflecting the hierarchical nature of prevention data, specifically testing the impact of varying levels of implementation of environmental change mechanisms; (c) prevention audience profiling, including methodologies appropriate for the identification of individuals at risk for future abuse and dependence; and, more broadly, (d) innovative multidisciplinary, multimethod, and multilevel research designs and methods for behavioral and social science research.

The need to answer increasingly complex substantive questions inspires the development of new statistical methods. These new analysis techniques have fundamentally altered how we conceptualize and study change. Methodology for the study of change has matured sufficiently now that researchers are beginning to identify larger frameworks in which to integrate knowledge. One such framework is latent variable growth modeling (LGM). The LGM makes available to a wide audience of researchers in prevention and treatment an analytical framework for a variety of analyses of growth and developmental processes.

A latent variable approach to growth curve modeling

The LGM approach differs from more traditional fixed-effects analytical approaches in at least three important ways. First, the approach allows for the modeling of not only the group statistics of interest but also the individual variation about the mean, representing inter-individual differences in intra-individual growth. Second, and perhaps the most compelling characteristic of LGM, is the capacity to estimate and test relationships among latent variables. The isolation of concepts from uniqueness and unreliability of their indicators increases the potential for detecting relationships and obtaining estimates of parameters close to their population values. Finally, the LGM approach permits a more comprehensive and flexible approach to research design and data analysis than any other single statistical model for longitudinal data in standard use by social and behavioral researchers. Paralleling the growth in complexity of the theoretical models guiding substance abuse research, methodologists have extended the latent variable framework to accommodate longitudinal models that include multivariate or higher-order specifications, multiple populations, the accelerated collection of longitudinal data, non-linear and interactive effects, multilevel or hierarchical structures, missingness, and complex relations, including mediation, moderation, recursive and non-recursive relationships, and reciprocal causation.

A comprehensive treatment of the LGM approach to studying substance use development is not possible in the context of a single chapter. Instead, this chapter focuses on several recent advances in latent variable growth curve methodology applicable to the study and treatment of substance use and abuse. The chapter begins by introducing an approach to growth analyses using a LGM specification that allows for complex representations of growth and correlates of change. This includes informal definitions and interpretations as well as formal specifications for the various model parameters. Subsequent sections build on the introduction, presenting various extensions to the basic LGM that address substance abuse treatment research questions such as (a) the detection of differences in treatment program effectiveness by attributes such as subgroup membership, content delivered, and content exposure (p. 60); (b) methodologies reflecting the hierarchical nature of prevention and treatment data (see p. 64); and (c) prevention audience profiling, including methodologies appropriate for the identification of individuals for whom an intervention was most efficacious or who are at increased risk for future abuse and dependence (see p. 69).

Typical approaches to studying change

Historically, the most prevalent type of longitudinal data in the behavioral and social sciences has been longitudinal panel data consisting of observations made on many individuals across pretest and post-test occasions. Traditional approaches to studying change within this context have been fixed-effects analysis of variance (ANOVA) and multiple regression techniques. However, these approaches analyze only mean changes, treating differences among individual subjects as error variance. Some of this error variance may contain valuable information about change. Recently, a host of methodological contributions have extended researchers' abilities to describe individual differences and the nature of change over time (e.g., random-effects ANOVA, random coefficient modeling, multilevel modeling, and hierarchical linear modeling). A strength of these random-effects approaches is that individual differences in growth over time are captured by random coefficients, enabling more realistic modeling of the growth process. A weakness is that statistical modeling within these methods has been largely limited to a single response variable. As such, these methods do not fully accommodate the complexity and analytical needs of current developmental theories (e.g., Conger, 1997).

A largely independent tradition to analysis of longitudinal data has been conducted within the latent variable framework of structural equation modeling (SEM). Although the estimation procedures are not yet well established for sufficiently general cases, the modeling framework has much more flexibility to examine more fully the types of question now posited by researchers in developmental and preventional intervention. Once the random coefficient model has been placed within the LGM framework, many general forms of longitudinal analyses can be studied. It has been suggested that the development of the LGM framework is perhaps the most important and influential statistical revolution to have occurred recently in the social and behavioral sciences (Cliff, 1983).

Toward an integrated developmental model

A recent resurgence of interest in statistical models for time-ordered data utilizing structural equation methodology has reintroduced the formative work of Rao (1958) and Tucker (1958). Such models can simultaneously incorporate information about the group or population and about the individual. These authors argued that individual differences are both meaningful and important, and proposed a procedure that included unspecified longitudinal growth curves or functions. The LGM is one strategy for modeling individual differences in growth curves.

Although strongly resembling the classic confirmatory factor analysis, the latent growth factors are actually interpreted as individual differences in attributes of growth trajectories over time (McArdle, 1988). For example, two potentially interesting attributes of growth trajectories are rates of change and initial status, which, for simple straight-line growth models, are the slope and intercept, respectively. Meredith and Tisak (1990) noted that models based on fixed-effects repeated measures polynomial ANOVA are actually special cases of LGMs in which only the factor means are of interest. In contrast, a fully expanded LGM analysis takes into account both factor means, which correspond to group level information, and variances, which correspond to individual differences. Heuristically, growth curve methodology can be thought of as consisting of two stages. In the first stage, a regression curve, not necessarily linear, is fitted to the repeated measures of each individual in the sample. In the second stage, the parameters for an individual's curve become the focus of the analysis rather than the original measures.

Beyond describing and summarizing growth at the group and individual level, the model can also be used to study predictors of individual differences and answer questions about which variables exert important effects on the rate of development. The latent growth curve approach is laid out in more technical detail in Duncan *et al.* (1999), Meredith and Tisak (1990), and Stoolmiller (1995). Applications of LGM may be found in Duncan and Duncan (1995, 1996), Duncan *et al.* (2001a, 2002a), Hix-Small *et al.* (2004), McArdle (1988), and McArdle and Epstein (1987).

Since LGM is carried out using SEM methodology, it shares many of the same strengths with regard to statistical methodology. Some of the strengths of LGM include the ability to test the adequacy of the hypothesized growth form, to incorporate both fixed and time-varying covariates, to correct for measurement error in observed indicators, to incorporate growth on several constructs simultaneously, and to develop from the data a common developmental trajectory, thus ruling out cohort effects.

Specification of the latent variable growth model

The simplest LGM involves one variable (e.g., a clinical diagnosis of adolescent substance abuse) measured the same way at two time points. However, two points in time are not ideal for studying development or for using growth curve methodology (Rogosa & Willett, 1985), as the collection of individual trajectories are limited to a collection of straight lines. Although two observations provide information about change, they poorly address some research questions (Rogosa, Brandt, & Zimowski, 1982). For example, two temporally separated observations of substance abuse allow for estimating the amount of change, but it is impossible to study the *shape* of the developmental trajectory of substance abuse or the rate of change in the individual. The shape of individual development in substance abuse between two observations may be of theoretical interest, either as a predictor or a sequela. Two-wave designs are appropriate only if the intervening growth process is considered irrelevant or is known to be linear.

Multiwave data offer important advantages over two-wave data. With more than two observations, the validity of the straight-line growth model for the trajectory can be evaluated (e.g., tests for non-linearity can be performed). In addition, the precision of parameter estimates will tend to increase with the number of observations for each individual. To introduce the LGM, a model with two time points is presented in Fig. 3.1.

Intercept

As can be seen from the diagram, the first factor is labeled "Intercept." The intercept is a constant for any given individual across time, hence the fixed values of 1 for factor loadings on the repeated measures. The intercept in this model for a given individual has the same meaning as the intercept of a straight line on a two-dimensional coordinate system: it is the point where the line "intercepts" the vertical axis. The intercept factor presents information in the sample about the mean (Mi) and variance (Di) of the collection of intercepts that characterize each individual's growth curve.

Slope

The second factor, labeled "Slope," represents the slope of an individual's trajectory (e.g., substance abuse). In this case, it is the slope of the straight line determined by the two repeated measures. The slope factor has a mean (Ms) and variance (Ds) across the whole sample that, like the intercept mean and variance, can be estimated from the data. The two factors, slope and intercept, are allowed to covary (Ris),

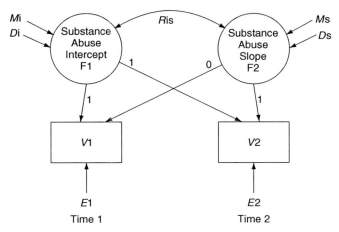

Fig. 3.1   The latent variable growth model for two time points. See the text for further details.
M, mean; *D*, Variance; i, intercept; s, slope; *R*, covariance; *F*, factor; *E*, residual
variance; *V*, observed variable; 0, 1, values of factor loading.

which is represented by the double-headed arrow between the factors. The error
variance terms ($E1$, $E2$) are shown in the diagram, but in the model based on two
points in time the error is assumed to be zero (i.e., $E1 = E2 = 0$). Although
the choice of factor loadings is somewhat arbitrary, the intercept factor is bound
to the time scale. Shifting the loadings on the slope factor alters the scale of time,
which affects the interpretation of Mi and Di.

For the slope factor, the fixed values of 0 and 1 for factor loadings on the
repeated measures simply starts the curve at the first time point and describes
a linear relationship of change in terms of linear differences from initial status at
time 1. The values Ms and Ds differ from Mi and Di in that changing the fixed
loadings, and thereby changing the time scale, rescales the former, in this case by
constants. Rescaling by constants does not change the fundamental meaning or
affect significance tests of the parameters. It also does not affect the correlations
between the slope factor and other predictors in the model. By expanding the
model to include error variance terms, the model parameters retain the same basic
interpretations but are now corrected for random measurement error.

Representing the shape of growth over time

With three or more points in time, the factor loadings carry information about the
shape of growth over time, providing the opportunity to test for non-linear
trajectories in substance abuse trajectories across time (e.g., during adolescence).
The most familiar approach to non-linear trajectories is probably the use of

polynomials. The inclusion of quadratic or cubic effects is easily accomplished by including more factors. The factor loadings can then be fixed to represent a quadratic function of the observed time metric.

However, polynomials with squared or higher-order terms are not the only way to model non-linear growth. Other plausible non-linear growth curves can be modeled with fewer than three factors. The two-factor model also can be used to model unspecified trajectories. For example, if the shapes of the substance abuse trajectories are not known, the data can determine their shape. This could be a starting point from which more specific types of trajectory (e.g., quadratic) are tested. In unspecified models, when there are enough time points to estimate freely factor loadings beyond the two required for identification of the model, the slope factor is better interpreted as a general shape factor.

Occasionally, interest centers on changes in substance abuse during distinct time periods (e.g., transitions from middle to high school or during treatment and follow-up phases of a treatment-outcome trial). As such, factors related to differences in change in one segment of the overall growth period may differ substantially from those in a different segment. Moreover, rates of change during one period may vary substantially among individuals, whereas in another period they may be fairly homogeneous. By subdividing a series of repeated measurements into meaningful segments and summarizing growth in each segment, piecewise growth models provide a means of examining (a) whether rates of change differ as a function of growth period, (b) whether individual variability in rates of change differ between periods of interest, and (c) important predictors of change unique to a particular developmental period. Applications of piecewise LGMs may be found in Sayer and Willet (1998) and Wang *et al.* (1999).

Including predictors and sequelae of change

Once the shape of growth is determined, the parameters for an individual's curve can be used to study predictors of individual differences and answer questions about which variables (e.g., family and/or peer influences) affect the rate of adolescent substance abuse development and about how development influences subsequent behaviors (e.g., transitions to adult roles or subsequent or continued substance use/abuse). Continuous covariates accommodated in an ANOVA allow for tests of both continuous predictors of change and change as a predictor, but not for the simultaneous inclusion of change as both an independent and dependent variable. The ability to use variables simultaneously as both independent and dependent variables in the same model, allowing for complex representations of growth and correlates of change, represents a major advantage of the LGM compared with more traditional approaches.

Multivariate and higher-order extensions

The first part of this chapter has described how LGMs can be used to model growth as a factor of repeated observations of one variable (e.g., alcohol abuse). Although development in a single behavior is often of interest, longitudinal studies often examine a number of behaviors simultaneously to clarify interrelationships in their development (e.g., abuse of multiple substances). To this end, multivariate or associative longitudinal models may be considered. The univariate longitudinal model is actually a special case of the general multivariate growth curve model. Multivariate LGMs provide a more dynamic view of correlates of change, as development in one variable may be associated with development in another variable. An example of the multivariate LGM for alcohol and marijuana use is shown in Fig. 3.2. Associative models are useful in determining the extent to which *pairs* of behaviors covary over time. However, McArdle (1988) has suggested two additional methods for conducting a *multivariate* analysis of the relations among numerous behaviors (e.g., alcohol, marijuana, cigarettes, illicit drugs). This second- or higher-order multivariate LGM approach includes two alternative methods, a *factor-of-curves* model and a *curve-of-factors* model (McArdle, 1988), which are discussed on p. 65. Examples of these multivariate models can be found in Curran, Stice, and Chassin (1997), Duncan and Duncan (1996), Duncan, Duncan, and Strycker (2001b), Ge *et al.* (1994), McArdle (1988), Tisak and Meredith (1990), and Wickrama, Lorenz, and Conger (1997).

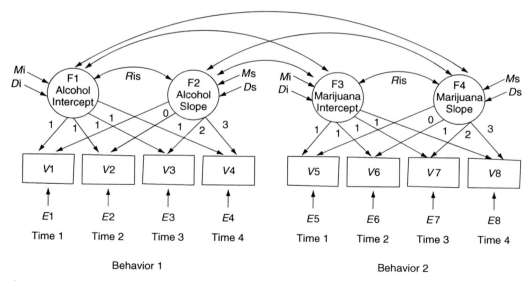

Fig. 3.2   Multivariate extension of the latent variable growth model. See Fig. 3.1 for abbreviations and text for further details.

In addition to modeling growth for a single population, LGMs allow researchers to analyze change in behavior among multiple groups (e.g., treatment and control conditions, age, and gender). Just as repeated measures ANOVA models can be considered special cases of the general LGM, so too can between-subjects repeated measures ANOVAs be considered a special case of the multiple-sample LGM approach.

Analyzing treatment effectiveness: modeling between-subjects effects

In the typical LGM application, individuals whose data are being analyzed are assumed to represent a random sample of observations from a single population. However, in practice, this assumption is not always reasonable. A powerful application of the general LGM is in the examination of substance abuse treatment effects within an experimental design. For example, individuals may be identified as belonging to certain groups, such as treatment or control conditions. In this case it is appropriate to test for the existence of multiple populations (treatment and control) rather than a single population, as well as multiple developmental pathways for each condition rather than a single underlying trajectory for all. Many studies involving multiple populations have examined separate models for each group and compared the results. Unfortunately, such procedures do not allow a test of whether a common developmental model exists, and whether there are multiple developmental pathways across groups.

Developmental hypotheses involving multiple populations can be evaluated simultaneously provided that data on the same variables over the same developmental period are available in multiple samples. For example, the multiple-sample growth model has clear relevance to randomized controlled trials where one group might involve a wait-list control or an alternative treatment condition. In many cases, populations may be indistinguishable as far as the measured variables are concerned. When this occurs, the same population moment matrix describes all populations, and different sample moment matrices obtained from the various samples would simply be estimates of the same single population moment matrix. Growth models generated from the different samples should describe the same underlying developmental process for the population, and the separate models should be identical except for chance variations.

In other cases, the populations may share the same population covariance matrix, but differ in the means obtained from the various samples. Growth models generated from these different samples would not be expected to describe the same underlying developmental process for the population, and the separate models would carry unique information concerning the growth trajectories for that population despite identical covariance structures (except for chance variations).

A variety of growth models can be generalized to the simultaneous analysis of substance abuse data from multiple populations. To some extent, population differences can be captured in single-population analyses by representing the different groups as dummy vectors used as time-invariant covariates. However, to achieve more generality in modeling as well as specificity in the examination of population differences, it is necessary to use the multiple-population approach. Collapsing across different populations may mask potential group differences that are important to the study of change. Multiple-sample LGM has the potential to test for similarities and differences in developmental processes across different populations, including differences in levels of behaviors, developmental trajectories, rates of change, and effects of predictors and outcomes. Therefore, when data from multiple populations are available, a multiple-sample LGM is likely to be advantageous in the study of numerous behavioral processes.

Added growth models

Conventional longitudinal multiple-population latent variable analyses specify a common growth model in multiple groups, testing for equality of parameters across the different populations. An alternative approach (Muthén & Curran, 1997) is shown in Fig. 3.3. Here, an "added growth factor" is introduced for one population (for example, the treatment condition in a program to reduce family substance use). Whereas the first two factors (i.e., intercept and slope) are the same in both groups (control and treatment conditions), the added growth factor, specified in one group (e.g., treatment condition), represents incremental/decremental growth that is specific to that group.

In Fig. 3.3, the linear slope factor captures normative growth that is common to both control and treatment groups, whereas the added growth factor is specified to capture linear differences between the two groups. For research into substance abuse, the multiple-sample LGM framework affords a powerful design for detecting differences in program effectiveness by attributes such as subgroup membership. Examples of the multiple-sample approach can be found in Duncan, Duncan, and Alpert (1997a), Jo and Muthén (2001), McArdle *et al.* (1991), Muthén and Curran (1997), Muthén *et al.* (2002), and Tisak and Tisak (1996).

Alternative approaches to analyzing treatment effects: interrupted time series models

Although randomized controlled trial designs are generally preferred in intervention settings and analyzed in a multiple-population framework (e.g., Muthén & Curran, 1997), interrupted time series (ITS) designs, although less common in treatment research, have been widely used in research into prevention, intervention, and

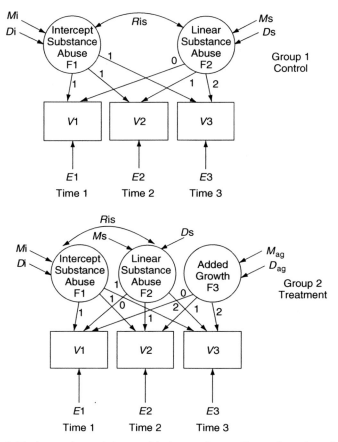

Fig. 3.3   Added growth model. ag, added growth; see Fig 3.1 for other abbreviations and text for futher details.

services, particularly in applied settings where randomized experiments are not feasible or indicated. Although considered quasi-experimental, the ITS design has been noted as representing one of the strongest alternatives to the randomized experiment. In the basic ITS design, measurements of the outcome variable (e.g., alcohol abuse) are collected at equally spaced intervals over an extended period of time, with an intervention implemented at a specific point within that period. ITS designs allow for assessments of the onset and duration of change in response to the implementation of an intervention for which the effects may be cumulative. These advantages make the ITS design highly appropriate for use in pilot studies, where the goal is to document the presence of effects that might warrant further evaluation in a large-scale randomized trial. Of particular relevance here is the fact that ITS designs permit assessment of the onset and duration of change in response to an intervention.

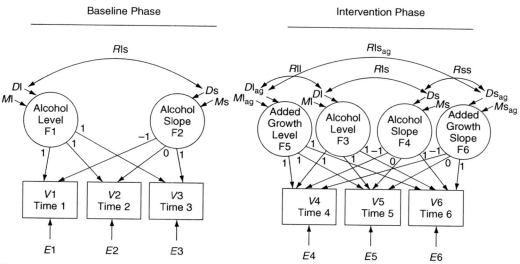

Fig. 3.4   Interrupted time series latent variable growth model. I, level (collection of intercepts); see Figs. 3.1 and 3.3 for other abbreviations and text for further details.

As can be seen from Fig. 3.4, the ITS LGM is similar to the added growth model, except that the ITS LGM model captures both intercept and slope differences in the outcome variable (e.g., alcohol abuse) over baseline and treatment intervention periods in a single sample. This allows researchers to examine specifically changes in level and slope of alcohol abuse over the intervention implementation phase compared with the baseline phase. Basis terms for the slope factors can be fixed at values of -1, 0, and 1, allowing for interpretation of the alcohol slope factors as linear change, and the alcohol level factors as average levels over time.

As can be seen from the diagram, the first factor is labeled "Level" and represents the average level of alcohol use over time. Just like the intercept factor, the level is a constant for any given individual across time, hence the fixed values of 1 for factor loadings on the repeated measures. For the slope factor, the fixed values of -1, 0, and 1 allow for interpretation of the alcohol slope factors as linear change, and the alcohol level factors as average levels over time. The level factor presents information in the sample about the mean (Ml) and variance (Dl) of the collection of intercepts that characterize each individual's substance abuse growth curve. The slope factor also has a mean (Ms) and variance (Ds) across the whole sample. The growth factors are allowed to covary (e.g., Rls, Rll, Rss), which are represented by the double-headed arrows between the factors.

As in the general LGM framework, ITS LGM allows the researcher to predict changes in treatment outcomes from time-invariant and time-varying covariates, and to use changes in treatment outcomes as predictors of subsequent outcomes.

Incorporating effects of the social context: hierarchical or multilevel designs

How individuals and social factors operate independently and interactively to shape development can be adequately studied only in the context of longitudinal and hierarchically structured research. While personal characteristics create propensities for specific types of developmental trajectory, these characteristics develop within the context of the social environment. There are several research designs for analysis of substance abuse in which it becomes essential to include social contextual effects in the analysis of longitudinal data. In many randomization trials, intact groups such as communities, families, or therapy groups, rather than individuals, are randomly assigned to experimental substance abuse treatments. Moreover, the treatments are administered to these intact groups rather than to individuals. It is assumed, therefore, that the responses of individuals in these groups will be similar by virtue of the experiences they share in those settings (Raudenbush, 1995).

Researchers have struggled for some time with such concepts as hierarchically nested observations, intraclass correlation, the unit of analysis, and random rather than fixed effects. Despite the assumption of somewhat homogeneous shared social environments, substance use researchers, until recently, have had few tools to accommodate the interdependence of such data. The absence of hierarchical methodologies for handling interdependence often led researchers to rely on analyses that assumed the data consisted of independent and identically distributed observations from a simple random sample in a single population. However, analyzing the data as a simple random sample ignores the potential interdependence within social or experimental clusters and increases the possibility of inflated test statistics for estimated parameters and overall model fit. A hierarchical approach to statistical modeling avoids these distortions. The analysis of data that has a hierarchical structure and contains measurements from different levels of the hierarchy requires techniques based on assumptions that are in agreement with the data structure.

Not only are the more traditional fixed-effects analytical methods (e.g., ANOVA) limited in their treatment of the technical difficulties posed by nested designs, they also are limited in the questions they are able to address. New analytic techniques that are more suited to the hierarchical data structure have recently emerged under the labels of hierarchical, or multilevel, models (e.g., Goldstein, 1986; Kreft, 1994; Longford, 1987; Raudenbush & Bryk, 1988). Muthén and Satorra (1989) emphasized that multilevel or hierarchical models take into account correlated observations and observations from heterogeneous populations with varying parameter values.

While appropriate analysis techniques of this kind are now widely available for standard regression and ANOVA situations, Muthén and Satorra (1989) highlighted the lack of techniques for covariance structure analyses. Just as ANOVA and multiple regression techniques can be considered special cases of the general SEM (Hoyle, 1995), so too can hierarchical linear models be viewed as special cases of the general multilevel covariance structure model. The multilevel covariance analysis (MCA) approach differs from more traditional hierarchical approaches in at least two important ways. First, and perhaps the most compelling, is its capacity to estimate and test relationships among latent variables. In much of the behavioral sciences, measurement of human behaviors is less than precise and fraught with measurement error given the sensitive nature of the data collected. The isolation of concepts from uniqueness and unreliability of their indicators increases the probability of detecting relationships and obtaining sound estimates of parameters close to their population values. Second, MCA allows for a more comprehensive and flexible approach to research design and data analysis than any other single statistical model for hierarchical data in standard use by social and behavioral researchers. Muthén (1989) has discussed the relationships of multilevel SEM to conventional SEM and pointed out the possibility of using conventional SEM software for multilevel SEM.

Full information maximum likelihood

McArdle (1988) presented two full information maximum likelihood (FIML) methods appropriate for hierarchical analyses with longitudinal substance abuse data. Originally formulated to model change in substance abuse for multiple variables or scales (e.g., different types of substance) over multiple occasions, these two methods are easily extended to modeling growth for multiple informants over multiple occasions (e.g., longitudinal and hierarchically nested data). These methods are termed the factor-of-curves and curve-of-factors models. The factor-of-curves model can be used to examine whether a higher-order factor adequately describes relationships among lower-order developmental functions (e.g., intercept and rate of change). Figure 3.5 depicts a factor-of-curves model for family members wherein substance abuse growth curves are applied to each family member separately. In this model, each first-order LGM is used to describe individual differences within each member series, and the second-order common factor model is used to describe family differences among the first-order LGMs. This FIML approach offers opportunities for evaluating the dynamic structure of both intra- and inter-individual change at multiple levels of the hierarchy.

Here, repeated measures within persons are viewed as the lowest level (level 1) with first-order observed variables, Vs, representing within-person change over time. Variables V1 through V4 represent observations for person 1 and variables V5 through V8 represent observations for person 2 from the same family or cluster. The basis terms, or factor loadings, are the coefficients for the influence of

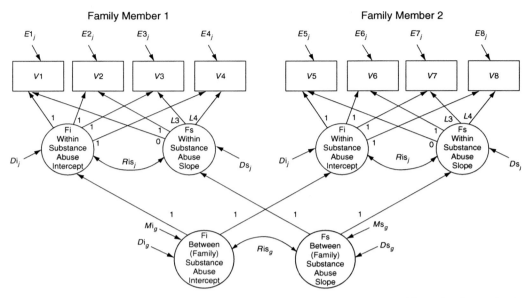

Fig. 3.5   Full information factor-of-curves model for family data. *L*, estimated factor loading or basic term; *j*, person; *g*, family; see Fig 3.1 for abbreviations and text for further details.

the intercept and slope factors on the observed V variables. It is possible to accommodate non-linear growth by estimating the third and fourth coefficients on the slope factor, *L3* and *L4*, holding the first two values fixed at 0 and 1, respectively. The growth curves are then applied to each family member separately, representing between-person change (level 2) with first-order latent factors, *Fi* and *Fs*, variance, Di_j *and* Ds_j, and measurement errors, E_j, for a two-member family. The growth factors are allowed to covary, Ris_j, which is represented by the double-headed arrows between the intercept and slope factors. The variation among families is captured at the highest level (level 3) second-order latent factors, *Fi* and *Fs*, means Mi_g *and* Ds_g and variance Di_g *and* Ds_g. The factor loadings for the influence of the family-level factors on the person-level factors are fixed at 1 so that the contribution to the family-level means and variances are the same for each family member. The second-order growth factors are allowed to covary, Ris_g.

The curve-of-factors method can be used to fit a growth curve to factor scores representing what the lower-order factors have in common at each point in time. Applications of these two methods can be found in Duncan and Duncan (1996). When there are many clusters of different size (e.g., unbalanced data), FIML estimation can be accomplished using a model-based extension of the multiple groups framework. For applications of these full information approaches see Duncan *et al.* (2001a) and McArdle (1988).

Limited information multilevel latent growth modeling

While FIML approaches can be used for multilevel longitudinal data, they can be computationally heavy and input specifications can be tedious if group sizes are large. Consequently, Muthén (1991, 1994) proposed a MCA approach to analyzing multilevel data using a limited information estimation approach that is simpler to compute than FIML. Muthén (1994) showed that the estimator provides full maximum likelihood estimation for balanced data (e.g., hierarchical clusters of the same size), and gives similar results to full maximum likelihood for data that is not too badly unbalanced. Within the Mplus SEM program (Muthén & Muthén, 2004), the ad hoc approach greatly simplifies model specification for unbalanced hierarchically nested longitudinal data. Therefore, with large groups of different sizes, little may be gained by the extra effort of FIML computation. The MCA model for family substance use can be illustrated by a diagram such as that in Fig. 3.6. In the MCA, the total covariance matrix is decomposed into two independent components, a between-level covariance matrix (e.g., family) and a within-level covariance matrix (e.g., individuals or family members). Conventional covariance structure analysis that ignores grouping or clustering assumes that all observations are independent. The part of the model below the squares refers to the within- or individual-level structure while the part above refers to the between- or family-level structure. The setup is a multiple-sample model in which the first group involves both between- and within-level structures and the second group involves only the within-level structure.

The model setup in the first group, using the between-level covariance matrix, S_B, as input, requires the creation of extra latent variables to capture the weighting by the constant, C. These extra latent variables are depicted as F1 through F4 and their contribution to the observed V variables is scaled by fixing the path (loading) to $\sqrt{C}$. The residual variances of F1 through F4 ($D1_B$ through $D4_B$) capture the between-level composite error variances. The mean structure, Mi_B and Ms_B, for the MLGM arises from the four observed variable means expressed as functions of the means of the Fi_B and Fs_B between-level factors. Between-level factor variances are shown as Di_B and Ds_B. The factors are allowed to covary, Ris_B. The means of the within-level growth factors, Fi_W and Fs_W, are fixed at zero. The third and fourth coefficients on the slope factor, $L3_B$ and $L4_B$, indicate it is possible to accommodate non-linear growth at the between level, holding the first two values fixed at 0 and 1, respectively. The second group in the multiple-group setup corresponds to the within-level variation. The within-level covariance structure, S_{PW}, is captured by using the same model structure as for the first group but fixing all between-level coefficients and variance–covariance parameters to zero. Within-level composite error variance is captured by residual error variances, $E1_W$ through $E4_W$, for the V variables. Within-level factor variances are shown as Di_W and Ds_W,

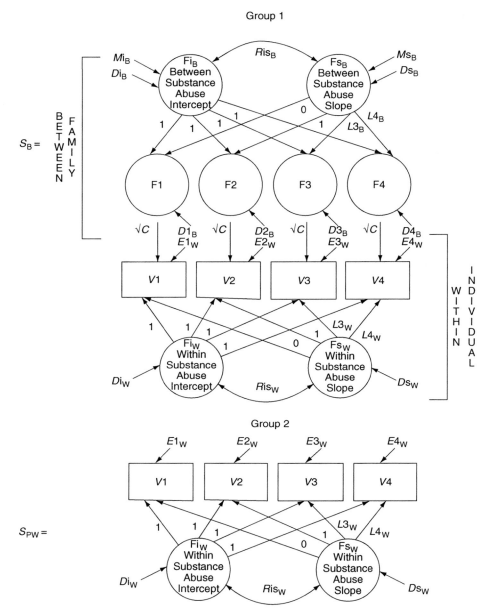

Fig. 3.6   Multilevel covariance structure model. *S*, covariance matrix; B, between level; W, within level; *C*, average group or cluster size; *D*, residual variance; see Fig. 3.1 for other abbreviations and text for further details.

and the factors are allowed to covary, Ris_W. As in the between-level case, non-linear growth can be accommodated with careful specification of the third and fourth coefficients on the slope factor, $L3_W$ and $L4_W$.

As in the general LGM framework, the MCA allows the researcher to specify the hierarchical structure in multiple populations (e.g., treatment and control conditions), to predict changes in treatment outcomes from time-invariant and time-varying covariates, and to use changes in treatment outcomes as predictors of subsequent outcomes.

Developments such as these make possible the construction, estimation, and testing of a variety of complex models involving hierarchically structured longitudinal substance abuse data. For applications of the MCA limited information approach, see Duncan *et al.* (1997a,b, 2001a, 2002b) Khoo and Muthén (2000), and Muthén (1997).

The use of LGMs that incorporate information from various levels of the hierarchy allows for potentially greater insight into the developmental nature, antecedents, and sequelae of a plethora of behavioral outcomes. The flexibility of these techniques makes them attractive tools for a variety of analyses investigating growth and development in multilevel substance use prevention and treatment data.

Modeling unobserved heterogeneity: treatment audience profiling

As previously stated, traditional implementation of latent growth methodology assumes data were collected from a single population. This assumption of sample homogeneity is often not met, which can result in seriously biased parameter estimates. Developmental hypotheses involving multiple populations can be evaluated simultaneously within a multiple-sample approach when the sample heterogeneity involves easily identified groups, such as males and females, age cohorts, ethnicities, or treatment and control conditions. But what can you do when the sample heterogeneity is not readily apparent? The following sections present the methodological and substantive issues surrounding the modeling of changes in substance abuse behavior within a finite mixture modeling framework that accounts for unobserved sample heterogeneity.

The underlying theory of finite mixture modeling assumes that the population analyzed is not homogeneous in its behavior (as measured by response probabilities) but consists of heterogeneous subpopulations with different behavior patterns in each latent class (component) (e.g., capturing qualitatively different growth trajectories in substance abuse). The methodological framework enables researchers to investigate a variety of substantive hypotheses concerning differences between the mixture components. The basic idea of mixture modeling is to partition the population into an unknown number of latent classes or subpopulations wherein each latent class membership is determined by specific parameters. The mixture modeling approach offers a distinct advantage to the intervention researcher who knows that not all interventions work for all people by facilitating the identification of those subjects who most benefit from the intervention.

Growth mixture modeling

Recently, Muthén (2001) proposed an extension of current LGM methodology that includes relatively unexplored mixture models, such as growth mixture models, mixture structural equation models, and models that combine latent class analysis and SEM. Fitting these models can be done through newly developed Mplus software (Muthén & Muthén, 2004).

Relevant to longitudinal substance abuse research is the growth mixture modeling approach, which combines categorical and continuous latent variables into the same model. Muthén and colleagues (Muthén & Muthén, 2000; Muthén & Shedden, 1999) described in detail the generalization of LGM to finite mixture latent trajectory models and proposed a general growth mixture modeling framework (GGMM). The GGMM strategy allows for unobserved heterogeneity in the sample, where different individuals defined by their growth trajectories or other responses to a treatment intervention can belong to different subpopulations. The model can be extended further to estimate varying class membership probability as a function of a set of covariates (i.e., for each class, the values of the latent growth parameters are allowed to be influenced by covariates) and to incorporate outcomes of the latent class variable.

Figure 3.7 displays a full growth mixture model representing Muthén and colleagues' framework for latent class/latent growth modeling. This model contains a combination of continuous latent growth variables (e.g., substance abuse intercept and slope) and a latent categorical variable, C, with k classes; C_i is 1 if individual i belongs to class k and zero otherwise. These latent attributes are represented by circles in the figure. The latent continuous growth variable portion of the model represents conventional growth modeling with multiple indicators, V, measured at four time points (e.g., Willett & Sayer, 1994). The categorical latent variable is used to represent latent trajectory classes underlying the latent growth variable. Both latent continuous and latent class variables can be predicted from a set of background variables or covariates, X, since the model allows the mixing proportions to depend on prior information and/or subject-specific variables. The growth mixture portion of the model, however, can have mixture outcome indicators (e.g., subsequent substance abuse-related outcomes), U. In this model, the directional arrow from the latent trajectory classes to the growth factors indicates that the intercepts of the regressions of the growth factors on $X1$ vary

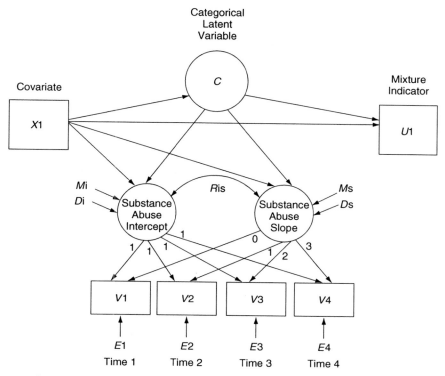

Fig. 3.7   Growth mixture model. *C*, categorical latent variable; *X*, covariate; *U*, mixture outcome indicator; see Fig. 3.1 for other abbreviations and text for further details.

across the classes of *C*. The directional arrow from *C* to *U*1 indicates that the probabilities of *U*1 vary across the classes of *C*.

The ability to detect different intervention effects for individuals belonging to different trajectory classes has important implications for designing future intervention strategies for substance abuse. It is possible to select different substance abuse interventions for individuals belonging to different trajectory classes using longitudinal screening procedures, or to classify individuals into their most likely trajectory class based on a set of initial repeated measurements taken before the intervention starts. For example, in a mixture analysis of alcohol and marijuana use, Hix-Small *et al.* (2004) found that individuals classified as having either elevated levels of use in both alcohol and marijuana or elevated levels of use in only alcohol had only marginally higher odds ratios for subsequent substance use problems than individuals with steep developmental trajectories for both alcohol and marijuana use. That is, individuals classified as high-rate substance users did not differ significantly in their subsequent behavioral outcomes compared with individuals on a delayed upward trajectory. It is possible that individuals in the delayed trajectory classes would be more receptive to intervention than their high-rate counterparts, given that their behavior may not yet be fully established. The strength of studies using randomized repeated measures is that they allow for the assessment of intervention effects on trajectories rather than focusing on overall intervention effects at a particular time point. The analysis capitalizes on this strength by allowing for a variety of growth forms of unobserved heterogeneity among treatment respondents, which is typically encountered in prevention and treatment research.

Muthén (2001) considered growth mixture modeling to be a second generation of SEM. Indeed, the general framework outlined by Muthén (2001) provides new opportunities for growth modeling and holds great promise as a modeling framework for longitudinal substance use studies in which individual growth trajectories are heterogeneous and belong to a finite number of unobserved groups. Researchers have already begun to use these techniques to aid them in the identification of individuals at risk for future drug abuse and dependence, potentially allowing for the development of targeted, rather than more global, intervention strategies. The application of mixtures to growth modeling also may be used as an alternative to cluster analytic techniques if the posterior probability of membership of an individual in a latent class is used to assign latent class membership. Examples of the mixture approach can be found in Muthén (2000, 2001) and Muthén and Muthén (2000).

Conclusions

Advantages of the latent variable growth model

Methodology based on the LGM provides a number of advantages for researchers in both the epidemiology of substance abuse and its prevention who are interested in change over time. The LGM describes a single individual's developmental trajectory and captures individual differences in these trajectories over time. Moreover, the LGM is able to include predictors of those individual differences to answer questions about which variables exert important effects on the rate of development of substance use and abuse. At the same time, the model is able to capture the important group statistics in a way that allows the researcher to study substance abuse development at the group level. Given more than two assessment points, LGMs are able to test both linear and non-linear growth functions. When appropriate, the LGM also allows the flexibility of including more than two factors to capture developmental trends through the use of specified growth functions and additional growth factors (e.g., quadratic, cubic growth). Another advantage of LGM methodology is its ability to incorporate time-varying covariates. Both static and time-varying variables can be included in models as predictors as well as outcomes of substance use growth functions, thus allowing the researcher to address questions related to the antecedents and consequences of substance use/abuse development. In practical terms, LGMs offer different opportunities for evaluating the dynamic structure of both intra- and inter-individual change, and they represent a logical progression in the paradigm of representing behavioral dynamics. In addition to the special cases of the LGM already presented, several other noteworthy extensions are possible.

Incorporating missing data in latent variable growth models

Because nearly all longitudinal data sets suffer from various missing data, analytic techniques must be able to handle planned "missingness" appropriately as well as missing data resulting from attrition and omissions. From a statistical point of view, the best missing data procedures do several things. First, they take into consideration all available causes of missingness. Second, they employ the same statistical model to handle the missing data that is used to perform the desired analysis. For example, if the final model is a LGM, the best approach also would use a LGM to handle the missing data. Finally, the best procedures provide consistent and efficient parameter estimates. Within LGM, model-based procedures can be used to analyze incomplete data using either multiple-sample SEM or raw maximum likelihood procedures. Both approaches allow the researcher to take into consideration all available causes of missingness, employ the same statistical model to handle the missing data that is used to perform the desired analysis, and provide consistent and efficient parameter estimates. For examples of the SEM approach to missing data, see Duncan and Duncan (1994) and Muthén, Kaplan, and Hollis (1987).

Design issues: sample size selection and power estimation

The LGM method described in this chapter also provides a power-estimation framework to aid researchers in making design decisions for a variety of intervention studies. From a statistical point of view, the best procedures for power estimation should (1) employ the same statistical model for power and sample size estimation as that used for the desired analysis (for example, if the final model is an LGM, the best approach for power estimation also would use an LGM); (2) cover the situations most commonly encountered by researchers; (3) be flexible enough to deal with new or unusual situations; (4) allow easy exploration of multiple values of input parameters; and (5) allow estimation of sampling variance from pilot data and from the statistics commonly reported in the literature.

Under the LGM approach, power estimation is directly related to the parameter values of a specified model. The relations among values of the level of significance, measures of effect size, the sample size, and the degrees of freedom are identical to those in more traditional techniques. However, LGM has the added advantage of accounting for measurement error, thus disattenuating the relationships among the variables of interest, which increases reliability and power and reduces sample size requirements. Examples of power analyses conducted within the SEM framework can be found in Muthén and Curran (1997), Muthén and Muthén (2003), and Duncan *et al.* (2002a).

Limitations of the latent variable growth model

Despite numerous attractions, LGM is not always the appropriate analytical choice for substance use/abuse prevention and treatment research. The more commonly cited limitations of SEM programs for estimating LGM include multinormally distributed variables and the necessity of large samples. However, recent Monte Carlo simulations have demonstrated that basic LGMs hold up well with relatively small numbers of data points (e.g., Muthén & Muthén, 2003). In fitting LGMs, inferences are made from observed data to the model thought to be generating those observations (Tanaka, 1987). In part, these inferences depend on the degree to which the information in the sample is representative of the same information in the complete population, which in turn depends on the adequacy of the sample size. Therefore, the requisite sample size largely depends on the specific empirical context (e.g., psychometric behavior of indicators, amount of missing data, size of effects) and design aspects such as the number of assessment points.

In terms of modeling flexibility, the LGM is also limited in its handling of randomly varying within-subjects designs, including unequal intervals of observations and varied within-person distributions of time-varying covariates having random effects. Although recent software developments have begun to address these limitations (e.g., Muthén & Muthén, 2003), LGM analyses do not yet allow the flexibility of the random coefficient approach conducted within the regression framework (Muthén & Curran, 1997).

Summary

The search for the best methods to address complex issues encountered in studies of substance abuse continues. As research in this field continues to develop, new and more complex research questions will be posed and these will continue to prompt the development of new statistical methods. Just as there are a plethora of substantive questions posed by researchers in substance abuse, so too is there a broad and varied assortment of newly developed statistical methods available to apply to these questions. The LGM approach presented here allows for a comprehensive and flexible approach to research design and data analysis that has the potential to answer an increased variety of questions on substance use posed by social and behavioral researchers by accommodating the complex integration of behavioral, social, genetic, and biomedical data required to determine intervention effectiveness.

ACKNOWLEDGEMENTS

This research was supported by grants DA11942 and DA09548 from the National Institute on Drug Abuse. Partial support in preparing this manuscript was provided by grant AA11510 from the National Institute on Alcohol Abuse and Alcoholism.

REFERENCES

Akers, R. L. & Cochran, J. E. (1985). Adolescent marijuana use: a test of three theories of deviant behavior. *Deviant Behavior*, **6**, 323–346.

Cliff, N. (1983). Some cautions concerning the application of causal modeling methods. *Multivariate Behavioral Research*, **18**, 115–126.

Collins, L. & Horn, J. L. (1991). *Best Methods for the Analysis of Change*. Washington, DC: American Psychological Association Press.

Collins, L. & Sayer, J. L. (2001). *New Methods for the Analysis of Change*. Washington, DC: American Psychological Association Press.

Conger, R. D. (1997). The social context of substance abuse: a developmental perspective. In E. B. Robertson, Z. Sloboda, G. M. Boyd, L. Beatty, & N. J. Kozel (eds.), *Rural Substance Abuse: State of Knowledge and Issues*. [*NIDA Research Monograph* No. 168, pp. 6–36.] Rockville, MD: National Institutes of Health.

Curran, P. J., Stice, E. & Chassin, L. (1997). The relation between adolescent alcohol use and peer alcohol use: a longitudinal random coefficients model. *Journal of Consulting and Clinical Psychology*, **65**, 130–140.

Duncan, S. C. & Duncan, T. E. (1994). Modeling incomplete longitudinal substance use data using latent variable growth curve methodology. *Multivariate Behavioral Research*, **29**, 313–338.
 (1996). A multivariate latent growth curve analysis of adolescent substance use. *Structural Equation Modeling*, **3**, 323–347.

Duncan, S. C., Duncan, T. E., & Strycker, L. A. (2001b). Qualitative and quantitative shifts in adolescent problem behavior development: a cohort-sequential multivariate latent growth modeling approach. *Journal of Psychopathology and Behavioral Assessment*, **23**, 43–50.
 (2002b). A multilevel analysis of neighborhood context and youth alcohol and drug problems. *Prevention Science*, **3**, 125–134.

Duncan, T. E. & Duncan, S. C. (1995). Modeling the processes of development via latent variable growth curve methodology. *Structural Equation Modeling*, **2**, 187–213.

Duncan, T. E., Duncan, S. C., Alpert, A., *et al.* (1997a). Latent variable modeling of longitudinal and multilevel substance use data. *Multivariate Behavioral Research*, **32**, 275–318.

Duncan, T. E., Duncan, S. C., & Alpert, A. (1997b). Multilevel covariance structure analysis of family substance use across samples and ethnicities. *Journal of Gender, Culture, and Health*, **2**, 271–286.

Duncan, T. E., Duncan, S. C., Strycker, L. A., Li, F., & Alpert, A. (1999). *An Introduction to Latent Variable Growth Curve Modeling: Concepts, Issues, and Applications*. Hillsdale, NJ: Lawrence Erlbaum.

Duncan, T. E., Duncan, S. C., Strycker, L. A., & Li, F. (2002a). A latent variable framework for power estimation and analyses within intervention contexts. *Journal of Psychopathology and Behavioral Assessment*, **24**, 1–12.

Duncan T. E., Duncan, S. C., Li, F., & Strycker, L. A. (2001a). A comparison of longitudinal multilevel techniques for analyzing adolescent and family alcohol use data. In D. S. Moskowitz & S. L. Hershberger (eds.), *Modeling Intra-individual Variability with Repeated Measures Data: Methods and Applications* (pp. 171–201). New York: Plenum Press.

Ge, X., Lorenz, F. O., Conger, R. D., & Elder, G. H. (1994). Trajectories of stressful life events and depressive symptoms during adolescence. *Developmental Psychology*, **30**, 467–483.

Goldstein, H. I. (1986). Multilevel mixed linear model analysis using iterative general least squares. *Biometrika*, **73**, 43–56.

Gottman, J. M. (1995). *The Analysis of Change*. Hillsdale, NJ: Lawrence Erlbaum.

Hix-Small, H., Duncan, T. E., Duncan, S. C., & Okut, H. (2004). A multivariate associative finite growth mixture modeling approach examining adolescent alcohol and marijuana use. *Journal of Psychopathology and Behavioral Assessment*, **26**, 255–269.

Hoyle, R. (1995). The structural equation modeling approach: basic concepts and fundamental issues. In R. H. Hoyle (ed.), *Structural Equation Modeling: Issues and Applications* (pp. 1–15). Thousand Oaks, CA: Sage.

Jo, B. & Muthén, B. (2001). Modeling of intervention effects with noncompliance: a latent variable approach for randomized trials. In G. A. Marcoulides & R. E. Schumacker (eds.), *New Developments and Techniques in Structural Equation Modeling* (pp. 57–87). Hillsdale, NJ: Lawrence Erlbaum.

Khoo, S. T. & Muthén, B. (2000). Longitudinal data on families: growth modeling alternatives. In J. Rose, L. Chassin, C. Presson, & J. Sherman (eds.), *Multivariate Applications in Substance Use Research* (pp. 43–78). Hillsdale, NJ: Lawrence Erlbaum.

Kreft, I. G. (1994). Multilevel models for hierarchically nested data: potential applications in substance abuse prevention research. In L. Collins & L. Seitz (eds.), *Advances in Data Analysis for Prevention Intervention Research*. [*NIDA Research Monograph* No. 142, pp. 140–183.] Rockville, MD: National Institutes of Health.

Longford, N. T. (1987). A fast scoring algorithm for maximum likelihood estimation in unbalanced mixed models with nested effects. *Biometrika*, **74**, 817–827.

McArdle, J. J. (1988). Dynamic but structural equation modeling of repeated measures data. In R. B. Cattell & J. Nesselroade (eds.), *Handbook of Multivariate Experimental Psychology*, 2nd edn (pp. 561–614). New York: Plenum Press.

McArdle, J. J. & Epstein, D. (1987). Latent growth curves within developmental structural equation models. *Child Development*, **58**, 110–133.

McArdle, J.J., Hamagami, F., Elias, M.F., & Robbins, M.A. (1991). Structural modeling of mixed longitudinal and cross-sectional data. *Experimental Aging Research*, **17**, 29–52.

Meredith, W. & Tisak, J. (1990). Latent curve analysis. *Psychometrika*, **55**, 107–122.

Muthén, B. (1989). Latent variable modeling in heterogeneous populations. *Psychometrika*, **54**, 557–585.

(1991). Multilevel factor analysis of class and student achievement components. *Journal of Educational Measurement*, **28**, 338–354.

(1994). Multilevel covariance structure analysis. *Sociological Methods and Research*, **22**, 376–398.

(1997). Latent variable modeling of longitudinal and multilevel data. In A. Raftery (ed.), *Sociological Methodology* (pp. 453–480). Boston, MA: Blackwell.

(2000). Methodological issues in random coefficient growth modeling using a latent variable framework: applications to the development of heavy drinking. In J. Rose, L. Chassin, C. Presson, & J. Sherman (eds.), *Multivariate Applications in Substance Use Research* (pp. 113–140). Hillsdale, NJ: Lawrence Erlbaum.

(2001). Second-generation structural equation modeling with a combination of categorical and continuous latent variables: new opportunities for latent class-latent growth modeling. In L. Collins & A. Sayer (eds.), *New Methods for the Analysis of Change* (pp. 291–322). Washington, DC: American Psychological Association Press.

Muthén, B. & Curran, P. (1997). General growth modeling of individual differences in experimental designs: a latent variable framework for analysis and power estimation. *Psychological Methods*, **2**, 371–402.

Muthén, B. & Muthén, L. (2000). Integrating person-centered and variable-centered analysis: growth mixture modeling with latent trajectory classes. *Alcoholism: Clinical and Experimental Research*, **24**, 882–891.

Muthén, B. & Satorra, A. (1989). Multilevel aspects of varying parameters in structural models. In R.D. Bock (ed.), *Multilevel Analysis of Educational Data* (pp. 87–99). San Diego, CA: Academic Press.

Muthén, B. & Shedden, K. (1999). Finite mixture modeling with mixture outcomes using the EM algorithm. *Biometrics*, **55**, 463–469.

Muthén, B., Kaplan, D., & Hollis, M. (1987). On structural equation modeling with data that are not missing completely at random. *Psychometrika*, **52**, 431–462.

Muthén, B., Brown, C.H., Masyn, K., *et al.* (2002). General growth mixture modeling for randomized preventive interventions. *Biostatistics*, **3**, 459–475.

Muthén, L.K. & Muthén, B. (2004). *Mplus: User's Guide* 3rd edn. Los Angeles, CA: Muthén & Muthén.

(2003). *Addendum to the Mplus User's Guide.* Los Angeles, CA: Muthén & Muthén.

Patterson, G.R., Reid, J.B., & Dishion, T.J. (1992). *A Social Learning Approach: IV. Antisocial Boys.* Eugene, OR: Castalia.

Rao, C.R. (1958). Some statistical methods for comparison of growth curves. *Biometrics*, **14**, 1–17.

Raudenbush, S.W. (1995). Statistical models for studying the effects of social context on individual development. In J. Gottman (ed.), *The Analysis of Change* (pp. 165–201). Hillsdale, NJ: Lawrence Erlbaum.

Raudenbush, S. & Bryk, A. (1988). Methodological advances in studying effects of schools and classrooms on student learning. In E. Z. Roth (ed.), *Review of Research in Education* (pp. 423–475). Washington, DC: American Educational Research Association.

Rogosa, D. & Willett, J. B. (1985). Understanding correlates of change by modeling individual differences in growth. *Psychometrika*, **50**, 203–228.

Rogosa, D. R., Brandt, D., & Zimowski, M. (1982). A growth curve approach to the measure of change. *Psychological Bulletin*, **92**, 726–748.

Sampson, R. J. (1988). Local friendship ties and community attachment in mass society: a multilevel systemic model. *American Sociological Review*, **53**, 766–779.

(1992). Family management and child development: insights from social disorganization theory. In J. McCord (ed.), *Advances in Criminological Theory*, vol. 3: *Facts, Frameworks and Forecasts* (pp. 63–93). New Brunswick: Transaction.

Sampson, R. J. & Laub, J. H. (1990). Crime and deviance over the life course: the salience of adult social bonds. *American Sociological Review*, **55**, 609–627.

Sayer, A. G. & Willet, J. B. (1998). A cross-domain model for growth in adolescent alcohol expectancies. *Multivariate Behavioral Research* **33**, 509–543.

Stoolmiller, M. (1995). Using latent growth curve models to study developmental processes. In J. M. Gottman (ed.), *The Analysis of Change* (pp. 103–138). Hillsdale, NJ: Lawrence Erlbaum.

Tanaka, J. S. (1987). How big is big enough? Sample size and goodness of fit in structural equation models with latent variables. *Child Development*, **58**, 134–146.

Tisak, J. & Meredith, W. (1990). Descriptive and associative developmental models. In A. von Eye (ed.), *Statistical Methods in Developmental Research*, Vol. 2 (pp. 387–406). San Diego, CA: Academic Press.

Tisak, J. & Tisak, M. S. (1996). Longitudinal models of reliability and validity: a latent curve approach. *Applied Psychological Measurement*, **20**, 275–288.

Tucker, L. R. (1958). Determination of parameters of a functional relation by factor analysis. *Psychometrika*, **23**, 19–23.

Wang, J., Siegal, H., Falck, R., Carlson, R., & Rahman, A. (1999). Evaluation of HIV risk reduction intervention programs via latent growth curve model. *Evaluation Review: A Journal of Applied Social Research*, **23**, 649–663.

Wickrama, K. A. S., Lorenz, F. O., & Conger, R. D. (1997). Parental support and adolescent physical health status: a latent growth-curve analysis. *Journal of Health and Social Behavior*, **38**, 149–163.

Willett, J. B. & Sayer, A. G. (1994). Using covariance structure analysis to detect correlates and predictors of individual change over time. *Psychological Bulletin*, **116**, 363–381.

4

Clinical course of youth following treatment for alcohol and drug problems

Sandra A. Brown and Danielle E. Ramo

Veterans' Affairs San Diego Healthcare System, University of California, San Diego, CA, USA
San Diego State University/University of California, San Diego, USA

Alcohol and drug abuse by adolescents is a problem of critical importance in the USA. Treatment facilities are now providing programs specifically for substance use disorders (SUDs) among adolescents, and research has begun to examine long-term outcomes for these youth. This chapter examines the clinical course of youth following alcohol and/or drug treatment. It considers the use patterns observed after treatment in community treatment programs and through clinical trials, the personal and environmental factors that may influence these outcomes, and the important distinctions between adolescent and adult relapse patterns. A revised cognitive–behavioral model of relapse is presented that incorporates the factors found to be particularly important in understanding the adolescent relapse process. Special challenges for youth are explored, including the prevalence and impact of psychiatric comorbidity, the neurocognitive impact of early alcohol and drug involvement, and the developmental transitions associated with elevated risk for youth with a history of substance abuse.

Adolescent alcohol and drug use is a major social and public health concern. *Monitoring the Future*, a study funded by NIDA, indicated that 80% of high school students have used alcohol and 54% have used other drugs at least once (Johnston, O'Malley, & Bachman, 2002). Hazardous drinking (five or more drinks on one occasion) is also a frequent occurrence, with 30% of all adolescents nationwide in the USA reporting episodes of binge drinking (Grunbaum *et al.*, 2002). Alcohol and drug use in adolescence is associated with substantial adverse consequences, such as drinking and driving (Walsh, 1985), risky sexual behaviors (Staton *et al.*, 1999), criminal activity (Temple & Ladouceur, 1986), and delinquency (Brown *et al.*, 1996). The severity of consequences from alcohol and drug use among teenagers is further demonstrated by the prevalence of problems among adolescents receiving treatment (Brown, Vik, & Creamer, 1989a). Successful treatment outcomes for adolescents have eluded both researchers and clinicians in this field,

Adolescent Substance Abuse: Research and Clinical Advances, ed. Howard A. Liddle and Cynthia L. Rowe.
Published by Cambridge University Press. © Cambridge University Press 2006.

with approximately half of the adolescents receiving community-based treatment for SUDs relapsing within the first 3 months following treatment (Brown, Mott, & Myers, 1990) and two thirds to four fifths of youth relapsing after 6 months (Brown *et al.*, 2001; Cornelius *et al.*, 2001).

A growing body of longitudinal research has examined the clinical course of youth after treatment for alcohol and drug problems. According to this work, outcomes after treatment are not the same for adolescents as for adults. Specifically, there are differences in environmental influences, cognitions, and coping mechanisms used by adolescents that help to explain their relapse patterns following treatment (Myers & Brown, 1990a,b; Myers, Brown, & Mott, 1993). The variability of circumstances of relapse across the developmental spectrum has broad implications for treatment and research in the field of adolescent substance abuse. This chapter will focus on three topics related to outcomes in treatment of adolescent substance abuse. First, we will review the patterns and processes of relapse or reinstatement of drug use following treatment as adolescents transition into young adulthood. Next, we will discuss the factors that are associated with successful behavior change, highlighting strategies that work well for particular groups. Finally, we will consider developmentally specific challenges to sustained improvement following treatment for youth. The reader will have a greater understanding of the variability in outcomes associated with treatment for SUDs in youth, as well as some of the personal and environmental characteristics associated with these patterns. This will greatly inform the work of those seeking to adapt substance abuse treatment to the individual characteristics of its recipients.

Adolescent relapse patterns following drug and alcohol treatment: treatment outcome studies

Compared with outcome research for adult drug treatments, less is known about what happens to adolescents after treatment for alcohol or drug abuse (Brown, 1999). Of note, a sizable portion of available data comes from outcome studies conducted during the 1970s and 1980s, when adolescents with SUDs were treated in adult programs. Among initial attempts to evaluate the effectiveness of substance abuse treatment for adolescents were the Drug Abuse Reporting Program (Sells & Simpson, 1979), the Pennsylvania Data Collection System (Rush, 1979), and the Treatment Outcome Prospective Study (Hubbard *et al.*, 1983). Many early investigations did not have control or comparison groups, had little information on reliability of data, and the variables measured reflected evaluation of characteristics specific to adults rather than adolescents. Finally, while contemporary community-based adolescent drug treatment programs have designed treatment better matched to the needs of younger adolescents, many of the data in these studies were derived from older teenagers in adult treatment programs. Consequently, much of the early research on adolescent treatment outcome has been compromised by methodological limitations and a lack of direct applicability to current practices.

Since the mid-1990s, longitudinal studies have begun to examine the outcomes of adolescents following treatment in community-based facilities for adolescents. The Drug Abuse Treatment Outcome Study for Adolescents (DATOS-A) (discussed in detail in Ch. 6; Bennett & Grella, 2001), is the largest NIDA-funded adolescent treatment outcome study to date. This study evaluates outcomes of youth treated in 37 community-based treatment programs across six USA cities. The treatment modalities studied include short-term inpatient, therapeutic community or residential, and outpatient drug-free. Preliminary outcomes in a subset of youth (1167) suggested that over half (54%) of participants reduced their use of alcohol from pretreatment levels; 22% increased use over the year; 18% did not change use; and 6% reported abstinence both pre-and post-treatment (Chung et al., 2003).

A number of studies since DATOS-A have followed adolescents after drug and alcohol treatment using demographically matched comparison groups. In a series of studies in our group (Brown, 1993; Brown et al., 1994, 2001), two clinical cohorts of youth who met criteria for a SUD (abuse or dependence) were assessed following inpatient treatment modeled after the Alcoholics Anonymous (AA) 12-step approach. As shown in Figs. 4.1 and 4.2, adolescent addiction relapse rates were similar to those observed by adult addicts 1 year following treatment (Brown, 1999). Similar to adults, approximately one third of adolescents used alcohol or another drug in the first month after treatment, with up to three quarters of youth having at least one alcohol or drug experience by 1 year after discharge. Six months after treatment, three general relapse patterns began to emerge: 27% of adolescents abstained completely or had only one minor use episode ("abstainers"); 30% had limited alcohol or drug use episodes (fewer than 3 consecutive days in the time period), without bingeing and with no identifiable problems associated with their substance use ("minor relapsers"); 42% had returned to more severe alcohol or drug involvement ("major relapsers").

Data from these samples also demonstrated prevalence rates for extended periods following treatment (Brown et al., 2001) that could be compared with national rates in individuals aged 18–25 years surveyed as part of the National Household Survey of Drug Abuse (NHSDA; SAMHSA, 2000). As shown in Table 4.1, alcohol was the most common substance adolescents used when entering treatment (intake), and 1-month prevalence rates of alcohol use at all follow-up time points were similar to those reported in the NHSDA. Marijuana use rates ranged from 2.5 to 3.0 times higher than the national prevalence rates through

Table 4.1 Substance use prevalence rates and average days using per month for treated youth compared with young adults from the household drug abuse survey

| | Treated youth at | | | | | | | | | | Comparison group: using drugs (%) |
| | Intake | | 6 months | | 1 year | | 2 years | | 4 years | | |
	% using	Days/month[a]	% using	Days/month	% using	Days/month	% using	Days/month	% using	Days/month	
Alcohol	91.4	12.3	50.7	7.8	50.7	8.7	53.6	12.0	66.0	14.4	56.9
Cigarettes	85.4	28.2	87.1	26.5	78.1	28.1	79.5	27.5	77.3	26.5	29.2
Marijuana	84.0	19.5	35.0	11.1	38.8	13.6	42.7	12.2	44.4	14.9	15.8
Stimulants	84.6	21.5	26.1	9.4	30.2	10.2	23.7	10.7	19.5	12.0	0.8
Other drugs	32.3	5.5	11.7	3.3	19.5	4.0	11.9	2.1	15.5	6.0	–

Source: Youth data from Brown *et al.* (2001). Comparison group is information taken from the National Household Survey of Drug Abuse, for individuals aged 18–25 years (SAMHSA, 2000).

[a] Days per month are calculated only for those who reported past month use of the substance during the follow-up time period.

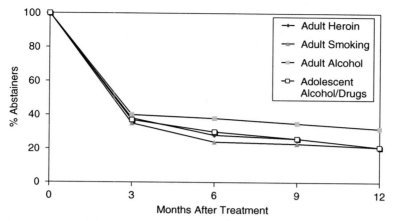

Fig. 4.1   Survival rates adults and adolescents. (From Brown *et al.*, [1989a] and Hunt, Barnett, & Branch [1971], adapted with permission.)

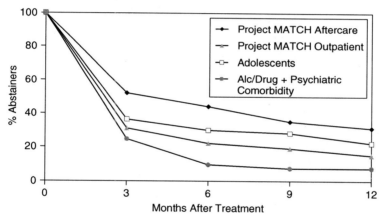

Fig. 4.2   Survival rates in Project MATCH for treated adolescents. (From Tomlinson *et al.* [2004] and Project MATCH Research Group [1997], with permission.)

the first 4 years following treatment. In the first 6 months following treatment, there was a 40% fall in the proportion of youth using alcohol (from 91% to 51%) and marijuana (from 84% to 35%), and a 58% reduction in stimulant use. Following the initial post-treatment drop in prevalence, both alcohol and marijuana prevalence increased at each follow-up, although the proportion of users remained below intake levels at the 4-year time point (25% lower for alcohol; 40% lower for marijuana). Although stimulant prevalence modestly increased at the 1-year follow-up, prevalence rates fell to 64% below intake rates at 4 years after treatment. At the 4-year time point, prevalence rates of the clinical sample were

10% higher than the NHSDA sample for alcohol (66% vs. 56.9%), three times higher for marijuana (44.4% vs. 15.8%), and substantially higher for stimulants (19.5 vs. 0.8%).

Based on these 4-year prevalence rates and relapse categories determined at each time point (abstainer, minor relapser, major relapser), youth could be categorized into five longitudinal trajectory groups (Brown *et al.*, 2001). *Continuous heavy users* (48%), consisting of the major relapsers category at all follow-ups, used alcohol and/or drugs between 18 and 25 times per month. Another group of youth (27%) initially improved with treatment but failed to maintain this in late adolescence. This *worse with time* group were abstainers or minor relapsers categories at the 6-month and 1-year assessments and major relapsers category at the 2 and 4 year assessments. Their average use range was 2–25 episodes per month. *Slow improvers* (10%) were youth classified as major relapsers at 6 or 12 months, and either minor relapsers or abstainers at all subsequent time periods (1–8 alcohol or marijuana use episodes per month). *Non-problem drinkers* (8%) were either abstainers or minor relapsers at all time points and averaged 1–7 use episodes per month. *Abstainers* (7%) consisted of those classified as abstainers at all follow-up time points.

A number of other studies have similarly tracked substance use outcomes in youth following treatment. Chung and colleagues (2003) followed 144 adolescents for 3 years after treatment for alcohol abuse in abstinence-promoting outpatient, inpatient, and residential treatment programs. Three years after treatment, they were classified as *chronic problem drinkers* (37%), *stable non-problem drinkers* (21%), *worse* (in the abstainer or non-problem drinker categories at the 1-year follow-up but lapsed into problem drinking after 3 years [15%]), *better* (had problem drinking until 1-year follow-up and then transitioned into abstinence or non-problem drinking [14%]), and *abstainer/non-problem drinkers* (12%).

In another longitudinal study, Chung *et al.* (2003) reported on 5-year outcomes of 179 adolescents diagnosed with substance dependence while receiving an evaluation at a 12-step treatment program (Chung *et al.*, 2003). Use rates at various time points were calculated using "lapse" (use of alcohol or drugs on one or two occasions in the follow-up period) and "relapse" (use of alcohol or drugs on three or more occasions in the follow-up period) criteria. Six months following treatment, lapse and relapse rates were 25% and 46%, respectively. Five years after treatment, lapse rates were 9%, while relapse rates were 85%. Therefore, 94% of the youth in this sample had used alcohol or drugs at least once in the 5 years following treatment. The study also looked at *clinical improvement*, defined as either no alcohol or drug use, or as alcohol and drug use with zero or one symptom of SUD. The *non-clinical improvement* group consisted of youth exhibiting two or more symptoms of SUD, regardless of use pattern. One year following treatment, 58% of the youth in this sample exhibited clinical improvement, while 36% improved after 5 years. Another group of adolescents who were assessed and given a recommendation for treatment but did not receive treatment at the time of initial assessment ("no treatment" group) had higher lapse and relapse rates after 5 years and showed lower rates of improvement. The history of substance abuse treatment experience and the absence of externalizing personality characteristics were found to be associated with improved outcomes into young adulthood.

Crowley and colleagues (1998) reported on the 2-year outcomes of 89 male adolescents diagnosed with SUD and conduct disorder, all completing community-based inpatient treatment. There were no differences in the use of drugs in the sample between intake and follow-up from self-report measures; however, the proportion of the sample testing positive for any drug use using a urine toxicology screen increased significantly from 19.4% at intake to 50.0% at 2 years following treatment.

Together, these findings suggest an overall reduction in problem use among adolescents following treatment for alcohol and drug abuse. However, substance involvement in these clinical samples remains substantially higher than national rates for this age range. While the vast majority of youth with SUD receiving treatment do use alcohol or drugs at least occasionally in the first few years following treatment, it is clear that distinct patterns exist such that some youth show extensive use throughout follow-up, some get worse over time, some improve significantly, while others remain abstinent or at low levels of use.

Many of the data available on the long-term relapse patterns of youth after treatment refer to standard community-based treatment programs. However, a number of recent studies have begun to explore youth outcomes up to 1 year after treatment through randomized, controlled clinical trials. Among the treatments found to show at least some improvement in alcohol or drug use outcomes in the long term are multisystemic therapy and family, group, or individual cognitive and behavioral therapies.

In a study with one of the longest follow-up periods to date, Henggeler et al. (2002) reported on 4-year outcomes of adolescents treated with either multisystemic therapy or usual community services. While self-reported rates of drug use did not differ significantly between the two groups, two biological indices indicated that those treated with the former had a significantly higher rate of abstinence from marijuana at the 4-year follow-up. Participants in multisystemic therapy also evidenced lower rates of aggressive behavior and convictions for aggressive behavior than those in the usual treatment condition.

A number of other studies have reported on youth outcomes up to 1 year following treatment through a clinical trial. For example, Azrin and colleagues (2001) demonstrated that 6 months of either family behavior therapy or individual cognitive problem-solving therapy resulted in similar and significant decreases in substance use 6 months following treatment in a sample of 56 youth with SUD and conduct disorder. Almost half of the youth in each treatment condition (45% for family behavior therapy and 44% for individual cognitive problem-solving therapy) were abstinent at the 6-month follow-up. Another study comparing cognitive–behavioral coping skills with psychoeducation therapies in a sample of 88 adolescents showed no difference in treatment outcomes between the two groups at a 9-month follow-up (Kaminer, Burleson, & Goldberger, 2002). A clinical trial comparing Cognitive–Behavioral Therapy (CBT), Functional Family Therapy (FFT), a combination of both, and a group intervention considered outcomes for adolescents up to 7 months after treatment (Waldron *et al.*, 2001). Youth in the joint and group conditions had significantly fewer days of marijuana use from intake to 7 months, while there was no change for the youth in the CBT or FFT groups. There was also a clinically significant change from heavy marijuana use to minimal use (abstinence or near abstinence) in the FFT, FFT plus CBT, and group intervention sets at the 7-month follow-up.

In another large clinical trial, the Cannabis Youth Treatment Randomized Field Experiment (Dennis *et al.*, 2002), youth aged 12–18 years who meet criteria for cannabis abuse or dependence were randomized to one of three outpatient treatment conditions incorporating Motivational Enhancement Therapy (MET), CBT, Family Support Network (FSN) treatment, Multidimensional Family Therapy (MDFT), and the Adolescent Community Reinforcement Approach (ACRA). Preliminary results show that in the incremental arm of the study, 5 weeks of CBT/MET and 12 weeks of CBT/MET with FSN resulted in fewer past-month substance problems than 12 weeks of MET/CBT after treatment, but that these differences were not significant 1 year after treatment. In the other arm of the study, 5 weeks of MET/CBT resulted in fewer problems associated with past-month substance use immediately after treatment than ACRA or MDFT, although this difference was also non-significant after 1 year.

Brief Strategic Family Therapy (BSFT) is another treatment and has been linked to improvement in substance use outcomes in Hispanic youth (Szapocznik & Williams, 2000). This therapy is geared toward identifying and understanding maladaptive family interactions and their relationship with adolescent behavior problems (including substance use/abuse). While long-term follow-up data of BSFT clinical trials have yet to be gathered, short-term outcomes suggest BSFT is effective in reducing marijuana use compared with a control condition (D. A. Santisteban *et al.*, 2003).

The body of outcome literature has demonstrated promising therapies for adolescent substance abuse. However, long-term outcome studies of adolescents treated together in hospitals or clinical trials have still shown marked variability in substance use patterns after treatment. Consequently, it is important to establish personal, environmental, and therapy-specific factors that account for these different patterns in order to identify the youth who are at high risk for early adverse outcomes and those more likely to return to substance use in a delayed fashion.

The process of relapse for adolescents

The dominant model of addiction relapse since the early 1980s has been the Cognitive–behavioral model (Fig. 4.3 Marlatt & Gordon, 1980). Although modifications have been suggested (e.g., incorporating craving, cue reactivity), the basic premise is that individuals self-select or unexpectedly find themselves in situations with elevated risk for relapse. When the abusers adequately cope with these situations without using addictive substances, they experience more confidence in their ability to abstain (increased self-efficacy) and are more likely to do so in the future when facing similar situations. By contrast, if the individual fails to employ an effective coping strategy, and there are strong expectations of substance use expectations, the likelihood of substance use in these situations is high. If drinking or drug use is initiated, negative cognitive states (e.g., guilt, self-blame) ensue such that self-efficacy is decreased and likelihood of future or sustained substance involvement is elevated.

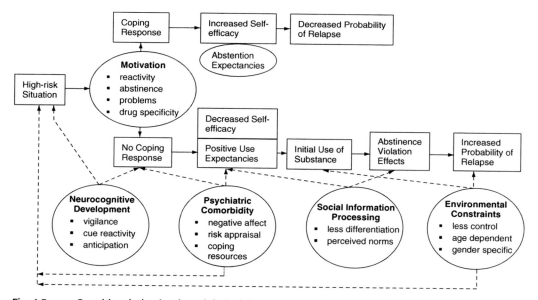

Fig. 4.3   Cognitive–behavioral model of adolescent addiction relapse with suggested revisions. (From Brown [2004] and Marlatt and Gordon [1985], Marlatt, with permission.)

Studies of adolescent relapse into substance abuse suggest that, while components of the model are relevant to adolescent relapse (e.g., coping predicts post-treatment substance use), there are significant differences in both content and process of youth relapse compared with adults. As highlighted in Fig. 4.3, important developmental specificity is needed to enhance the model's applicability to youth (Brown, 2004; Brown & D'Amico, 2001; Deas et al., 2000). For example, dominant contextual features of high-risk situations are substantially different for teenagers than for adults. Immediate risks for teenagers are social situations paired with strong positive affect compared with those associated with negative emotional states in adults (Brown, Stetson, & Beatty, 1989b). Further, substantial portions of substance-dependent youth either do not anticipate the risk situations (reduced vigilance) or are unprepared for their reactivity to the substance cues in such situations (Myers & Brown, 1990a). These differences may, in part, reflect neuroanatomical development. Specifically, frontal and prefrontal regions of the brain are the last to myelinate but are most critical for such cognitive activities as planning and anticipating sequences.

Perhaps one of the most important modifications of this model for youth is the key role of motivation. Youth entering treatment programs commonly have little motivation to abstain even though they may be motivated to resolve substance-related problems (Brown, 1999). Youth also exhibit marked differences in the factors determining initial use of a substance (relapse) in that motivation for abstinence varies across substances (Brown et al., 2000a). Motivation will dictate the extent to which they make effortful coping responses in risk situations. Youth are further constrained by their mobility in their environment and control over exposure to substances. Finally, developmental differences in social information processing may result in perceptions of greater use than is the norm and less differentiation of options to manage the emotional consequences of initial use (Brown et al., 1989b).

Follow-up studies have provided rich information about the processes of addiction relapse in youth. For example, the majority of episodes of adult alcoholic relapse are precipitated by situations of anger or frustration, social pressure to drink, or interpersonal conflict (Litman et al., 1977; Marlatt & Gordon, 1985). In contrast, adolescents appear to relapse most often in unsupervised social settings in which there is direct social pressure to drink, while negative affect or interpersonal conflict is seldom reported (Brown et al., 1989b). Myers and Brown (1990b) found that situations in which adolescents felt social pressure to drink or use were reported by over 90% of adolescent substance abusers interviewed following treatment. Exposure to substances in the environment, particularly through peer networks, is associated with reduced length of initial abstinence and measures of severity of post-treatment use (Vik, Grissel, & Brown, 1992).

Because risk situations differ, adolescents may also require different coping skills than adults to sustain abstinence. Myers and Brown (1990a) found that better outcome for adolescents in the 6 months following treatment was associated with more problem-focused and social-support strategies and less wishful thinking in response to a relapse risk situation. The same study found that teenagers abstinent for 6 months following treatment generated more types of behavioral coping and a larger total number of coping strategies than those who relapsed. Whereas cognitive coping strategies have been associated with successful outcomes for adult alcoholics (Ito & Donovan, 1990), this was not the case with adolescents. Rather, differences have been found between those who have a major relapse after treatment versus those who have a minor relapse, in that major relapsers more often report little or no forethought prior to the initial use episode following treatment, while minor relapsers report heightened awareness prior to a relapse episode (Brown *et al.*, 1989b). This cognitive vigilance observed among minor relapsers is consistent with the findings of Myers and Brown (1990a) that minor relapsers are more likely than major relapsers to identify a potential relapse scenario as an important and difficult situation, possibly leading to the avoidance of such situations. Unlike adults, behavioral rather than cognitive strategies are associated with better outcomes for adolescents with SUD. For example, Myers and colleagues (1993) found that less wishful thinking and use of more social supports predicted fewer days of alcohol and drug use 6 months following treatment.

Not only are there considerable differences in relapse situations and coping responses between adolescents and adults, but there are also differences in the substances used during relapse. Gateway substances appear to play a substantial role in relapse for youth. Brown *et al.* (2000a) examined 157 youth who had received inpatient treatment for alcohol or drug abuse. Although only 1% reported alcohol as their substance of choice upon admission to treatment, alcohol was involved in 46% of initial use episodes following treatment. Marijuana was involved in initial use episodes at rates comparable to pretreatment preference (47%), while stimulants (27%) and other drugs (5%) were less frequently consumed in initial relapse situations of youth. The use of alcohol and marijuana in the majority of adolescent post-treatment initial use episodes was associated with a more gradual return to use of other substances by youth in the first year after treatment. In contrast, use of one's drug of choice resulted in a more rapid return to abusive substance involvement. In summary, relapse for youth treated for SUDs is mediated by motivation and occurs under quite different contexts (situations, coping mechanisms, substances used) than relapse for adults, which has wide implications for treatment programs that include a relapse prevention component.

Factors that predict success for adolescents following drug and alcohol treatment

Self-help group attendance

Just as the determinants of relapse differ for adolescents and adults, there are also important distinctions in success strategies. For example, developmental factors (e.g., motivation, source of social support) lead to differences in the ways adolescents respond to traditional 12-step-based support groups compared with adults. Alcoholics Anonymous (AA) is by far the most prominent of these, with over 90% of adolescent alcohol and drug treatment programs currently including these 12-step groups as a facet of treatment (Kelly, Myers, & Brown, 2002). Evidence is mounting that AA programs lead to higher levels of commitment to abstinence and improved outcomes for adults (Morgenstern *et al.*, 1997) and for youth (Brown, 1993), both during and after treatment.

Brown (1993), in a study of adolescents who received inpatient treatment for alcohol abuse or dependence, found that 57% reported that they attended 12-step meetings regularly in the year following treatment. Of these, 69% had positive alcohol outcomes during the first year after treatment. In contrast, only 31% of those who did not attend meetings regularly (i.e., 0–10 sessions during the year after treatment) had a positive outcome. Hohman and LeCroy (1996) examined characteristics of adolescents who affiliated with AA following treatment versus those that did not. They found AA affiliation to be associated with prior alcohol or drug treatment, having friends who did not use drugs, less parental involvement in treatment, and more feelings of hopelessness. AA attendance has also been associated with enhanced motivation for abstinence in the first 3 months following treatment, which predicts better subsequent success (abstinence or lower use) by teens. For adolescents, attendance at a 12-step group appears to influence outcomes by enhancing factors critical for self-regulation, such as motivation for abstinence and use of abstinence-focused coping strategies, rather than immediately improving self-efficacy or coping skills for risk situations (Kelly, Myers, & Brown, 2000).

Personal/environmental characteristics

Certain personal and environmental factors contribute to success for adolescents following treatment for a SUD. Of significance, treatment length has been shown to lead to better outcomes in adolescents, independent of problem severity (Hser *et al.*, 2001). In the domain of family factors, greater expressiveness in the family (communication) the adolescent's perception of family support, and less exposure to substance-abusing family member models are associated with more positive outcomes following treatment (Brown *et al.*, 1990). Similarly, identification with abstaining peers and a greater proportion of non-users in the social resource network are associated with less substance use after treatment (Richter, Brown, & Mott, 1991; Vik *et al.*, 1992). Personal characteristics such as higher self-esteem and fewer conduct disorder-type behaviors have also been linked to more positive outcomes (Brown *et al.*, 1996; Richter *et al.*, 1991). Friedman, Terras, and Ali (1998) found that predictors of successful outcome from inpatient treatment for adolescents with SUD were younger age, greater years of education, not dropping out of high school, not being expelled from school, not being Catholic, and not being court referred to treatment. In the outpatient sample, better outcomes were associated with being female, not having been expelled from school, a high level of job for the head of household, and being self-referred.

It is expected that treatment-provoked reductions in substance use would be associated with improvement in other areas of adolescent functioning. Brown *et al.* (1994) examined the correlates of youth success 2 years following treatment for substance abuse and found marked differences in psychosocial functioning as a function of substance use patterns following treatment (*abstainers, non-problem users, slow improvers, worse with time*, and *abusers*). Abstainers were found to have better functioning in the areas of interpersonal problems, family relations, emotional well-being, social activities, and school performance. Greater post-treatment substance involvement was related to poorer school performance, with abstainers and non-problem drinkers consistently evidencing better school performance. Slow improvers changed their school performance over time to resemble the abstainers and non-problem users 2 years following treatment, while the worse with time group showed diminished school performance over time.

It is evident that a large number of individual factors contribute to success following treatment for SUD in adolescents, including attendance at self-help group meetings as well as personal and environmental characteristics, most notably school involvement and a social network that promotes abstinence. An important matter for further investigation involves how youth succeed who are not involved with treatment-recommended abstinence-focused support groups such as AA.

Alternative pathways to success

A number of strategies have been identified for maintenance of lifestyle change after substance abuse treatment that do not include sustained treatment involvement (e.g., after-care, 12-step groups, religious groups). Brown *et al.* (1990) reported on adolescents who did not attend self-help groups on a regular basis following treatment, using discriminant function analyses. Two improved groups (i.e., abstainers and minor relapsers) were found to differ from youth with poorer outcomes both in client characteristics (personal and environmental resources) and in their approach to success following treatment (behavioral efforts). In particular, some adolescents were able to establish abstinent lifestyles following alcohol and drug treatment despite little involvement with self-help groups; these tended to be younger (mean age 15.0 years), came from families with no drug use other than modest alcohol consumption, and had less exposure to drug use in their environment, especially among their closest friends. They were also more likely to persist in school and other structured activities. These teens reported higher levels of anxiety in the first 6 months following treatment, as families experienced significantly more conflict and pressure existed for them to establish new groups of friends and extracurricular activities. Symptoms of distress appear to abate after 1 year, however, when adolescents once again became actively involved in school and other activities. These successful youth used the strength of their families rather than formal treatment procedures to help them to master their lifestyle changes. They often reported distress immediately after treatment, mainly surrounding the adolescent's past drug involvement; however, at 2 years after treatment, these families report lower levels of conflict and higher levels of cohesion and expressiveness (Stewart & Brown, 1993). Consequently, one alternative road to success following treatment for adolescents with little family history of drug abuse and minimal drug exposure in their environment is through family support and involvement. While this approach may initially be more stressful, the long-term outcomes are positive if the adolescent has the personal and familial resources available to persist in reduced use for 1 year.

A second group of teenagers who exhibited marked improvement in post-treatment functioning despite minimal involvement with traditional self-help groups tended to be older and have higher levels of parental alcohol and drug problems. These adolescents perceived their families as less helpful in their attempts to make post-treatment lifestyle changes and so did not generally rely on family support. Instead they appeared to become more independent, involved in school or recreational activities and work. These experiences afforded them less exposure to risks at home and the opportunities to participate in self-esteem-enhancing activities outside of the family. Such individuals were more likely to persist in school and be connected with an adult at or outside of school. Consequently, these youth had better grades 1 year after treatment and reported that they had a teacher that they really liked. They did not show the same elevation in anxiety as the other group, perhaps because they tended not to change their friends. Typically, though, there was only limited substance use among their peer group. This subgroup of teenagers, in general, may evidence intermittent substance use, typically limited to alcohol, but do not exhibit any ongoing alcohol- or drug-related problems. Consequently for a portion of teenagers in treatment for alcohol and drug abuse, reduced family involvement and purposeful engagement in developmentally appropriate and self-esteem-enhancing activities outside the home appear to play a protective role in sustaining behavioral changes after treatment.

A major conclusion from the research examining the patterns exhibited after treatment by youth with SUD is that there are widely varying strategies employed in order to sustain major lifestyle changes critical for abstinence. Evidence is mounting that 12-step programs are effective for a portion of youth. Involvement of fellow teenagers appears to help to sustain 12-step attendance. These programs benefit youth by sustaining motivation to abstain. However, almost half of adolescents choose not to sustain 12-step involvement and not all these teens fail. In fact, there is evidence that they can use resources such as strong family ties, environmental and activity changes, and social relationships with non-using teens to help to sustain their success after treatment.

Special challenges youth face in controlling drug and alcohol use after treatment

Comorbidity

Consonant with adults with SUDs, comorbid psychiatric disorders are prevalent among adolescents who present to treatment with alcohol- or drug-related disorders. In studies examining the prevalence of SUDs in mental health treatment settings, estimates range from 19% to 83% (Aarons *et al.*, 2001; Deas-Nesmith, Campbell, & Brady, 1998), depending on the sector of care.

Evidence is mounting that adolescents with comorbid substance use and psychiatric diagnoses have poorer outcomes after treatment than substance-abusing youth without concomitant mental health disorders. Compared with non-comorbid teens, comorbid teens entering community-based substance abuse treatment have been found to be more likely to start using alcohol or marijuana at an earlier age, be dependent on marijuana, alcohol, or cocaine before treatment, and have had previous treatment (Grella *et al.*, 2001). In the DATOS-A study, comorbid youth were also more likely to have a parent with a SUD, reported higher rates of family problems and physical or sexual abuse, and evidenced more substance abuse after treatment. In particular, substance-abusing youth with a psychiatric diagnosis were found to be more likely to use marijuana regularly, use hallucinogens, engage in illegal acts, or be arrested following treatment (Grella *et al.*, 2001).

Tomlinson, Brown, and Abrantes (2004) compared a cohort of substance-abusing adolescents with comorbid axis I psychiatric disorders with adolescents with SUD but no concomitant psychopathology. The former were treated in inpatient psychiatric hospitals with a substance abuse program, while the latter were recruited from abstinence-based inpatient substance abuse treatment. They found that during the first 6 months following treatment, youth with and without comorbid psychiatric disorders substantially decreased the number of substance use episodes they had per month (79% and 73% reductions, respectively). The latter, however, were more likely to return to alcohol or drug use in the 6 months following treatment (87% vs. 74%), and to do so more rapidly after treatment discharge than adolescents without a comorbid disorder (61.44 vs. 82.78 days). Furthermore, there were differences in outcomes across mental health disorders. Consistent with other studies of substance-abusing adolescents with a diagnosis of conduct disorder or oppositional defiant disorder (e.g., Myers, Brown, & Mott, 1995; Myers, Stewart, & Brown, 1998), adolescents with SUD and an externalizing disorder returned to substance use more rapidly after treatment than youth with both an internalizing and externalizing disorder. Youth with only internalizing disorders evidenced fewer substance-dependence symptoms as defined by DSM-III-R (American Psychiatric Association, 1987) and used substances fewer days per month in the 6 months following treatment than those with both internalizing and externalizing disorders.

Comorbidity seems to pose a unique threat to the well-being of adolescents after substance abuse or psychiatric treatment. Not only are comorbid youth more likely to relapse and have substance-related problems after treatment, but they are at higher risk for problems such as suicide, violence, or pregnancy. Since comorbid youth have a harder time engaging in treatment for substance abuse (Riggs *et al.*, 1995), a strong argument can be made for substance abuse treatment programs (regardless of size or treatment modality) to move toward the assessment of psychiatric disorders and integration of mental health treatment and substance abuse treatment for adolescents (Riggs & Davies, 2002).

Neurocognitive factors

Another unique challenge for youth with SUDs is the connection between neuro-cognitive dysfunction and heavy substance involvement at an early age (Tapert & Brown, 1999). Neurocognitive deficits, in particular attention and executive functioning, are risk factors for the development of substance use disorders. Adolescents with attention-deficit hyperactivity disorder evidence higher rates and earlier onset of SUDs than those without this disorder (Milberger *et al.*, 1997). Also, deficits on a neurocognitive attention task predicted substance use frequency at an 8-year follow-up of a community sample of adolescents above and beyond effects accounted for by preexisting substance use levels, gender, education, conduct disorder symptoms, family history, and school placement for learning disabilities (Tapert *et al.*, 2002a).

Cognitive deficits are also known to result from alcohol and drug use in adolescents. Alcohol-abusing adolescents have displayed significantly poorer language skills than controls, and alcohol-abusing girls have performed worse on a test of perseveration and problem solving (Moss *et al.*, 1994). Brown *et al.* (2000b) looked at the effects of protracted alcohol use on adolescents following 3 weeks of alcohol detoxification. Alcohol-dependent adolescents performed more poorly than non-abusing adolescents matched for age, gender, and family history using the Wechsler Intelligence Scale for Children, revised (WISC-R) verbal comprehension subtests, and evidenced poorer retention rates of verbal and non-verbal information. Recent alcohol-withdrawal symptoms among adolescents were associated with poorer visuospatial functioning, whereas lifetime alcohol withdrawal was associated with poorer retrieval of verbal and non-verbal information. In female adolescents with SUD, severity of substance involvement has been associated with impairment of verbal functioning, school achievement, attention, and perceptual efficiency (Tarter *et al.*, 1995). This pattern supports the association between substance use and impulsivity found in epidemiological and etiological research on SUDs in adolescents. Studies of young adult abusers of inhalants provide the strongest evidence for cognitive deficits related to substance use: verbal abilities appear intact, but attention, memory, and fine motor and visuospatial skills are impaired relative to demographically matched controls (Allison & Jerrom, 1984; Berry, Heaton, & Kirby, 1978; Bigler, 1979). Poorer performance on cognitive tests could reflect either temporary states or serious underlying damage or delay in development. For example, youth with a history of alcohol abuse have been shown to have a smaller hippocampus than age- and gender-matched non-abusing peers (DeBellis *et al.*, 2000).

Using longitudinal analyses with a cohort of youth examined in middle adolescence, Tapert and Brown (1999) examined causal relations between adolescent substance abuse and neuropsychological functioning. The relationship between neuropsychological functioning and alcohol and drug use patterns over 4 years was evaluated in adolescents with a history of treatment for SUDs. Youth with continued heavy substance involvement showed increasing deficits in attentional functioning compared with those with improved substance use outcomes. Since adolescents did not differ on these measures at intake, attentional differences indicate that adolescents with more protracted alcohol or other drug use during the 4 years after treatment had modest but significant neurocognitive deficits by late adolescence or young adulthood. A subset of this sample was also evaluated 8 years after treatment (Tapert *et al.*, 2002b). Substance use, particularly if followed by withdrawal symptoms, predicted poorer visuospatial, attention, and verbal learning and memory performance. In contrast, language functioning appeared more robust and less adversely impacted by substance use or withdrawal history during this period.

Cognitive deficits appear to influence the onset of SUDs among youth and also result from use at a young age (Brown & Tapert, 2004). This line of research highlights the importance of prioritizing treatments with youth that address cognitive dysfunction, such as cognitive rehabilitation (Fals-Stewart & Shafer, 1992).

Developmental transitions

Many challenges for youth following substance abuse treatment reflect normal developmental transitions and environmental influences associated with the progression from adolescence to young adulthood. Factors associated with major fluctuations in alcohol and drug involvement after treatment may reflect both pretreatment risks for alcohol and drug use (e.g., exposure to substance-abusing peers, low motivation for abstinence) and post-treatment environmental factors that have been shown to influence the progression of substance involvement over time. For example, changes associated with increased independence and autonomy, such as getting a driver's license or moving out of the family home, may accelerate risk for alcohol and drug involvement (Brown, 1999). This is particularly threatening for teenagers in that motor vehicle accidents are the leading cause of death for this age group in the USA, where there were over 5000 alcohol-related deaths in the 15–19 age group during 2000 (NHTSA, 2000).

Kypri *et al.* (2004) evaluated changes in alcohol and drug use as adolescents initially moved from living with their families of origin to more independent environments. Two samples, one of 102 adolescents who had been previously treated for alcohol and drug problems and one of 70 non-abusing youths with comparable socioeconomic backgrounds and family history of alcohol and drug dependence, were assessed prior to and following the transition to their first independent living environment. There was a 35% increase in the number of monthly drinking episodes across this transition to independent living, and a 46% increase in the number of drinks per week. Drug involvement appeared less affected by this important personal and environmental transition; however, a larger proportion of teenagers with a history of substance abuse problems reported use of drugs (48% vs. 31%) following transition to independent living. Both level of exposure to substances in the new environment and peer substance use were significant predictors of post-treatment substance involvement. These findings have highlighted how changes in risk and protective factors associated with developmental transitions of late adolescence and young adulthood influence alcohol and drug involvement of young people.

Conclusions

This chapter has outlined the findings from a growing body of research evaluating adolescents during and after treatment for alcohol and drug abuse, and as they mature into young adulthood. It is clear from these longitudinal studies that the course of substance involvement for youth is both diverse and developmentally unique. There appear to be fundamental differences in the clinical course for adolescents and adults, which, in part, reflect developmental stage transitions.

The extant research on adolescent treatment and outcome shows that much needs to be done to increase the effectiveness of treatment for youth, and that youth succeed in a variety of ways following treatment depending on both personal and environmental resources. Studies on the relapse process have shown that the potential relapse situations adolescents encounter, resources at their disposal, and factors that influence their successful coping vary from those of adults. Furthermore, clinical samples of youth with SUDs exhibit high rates of psychiatric comorbidity that adversely impact their outcomes following treatment. Neurocognitive functioning both preceding substance involvement and conse-quential to early exposure to alcohol and other drugs also appears to influence the process and maintenance of behavioral change for youth following treatment. Developmental challenges unfolding across adolescence and into adulthood pro-voke periods of accelerated risk for substance involvement and exacerbate the difficulty of remaining abstinent even when motivation exists.

These distinctions between adolescents and adults in clinical presentation for treatment and course following treatment suggest several arenas of potential improvement in our efforts to treat alcohol and drug problems. For example, there is a clear need for innovative programs targeted to the developmental level, concerns, language, and lifestyle of substance-abusing youth (D'Amico & Fromme, 2000; Fromme & Brown, 2000; Henggeler, Menton, & Smith, 1992). Monti *et al.* (1999) have identified a unique niche for successfully applying a motivational interviewing intervention with older adolescents (ages 17–19 years) who were treated in an emergency room after an alcohol-related problem. At a 6-month follow-up, adolescents who received this intervention reported fewer injuries involving alcohol and were less likely to drive after drinking compared with adolescents who received standard emergency room care. Similar innovative approaches that focus on earlier intervention and target motivating concerns of youth (e.g., Brown, 2001) and that cater to the needs of more severely affected populations are needed to reach youth who may not prefer or seek traditional treatments.

While great strides have been made in the field of adolescent substance abuse treatment, many critical research and clinical questions remain unanswered. For example, more work is needed to understand the specific intervention needs and process of change for youth, as suggested in our revised Cognitive–behavioral model of addiction relapse. This model of youth relapse, based on empirical findings in treatment outcome research, has proven to be an innovative way to understand the known differences between relapses in adolescents and adults. Our laboratory at the University of California, San Diego has begun to test this model in a newly recruited cohort of youth with SUD and receiving treatment in a variety of inpatient and outpatient settings. Specific inquiries will be related to understanding the role of moderating and mediating factors in the adolescent relapse process and making specific treatment recommendations based on these findings.

Extended follow-up studies have proven to be a wealth of information on the impact of protracted substance involvement on youth development. Most of the long-term follow-up data to date have been taken from studies of youth in standard community-based treatment settings. Future studies that track youth for extended periods after treatment through randomized controlled clinical trials will allow for direct comparisons between these treatment modalities and standard or current treatments. As models of clinical course unfold, future outcome studies should incorporate hypothesized moderating and mediating variables from the revised cognitive–behavioral model of youth substance relapse to examine fit across various treatment modalities. This will allow for progress in our understanding of which treatments work best for youth with a variety of personal and environmental characteristics.

REFERENCES

Aarons, G. A., Brown, S. A., Hough, R. I., Garland, A. F., & Wood, P. A. (2001). Prevalence of adolescent substance use disorders across five sectors of care. *Journal of the American Academy of Child and Adolescent Psychiatry*, **40**, 419–426.

Allison, W. M. & Jerrom, D. W. (1984). Glue sniffing: a pilot study of the cognitive effects of long-term use. *International Journal of the Addictions*, **19**, 453–458.

American Psychiatric Association (1987). *Diagnostic and Statistical Manual III-Revised*. Washington, DC: American Psychiatric Press.

Azrin, N. H., Donohoe, B., Teicher, G. A., *et al.* (2001). A controlled evaluation and description of individual-cognitive problem solving and family-behavior therapies in dually diagnosed conduct-disordered and substance-dependent youth. *Journal of Child and Adolescent Substance Abuse*, **11**, 1–43.

Bennett, W. F. & Grella, C. E. (2001). The Drug Abuse Treatment Outcome Studies for Adolescents. *Journal of Adolescent Research*, **16** (Special issue 6), 537–702.

Berry, G. J., Heaton, R., & Kirby, M. (1978). Neuropsychological assessment of chronic inhalant abusers: a preliminary report. In C. W. Sharp & L. T. Caroll (eds.), *Voluntary Inhalation of Industrial Solvents* (pp. 111–136). Rockville, MD: National Institute on Drug Abuse.

Bigler, E. D. (1979). Neuropsychological evaluation of adolescent patients hospitalized with chronic inhalant abuse. *Clinical Neuropsychology*, **1**, 8–12.

Brown, S. A. (1993). Recovery patterns in adolescent substance abuse. In J. S. Baer, G. A. Marlatt, & R. J. McMahon (eds.), *Addictive Behaviors across the Lifespan: Prevention, Treatment and Policy Issues* (pp. 161–183). Beverly Hills, CA: Sage.

(1999). Treatment of adolescent alcohol problems: research review and appraisal. In Extramural Scientific Advisory Board (ed.), *Treatment* (pp. 1–26). Bethesda, MD: National Institute on Alcohol Abuse and Alcoholism.

(2001). Facilitating change for adolescent alcohol problems: a multiple option approach. In E. F. Wagner & H. B. Waldron (eds.), *Innovations in Adolescent Substance Abuse Interventions* (pp. 169–187). Oxford: Elsevier.

(2004). Measuring youth outcomes from alcohol and drug treatment. *Addictions*, **99**, 38–46.

Brown, S. A. & D'Amico, E. J. (2001). Outcomes for alcohol treatment for adolescents. In M. Galanter (ed.), *Recent Developments in Alcoholism*, Vol. XV: *Services Research in the Era of Managed Care* (pp. 307–327). New York: Plenum Press.

Brown, S. A. & Tapert, S. F. (2004). Health consequences and costs of adolescent alcohol use. In *Reducing Underage Drinking: A Collective Responsibility* (pp. 383–401). Washington, DC: National Academy Press.

Brown, S. A., Vik, P. W., & Creamer, V. A. (1989a). Characteristics of relapse following adolescent substance abuse treatment. *Addictive Behaviors*, **14**, 291–300.

Brown, S. A., Stetson, B. A., & Beatty, P. (1989b). Cognitive and behavioral features of adolescent coping in high risk drinking situations. *Addictive Behaviors*, **14**, 43–52.

Brown, S. A., Mott, M. A., & Myers, M. G. (1990). Adolescent alcohol and drug treatment outcome. In R. R. Watson (ed.), *Drug and Alcohol Abuse Prevention* (pp. 373–403). Clifton, NJ: Human Press.

Brown, S. A., Myers, M. G., Mott, M. A., and Vik, P. W. (1994). Correlates of success following treatment for adolescent substance abuse. *Applied and Preventive Psychology*, **3**, 61–73.

Brown, S. A., Gleghorn, A., Schuckit, M. A., Myers, M. G., & Mott, M. A. (1996). Conduct disorder among adolescent alcohol and drug abusers. *Journal of Studies on Alcohol*, **57**, 314–324.

Brown, S. A., Tapert, S. F., Tate, S. R., & Abrantes, A. M. (2000a). The role of alcohol in adolescent relapse and outcome. *Journal of Psychoactive Drugs*, **32**, 107–115.

Brown, S. A., Tapert, S. F., Granholm, E., & Delis, D. C. (2000b). Neurocognitive functioning of adolescents: effects of protracted alcohol use. *Alcoholism: Clinical and Experimental Research*, **24**, 164–171.

Brown, S. A., D'Amico, E. J., McCarthy, D. M., & Tapert, S. F. (2001). Four year outcomes from adolescent alcohol and drug treatment. *Journal of Studies on Alcohol*, **62**, 381–388.

Chung, T., Martin, C. S., Grella, C. E., *et al.* (2003). Course of alcohol problems in treated adolescents. *Alcoholism: Clinical and Experimental Research*, **27**, 253–261.

Cornelius, J. R., Maisto, S. A., Pollock, N. K., *et al.* (2001). Rapid relapse generally follows treatment for substance use disorders among adolescents. *Addictive Behaviors*, **27**, 1–6.

Crowley, T. J., Mikulich, S. K., MacDonald, M., Young, S. E., & Zerbe, G. O. (1998). Substance-dependent, conduct-disordered adolescent males: severity of diagnosis predicts 2-year outcome. *Drug and Alcohol Dependence*, **49**, 225–237.

D'Amico, E. J. & Fromme, K. (2000). Implementation of the risk skills training program: a brief intervention targeting adolescent participation in risk behaviors. *Cognitive and Behavioral Practice*, **7**, 101–117.

Deas-Nesmith, D., Campbell, S., & Brady, K. T. (1998). Substance use disorders in adolescent inpatient psychiatric population. *Journal of the National Medical Association*, **90**, 233–238.

Deas, D., Riggs, P., Langenbucher, J., Goldman, M., & Brown, S. (2000). Adolescents are not adults: developmental considerations in alcohol users. *Alcoholism: Clinical and Experimental Research*, **24**, 232–237.

DeBellis, M. D., Clark, D. B., Beers, S. R., *et al.* (2000). Hippocampal volume in adolescent-onset alcohol use disorders. *American Journal of Psychiatry*, **157**, 737–744.

Dennis, M. L., Godley, S. H., Diamond, G. S., *et al.* (2002). Main findings of the Cannabis Youth Treatment (CYT) randomized field experiment. In *the American Psychiatric Association Annual Conference: A Symposium on State-of-the-Art Adolescent Substance Abuse Prevention and Treatment*, Philadelphia, PA.

Fals-Stewart, W. & Shafer, J. (1992). Using neuropsychological assessment with adolescent substance abusers: a review of findings and treatment implications. *Comprehensive Mental Health Care*, **2**, 179–199.

Friedman, A. S., Terras, A., & Ali, A. (1998). Differences in characteristics of adolescent drug abuse clients that predict to improvement: for inpatient treatment versus outpatient treatment. *Journal of Child and Adolescent Substance Abuse*, **7**, 97–119.

Fromme, K. & Brown, S. A. (2000). Empirically based prevention and treatment approaches for adolescents and young adult substance use. *Cognitive and Behavioral Practice*, **7**, 61–64.

Grella, C. E., Hser, Y., Joshi, V., & Rounds-Bryant, J. (2001). Drug treatment outcomes for adolescents with comorbid mental and substance use disorders. *Journal of Nervous and Mental Disease*, **189**, 384–392.

Grunbaum, J. A., Kann, L., Kinchen, S. A., *et al.* (2002). Youth Risk Behavior Surveillance – United States 2001. *Morbidity and Mortality Weekly Report*, **51**, 1–64.

Henggeler, S. W., Menton, G. B., & Smith, L. A. (1992). Family preservation using multi-systemic therapy: an effective alternative to incarcerating serious juvenile offenders. *Journal of Consulting and Clinical Psychology*, **60**, 953–961.

Henggeler, S. W., Clingempeel, W. G., Brondino, M. J., & Pickrel, S. G. (2002). Four-year follow-up of multisystemic therapy with substance-abusing and substance-dependent juvenile offenders. *Journal of the American Academy of Child and Adolescent Psychiatry*, **41**, 868–874.

Hohman, M. & LeCroy, C. W. (1996). Predictors of adolescent AA affiliation. *Adolescence*, **31**, 339–352.

Hser, Y.-I., Grella, C. E., Hubbard, R. L., *et al.* (2001). An evaluation of drug treatment for adolescents in four USA cities. *Archives of General Psychiatry*, **58**, 689–695.

Hubbard, R. L., Cavanaugh, E. R., Graddock, S. G., & Rachel, J. V. (1983). *Characteristics, Behaviors, and Outcomes for Youth in TOPS Study*. [Report submitted to the National Institute on Drug Abuse, Contract No. 271-79-3611.] Research Triangle Park, NC: Research Triangle Institute.

Hunt, W. A., Barnett, L. W., & Branch, L. G. (1971). Relapse rates in addiction programs. *Journal of Clinical Psychology*, **27**, 455–456.

Ito, J. R. & Donovan, D. M. (1990). Predicting drinking outcome: demography, chronicity, coping and after-care. *Addictive Behaviors*, **15**, 553–559.

Johnston, L. D., O'Malley, P. M., & Bachman, J. G. (2002). *The Monitoring the Future National Results on Adolescent Drug Use: Overview of Key Findings, 2001*. [NIH Publication No. 02-5105] Bethesda, MD: National Institutes of Health.

Kaminer, Y., Burleson, J. A., & Goldberger, R. (2002). Cognitive–behavioral coping skills and psychoeducation therapies for adolescent substance abuse. *Journal of Nervous and Mental Disease*, **190**, 737–745.

Kelly, J. F., Myers, M. G., & Brown, S. A. (2000). A multivariate process model of adolescent 12-step attendance and substance use outcome following inpatient treatment. *Psychology of Addictive Behaviors*, **14**, 376–389.

(2002). Do adolescents affiliate with 12-step groups? A multivariate process model of effects. *Journal of Studies on Alcohol*, **63**, 293–304.

Kypri, K., McCarthy, D. M., Coe, M. T., & Brown, S. A. (2004). Transition to independent living and substance involvement of treated and high risk youth. *Journal of Child and Adolescent Substance Abuse*, **13**, 85–100.

Litman, G. K., Eiser, J. R., Rawson, N. S. B., & Oppenheim, A. N. (1977). Towards a typology of relapse: a preliminary report. *Drug and Alcohol Dependence*, **2**, 157–162.

Marlatt, G. A. & Gordon, J. R. (1980). Determinants of relapse: implications for the maintenance of behavior change. In P. Davidson & S. M. Davidson (eds.), *Behavioral Medicine: Changing Health Lifestyles* (pp. 410–452). Elmsford, NY: Pergamon.

(1985). *Relapse Prevention: Maintenance Strategies in the Treatment of Addictive Behaviors.* New York: Guilford Press.

Milberger, S., Biederman, J., Faraone, S. V., Wilens, T., & Chu, M. P. (1997). Associations between ADHD and psychoactive substance use disorders: findings from a longitudinal study of high-risk siblings of ADHD children. *American Journal on the Addictions*, **6**, 318–329.

Monti, P. M., Colby, S. M., Barnett, N. P., *et al.* (1999). Brief intervention for harm reduction with alcohol-positive older adolescents in a hospital emergency department. *Journal of Consulting and Clinical Psychology*, **67**, 989–994.

Morgenstern, J., Labouvie, E., McCrady, B. S., Kahler, C. W., & Frey, R. M. (1997). Affiliation with Alcoholics Anonymous after treatment: a study of its therapeutic effects and mechanisms of action. *Journal of Consulting and Clinical Psychology*, **65**, 768–777.

Moss, H. B., Kirisci, L., Gordon, H. W., & Tarter, R. E. (1994). A neuropsychologic profile of adolescent alcoholics. *Alcoholism: Clinical and Experimental Research*, **18**, 159–163.

Myers, M. G. & Brown, S. A. (1990a). Coping and appraisal in relapse risk situations among adolescent substance abusers following treatment. *Journal of Adolescent Chemical Dependency*, **1**, 95–115.

(1990b). Coping responses and relapse among adolescent substance abusers. *Journal of Substance Abuse*, **2**, 177–189.

Myers, M. G., Brown, S. A., & Mott, M. A. (1993). Coping as a predictor of adolescent substance abuse treatment outcome. *Journal of Substance Abuse*, **5**, 15–29.

(1995). Pre adolescent conduct disorder behaviors predict relapse and progression of addiction for adolescent alcohol and drug abusers. *Alcoholism: Clinical and Experimental Research*, **19**, 1528–1536.

Myers, M. G., Stewart, D. G., & Brown, S. A. (1998). Progression from conduct disorder to antisocial personality disorder following treatment for adolescent substance abuse. *American Journal of Psychiatry*, **155**, 479–485.

NHTSA (National Highway Traffic Safety Administration) (2000). *Traffic Safety Facts 2000: Alcohol.* [DOT HS 809 323] Washington, DC: US Department of Transport, National Center for Statistics and Analysis, Research and Development.

Project Match Research Group (1997). Matching alcoholism to client heterogeneity: Project MATCH post-treatment drinking outcomes. *Journal of Studies on Alcohol,* **58**, 7–30.

Richter, S. S., Brown, S. A., & Mott, M. A. (1991). The impact of social support and self esteem on adolescent substance abuse treatment outcome. *Journal of Substance Abuse,* **3**, 371–386.

Riggs, P. D. & Davies, R. D. (2002). A clinical approach to integrating treatment for adolescent depression and substance abuse. *Journal of the American Academy of Child and Adolescent Psychiatry,* **41**, 1253–1255.

Riggs, P. D., Baker, S., Mikulich, S. K., Young, S. E., & Crowley, T. A. (1995). Depression in substance-dependent delinquents. *Journal of the American Academy of Child and Adolescent Psychiatry,* **34**, 764–771.

Rush, T. V. (1979). Predicting treatment outcomes for juvenile and young adult clients in the Pennsylvania substance-abuse system. In G. M. Beschner & A. S. Friedman (eds.), *Youth Drug Abuse: Problems, Issues and Treatment.* Lexington, MA: Lexington Books.

SAMHSA (Substance Abuse and Mental Health Services Administration) (2000). *National Household Survey of Drug Abuse: Main Findings 1998.* [DHHS Publication No. (SMA) 00–3381.] Rockville, MD: Department of Health and Human Services, Substance Abuse and Mental Health Services, Administration Office of Applied Studies.

Santisteban, D. A., Coatsworth, J. D., & Perez-Vidal, A. (2003). Efficacy of brief strategic family therapy in modifying hispanic adolescent behavior problems and substance use. *Journal of Family Psychology,* **17**, 121–133.

Sells, S. B. & Simpson, D. D. (1979). Evaluation of treatment outcome for youths in the Drug Abuse Reporting Program (DARP): a followup study. In G. M. Beschner & A. S. Friedman (eds.), *Youth Drug Abuse: Problems, Issues and Treatment.* Lexington, MA: Lexington Books.

Staton, M., Leukefeld, C., Logan, T. K., *et al.* (1999). Risky sex behavior and substance use among young adults. *Health and Social Work,* **24**, 147–154.

Stewart, M. A. & Brown, S. A. (1993). Family functioning following adolescent substance abuse treatment. *Journal of Substance Abuse,* **5**, 327–339.

Szapocznik, J. & Williams, R. A. (2000). Brief strategic family therapy: twenty five years of interplay among theory, research and practice in adolescent behavior problems and drug abuse. *Clinical Child and Family Psychology Review,* **3**, 117–135.

Tapert, S. F. & Brown, S. A. (1999). Neuropsychological correlates of adolescent substance abuse: four-year outcomes. *Journal of the International Neuropsychological Society,* **5**, 481–493.

Tapert, S. F., Granholm, E., Leedy, N. G., & Brown, S. A. (2002a). Substance use withdrawal: neuropsychological functioning over 8 years in youth. *Journal of the International Neuropsychological Society,* **8**, 873–883.

Tapert, S. F., Baratta, M. V., Abrantes, A. M., & Brown, S. A. (2002b). Attention dysfunction predicts substance involvement in community youths. *Journal of the American Academy of Child and Adolescent Psychiatry,* **41**, 680–686.

Tarter, R. E., Mezzich, A. C., Hsieh, Y.-C., & Parks, S. M. (1995). Cognitive capacity in female adolescent substance abusers. *Drug and Alcohol Dependence*, **39**, 15–21.

Temple, M. & Ladouceur, P. (1986). The alcohol–crime relationship as an age-specific phenomenon: a longitudinal study. *Contemporary Drug Problems*, **13**, 89–115.

Tomlinson, K. L., Brown, S. A., & Abrantes, A. M. (2004). Psychiatric comorbidity and substance use treatment outcomes of adolescents. *Psychology of Addictive Behaviors*, **18**, 160–169.

Vik, P. W., Grissel, K., & Brown, S. A. (1992). Social resource characteristics and adolescent substance abuser relapse. *Journal of Adolescent Chemical Dependency*, **2**, 59–74.

Waldron, H. B., Slesnick, N., Brody, J. L., Turner, C. W., & Peterson, T. R. (2001). Treatment outcomes for adolescent substance abuse at 4- and 7-month assessments. *Journal of Consulting and Clinical Psychology*, **69**, 802–813.

Walsh, J. M. (1985). Polydrug and alcohol use. *Alcohol, Drugs, & Driving*, **1**, (1–2), 115–119.

5

Cannabis Youth Treatment intervention: preliminary findings and implications

Janet C. Titus and Michael L. Dennis

Chestnut Health Systems, Bloomington, IL, USA

Cannabis (including marijuana, hashish, and other forms of tetrahydrocannabinol) is the most prevalent psychoactive substance used by adolescents in the USA (Coffey *et al.*, 2002; Dennis *et al.*, 2002a; Hall & Babor, 2000; Institute of Medicine [IOM], 1999; Kraus & Bauernfeind, 1998; SAMHSA, 2000a; Swift, Copeland, & Hall, 1998). In 2002, it was estimated that nearly one half of all adolescents in 12th grade in the USA had used cannabis; nearly 40% of those in 10th grade and close to 20% of those in 8th grade reported the same (Johnston, O'Malley, & Bachman, 2003). Although they have leveled off, the rates of adolescent cannabis use continue to be approximately twice as high as they were in the early 1990s (Johnston *et al.*, 2003; SAMHSA, 2002). In addition, the number of adolescents starting use before the age of 15 grew throughout the 1990s, continuing a trend that has been unfolding since the 1980s, and its use and dependence are comorbid with a wide variety of psychological and behavioral conditions (reviewed at length in Dennis *et al.*, (2002b)). Cannabis is the leading substance mentioned in arrests and emergency room admissions of adolescents in the USA, and the second leading substance mentioned in autopsies (Bureau of Justice Statistics, 2000; SAMHSA, 2000b,c,d). From 1992 to 1998, the number of adolescents presenting for treatment for cannabis use rose by 53%; currently over two thirds of the adolescents in publicly funded treatment are being seen for cannabis-related problems, with 80% being seen in outpatient settings (Dennis *et al.*, 2003).

Evaluations of existing outpatient treatment practices for adolescent cannabis users in the USA have produced mixed results. While some studies have reported increases in cannabis use ranging from 3 to 13% following outpatient treatment (Hubbard *et al.*, 1985; Sells & Simpson, 1979; SAMHSA, 1995), others have reported decreases of 12–25% (Hser *et al.*, 2001). A recent study of 445 adolescents who attended outpatient treatment found a 21–25% reduction in cannabis use between the years before and after treatment (Grella *et al.*, 2001; Hser *et al.*, 2001).

These multisite evaluations typically used a standard of 3 or more months of treatment to determine an "adequate" dosage of treatment. However, less than 20% of the adolescents studied remained in treatment this long, the median length of staying being 1.5 months.

In 1997, there were no manual-guided therapies that were explicitly designed for short-term (less than 3 months) outpatient treatment of adolescent cannabis users that had been field tested and that could be readily used to support this expansion of the treatment system. In response to this gap CSAT created the Cannabis Youth Treatment (CYT) cooperative agreement (Clark *et al.*, 2002; Dennis *et al.*, 2002b). The goals of CYT were to (a) learn more about the characteristics and needs of adolescents presenting to short-term outpatient treatment, (b) produce developmentally appropriate treatment manuals for promising approaches to short-term outpatient treatment that could be readily disseminated to the field, and (c) field test their clinical effectiveness, cost, cost-effectiveness, and benefit cost. The aims of this chapter are to introduce the CYT interventions and study, to summarize some of the preliminary findings, and to discuss their implications for the field.

Treatments and their rationale

After a national competition, review of preliminary evidence and expert recommendations, and review by an external advisory board, the CYT steering committee identified five brief treatment conditions (completed within 7 to 14 weeks) that varied in theoretical orientation, delivery format (individual, group, family), service components, and duration. A team (including a clinical expert, researcher, and day-to-day clinical supervisor) was assigned to create manuals and to oversee each intervention. Each manual was revised after the study to incorporate examples of actual dialogue and practice, and these were submitted to an independent field review to identify any areas in need of further explanation or any issues related to disseminability and replicability. The final manuals included the background, specific procedures, all forms and worksheets, and an appendix on the supervision of the protocols. More detailed comparisons of the treatments are given in Diamond *et al.* (2002) and the manuals themselves have been put in the public domain (www.chestnut.org/li/bookstore or www.health.org). Below is a brief overview of each of the five CYT therapies.

Motivational enhancement treatment/Cognitive–Behavior Therapy 5 sessions

The first therapy (Sampl & Kadden, 2001) involved Motivational Enhancement Treatment (MET) sessions delivered individually and three sessions of Cognitive–Behavioral Therapy (CBT) in groups, with the total duration of treatment lasting 6–7 weeks. The therapy was known as MET/CBT5 and was designed to be an inexpensive first-tier intervention that would deliver its impact within the 6-week median length of stay that occurs in much of the USA treatment system. It was also believed that a shorter intervention would actually be more desirable to many adolescents, parents, and insurers for a first time intervention. The MET component proceeds from the assumptions that adolescents need both to resolve their ambivalence about whether they have a problem with cannabis and other substances and to increase their motivation for changing it. It seeks to help adolescents to see the relationship between their use and other problems they care about in order to conclude that the costs of cannabis use outweigh its benefits. The CBT sessions were added out of concern that problem recognition and motivation alone would not be sufficient for adolescents who had yet to develop the necessary coping skills to initiate and sustain change (see Baer, Kivlahan, & Donovan [1999] or Dunn, Deroo, & Rivara [2001] for a general discussion of the need to supplement MET). Earlier research had demonstrated efficacy of CBT strategies for adult substance abuse in general (Annis, 1990; Carroll, 1997; Rawson *et al.*, 1993, 1994) and cannabis problems in particular (Stephens, Roffman, & Simpson, 1993). CBT (particularly relapse prevention), in addition, has a history of being well received by community practitioners (Morgenstern & McCrady, 1992). The CBT component of this particular intervention teaches basic skills for (a) refusing offers of cannabis, (b) establishing a social network supportive of recovery and developing a plan for pleasant activities to replace cannabis-related activities, and (c) coping with unanticipated high-risk situations, problem solving, and recovering from relapse, should one occur. Although there had been no direct tests of MET/CBT5 with adolescents prior to CYT, several studies with adult cannabis users had demonstrated that one to two sessions of MET were more effective in reducing substance use than a no-treatment control group (Copeland *et al.*, 2001; Stephens, Roffman, & Curtis, 2000; the Marijuana Treatment Project [MTP], unpublished data), and that MET plus CBT was better than a control group or MET alone (Copeland *et al.*, 2001; MTP, unpublished data). While the CYT research group did consider a "CBT only" model, earlier adolescent studies suggested that it provided little or no advantage over minimal interventions or education only (Kaminer & Burleson, 1999; Kaminer, Burleson, & Goldberger, 2002). Consequently, it was considered that a combined version of MET and CBT (like the one that had been successful with adults) would have the best prospects of working with adolescents.

Motivational enhancement treatment/cognitive–behavior therapy 12 sessions

Supplementing the initial MET/CBT5 program with an additional seven CBT group sessions (Webb *et al.*, 2002) for a total therapy duration of 12 to 14 weeks produced the MET/CBT12 program. This intervention was designed to approximate more closely the kind of interventions that are in use in many existing treatment programs. These additional CBT sessions teach adolescents to use coping in place of cannabis as an alternative response to interpersonal problems, negative affect, and psychological dependence. The specific groups are on problem solving, anger awareness, anger management, communication skills, resistance to craving, depression management, and management of thoughts about cannabis. In addition to being closer to practice, this dosage of MET/CBT was closer to the combined dosage used in the earlier adult studies that had proven to be more effective than a control group or MET alone (Copeland *et al.*, 2001; MTP, unpublished data). A key assumption behind the use of a group format is that adolescent skill deficits are typically interpersonal in nature and need to be practiced in order to work. Groups offer a realistic yet "safe" setting (if well managed) in which to practice these skills. It should be noted that potential concerns about the risk of interclient problems were raised in this (as well as other conditions), and the clinical supervisors developed guidelines for avoiding and handling them. These guidelines are documented in the appendix to all CYT manuals (Angelovich *et al.*, 2001).

Family Support Network

The family support network (FSN; Bunch *et al.*, 1998) used MET/CBT12 to provide basic treatment for substance abuse but then wrapped additional services around it, including six parent education group meetings (to improve parent knowledge and skills relevant to adolescent problems and family functioning), four therapeutic home visits, referral to self-help support groups, and case management (to promote adolescent/parent engagement in the treatment process). The FSN was designed to approximate more closely the kind of "comprehensive treatment" recommended by experts in CSAT's (1992a, 1992b, 1993) Treatment Improvement Protocols for adolescents. The parent education groups addressed (a) adolescent development and parents' role, (b) substance abuse/dependence, (c) recovery process and relapse signs, (d) family development and functioning (boundaries, limits, etc.), (e) family organization and communication, and (f) family systems and roles. The home visits focused on (a) initial assessment and motivation building, (b) family roles and routines, (c) assessing progress and building commitment to change, and (d) continuing to assess progress and build commitment. Case management focused on facilitating treatment attendance (reminders, transportation, childcare), assessment of family needs, and referrals to other community services. Developed by a committee of leading researchers and clinicians, the original CSAT Treatment Improvement Protocols suggested several components of comprehensive care for adolescents but did not actually provide specific curriculum, procedures, or forms for implementation. They were based on early evidence that treatment outcomes were improved when parent education was provided for at-risk adolescents, family support interventions were added to treatment, and families were actively engaged in treatment (Barrett, Simpson, & Lehman, 1988; Brown *et al.*, 1994; Henggeler *et al.*, 1991, 2002; Liddle *et al.*, 2001). The key assumption is that problem recognition, motivation, and even individual coping skills may not be enough because adolescents are often dependent on their families in terms of managing their recovery environment, dealing with other systems (e.g., school, welfare, and juvenile justice), and even logistically getting to treatment. Making families effective assets to the recovery process required education, specific family management skills, social support, and direct assistance with case management.

The adolescent community reinforcement approach (ACRA)

The adolescent community reinforcement approach (ACRA) (Godley *et al.*, 2001a) is composed of 10 individual sessions with the adolescent, four sessions with caregivers (two of which are with the whole family), and a limited amount of case management provided over a period of 12 to 14 weeks. The therapy is procedure based (in contrast to the three session or curriculum-based manuals above) and designed to represent a more behavioral approach to treatment incorporating elements of operant condition, skills training, and a social systems approach. The three core procedures used in most ACRA sessions are (a) a functional analysis to identify the antecedents and consequences of substance use; (b) identifying and reviewing clear, simple, and obtainable "goals of counseling"; and (c) teaching self-monitoring through the use of a happiness scale to track progress. Some of the other procedures involve identifying and reinforcing pro-social behaviors that compete with substance use and the use of skills training related to relapse prevention and problem solving. The caregiver sessions focus on the above and key parenting practices, including increasing positive communication, modeling good behaviors, involvement in the adolescent's life outside of the home, and monitoring the adolescent's whereabouts. Community reinforcement approaches have been demonstrated to be effective with adult substance users (Azrin *et al.*, 1982; Hunt & Azrin, 1973; Meyers & Godley, 2001; Meyers & Smith, 1997; Meyers *et al.*, 1999), have been recommended as one of the most promising approaches to treatment by several expert panels from the IOM (1980, 1989, 1990, 1998), and have been successfully combined with other approaches including disulfiram (Azrin *et al.*, 1982), contingency contracting (Azrin *et al.*, 1994; Budney & Higgins, 1998), and family therapy (Hennegler *et al.*, 2002; Randall *et al.*, 2001; Sisson & Azrin, 1993). Though this approach had not been formally used with adolescents prior to CYT, it was one of the underlying approaches used in a behavioral therapy study (without a guidance manual) with adolescents that produced significant improvements relative to a control group (which actually deteriorated significantly)(Azrin *et al.*, 1994). In adapting the community reinforcement approach for adolescents, the ACRA team also drew on other work related to effective parenting practices (Ary *et al.*, 1999; Bry *et al.*, 1998; Melidonis & Bry, 1995). Two key assumptions of ACRA are that parts of the adolescent's social environment are probably supporting continued substance use and that it is more effective to reinforce competing prorecovery behaviors (e.g., going to a dry dance or other substance-free structured or prosocial activities) than to try to punish risk behaviors or environmental situations. The therapist needs to help the adolescent to (a) recognize that his/her drug use is incompatible with other short- or long-term reinforcers (e.g., parental approval, staying out of criminal justice system, having a girlfriend or boyfriend); (b) maximize family/peer/community resources and activities to reward non-drug using behavior and to increase alternative positive, non-drug-related social/recreational activities; and (c) develop social skills (e.g., problem solving, drug refusal, etc.) that will increase the likelihood of success in these endeavors.

Multidimensional family therapy

Multidimensional Family Therapy (MDFT; Liddle, 2002) is composed of 12 to 15 sessions (typically six with the adolescent, three with parents, and six with the whole family) and case management provided over a period of 12 to 14 weeks. Therapy proceeds in three phases: (a) setting the stage (engage adolescent, engage parents, build alliances with all members of system, identify goals of treatment), (b) working the themes for adolescents (trust/mistrust, abandonment and rejection, disillusionment and past hurts, motivation and self-agency, hope or lack of hope for future, credibility) and families (preparing for parent–adolescent communications, managing conversation in session, shifting from high conflict to affective issues, developing positive experiences/interactions with each other, tying conversation and themes to drug use), and (c) sealing the changes (preparing for termination, reviewing treatment work, preparing for future challenges ["What will you do when …"]). The MDFT approach is based on research linking reductions in adolescents' drug and behavior problem with changes in parenting practices (Schmidt, Liddle, & Dakof, 1996), therapist–adolescent alliance (Diamond & Liddle, 1996), and the use of culturally specific themes to engage African-American males (Jackson-Gilfort *et al.*, 2001) and females (Dakof, 2000). Unlike FSN (that layered family therapy on to substance abuse treatment), MDFT integrates substance abuse treatment into family therapy. A key assumption of MDFT is that adolescents are involved in multiple systems (e.g., family, peers, school, welfare, and legal), producing multiple risk and protective factors that can be best addressed in a family-based, developmental–ecological, multiple systems approach to treating adolescent substance abuse. The MDFT approach had generated promising pilot data prior to CYT and (concurrent to CYT) has been demonstrated to be as or more effective than multi-family education, adolescent group therapy, or CBT alone (Dakof, Tejeda, & Liddle, 2001; Liddle *et al.*, 2001). It has also been identified as an effective drug abuse treatment approach by NIDA's Behavioral Therapies Development Program (NIDA, 1993).

Overview of field trials

The five CYT therapies were field tested in two randomized trials conducted in four USA sites: University of Connecticut Health Center in Farmington, CT; Operation PAR in St. Petersburg, FL; Chestnut Health Systems in Madison County, IL; and the Children's Hospital of Philadelphia in Philadelphia, PA. The study was broken into two trials because it was not feasible to implement more than three therapies in a single site. In the first trial (conducted at Farmington and St. Petersburg), adolescents were randomly assigned to MET/CBT5, MET/CBT12, or FSN. In the second trial (conducted in Madison County and Philadelphia), adolescents were randomly assigned to MET/CBT5, ACRA, or MDFT. Randomization was carried out within sites so that data could be analyzed within or across the pair of sites. Across both trials, adolescents were eligible for CYT if they were between the ages of 12 and 18 years, reported one or more DSM-IV criteria for cannabis abuse or dependence, had used cannabis in the past 90 days (or 90 days prior to being in a controlled environment), and were appropriate for outpatient or intensive outpatient treatment (American Society of Addiction Medicine [ASAM], 1996). Participants were considered too severely affected and ineligible if they (a) reported use of alcohol 45 or more of the 90 days prior to intake, (b) reported use of other drugs 13 or more of the 90 days prior to intake, (c) reported an acute medical or psychological problem that was likely to prohibit full participation in treatment, (d) had insufficient mental capacity to understand the consent procedure or participate in treatment, (e) lived outside of the program's catchment area, or (f) had a history of repeated, violent behavior or severe conduct disorder that might put other participants at risk. Of the 1244 adolescents screened, 54% were eligible (with over 20% being too severely affected for outpatient treatment and 26% needing only early intervention). Of the 702 who were eligible, 600 (85%) agreed to participate. Interviews at intake and at follow-up at 3, 6, 9, and 12 months were conducted by independent research staff who were trained and certified in the assessment administration. Of the 600 adolescents randomized, one or more follow-up interviews were conducted with 99% of them (with 94% or more at each wave). A more detailed discussion of the design is available elsewhere (Dennis *et al.*, 2002b).

The participant characteristics and primary outcomes were measured with the Global Appraisal of Individual Needs (Dennis, 1999; Dennis et al., 2002c), a comprehensive, structured interview that has eight main sections (background, substance use, physical health, risk behaviors, mental health, environment, legal, and vocational). The intake version requires approximately 90–120 minutes to complete, and the follow-up version usually requires 30–45 minutes. The majority of the 600 participating adolescents were male (83%), in school (87%), started using under the age of 15 (85%), were currently over the age of 15 (85%), white (61%), and/or were from single parent families (50%). Their patterns of weekly substance use were dominated by cannabis smoking (71%) and alcohol consumption (17%), with use of other drugs being only 1%. Lifetime injection drug use was less than 1%. Though 48% met criteria for dependence based on their own self-reports, only 26% had ever been in treatment. This is comparable to or, actually, slightly more severe than found when looking at the characteristics of adolescents with cannabis-related problems presenting to publicly funded outpatient treatment in the USA (Tims et al., 2002).

Highlights of findings

Co-occurring problems are the norm

Besides cannabis use disorders, 95% of the CYT adolescents reported one or more other major problems (83% had three or more), such as alcohol use disorders (37%), other substance use disorders (25%), internal disorders (14% major depression, 13% generalized anxiety, 9% suicidal thoughts or actions, 14% traumatic stress disorders), and external behavioral disorders (53% conduct disorder, 38% attention-deficit hyperactivity disorder, including 30% with both). Over 83% reported illegal activity other than just drug possession or use, and 66% reported engaging in acts of physical violence such as assault. Not surprisingly, 62% were involved in the criminal justice system at the time of intake, including 42% who were on probation, 21% awaiting a trial, 17% assigned to the Treatment Accountability for Safer Communities (TASC) program or another diversion program, and 7% awaiting sentencing. Many were sexually active (72%, including 39% with multiple sexual partners), employed (47%), coming from a controlled environment (25%), or recently home-less/run away (7%). Most faced one or more potential negative environmental influences on recovery, including regular peer use of drugs (89%) or alcohol (64%) and weekly use in the home of drugs (11%) or alcohol (23%); 57% had a history of victimization. The prevalence of these co-occurring problems or risk factors went up as the number of abuse/dependence symptoms went up (see Tims et al. [2002] or Diamond, Leckrone, & Dennis [2005] for more details on these co-occurring problems).

Problem recognition and low motivation are endemic

Though 96% of the adolescents reported sufficient symptoms to meet criteria for abuse or dependence, only 20% saw their substance use as a "problem." This is *not* "denial" since they do acknowledge symptoms of drug abuse and dependence when asked in behavioral terms. However, developmentally they do not always recognize the more abstract concept of "problems," which requires a recognition of how certain problematic behaviors are related to substance use, dependence, each other, as well as to a class of problems. Compounding matters further, treatment motivation at intake was moderately low, though higher levels of motivation predicted reduction in both use and use problems at the 3-month follow-up (S. H. Godley, R. R. Funk, & M. L. Dennis, 2001, unpublished data for Chestnut Health Systems). Interestingly, by the 30-month follow-up, adolescents' motivations to quit cannabis were gained only at a price, as the two most common reasons for quitting were "damage to body and mind" and "getting into trouble" (Titus *et al.*, 2002). These results are in line with those found by Battjes and colleagues (2003): motivation to change at intake was low, but experiencing various negative consequences of substance use were strong predictors for changing one's behavior.

Common subtypes are related to changes in substance use and problems

Analyses were conducted on six common subtypes: gender, age of onset, family history of substance use, externalizing disorders, internalizing disorders, and temperament. Subgroups were compared in terms of substance use frequency, substance abuse problems, social support for substance use, family conflict, school problems, and negative peer associations (Babor *et al.*, 2002). The construct validity of each of these subtypes and their general relationship to outcomes were verified after controlling for demographic factors, thereby indicating that each has valuable explanatory power from a theoretical perspective. Externalizing disorders, onset age, difficult temperament, and internalizing disorders continued to add unique variance to discrimination after the effects of the other subtypes had been removed. At 12-month follow-up, there were no differences between subtypes on substance use frequency, but adolescents with higher levels of externalizing disorders and internalizing disorders continued to experience more substance use problems. Babor and colleagues are currently doing work to see whether and how these subtypes interact with the specific CYT interventions.

Treatment participation was high

While 90 days of treatment has historically been used as a benchmark of sufficient treatment in national studies of treatment practice (Hser *et al.*, 2001; Hubbard *et al.*, 1985; SAMHSA, 1995, 1998; Sells & Simpson, 1979), less than 20% of adolescents in these studies met these criteria for sufficient treatment, and the median length of stay was 6–8 weeks. Of the adolescents assigned to one of the four 12- to 14-week treatment interventions, the mean length of stay (from intake to last formal therapy session) was 80 days, with 52% staying just over 90 days and 86% staying 6 or more weeks. For the MET/CBT5 condition, an intervention lasting 6–7 weeks, the mean length of stay was 43 days, with 62% staying in treatment for 6 or more weeks. If we focus on number of sessions, 71% of the adolescents completed three quarters or more of their prescribed sessions, 22% received partial dosages, and 5% never returned to treatment after randomization (see Dennis *et al.* (2004) for more details on the treatment received).

Treatments reduced use and problems

On average, the five CYT treatments had a significant positive impact on the adolescents and their families. From intake to 3–6 months, there were significant increases in the number of adolescents reporting no past month use and no past month substance-related problems. Significant increases were also observed for clean urine tests and no past-month symptoms of abuse or dependence. By 6 months after intake, the rate of any use decreased even more and the rate of early remission increased dramatically. Increases were observed in the number of adolescents not involved in criminal justice in the past month and the number of adolescents attending school and/or work. In addition, the impact of CYT on negative behaviors showed significant decreases in weekly attention/behavior problems, family problems, school problems, illegal activity, fighting and/or violence, and illegal activities for money.

Trial 1

While adolescents in all three intervention conditions in trial 1 (i.e., MET/CBT5, CBT7, and FSN) reduced their days of cannabis use, there were no significant differences in the rate of change by treatment. At 3 months, the number of past-month substance-related problems was reduced. The size of the reductions varied significantly by intervention, with the greatest change observed for FSN followed by MET/CBT5 and MET/CBT12. The range of these differences, however, narrowed and were no longer significant at 6 months. The individuals' severity of problems (i.e., level of drug use and/or number of problems) at intake was also a factor in outcomes associated with past month substance-related problems. At 3 months, MET/CBT5 produced greater reductions than the other two interventions in past month symptom counts for adolescents with problems of low severity, while FSN produced greater reductions for those with problems of high severity. The pattern of outcomes changed at 6 months. The latter group continued to reduce past month symptom counts in all three treatment groups. For those with less severe problems, adolescents assigned to FSN made further reductions, while the other two treatment groups maintained their previous reductions. Part of the further reductions by the FSN group was probably a consequence of significantly higher rates of being in a controlled environment (both inpatient treatment and detention). After a slight reduction from intake to 3 months, the average number of days in a controlled environment for FSN adolescents jumped dramatically compared with the other two treatments.

Trial 2

The number of days of cannabis use was reduced in all three of the interventions evaluated in trial 2 (i.e., MET/CBT5, ACRA, MDFT). The rate of reduction varied significantly by condition. The greatest reduction was observed for ACRA, followed by MET/CBT5 and MDFT. Days of substance use continued to decline from 3 to 6 months and the differences across treatments were no longer significant. While the number of substance-related problems was reduced in all three conditions, there were no significant differences by condition. There were no significant differences in the above outcomes by clinical severity. The participants with low severity, however, did increase their days in a controlled environment from 0 to 3 to 6 months, while the adolescents with severe clinical problems reduced them at 3 months and increased them by the 6-month follow-up (ending up higher than baseline). ACRA had the smallest reductions in number of days of being in a controlled environment at 3 months, but also had the smallest increases at 6 months.

Treatments are affordable

Since CYT was designed to produce "disseminable" models of effective short-term treatment, the "economic" costs and benefits of each intervention episode were evaluated (French *et al.*, 2002, 2003). In trial 1, the average cost per treatment episode was $1089 for MET/CBT5, $1256 for MET/CBT12, and $3920 for FSN. In trial 2, the average cost per treatment episode was $1445 for MET/CBT5, $1459 for ACRA, and $2105 for MDFT. Higher costs were partially a function of increased patient contact hours and actual staff time. However, site differences (e.g., cost of living, staffing patterns, minimization of excess capacity) explained as much or more than the variation by condition in the second trial, ranging from an average of $1167 per episode (across conditions) at Chestnut Health Systems to $2128 at the Children's Hospital of Philadelphia. This said, it should be noted that episode costs of all five CYT treatments were below the inflation-adjusted costs reported by program directors in the USA National Treatment Improvement Evaluation Study and prorated for the longer lengths of stay observed here ($356/week; $2136 for 6–7 weeks of MET/CBT5; $4272 for 12–14 weeks of other treatment conditions).

(See French *et al.* [2002] for a more detailed discussion of the costs and French *et al.* [2003] for the impact of the interventions on costs to society.)

Therapists overall reacted positively to treatment manuals

Many have questioned whether treatment manuals can address individual needs of patients, can be applied to patients with complex comorbidities, and whether manuals will restrict therapists' necessary creative application of psychotherapy (Addis, 1997; Silverman, 1996). To explore these issues from the therapist's perspective, 25 CYT providers were interviewed at the end of the treatment phase (Godley *et al.*, 2001b). Three quarters of the therapists felt that they were able to attend to the individual needs of each client. Modifications (e.g., using participants' stories as examples) were not viewed as deviations from the manual but rather as appropriate applications of the treatment approach. The MET/CBT and FSN psychoeducation therapists felt the most restricted by the manuals, but many of these therapists reported feeling easily able to adapt the material to the client's needs. In terms of restricting creativity, few therapists felt overly confined by the manuals. In fact, most welcomed the structure and organization. Many reported that the manuals provided guidance and focus. In the more structured treatments, therapists accepted the restrictions because they believed the information they were teaching was valuable. In terms of treating comorbidity, the outcome data suggest that the individuals with the most-complex and severe problems showed similar retention rates and magnitudes of change on key outcome variables to those with less-complex problems (although those with more-complex problems were often still worse off at post-treatment). Overall, exploration of the therapists' reactions to the manuals suggested that the 25 therapists predominately had positive experiences. Interestingly, many of the therapists pointed to the intensive supervision that accompanied the manuals as the greatest benefit, suggesting that manuals by themselves may not have as much impact on the practice community if not accompanied by training and supervision.

Implications and next steps

Although CYT has added to the knowledge base and application in the field of adolescent substance abuse treatment, many questions surfaced during the study, adding to the already rich collection of questions to explore and spawning additional research efforts for the answers. What have we learned from CYT and where do we go from here?

When the CYT study began in late 1997, the prevailing view was that short-term outpatient substance abuse treatment for adolescents generally did not work, but that some experimental family therapies had promise. This impression was not necessarily misguided given the history of equivocal and non-sustained reductions reported in major research efforts prior to CYT. What CYT demonstrates is that a wide range of short-term outpatient treatment approaches (both family and non-family) can help to reduce substance use, substance-related problems, and a variety of other problems. The reductions reported across interventions in the CYT field trials are larger than those reported in regional and national studies of treatment practice (e.g., Dennis *et al.*, 2003; Gerstein & Johnson, 1999; Hser *et al.*, 2001; Hubbard *et al.*, 1985; SAMHSA, 1995; Sells & Simpson, 1979) and are comparable to the reductions reported in more controlled "efficacy" studies of these and other interventions (Azrin *et al.*, 1994; Heneggler *et al.*, 1991, 2002; Kaminer *et al.*, 2002; Latimer *et al.*, 2003; Liddle *et al.*, 2001; Waldron *et al.*, 2001). Multiple efforts to replicate CYT outcomes are currently underway and may provide support for their validity and point to several active ingredients that are at least partially responsible for the study's observed effects. Here we will speculate on the implications of the findings for these and other future efforts, as well as the primary factors that we believe accounted for the CYT findings.

Why were retention rates so high?

Rates of treatment retention in CYT were higher than those reported in the literature for longer therapy conditions and were not significantly different by condition among those planned for 12 to 14 weeks. Success in this arena is most likely attributable to explicit efforts to encourage treatment retention. While the procedures varied somewhat by condition and site, each site tried to schedule regular meeting times, send out reminders by mail/phone, review transportation and childcare issues with the adolescent and caregivers, and call back those who missed an appointment to encourage them to return. The more intensive interventions devoted more time, energy, and case management resources to treatment retention. This is much more assertive than the path followed in many community treatment programs; however, the cost of this approach was included in the total treatment costs and hence it is, at least theoretically, feasible in practice.

Why were the clinical outcomes so similar?

Greater differences were expected in the relative effectiveness of the various therapies. Specifically, we had expected that longer and family-based therapies would do better. However, the observed differences were small and unrelated to dosage or family orientation. Why? It is possible this happened because over a third of the adolescents went on to get additional treatment in the 3 months following the end of CYT treatment. On average, adolescents received twice as many days of subsequent treatment in the 9 months after discharge as they did during the 3-month CYT treatment phase. Since obtaining subsequent treatment was *not* related to CYT condition, any influence from it was averaged over the conditions (causing more similar outcomes). Two other possibilities are that the CYT interventions were all developmentally appropriate and involved higher than average levels of clinical supervision (which had previously primarily been associated only with family and longer-term approaches). Comparing characteristics and outcomes of those who sought and did not seek subsequent treatment could generate a fuller understanding of this phenomenon. It is also possible that one or more of the treatments had progressively diminishing effects while other(s) had delayed benefits that came out as time went on. Relatively small between-treatment differences provoke further questions. Would experiments on matching subtypes of adolescents to differing treatments generate greater differences between treatment outcomes? CYT treatments were carried out in community-based treatment and research settings; perhaps differences between treatments would be more distinct in alternative settings such as in juvenile detention facilities or schools.

If treatments were effective, why was there a need for continuing care?

Despite the reductions in use and problems achieved by these short-term therapies, nearly a third of adolescents who completed a CYT treatment relapsed during the 3 months following treatment, and over two thirds relapsed one or more times over 12 months. Too many adolescents in CYT, as well as in other outpatient treatment programs, continue to have problems after treatment or move in and out of recovery and relapse. What is needed is a better understanding of the mediators of longer-term treatment outcomes and the development of after-care programs that impact these mediators more effectively. Two of the most promising mediators that the CYT team is investigating include the recovery environment (e.g., substance use in the home, homelessness, violence, victimization, self-help group participation, availability of structured activities) and peer group risks (e.g., the extent to which one's friends are involved in substance use, illegal activity, violence, treatment, recovery, and vocational activities). Across multiple databases, these two factors consistently come up as mediators between treatment and changes in substance use and problems (e.g., Godley *et al.*, 2005). The CYT team believes that better outcomes will be achieved if primary-treatment and continuing-care protocols are developed and refined to address these factors.

Would therapists in the community accept and/or use manual-guided therapies?

There is some debate already about the use of manual-guided therapies, and it is not clear if creating manuals for further treatment modalities would be successful, or whether therapists outside of research studies would even accept them. Despite early skepticism, CYT therapists overwhelmingly favored the treatment manuals because they provided structure to their therapeutic work, with a shift away from paperwork to more clinical practice. Most therapists did not feel rigidly bound by the structure and were able to address individual patient needs successfully (Godley *et al.*, 2001b). The manuals also did very well in field review, with therapists liking the clarity, experienced therapists liking the off-the-shelf nature of developmentally appropriate versions of family materials, and supervisors liking the ease with which they could be used to deal with staff turnover, training, and supervision. There are a number of questions still to be answered. What effect does manual-guided treatment have on the quality of treatment? Can all therapists be trained to successfully deliver a manual-guided therapy successfully, or do some therapists fare better with some therapies while others do not?

Would the level of therapist supervision utilized in the program be realistic or even necessary in a community setting?

Despite the recent emphasis on better supervision of therapists working in the field (see www.jcaho.org or www.carf.org), in practice there is often minimal supervision and much of it is focused on paperwork and personnel issues. Arguments against intensive supervision are that it is not affordable or practical given budget constraints and already heavy caseloads. An important finding from CYT is that good clinical supervision is affordable and is indeed important, and may very well be directly related to some of the most important factors behind the success of the CYT treatments (e.g., quality assurance of treatment delivery, therapeutic alliance). Intensive supervision is common practice in clinical trial research studies and may indeed be the most active ingredient in obtaining positive outcomes. Cost estimates for CYT interventions (French *et al.*, 2002) *included* expenses related to the provision of intensive supervision (e.g., training of supervisors, provision of intensive supervision) and were still lower, on average, than those of the average episode cost as reported in a survey of outpatient program directors. In addition, caseloads of CYT therapists compared with those of therapists in community settings were not significantly different, with the CYT therapists taking on similar caseloads, despite providing more treatment on an hour for hour basis. Most importantly, without intensive supervision in regular settings of substance abuse treatment, manuals may not produce expected results. Many of the CYT therapists pointed to the intensive supervision that accompanied the manuals as the greatest benefit, suggesting that manuals by themselves may not have as much impact on the practice community as manuals accompanied by training and supervision. Studies of the relationship between supervision, treatment fidelity, and ongoing monitoring of the therapists' delivery are needed to address more fully the role of supervision in the workplace. Consequently, we believe that provision of manuals and good clinical supervision creates a symbiosis that improves outcomes.

Why have reactions to the Cannabis Youth Treatment experiments been mixed?

The research field, in general, has applauded the methodological gains in measurement, retention, and follow-up completion achieved by CYT. However, many have had difficulty interpreting findings because there was no "untreated control" group or clear "winner." Those working in health services research and clinical treatment, however, have embraced the findings as a key study of treatment effectiveness that addressed a number of major gaps in the system. CYT addressed the need for manual-guided, affordable, and empirically validated treatments. Manuals and documented procedures have allowed for rapid dissemination of therapies into active treatment settings and have encouraged the establishment of treatment programs in community settings outside formal treatment settings (such as in juvenile justice and student assistance programs). Documented, standard treatments add to treatment efficiency, provide a standard for treatment quality assurance, and aid in staff training – a key advantage in a field with high turnover. The treatments themselves are more affordable than current practice, and their variability in content and structure allows for the tailoring of treatment offerings to a program's characteristics and resources. The CYT treatments' components are not new: cognitive–behavioral, family-based, environmentally based, and motivational treatments have been around for years. What is distinctive about CYT is that it unifies a variety of treatment approaches, providing structure and standard definitions of treatment centered on empirically supported therapies rather than the common "anything goes" found in many community-based clinics. Whether CYT treatments and outcomes will generalize to additional community settings remains to be seen, and current studies of several CYT treatments are examining their effectiveness in alternative settings such as juvenile detention and schools.

What is happening with the manuals?

CYT treatments, measurements, and procedures have been adopted and are currently used in over 100 adolescent treatment studies in the field (more than twice as many studies as the total number carried out before 1997, the year CYT started). The CYT manuals are being distributed by the National Clearinghouse on Alcohol and Drug Information (NCADI; www.health.org or see www.chestnut.org/li/bookstore for free downloadable electronic copies) and have required multiple printings of 50,000 copies within 4 years from publication. All of the CYT interventions have received national attention, and over 100 studies have already started replicating them (some in experiments). For example, CSAT is currently completing a replication of the MET/CBT5 intervention in 38 sites. Several state and regional systems are using the treatments to set minimum standards of care or to expand services, and some student assistance programs and juvenile justice programs have adopted MET/CBT5 for use as an early intervention. Collaboration between researchers and clinical providers and the focus on practical approaches that are quickly adaptable for use in the field likely contributed to the relatively fast absorption of the CYT treatments into the world of active treatments.

What are our plans for the future?

During the coming years, more information on the study's 12- and 30-month findings will be released, as well as more detailed examinations of specific subpopulations or issues. The CYT research group has produced and continues to produce dozens of articles, presentations, and other professional publications, conducting trainings and providing supervision in the treatments. Topics explored so far are wide ranging and, among many more, include questions on the characteristics of adolescent clients and their outcomes, treatment matching, comorbidities, and health status; costs, cost-effectiveness, and cost–benefits of the treatments; prediction and patterns of relapse and recovery; outcomes for adolescents by source of referral, including the criminal justice system; the relationship between motivations to use and outcomes; mediators of behavior change; topics in research methodology; and treatment transfer. Comparisons of the CYT results with those of other projects replicating these interventions and/or comparing them with other treatment approaches will further our understanding of their robustness and limitations. Clearly, CYT marked the beginning of a major renaissance in adolescent treatment research. However, the field is expanding rapidly and promises to go much further in the years to come.

REFERENCES

Addis, M. E. (1997). Evaluating the treatment manual as a means of disseminating empirically validated psychotherapies. *Clinical Psychology: Science and Practice*, **4**, 1–11.

American Society of Addiction Medicine (1996). *Patient Placement Criteria for the Treatment of Psychoactive Substance Disorders*, 2nd edn. Chevy Chase, MD: American Society of Addiction Medicine.

Angelovich, N., Karvinen, T., Panichelli-Mindel, S., *et al.* (2001). *The Clinical Management of a Multisite Field Trial of Five Outpatient Treatments for Adolescent Substance Abuse*. Rockville, MD: Center for Substance Abuse Treatment, Substance Abuse and Mental Health Services Administration.

Annis, H. M. (1990). Relapse to substance abuse: empirical findings within a cognitive learning approach. *Journal of Psychoactive Drugs*, **22**, 117–124.

Ary, D. V., Duncan, T. E., Duncan, S. C., & Hops, H. (1999). Adolescent problem behavior: the influence of parents and peers. *Behaviour Research and Therapy*, **37**, 217–230.

Azrin, N. H., Sisson, R. W., Meyers, R. J., & Godley, M. D. (1982). Outpatient alcoholism treatment by community reinforcement and disulfiram therapy. *Journal of Behavior Therapy and Experimental Psychiatry*, **13**, 105–112.

Azrin, N. H., McMahon, P., Donohue, B., *et al.* (1994). Behavior therapy for drug abuse: a controlled treatment-outcome study. *Behaviour Research and Therapy*, **32**, 857–866.

Babor, T. F., Webb, C., Burleson, J. A., & Kaminer, Y. (2002). Subtypes for classifying adolescents with marijuana use disorders: construct validity and clinical implications. *Addiction*, **97**(Suppl. 1), 58–69.

Baer, J. S., Kivlahan, D. R., & Donovan, D. M. (1999). Integrating skills training and motivational therapies: implications for the treatment of substance dependence. *Journal of Substance Abuse Treatment*, **17**, 15–23.

Barrett, M. E., Simpson, D. D., & Lehman, W. E. (1988). Behavioral changes of adolescents in drug abuse intervention programs. *Journal of Clinical Psychology*, **44**, 461–473.

Battjes, R. J., Gordon, M. S., O'Grady, K. E., Kinlock, T. W., & Carswell, M. A. (2003). Factors that predict adolescent motivation for substance abuse treatment. *Journal of Substance Abuse Treatment*, **24**, 221–232.

Brown, S. A., Myers, M. G., Mott, M. A., & Vik, P. W. (1994). Correlates of success following treatment for adolescent substance abuse. *Applied and Preventive Psychology*, **3**, 61–73.

Bry, B. H., Catalano, R. F., Kumpfer, K. L., Lochman, J. E., & Szapocznik, J. (1998). Scientific findings from family prevention intervention research. In R. Ashery, E. B. Robertson, & K. L. Kumpfer (eds.), *Drug Abuse Prevention through Family Interventions* (pp. 103–129). Rockville, MD: Center for Substance Abuse Treatment, Substance Abuse and Mental Health Services Administration.

Budney, A. J., & Higgins, S. T. (1998). *A Community Reinforcement plus Vouchers Approach: Treating Cocaine Addiction*. Rockville, MD: National Institute on Drug Abuse.

Bunch, L., Hamilton, N., Tims, F., Angelovich, N., & McDougall, B. (1998). *CYT: A Multisite Study of the Effectiveness of Treatment for Cannabis Dependent Youth, Family Support Network*. St. Petersburg, FL: Operation PAR, Inc.

Bureau of Justice Statistics (2000). *Sourcebook of Criminal Justice Statistics 1999*, 27th edn. Washington, DC: US Department of Justice.

Carroll, K. M. (1997). New methods of treatment efficacy research: bridging clinical research and clinical practice. *Alcohol Health and Research World*, **21**, 352–359.

Clark, H. W., Horton, A. M., Jr., Dennis, M. L., & Babor, T. F. (2002). Moving from research to practice just in time: the treatment of cannabis use disorders comes of age. *Addiction*, **97**(Suppl. 1), 1–3.

Coffey, C., Carlin, J. B., Degenhardt, L., *et al.* (2002). Cannabis dependence in young adults: an Australian population study. *Addiction*, **97**, 187–194.

Copeland, J., Swift, W., Roffman, R., & Stephens, R. (2001). A randomized controlled trial of brief Cognitive–behavioral interventions for cannabis use disorder. *Journal of Substance Abuse Treatment*, **21**, 55–64.

CSAT (Center For Substance Abuse Treatment) (1992a). *Empowering Families, Helping Adolescents: Family-Centered Treatment of Adolescents with Alcohol, Drug Abuse, and*

Mental Health Problems. [*Technical Assistance Publication Series*, No. 6.] Rockville, MD: Center for Substance Abuse Treatment.

(1992b). *Guidelines for the Treatment of Alcohol- and Other Drug-abusing Adolescents.* [*Treatment Improvement Protocol Series*, No. 4.] Rockville, MD: Center for Substance Abuse Treatment.

(1993). *Screening and Assessment of Alcohol and Other Drug-abusing Adolescents.* [*Treatment Improvement Protocol Series*, No. 3.] Rockville, MD: Center for Substance Abuse Treatment.

Dakof, G. A. (2000). Understanding gender differences in adolescent drug abuse: issues of comorbidity and family functioning. *Journal of Psychoactive Drugs*, **32**, 25–32.

Dakof, G. A., Tejeda, M., & Liddle, H. A. (2001). Predictors of drop-out in family based treatment for adolescent drug abuse. *American Journal of Child and Adolescent Psychiatry*, **40**, 274–281.

Dennis, M. L. (1999). *Global Appraisal of Individual Needs (GAIN): Administration Guide for the GAIN and Related Measures, version 1299.* Bloomington, IL: Chestnut Health Systems.

Dennis, M. L., Babor, T., Roebuck, C., & Donaldson, J. (2002a). Changing the focus: the case for recognizing and treating marijuana use disorders. *Addiction*, **97**(Suppl. 1), 4–15.

Dennis, M. L., Titus, J. C., Diamond, G., *et al.* For the CYT Steering Committee (2002b). The Cannabis Youth Treatment (CYT) experiment: rationale, study design and analysis plan. *Addiction*, **97**(Suppl. 4), 16–34.

Dennis, M. L., Titus, J. C., White, M. K., Unsicker, J. L., & Hodgkins, D. (2002c). *Global Appraisal of Individual Needs: Administration Guide for the GAIN and Related Measures*, version 5. Bloomington, IL: Chestnut Health Systems. Available at: http://www.chestnut.org/li/gain/gadm1299.pdf.

Dennis, M. L., Dawud-Noursi, S., Muck, R. D., & McDermeit, M. (2003). The need for developing and evaluating adolescent treatment models. In S. J. Stevens & A. R. Morral (eds.), *Adolescent Substance Abuse Treatment in the United States: Exemplary Models from a National Evaluation Study* (pp. 3–34). Binghamton, NY: Haworth Press.

Dennis, M. L., Godley, S. H., Diamond, G., *et al.* (2004). The Cannabis Youth Treatment (CYT) study: main findings from two randomized trials. *Journal of Substance Abuse Treatment*, **27**, 197–213.

Diamond, G. S. & Liddle, H. A. (1996). Resolving a therapeutic impasse between parents and adolescents in multidimensional family therapy. *Journal of Consulting and Clinical Psychology*, **64**, 481–488.

Diamond, G., Godley, S. H., Liddle, H., *et al.* (2002). Five outpatient treatment models for adolescent marijuana use: a description of the Cannabis Youth Treatment interventions. *Addiction*, **97**(Suppl. 1), 70–83.

Diamond, G. S., Leckrone, J., & Dennis, M. L. (2005). The Cannabis Youth Treatment study: clinical and empirical developments. In R. Roffman & R. Stephens (eds.), *Cannabis Dependence: Its Nature, Consequences, and Treatment.* Cambridge, UK: Cambridge University Press, in press.

Dunn, C., Deroo, L., & Rivara, F. P. (2001). The use of brief interventions adapted from motivational interviewing across behavioral domains: a systematic review. *Addiction*, **96**, 1725–1742.

French, M. T., Roebuck, M. C., Dennis, M. L., *et al.* (2002). The economic cost of outpatient marijuana treatment for adolescents: findings from a multisite field experiment. *Addiction,* **97**(Suppl. 1), 84–97.

(2003). Outpatient marijuana treatment for adolescents: economic evaluation of a multisite field experiment. *Evaluation Review,* **27,** 421–459.

Gerstein, D. R. & Johnson, R. A. (1999). *Adolescents and Young Adults in the National Treatment Improvement Evaluation Study.* Rockville, MD: Center for Substance Abuse Treatment.

Godley, M. D., Kahn, J. H., Dennis, M. L., Godley, S. H., & Funk, R. R. (2005). The stability and impact of environmental factors on substance use and problems after adolescent outpatient treatment for cannabis use and dependence. *Psychology of Addictive Behaviors,* **19,** 62–70.

Godley, S. H., Meyers, R. J., Smith, J. E., *et al.* (2001a). *Cannabis Youth Treatment (CYT) Series,* Vol. 4: *The Adolescent Community Reinforcement Approach for Adolescent Cannabis Users.* Rockville, MD, Center for Substance Abuse Treatment, Substance Abuse and Mental Health Services Administration. Retrieved from http://www.samhsa.gov.csat.csat.htm.

Godley, S. H., White, W. L., Diamond, G., Passetti, L., & Titus, J. C. (2001b). Therapist reactions to manual-guided therapies for the treatment of adolescent marijuana users. *Clinical Psychology Science and Practice,* **8,** 405–417.

Grella, C. E., Hser, Y. I., Joshi, V., & Rounds-Bryant, J. (2001). Drug treatment outcomes for adolescents with comorbid mental and substance use disorders: findings from the DATOS-A. *Journal of Nervous and Mental Disease,* **189,** 384–392.

Hall, W. & Babor, T. F. (2000). Cannabis use and public health: assessing the burden. *Addiction,* **95,** 485–490.

Henggeler, S. W., Borduin, C. M., Melton, G. B., *et al.* (1991). Effects of multisystemic therapy on drug use and abuse in serious juvenile offenders: a progress report from two outcome studies. *Family Dynamics of Addiction Quarterly,* **1,** 40–51.

Henggeler, S. W., Clingempeel, W. G., Brondino, M. J., & Pickrel, S. G. (2002). Four-year follow-up of multisystemic therapy with substance-abusing and substance-dependent juvenile offenders. *Journal of the American Academy of Child and Adolescent Pyschiatry,* **41,** 868–874.

Hser, Y. I., Grella, C. E., Hubbard, R. L., *et al.* (2001). An evaluation of drug treatments for adolescents in four USA cities. *Archives of General Psychiatry,* **58,** 689–695.

Hubbard, R. L., Cavanaugh, E. R., Craddock, S. G., & Rachel, J. V. (1985). Characteristics, behaviors, and outcomes for youth in the TOPS: treatment Services for Adolescent Substance Abusers. In A. S. Friedman & G. M. Beschner (eds.), *Treatment Services for Adolescent Substance Abusers* (pp. 49–65). Rockville, MD: National Institute on Drug Abuse.

Hunt, G. M. & Azrin, N. H. (1973). A community-reinforcement approach to alcoholism. *Behavior Research and Therapy,* **11,** 91–104.

Institute of Medicine (1980). *Alcoholism, Alcohol Abuse, and Related Problems: Opportunities for Research.* Washington, DC: National Academy Press.

(1989). *Prevention and Treatment of Alcohol Problems: Research Opportunities.* Washington, DC: National Academy Press.

(1990). *Broadening the Base of Treatment for Alcohol Problems.* Washington, DC: National Academy Press.

(1998). *Bridging the Gap between Practice and Research: Forging Partnerships with Community-based Drug and Alcohol Treatment*. Washington, DC: National Academy Press.

(1999). *Marijuana and Medicine: Assessing the Science Base*. Washington, DC: National Academy Press.

Jackson-Gilfort, A., Liddle, H. A., Tejeda, M. J., & Dakof, G. A. (2001). Facilitating engagement of African-American male adolescents in family therapy: a cultural theme process study. *Journal of Black Psychology*, **27**, 321–340.

Johnston, L. D., O'Malley, P. M., & Bachman, J. G. (2003). *The Monitoring the Future National Results on Adolescent Drug Use: Overview of Key Findings, 2002*. Bethesda, MD: National Institute on Drug Abuse.

Kaminer, Y. & Burleson, J. A. (1999). Psychotherapies for adolescent substance abusers: 15-month follow-up of a pilot study. *American Journal on Addictions*, **8**, 114–119.

Kaminer, Y., Burleson, J. A., & Goldberger, R. (2002). Cognitive–behavioral coping skills and psychoeducation therapies for adolescent substance abuse. *Journal of Nervous and Mental Disease*, **190**, 737–745.

Kraus, L. & Bauernfeind, R. (1998). Konsumtrends illegaler drogen in Deutschland: Daten aus bevolkerungssurveys 1990–1995. *Sucht*, **44**, 169–182.

Latimer, W. W., Winters, K. C., D'Zurilla, T., & Nichols, M. (2003). Integrated family and Cognitive–behavioral therapy for adolescent substance abusers: a stage I efficacy study. *Drug and Alcohol Dependence*, **71**, 303–317.

Liddle, H. A. (2002). *Cannabis Youth Treatment (CYT) Manual Series*, Vol. 5: *Multidimensional Family Therapy for Adolescent Cannabis Users*. Rockville, MD, Center for Substance Abuse Treatment, Substance Abuse and Mental Health Services Administration. Retrieved from http://www.samhsa.gov.csat.csat.htm.

Liddle, H. A., Dakof, G. A., Parker, K., Diamond, G. S., Barrett. K., & Tejeda, M. (2001). Multidimensional family therapy for adolescent substance abuse: results of a randomized clinical trial. *American Journal of Drug and Alcohol Abuse*, **27**, 651–688.

Melidonis, G. G. & Bry, B. H. (1995). Effects of therapist exceptions questions on blaming and positive statements in families with adolescent behavior problems. *Journal of Family Psychology*, **9**, 451–457.

Meyers, R. J. & Godley, M. D. (2001). The community reinforcement approach. In R. Meyers & W. Miller (eds.), *A Community Reinforcement Approach to Addition Treatment* (pp. 1–7). Cambridge, UK: Cambridge University Press.

Meyers, R. J. & Smith, J. E. (1997). Getting off the fence: procedures to engage treatment-resistant drinkers. *Journal of Substance Abuse Treatment*, **14**, 467–472.

Meyers, R. J., Miller, W. R., Hill, D. E., & Tonigan, J. S. (1999). Community reinforcement and family training (CRAFT): engaging unmotivated drug users in treatment. *Journal of Substance Abuse*, **10**, 291–308.

Morgenstern, J. & McCrady, B. S. (1992). Curative factors in alcohol and drug treatment: behavioral and disease model perspectives. *British Journal of Addiction*, **87**, 901–912.

Randall, J., Henggeler, S. W., Cunningham, P. B., Rowland, M. D., & Swenson, C. C. (2001). Adapting multisystemic therapy to treat adolescent substance abuse more effectively. *Cognitive and Behavioral Practice*, **8**, 359–366.

Rawson, R. A., Obert, J. L., McCann, M. J., & Marinelli, C. P. (1993). Relapse prevention strategies in outpatient substance abuse treatment. *Psychology of Addictive Behaviors*, **7**, 85–95.

Rawson, R. A., Obert, J. L., McCann, M. J., & Marinelli, C. P. (1994). Relapse prevention models for substance abuse treatment. *Psychotherapy: Theory, Research, Practice, Training*, **30**, 284–298.

Sampl, S. & Kadden, R. (2001). *Cannabis Youth Treatment (CYT) Manual Series*, Vol. 1: *Motivational Enhancement Therapy and Cognitive Behavioral Therapy (MET-CBT-5) for Adolescent Cannabis Users.* Rockville, MD: Center for Substance Abuse Treatment, Substance Abuse and Mental Health Services Administration. Retrieved from http://www.chestnut.org/li/cyt/products/mcb5_cyt_v1.pdf.

SAMHSA (1995). *National Household Survey on Drug Abuse.* Rockville, MD: Substance Abuse and Mental Health Services Administration Office of Applied Studies.

(1998). *Behavioral Therapies Development Program.* Rockville, MD: National Institutes of Health. Retrieved May 15, 2004 from http://grants.nih.gov/grants/guide/rfa-files/RFA-DA-94-002.html.

(2000a). *National Household Survey on Drug Abuse: Main Findings 2000.* Rockville, MD: Substance Abuse and Mental Health Services Administration. Retrieved from http://www.samhsa.gov/statistics.

(2000b). *National Household Survey on Drug Abuse: Main Findings 1998.* Rockville, MD: Substance Abuse and Mental Health Services Administration. Retrieved from http://www.samhsa.gov/statistics.

(2000c). *Mid-Year 2000 Emergency Department Data From the Drug Abuse Warning Network (DAWN).* [DHHS Publication No. (SMA) 01–3502, DAWN Series D-17.] Rockville, MD: Substance Abuse and Mental Health Services Administration. Retrieved from http://www.samhsa.gov/statistics.

(2000d). *Year-End 1999 Medical Examiner Data From the Drug Abuse Warning Network (DAWN).* [DHHS Publication No. (SMA) 01–3491, DAWN Series D-16.] Rockville, MD: Substance Abuse and Mental Health Services Administration.

(2002). *Summary of National Findings*, Vol. I: *Prevalence and Correlates of Alcohol, Tobacco, and Illegal Drug Use.* Rockville, MD: Substance Abuse and Mental Health Services Administration. Retrieved from http://www.samhsa.gov/oas/nhsda/2k1nhsda/vol1/toc.htm.

Schmidt, S. E., Liddle, H. A., & Dakof, G. A. (1996). Changes in parenting practices and adolescent drug abuse during multidimensional family therapy. *Journal of Family Psychology*, **10**, 12–27.

Sells, S. B. & Simpson, D. D. (1979). Evaluation of treatment outcome for youths in the Drug Abuse Reporting Program (DARP): a follow-up study. In G. M. Beschner & A. S. Friedman (eds.), *Youth Drug Abuse: Problems, Issues, and Treatment* (pp. 571–628). Lexington, MA: DC Heath.

Silverman, W. H. (1996). Cookbooks, manuals, and paint-by-numbers: Psychotherapy in the 90s. *Psychotherapy*, **33**, 207–215.

Sisson, R. W. & Azrin, N. H. (1993). Community reinforcement training for families: a method to get alcoholics into treatment. In T. J. O'Farrell (ed.), *Treating Alcohol Problems: Marital and Family Interventions* (pp. 34–53). New York: Guilford Press.

Stephens, R. S., Roffman, R. A., & Simpson, E. E. (1993). Adult marijuana users seeking treatment. *Journal of Consulting and Clinical Psychology*, **61**, 1100–1104.

Stephens, R. S., Roffman, R. A., & Curtin, L. (2000). Comparison of extended versus brief treatments for marijuana use. *Journal of Consulting and Clinical Psychology*, **61**, 1100–1104.

Swift, W., Copeland, J., & Hall, W. (1998). Choosing a diagnostic cut-off for cannabis dependence. *Addiction*, **93**, 1681–1692.

Tims, F. M., Dennis, M. L., Hamilton, N., et al. (2002). Characteristics and problems of 600 adolescent cannabis abusers in outpatient treatment. *Addiction*, **97**(Suppl. 1), 46–57.

Titus, J. C., Dennis, M. L., White, M., et al. (2002). An examination of adolescents' reasons for starting, quitting, and continuing to use drugs and alcohol following treatment. *Drug and Alcohol Dependence*, **66**, S183.

Waldron, H. B., Slesnick, N., Brody, J. L., Turner, C. W., & Peterson, T. R. (2001). Treatment outcomes for adolescent substance abuse at four- and seven-month assessments. *Journal of Consulting and Clinical Psychology*, **69**, 802–812.

Webb, C., Scudder, M., Kaminer, Y., Kadden, R., & Tawfik, Z. (2002). *Cannabis Youth Treatment (CYT) Manual Series*, Vol. 2: *The MET/CBT 5 Supplement: 7 Sessions of Cognitive Behavioral Therapy (CBT 7) for Adolescent Cannabis Users*. Rockville, MD: Center for Substance Abuse Treatment, Substance Abuse and Mental Health Services Administration. Retrieved from http://www.samhsa.gov/csat/csat.htm.

Part II

Practice and policy trends in treatment for adolescent substance abuse

6

Epidemiological trends and clinical implications of adolescent substance abuse in Europe

Cecilia A. Essau

Whitelands College, Roehampton University, London, UK

Substance use and abuse are considered to be among the most common public health problems among adolescents in Europe (European Monitoring Centre for Drugs and Drug Addiction [EMCDDA], 2002). As shown by numerous studies, substance abuse is strongly associated with delinquency, poor scholastic attainment, suicide, and traffic accidents (e.g., BzgA [Federal Centre for Health Education] 2001; EMCDDA, 2002). The negative impact of drug and alcohol use in Europe has become increasingly more apparent in recent years. According to a recent report of the EMCDDA (2002), each year there are about 7000 to 8000 acute drug-related deaths in the European Union (EU). The estimated direct health-care cost of drug dependence and harmful use in the EU is enormous, with figures in the hundreds of millions of euros. Furthermore, a few million euros have been spent in preventing drug consumption and addiction. For example, during the fiscal year 2000, the German government allocated a total of 13.9 million euro for measures against the misuse of drugs and narcotics (Simon et al., 2001). In 2002, the budget spent on treatment, education, and model projects in the area of drugs and addiction in Germany was about 1 billion euro (Simon et al., 2001).

The increase in the prevalence and associated problems of substance abuse has prompted government support for several large-scale surveys of substance use and abuse. Most studies to date have, however, focused on adults and, less frequently, on adolescents (reviewed by Essau, Barrett, & Pasquali, 2002). One possible explanation for this is that not all adolescent substance users progress to substance abuse and dependence (Boys et al., 1999). Yet, a substantial number of adult substance abusers began using during their adolescent years (Kessler et al., 1994).

In this chapter, some recent large-scale studies conducted in some European countries will be presented, followed by findings on the factors related to substance consumption and to the progression from substance use to abuse. Clinical implications of the epidemiological data on substance abuse and political trends that influence policy decisions about prevention efforts and treatment services in the EU in general, and in Germany specifically, will also be discussed. This chapter is intended to provide readers with contemporary epidemiological trends of substance use and abuse in Europe, as well as their clinical and political implications.

Prevalence of substance use

A number of epidemiological studies have been conducted in Europe that provide information on the prevalence of substance use, abuse, and dependence in adolescents. Because of methodological differences, such as differences in the case definition, assessment instruments, time frame (lifetime, 6 months, current), and age groups, it is difficult to make a direct comparison of findings across studies. Therefore, the main findings from selected studies in some European countries will be presented.

Across Europe

Two major surveys that have examined the prevalence of substance use and abuse across Europe are the European Schools Project on Alcohol and other Drugs (ESPAD) and the Health Behaviour in School-aged Children Survey (HBSC).

European Schools Project on Alcohol and other Drugs

The ESPAD is similar to the USA Monitoring the Future (MTF) study. Its main aim was to examine the frequency and risk factors of substance use in over 50 000 16 year olds across Europe (Morgan *et al.*, 1999). Two surveys have been conducted: the first in 1995 involving 26 European countries and the second in 1999 involving 30 countries (Hibell *et al.*, 2000).

The results of the two ESPAD surveys can be summarized as follows (Hibell *et al.*, 2000; Morgan *et al.*, 1999). (a) Up to 42% of the adolescents in the ESPAD indicated that they had smoked during the past month. (b) The use of cannabis was common, especially in the Czech Republic, France, Ireland, and the UK. (c) In terms of alcohol beverages, more beer was drunk than wine. Wine was commonly drunk (three times or more in the last 30 days) in countries with a wine-drinking culture, such as the Czech Republic, Greece, Italy, Slovak Republic, and Slovenia. (d) In comparison with the first ESPAD survey, the second survey demonstrated an increase in all illegal drug use, smoking, and wine consumption in many countries, especially in central and eastern European countries. (e) Risk perception played an important role in the actual behaviors that involved heavy drinking, getting drunk, and drug use.

When comparing the ESPAD data with that of the MTF significant differences were found in terms of alcohol and illicit drug consumption, and cigarette smoking (Hibell *et al.*, 2000). Compared with adolescents in 10th grade in the USA (26%), more adolescents of this age group in almost all ESPAD countries (37%) reported smoking cigarettes and consuming alcohol (MTF, 40%; ESPAD, 61%) in the past 30 days. The lifetime use of cannabis and any illicit drug use was much higher in the MTF study (cannabis, 41%; other illicit drug, 23%) than in the ESPAD (cannabis, 17%; other illicit drug, 6%).

The Health Behaviour in School-aged Children Survey

The HBSC was originally initiated by a group of researchers in England, Finland and Norway in 1982 to investigate health issues of 13 and 15 year olds both within and across the participating countries (Currie *et al.*, 2000). The project was later adopted by the World Health Organization (WHO) for Europe as a WHO Collaborative Study. Since its initiation, four surveys have been conducted at 4-year intervals, with an increasing number of countries participating with each survey. In the latest survey, conducted in 1997–1998, 29 countries participated including Canada and the USA. The main aim of the HBSC was to collect information on health behavior, lifestyles, and their context in young people. An additional aim was to inform and influence policy on health promotion and health education. Alcohol and tobacco were the only substances examined in the HBSC.

Although more than 50% of the 11 year olds in most European countries had drunk alcoholic beverages, only a few used alcohol on a regular basis (Settertobulte, Jensen, & Hurrelmann, 2001). The rates of alcohol consumption increased from low to moderate levels among the 13 year olds, and became customary among the 15 year olds in all countries. The rate of drunkenness differed across countries. Those from Mediterranean countries reported low rates of drunkenness, while high rates of drunkenness were found in countries of the UK. In terms of smoking, both the rates of tobacco experimentation and the rate of daily smoking increased significantly with age, with the largest increases between the ages of 13 and 15 (Gabhainn & Francois, 2000).

European Monitoring Centre for Drugs and Drug Addiction

Information about the prevalence and trends of substance use in Europe can also be obtained from the EMCDDA (www.emcdda.eu.int). Since 1995, the EMCDDA has published an annual report containing information about the drug situation (e.g., drug use in the general population, problem drug use, drug-related crime, drug markets, and drug availability) and responses to drug problems (e.g., drug strategies, demand and supply reduction). According to the EMCDDA annual report for 2002, the use of cannabis among those aged 15–35 years increased significantly in almost all EU countries during the 1990s, but had appeared to level off, or even decrease, in recent years.

Specific European countries

United Kingdom

Several surveys have been conducted that provide information about the frequency of substance use among adolescents in the UK. These included the British Crime Survey (BCS), the Youth Lifestyles Survey, and the Health Survey for England. The BCS is an annual large-scale national survey of adults, aged 16 to 59 years, in England and Wales. The main aim of the BCS orginally was to obtain information about experience of crime and other-related issues; however, since 1994, information about drug misuse was also collected. According to the 2001–2002 BCS, those aged 16–24 years have significantly higher prevalence of any drug use compared with older age groups (Aust, Sharp, & Goulden, 2002). The 1998–1999 Youth Lifestyles Survey (Pudney, 2002) was based on a nationally representative sample of about 4000 individuals aged 12–30 years who lived in private households in England and Wales. The main aim of this survey was to get information about lifestyles, including drinking, smoking, use of and attitudes towards illegal drugs, and offending. The Health Survey for England was an annual survey aimed at monitoring trends in the nation's health (Prescott-Clarke & Primatesta, 1997). The target sample in the 1997 Health Survey for England consisted of those aged 2–24 years.

The findings of these three studies can be summarized as follows. (a) The most commonly used drug in the BCS was cannabis; in the Youth Lifestyles Survey, it was glue/solvent. (b) Significantly fewer adolescents and young adults reported using different types of drug (e.g., amphetamine, LSD, magic mushrooms, glue, and methadone) in the 2001–2002 BCS compared with the 1998 BCS, except for cocaine and ecstasy (Aust *et al.*, 2002). The significant increase in the 2001–2002 BCS in cocaine and ecstasy use may be related to their cheaper supply compared with other stimulants and hallucinants. (c) Approximately 85% of the adolescents reported having drunk alcohol and 61% had had some experience with cigarettes sometime in their lives (Aust *et al.*, 2002). (d) Both the onset and the persistent use of drugs were associated with the extent to which the drugs were easily accessible (Aust *et al.*, 2002). (e) There was a strong relationship between parental and adolescent smoking, and between the amount of money spent and the number of offenses. The age of onset for using drugs differed slightly depending on the substance. The age of onset for glue was the lowest (14.1 years), followed by cannabis (approximately 15 years). The age of onset for most hard drugs, such as heroin, crack, ecstasy, methadone, and cocaine was much later, ranging from 17 to 20 years (Pudney, 2002).

Germany

The Drug Affinity Study (Drogenaffinitätsstudie) is a representative survey of substance use among young people in Germany. It has been carried out since 1973 by the Federal Centre for Health Education (BzgA, 2001) at 3- to 4-year intervals. The first six studies (1973, 1976, 1979, 1982, 1986, 1990) were conducted in West Germany, and the last three studies (1993, 1997, 2001) also included adolescents from former East Germany. The main aim of the survey was to examine the frequency of substance use (alcohol, tobacco, and illegal drugs) and factors related to the motives and attitudes towards substance use.

As a whole, the rate of consumption of illegal drugs (particularly cannabis) increased among those aged 12–25 years in West and former East Germany, whereas the rate of smoking and alcohol consumption decreased from 1973 to 2001. The increased use of cannabis was notable among adolescents in the former East Germany between 1993 and 1997, and among girls in West and former East Germany. The age at which adolescents first tried most types of illegal drug had remained stable, except for cannabis, for which a lower age of onset has been noted in more recent studies. Almost all adolescents (92%) have drunk alcoholic beverages (BzgA, 2001) sometime in their lives, with 60% of them having already experienced alcohol intoxication. In terms of smoking, no significant differences could be noted among adolescents in East and West Germany, nor were there any gender differences. The average age at which the adolescents first tried cigarettes was 13.6 years, with most adolescents (80%) having their first cigarette experience between the ages of 11 and 16 years.

In addition to the Drug Affinity Study, information on the frequency and patterns of substance use has been provided by two epidemiological studies: the Early Development Stages of Psychopathology (EDSP; Wittchen, Nelson, & Lachner, 1998) and the Bremen Adolescent Study (Essau, Karpinski, Petermann, & Conradt, 1998). In both epidemiological studies, a large percentage of adolescents and young adults reported having consumed alcoholic beverages sometime in their lives (77–95%; Essau *et al.*, 1998; Holly *et al.*, 1997). Drug consumption was also common, with cannabis being the most widely used substance (23.7–34.9%). Opioid use, including prescription drugs such as codeine and methadone, was reported by 3.4% of the participants (Perkonigg, Lieb, & Wittchen, 1997).

Austria

In the Styrian study (Gasser-Steiner & Stigler, 1997), 12% of the adolescents reported having tried illegal drugs sometime in their lives. Stimulants (13.3%) were the most commonly used substance, followed by marijuana (12.1%) and medication in combination with alcohol (8.8%). Drug use increased with age until it reached a plateau around the ages of 18 to 20 years. Up to 58% of the adolescents reported regular consumption of alcohol. About 40% of the adolescents reported having smoked, with about one quarter of them smoking daily. Their findings also showed alcohol consumption and smoking to be related to adolescent educational status, with apprentices being at the highest risk. Significantly more males than females consumed alcoholic beverages and smoked on a regular basis. First contact with alcohol was generally made in a family context, whereas smoking tended to be initiated not through family but with friends. Cigarette and alcohol consumption are socially tolerated and reflect culturally accepted behaviour. For example, 60% of the 16 year olds regarded alcohol as an integral part of their everyday life.

Switzerland

In the Zurich Adolescent Psychopathology Project (Steinhausen & Metzke, 1998), 28.5% of youth aged 10–17 years had consumed at least one glass of alcohol, and about 9.5% reported having been drunk at least once in their lifetime. The most common factors associated with alcohol drinking included getting together with friends and family members, or attending parties. For 9% of the alcohol users, drinking was associated with personal problems, feelings of loneliness, or boredom. The frequency of drinking was also associated with parental substance use. That is, the more the parents drank and smoked, the more likely it was that their children also used alcohol and cigarettes. As reported in other countries, the use of illicit drugs, such as hallucinogens, heroin or cocaine, and non-prescribed drugs (e.g., barbiturates, codeine, amphetamines, and anticholinergic drugs) were less common (Konings *et al.*, 1995; Madianos *et al.*, 1995).

Finland

In Finland, the prevalence of and factors related to substance use have been reported by two research groups, one at the University of Kuopio (Kumpulainen & Roine, 2002; Kumpulainen *et al.*, 2000) and another at the Finnish Foundation of Alcohol Studies (Poikolainen *et al.*, 2001a,b). The study by Kumpulainen and colleagues was a 5-year follow-up of a longitudinal study conducted in Kuopio, Eastern Finland since 1989. Following the initial data collection, the children (born in 1981) have been assessed twice, at 12 and 15 years of age. The Foundation of Alcohol Studies (Aalto-Setäla *et al.*, 2001; Poikolainen *et al.*, 2001a,b) started in 1990, with a follow-up investigation in 1995 when the subjects were 20–25 years of age.

In the Kuopio study (Kumpulainen *et al.*, 2000), 78% of the adolescents had drunk alcohol beverages during the last 12 months. Among those who had been intoxicated more than three times during the past 30 days (i.e., heavy users of alcohol), 61% were girls. The finding that more girls than boys were heavy users of alcohol has been interpreted as a function of age, social development, changes in traditional values, and societal expectations about behavior. According to parental report, heavy users were significantly more hyperactive and had more relationship difficulties, psychosomatic symptoms, and externalizing behaviors compared with other adolescents. Based on teacher reports, heavy users had higher scores on hyperactivity, relationship difficulties, and internalizing and externalizing behavior compared with other adolescents. Heavy use of alcohol was associated with the presence of various types of psychiatric symptom in the home. That is, the probability of being a heavy alcohol user was 3.6 times greater if the adolescent was depressed and hyperactive, and 3.9-fold if he/she demonstrated externalizing behaviors. Predictors of later heavy alcohol use differed significantly across gender (Kumpulainen & Roine, 2002). In girls, heavy alcohol use at the age of 15 years was related to perceiving oneself as failing to perform on an expected level at school and having low self-esteem. Among boys, heavy alcohol use was related to interpersonal problems with aggressive tendencies.

In the study of Poikolainen *et al.* (2001b), 21.4% of those aged 15–19 years reported having tried cannabis sometime in their lives. Initiation to cannabis use was related to being male, absence of mother, grade-point average 1–3 years before the baseline examination, lack of motivation, and an early age of first sexual intercourse. The significant association between the mother's absence from home and cannabis consumption may suggest a lack of control and care received by the adolescent at home. That is, adolescents with low attachment to home and their family generally depend on the support of their peers and friends and conform to the norms of the peer group. Another explanation is that initiation to cannabis could be explained as a way of coping with the mother's absence or loss. Alcohol intake or heavy drinking (defined as at least 13 drinks on one occasion) 5 years later was predicted by being male, reporting frequent relief smoking and drinking, and by the interaction between relief drinking and relief smoking. Parental alcohol problems, social group, perceived degree of social support, trait anxiety, number of negative life events, self-esteem, grade-point average, somatic symptoms score, and defence style (i.e., immature, neurotic, and mature) assessed during the index investigation failed to predict alcohol intake.

Prevalence of substance abuse and dependence

The Netherlands and Spain

Information on the prevalence of substance abuse in the Netherlands is based on the study by Verhulst and colleagues (1997), a two-phase survey to estimate the 6-month prevalence of substance use disorders (SUDs) and other psychiatric disorders in adolescents. The 6-month prevalence of SUDs varied based on the informant: according to parental report it was 0.4% and according to adolescent report it was 3.3%. Significantly more boys than girls met a diagnosis for an SUD.

The prevalence of SUDs among Spanish adolescents was based on the study by Canals *et al.* (1997). The main aims of their study were to estimate the prevalence, comorbidity rates, risk factors, and utilization of mental health services for SUDs and other psychiatric disorders. Their findings showed a relatively low rate of SUD (0.3%).

Germany

The Bremen Adolescent Study is a longitudinal large-scale school-based study of the epidemiology of psychiatric disorders among adolescents aged 12 to 17 years (Essau *et al.*, 1998). The aims of the study were to estimate the prevalence, risks, course, and comorbidity patterns of psychiatric disorders, as well as to examine the associated psychosocial impairment and service utilization. The 1035 participants were randomly selected from 36 schools in the province of Bremen, in the northern part of Germany. Psychopathological and diagnostic assessments were based on the computer-assisted version of the Munich-Composite International Diagnostic Interview (M-CIDI) to cover criteria of DSM-IV and the WHO *International Classification of Diseases*, 10th Draft (ICD-10) (Wittchen & Pfister, 1996).

The EDSP study sample of 3021 individuals was drawn from the 1994 Bavarian government registry of residents in Munich and the surrounding counties (Wittchen *et al.*, 1998). Two follow-up investigations were completed following the index baseline assessment, covering an overall period of 42 months. Most interviews, using the M-CIDI, took place at the time of first contact in the home of the probands.

The findings of these two German epidemiological studies can be summarized as follows. Of all the DSM-IV disorders covered in the EDSP, SUDs were the most common. In the Bremer Adolescent Study, about 12.3% of those aged 12–17 years met lifetime diagnosis for an SUD. Of the substances covered, the most commonly used was alcohol, with a rate of consumption of 9.3% (Essau *et al.*, 1998). Opiate, amphetamine, and hallucinogen use disorders occurred less frequently. The prevalence of SUDs was significantly higher in males than in females, with a ratio of 2:1.

Finland

The Finland Study by Aalto-Setälä *et al.* (2001) was a 5-year follow-up study designed to examine the prevalence and comorbidity rates of SUDs and psychiatric disorders among those aged 20–24 years. Other aims were to examine the degree of psychosocial impairment and estimated need of psychiatric treatment, and the impact of comorbidity on treatment.

The 1 month prevalence of SUDs based on DSM-IV criteria was 6.2%. Among those SUDs reported, the most common was cannabis abuse (2.7%), followed by alcohol abuse (2.1%) and alcohol dependence (1.4%). The prevalence rates of SUDs decreased when additional criteria were used in case definition. That is, the prevalence of SUDs was 6.0% and 3.0%, respectively, when the global assessment of functioning value was <71 (mild impairment) and <61 (moderate impairment) as additional criteria.

Summary

Recent studies have shown substance use to be a relatively common phenomenon among adolescents in Europe. The rates of substance use reported, however, varied across studies and countries, probably because of differences in methodological issues, the legal system, and societal views on the use of substances.

Comorbidity and temporal sequences of disorders

Both the Bremen Adolescent Study (Essau *et al.*, 1998) and the EDSP (Wittchen *et al.*, 1998) data indicated high comorbidity between SUDs and other disorders such as anxiety, affective, and somatoform disorders, as well as within the different types of SUD. For example, in the Bremen Adolescent Study, approximately a third of those with one type of SUD had at least one other type of abuse/dependence, with alcohol use disorders (AUDs) being the most frequent. Similarly, in a recent analysis of the EDSP data, Lieb *et al.* (2002) found that most ecstasy users were polydrug users: 53% met the criteria for nicotine dependence, 44% for illicit SUDs, and 53% for AUDs. Ecstasy users also used significantly more prescription medications than those who had never used an illicit substance (e.g., pain killers, sedatives, sleeping pills, stimulants), suggesting their likelihood to misuse prescription drugs.

Among those with comorbid disorders, other psychiatric disorders generally occurred prior to the SUD. For example, among ecstasy users with comorbid disorders, other psychiatric disorders began prior to the onset of the first use of ecstasy in 80.4% (Lieb *et al.*, 2002). The disorders that most commonly preceded the onset of first ecstasy use were phobias (55–98%, depending on the type of phobias), somatoform disorders (73%), and dysthymia (69%). This finding may indicate the role of substance use as a self-medication to cope with problems associated with other psychiatric disorders.

Although SUDs co-occur frequently with other disorders, the meaning of this finding in terms of classification and etiological mechanisms remains unknown. However, given the temporal sequencing of disorders (based on age of onset), current findings seem to suggest substance use or abuse as a "self-medication" to cope with other disorders such as anxiety, somatoform (e.g., pain disorder), and depressive disorders.

Risk factors

Given the number of existing review papers on risk factors for substance use and abuse (reviewed by Sullivan & Farrell, 2002), this section will only briefly cover some findings from European studies, focusing on factors related to the progression from substance use to abuse. Based on the risk factor typology of Hawkins, Catalano, and Miller (1992), the factors that are associated with the initiation of substance use in adolescents are outlined below.

Socioenvironmental factors (e.g., age and gender)

As shown in almost all studies (e.g., Essau *et al.*, 1998; Wittchen *et al.*, 1998), males have higher rates of substance use and abuse than females. The age of peak usage for different substances varies, suggesting age as a significant risk factor for the use of different substances. For example, the use of alcohol and marijuana peaks around the age of 16–17 years and declines after the age of 20 years, while many other illicit drugs peak around 18 and decline after 21 years.

Substance-related factors (e.g., attitudes toward drug use and peer drug use)

During adolescence, peers become increasingly more important. With parental influence declining, adolescents begin to be highly influenced by the peers they choose to associate with (reviewed by Adams, Cantwell, & Mathies, 2002). As such, adolescents who involves themselves with peers who are using alcohol and other drugs are more likely to become involved with substance use themselves (Morgan *et al.*, 1999). As argued by Beman (1995), peers shape attitudes about drugs, provide drugs and social context for drug use, and share ideas and beliefs that form the rationale for drug use.

Intrapersonal factors

Intrapersonal factors, such as poor temperament, early conduct problems, and a risk-taking orientation, are also important risk factors for substance use (reviewed by Adams *et al.*, 2002; Sullivan & Farrell, 2002). Poor academic performance, low aspirations for academic achievement, and low self-esteem are also common risk factors for the initiation and continued use and abuse of substances (reviewed by Adams *et al.*, 2002; Sullivan & Farrell, 2002). In a longitudinal study by a Swedish group (Wennberg *et al.*, 2002), hazardous alcohol consumption prior to age 21 and at age 36 was predicted by attention problems and poor school achievement at age 10.

Interpersonal factors

Interpersonal factors (e.g., familial factors such as impaired parent–child relationship, sexual abuse, and parental illicit drug use) are also among the most consistently cited risk factors for substance use (reviewed by Sullivan & Farrell, 2002). As shown by Lieb *et al.* (2002), children of parents with AUDs are more likely to engage in alcohol use and develop AUDs than children whose parents do not report these disorders. Parental AUD also predicts age of onset of alcohol use and AUDs in offspring. Having one or two affected parents increases the risk for early onset of hazardous use and dependence between the ages of 14 and 17 (compared with an average age of 24 among young people whose parents do not have AUDs). The risk of beginning problem use at younger ages and developing earlier-onset AUDs is increased among youngsters with two alcoholic parents. These findings also linked maternal AUD to the transition from occasional into regular use. Paternal AUD tended to increase the risk for transition from regular into hazardous use. It was argued that fathers demonstrate more excessive drinking than mothers, which, in turn, may provide a role model for the hazardous use of alcohol in their children.

Predictors of incident substance use seemed to differ from those of SUD. For example, in a recent publication of the EDSP data (von Sydow *et al.*, 2002), easy availability of drugs and peers' drug use predicted cannabis use, but not SUD. Adolescent attitudes toward future drug use were also important predictors for the incidence of cannabis use and for progression to abuse. Higher behavioral inhibition (social factor) in childhood and more frequent positive life events were protective against cannabis use. Factors that predicted progression into abuse included being male, the presence of positive attitudes toward future drug use, having a drug disorder at baseline, grandparental alcohol problems, and not having a good relationship with the father. A poor relationship with the mother tended to have a protective effect. It was concluded that "the same" maternal and paternal behaviors may have different implications for children. It may be that a very close parent–child relationship can be a strength, as well as an indicator of a problematic dynamic in the marital system, creating a parent–child coalition.

Political implications of adolescent substance abuse: a response from the European Union

In order to cope with the increasing drug problems in Europe, an organization of political coordination centered around the member states was proposed by the former French President, François Mitterrand, in 1989 (EMCDDA, 2002). His idea was to develop a drug-monitoring center in which the social and health aspects of the drug problem in Europe, and other related factors (e.g., drug trafficking), could be examined. Drug-related issues were mentioned for the first time in the Maastricht Treaty of the EU in 1993, with its provisions being strengthened in the Treaty of Amsterdam in 1999 (Council of the European Union, 2000). According to this treaty, the EU would complement its member states' actions to reduce harm related to drugs. The treaty also stressed the need to provide citizens with a high level of safety by preventing and combating crime (i.e., illicit drug trafficking).

The main targets of the EU Drug Strategy 2000–2004 were significantly to decrease over the 5 years the (a) prevalence of illicit drug use especially among 18 year olds and younger, (b) the number of drug-related health damages and deaths, (c) the availability of illicit drugs, (d) the number of drug-related crimes, and (e) the money-laundering and illicit trafficking of precursors (EMCDDA, 2002). Finally, it aimed to increase the number of successfully treated addicts. In order to put these strategies into concrete actions, the *EU-Action Plan on Drugs 2000–2004* (Council of the European Union, 2000) was developed in 2000. This outlined activities to be implemented by the EU by the end of 2004 and contained guidelines to evaluate the EU Drugs Strategy (2000–2004). The plan can be divided into five broad areas.

Coordination. This involves the use of a multidisciplinary approach towards drug programs and policies, and coordination at the national, regional and/or local level.

Information and evaluation. Some examples of these activities include the regular collection, analysis, and dissemination of epidemiological data related to the prevalence of drug use, drug-related deaths, and infectious diseases. Another activity was to launch "Eurobarometre" studies on public attitudes (especially young people) towards drugs at 2-year intervals.

Reduction of demand, prevention of drug use and of drug-related crime. An important aspect of this plan is to carry out drug-prevention programs in schools and to increase children's awareness of the risks associated with using drugs, alcohol, and tobacco. Another activity was to develop evidence-based strategies that would address the problems of the influence of drugs on road accidents.

Supply reduction. Some of the strategies intended to reduce the supply of drugs included the establishment of high levels of security at the external border of the EU, and the establishment of closer cooperation between police forces, customs, and other competent authorities, and between judicial and other competent authorities (e.g., rules on criminal matters in the member states).

International. This involves having a close collaboration with experts on substance use and abuse at the international level.

Consequently, in line with these plans, a number of activities in drug-related areas have been initiated in the member states. An example is the UK document

The Government's Ten Year Strategy for Tackling Drugs (UK Drug Strategy Directorate, 1998). The main aim is to help adolescents to resist misusing drugs and achieve their full potential in society. In order to achieve this aim, it is proposed that prevention should start early, with a broad life-skills approaches at primary school (aged 5–11 years), and build over time with age-appropriate programs through youth work, peer approaches, training, and wider community support. Another aim of this strategy is to protect communities from drug-related antisocial and criminal behavior, and to help drug-misusing offenders deal with their drug problems and become better integrated into society. This would involve targeting police resources to detecting drug-related crime and providing deterrence through punishment of drug dealers and suppliers. The final aim is to enable adolescents to overcome their drug problems and to live healthy and crime-free lives. Since serious drug problems are often associated with other problems (e.g., unemployment), it is important that substance abusers receive help in an appropriate and timely manner. Since this is an ongoing program, which is scheduled to finish in year 2008, no information is available regarding the implementation and achievements of these plans so far.

Clinical implications of adolescent substance abuse: response from Germany

Following the change of government in Germany in 1998, the Office of the Federal Drug Commissioner was moved from the Federal Ministry of the Interior to the Federal Ministry of Health (Simon *et al.*, 2001). This structural reorganization mirrors the importance of health and social aspects of the drug policy, with its emphasis on helping and treating instead of punishing those with drug problems. The Federal Drug Commissioner is responsible for the policy on addiction produced by the Federal Ministry of Health and for coordinating addiction and drug policy. Drug policy is both a national and a provincial (in German: Laender) affair in that the Federal Government is responsible for drug legislation, and its implementation is under the responsibility of the 16 provinces. Municipalities are responsible for funding those portions of counseling and social care not covered by other systems (e.g., pension, health, or unemployment insurance).

Addiction policy in Germany has concentrated on illegal substances. However, the recent Federal Drug Commissioner's report highlighted the intention to extend prevention to legal substances, alcohol and tobacco (e.g., establishing laws that forbid the sale of tobacco to those under 16 years). Dialogues have been carried out between the Federal Ministry of Health and the Tobacco Industry Association regarding financial contributions to protect children and adolescents from smoking. Furthermore, a new Action Plan on Drugs and Addiction was introduced in 2002, with goals to delay the start of substance consumption, to reduce high-risk use patterns, and to treat substance dependence with all available methods.

In addition to this new plan, numerous activities addressing specific drug-related issues have been introduced or strengthened at both national and local levels. These include model projects for children of addicted parents. Additionally, given a high number of drug-related deaths among ethnic German immigrants from Eastern Europe and other groups of immigrants (e.g., Turkey, ex-Yugoslavia), the Federal Government has produced videos in various languages about different therapy organizations in order to increase awareness of the available service systems. Another priority will be early intervention and prevention. In fact, numerous primary prevention programs have recently been implemented at the family (e.g., the publication of a series of brochures for parents on how to communicate with adolescents about drugs and how to prevent children from becoming addicted), school (e.g., introduction of prevention programs for substance abuse), and community levels. Some examples of prevention programs at the community level include telephone help lines, multimedia campaigns (e.g., poster, television, and advertisement), and use of electronic media to deliver information related to institutions that offer professional help for drug users and addicts. Furthermore, in the public houses, there is a legal obligation to sell at least one non-alcoholic drink for the same price as the cheapest alcoholic beverage of the same quantity. Another target agency for collaboration on drug prevention will be the German Federal Armed Forces. Their readiness for action and their legal obligation made a drug prevention effort necessary. With very few exceptions, most prevention studies are not methodologically sound and have not been systematically evaluated. Most prevention studies have little theoretical background, and the indicators to measure the efficacy of the prevention programs have been poorly operationalized.

In addition to these primary prevention programs, several intervention programs have been implemented, such as outreach work (e.g., "Street work", in which homeless drug users who stay at public streets/places are approached) and prevention of infectious diseases (i.e., free condoms and counseling to prevent infectious diseases). At the levels of treatment and health care, numerous programs have been introduced such as various substitution and maintenance programs (e.g., methadone substitution program), and after-care and reintegration services.

Conclusions

Recent studies have shown that a high number of adolescents in Europe have had some experience with alcohol, drugs, and tobacco. The most common drug used by young people throughout Europe is cannabis; its use is so common that it is often called an "illegal everyday drug." Recent trends have generally shown an increase in substance use and abuse in Europe, linked to youth culture and dance parties. In trying to understand the secular changes of substance abuse in Europe, it is important to consider significant social and political changes, especially in eastern Europe. It would be interesting to monitor the impact of increased mobility across different countries and the dissolution of social control in many eastern European countries on substance use and abuse.

The prevalence of use of different types of substance, however, varies tremendously across Europe. These differences may be partially accounted for by differences in laws regarding the purchase and consumption of alcoholic beverages across the European countries. The minimum legal age for buying alcohol varies across the EU, ranging from 15 years (in Denmark) to 21 years (in Lithuania). In most EU countries (i.e., Czech Republic, Finland, Greenland, Ireland, Norway, Poland, Russia Federation, Slovakia, and the UK), the minimum age is 18 years. These limits are enforced with different degrees of strictness in each country. Furthermore, regulations that govern to whom, where, and how alcohol and tobacco may be sold may also have an influence on the rates of substance use. In most European countries, alcohol is easily available in supermarkets, gas stations, grocery stores, and public facilities. As reported by Balding (1997), 25% of 15-year old pupils had bought alcohol from a supermarket in the previous week, and 10% had purchased alcohol in a public house. Further, laws regarding advertising for alcoholic beverages also differ across the EU. In some countries (e.g., Belgium, Lithuania, Norway, Poland, and Sweden), there are total bans on advertising except for sponsoring sports and cultural events, whereas in other countries (e.g., Denmark, France, Germany, Hungary, and Switzerland), there are regulations governing the content of the advertisements. In addition, cultural views regarding the use of certain substances (e.g., alcohol) may determine their accessibility and acceptance, and people in different parts of Europe differ in their drinking patterns. For example, in northern Europe, alcohol habits are characterized by high amounts of alcohol consumption during the weekends and holidays, whereas in southern European countries, it is distributed evenly over the week (Hupkens, Knibbe, & Drop, 1993). All these, together with methodological differences such as the sampling procedure and assessment instruments, make it difficult to compare findings across studies.

As mentioned above, numerous studies have been conducted in Europe that provide epidemiological data on substance use and abuse in adolescents. Ideally, these epidemiological data, such as information on the frequency, comorbidity, course, and risk factors of substance use and abuse, should be considered in the design of intervention strategies (see discussion by Dadds & McAloon [2002]). However, hardly any studies have taken this scientific-based information into consideration in their treatment designs. In this respect, the gap between worlds of the practitioner and the researcher world is still very wide.

In Germany, the treatment of SUDs in adolescents usually takes place in either inpatient or outpatient settings staffed by multidisciplinary teams consisting of physicians/psychiatrists, psychologists, nurses, and social workers. However, the effectiveness of these "usual" treatment strategies is unknown since, to my knowledge, there are no published evaluation studies for such interventions. Furthermore, the use of manual-guided interventions with empirically proven efficacy has been acknowledged with great reservation, as clearly indicated by the following comment (Strauss & Kaechele 1998, p. 158): "Reactions include uneasiness with respect to the potentially dangerous political tendency to declare a set of manualized treatments, dealing with specific disorders according to the DSM, as scientifically validated and recommendable to those who finance the health system." Consequently, one of the first steps in closing the gap between science and practice is to adapt the treatments that have been developed in research settings to fit real-world clinical settings. This would involve changing the behavior of practitioners from different disciplines. However, in order to make such adoption a success, we need to study the characteristics of the practice environment that hinder or facilitate the adoption process. As shown by Glisson and Himmelgarn (1998), the environment in which mental health providers work has an impact on the providers' attitudes, motivations, and behaviors. These, in turn, influence the child's outcomes. Therefore, our main task is to ensure the transfer of science-based information and services into everyday practice (i.e., dissemination and implementation) and to examine factors (such as organizational factors, training, and policy requirements necessary for successful adoption) that may hinder this process.

The next stage of research in Europe should be first to conduct methodologically sound treatment studies, using manual-guided interventions with established empirically validated efficacy (discussed elsewhere in this volume). Since these intervention strategies differ from usual care, educational efforts are needed to promote the acceptance of these new approaches. Second, treatment outcomes should be evaluated covering not only abstinence or relapse status but also the adolescents' psychosocial functioning in various life domains, such as school and leisure time activities. Third, the efficacy of different treatment strategies in different groups of adolescents (e.g., from different ethnic backgrounds, with comorbid disorders) requires evaluation and "treatment-matching" studies should be conducted: since not all adolescents respond equally to the same treatment, it is important to match each adolescent to a specific treatment modality (Bukstein, 1995). Therefore, in spite of the many advances that have been achieved in recent years, there is much more to be done in the future.

REFERENCES

Aalto-Setälä, T., Marttunen, M., Tulio-Henriksson, A., Poikolainen, K., & Lönnqvist, J. (2001). One-month prevalence of depression and other DSM-IV disorders among young adults. *Psychological Medicine*, **31**, 791–801.

Adams, G., Cantwell, A. M., & Matheis, S. (2002). Substance use and adolescence. In C. A. Essau (ed.), *Substance Abuse and Dependence in adolescence* (pp. 1–20). London: Brunner-Routledge.

Aust, R., Sharp, C., & Goulden, C. (2002). *Prevalence of Drug Use: Key findings from the 2001/2002 British Crime Survey*. London: Home Office.

Balding, J. (1997). *Young People and Illegal Drugs in 1996*. Exeter, UK: University of Exeter Press.

Beman, D. S. (1995). Risk factors leading to adolescent substance abuse. *Adolescence*, **30**, 201–208.

Boys, A., Marsden, J., Fountain, J., & Griffiths, P. (1999). What influences young people's use of drugs? A qualitative study of decision-making. *Drugs: Education, Prevention and Policy*, **6**, 373–385.

BzgA (Federal Centre for Health Education) (2001). *Die Drogenaffinität Jugendlicher in der Bundesrepublik Deutschland 2001*. Köln: Bundeszentrale für gesundheitliche Aufklärung.

Bukstein, O. G. (1995). *Adolescent substance abuse*. New York: John Wiley.

Canals, J., Domenech, E., Carbajo, G., & Blade, J. (1997). Prevalence of DSM-III-R and ICD-10 psychiatric disorders in a Spanish population of 18-year-olds. *Acta Psychiatrica Scandinavica*, **96**, 287–294.

Council of the European Union (2000). *EU-Action Plan on Drugs 2000–2004*. Brussels: Council of the European Union.

Currie, C., Hurrelmann, K., Settertobulte, W., Smith, R., & Todd, J. (2000). *Health and Health Behaviour among Young People*. Copenhagen: World Health Organization. www.ruhbc.ed.ac.uk/hbsc/download/hbsc.pdf.

Dadds, M. R. & McAloon, J. (2002). Prevention. In C. A. Essau (ed.), *Substance Abuse and Dependence in Adolescence*. London: Brunner-Routledge.

EMCDDA (European Monitoring Centre for Drugs and Drug Addiction) (2002). *Annual report on the State of the Drug Problem in the European Union and Norway*. Luxembourg: European Monitoring Centre for Drugs and Drug Addiction. http://www.emcdda.eu.int.

Essau, C. A., Karpinski, N. A., Petermann, F., & Conradt, J. (1998). Häufigkeit und Komorbidität von Störungen durch Substanzkonsum. *Zeitschrift Kindheit und Entwicklung*, **7**, 199–207.

Essau, C. A., Barrett, P., & Pasquali, K. (2002). Concluding remarks. In C. A. Essau (ed.), *Substance Abuse and Dependence in Adolescence* (pp. 225–238). London: Brunner-Routledge.

Gabhainn, S. & François, Y. (2000). Substance use. In C. Currie, K. Hurrelmann, W. Settertobulte, R. Smith, & J. Todd (eds.),. *WHO Policy Series: Health Policy for Children and Adolescents (HEPCA)*, No. 1: *Health and Health Behaviour Among Young People*. Copenhagen: World Health Organization Regional Office for Europe.

Gasser-Steiner, P. & Stigler, H. (1997). *Jugendlicher Drogenkonsum: Epidemiologische Befunde und sozialwissenschaftliche Modelle. Zur Verbreitung des Konsums legaler und illegaler Drogen in der Steiermark.* Graz: Karl-Franzens University.

Glisson, C. & Hemmelgarn, A. (1998). The effects of organizational climate and interorganizational coordination on the quality and outcomes of children's service systems. *Child Abuse and Neglect,* **22**, 401–421.

Hawkins, J. D., Catalano, R. F., & Miller, J. Y. (1992) Risk and protective factors for alcohol and other drug problems in adolescence and early adulthood: implications for substance abuse prevention. *Psychological Bulletin,* **112**, 64–105.

Hibell, B., Andersson, B., Ahlstrom, S., *et al.* (2000). *The ESPAD (European School Survey Project on Alcohol and Other Drugs) Report: Alcohol and Other Drug Use Among Students in 30 European Countries.* Stockholm: CAN.

Holly, A., Türk, D., Nelson, B., Pfister, H., & Wittchen, H.-U. (1997). Prävalenz von Alkoholkonsum, Alkoholmissbrauch und abhängigkeit bei Jugendlichen und jungen Erwachsenen. *Zeitschrift für Klinische Psychologie,* **26**, 171–178.

Hupkens, C. L. H., Knibbe, R. A., & Drop, M. J. (1993). Alcohol consumption in the European Community: uniformity and diversity in drinking patterns. *Addiction,* **88**, 1391–1404.

Lieb, R., Merikangas, K. R., Höfler, M., *et al.* (2002). Parental alcohol use disorders and alcohol use and disorders in offspring: a community study. *Psychological Medicine,* **32**, 63–78.

Kessler, R. C., McGonagle, K. A., Zhao, S., *et al.* (1994). Lifetime and 12-month prevalence of DSM-III-R psychiatric disorders in the United States: results from the National Comorbidity Survey. *Archives of General Psychiatry,* **51**, 8–19.

Konings, E., Dubois-Arber, F., Narring, F., & Michaud, P. (1995). Identifying adolescent drug users: results of a national survey on adolescent health in Switzerland. *Journal of Adolescence Health,* **16**, 240–247.

Kumpulainen, K. & Roine, S. (2002). Depressive symptoms at the age of 12 years and future heavy alcohol use. *Addictive Behaviors,* **27**, 425–436.

Kumpulainen, K., Rasanen, E., Roine, S., & Hamalainen, M. (2000). Heavy alcohol use and psychiatric deviance among 15-year-olds. *Journal of Substance Use,* **4**, 203–210.

Madianos, M. G., Gefou-Madianou, D., Richardson, C., & Stefanis, C. N. (1995). Factors affecting illicit and licit drug use among adolescent and young adults in Greece. *Acta Psychiatrica Scandinavia,* **91**, 258–264.

Morgan, M., Hibell, B., Andersson, B., *et al.* (1999). The ESPAD study: implications for prevention. *Drugs: Education, Prevention and Policy,* **6**, 243–256.

Perkonigg, A., Lieb, R., & Wittchen, H. U. (1997). Prevalence of use, abuse and dependence of illicit drugs among adolescents and young adults in a community sample. *European Addiction Research,* **134**, 1–15.

Poikolainen, K., Tuulio-Henriksson, A., Aalto-Setäla, T., Marttunen, M., & Lönnqvist, J. (2001a). Predictors of alcohol intake and heavy drinking in early adulthood: a 5-year follow-up of 15–19 year old Finnish adolescents. *Alcohol and Alcoholism,* **36**, 85–88.

Poikolainen, K., Tuulio-Henriksson, A., Aalto-Setäla, T., *et al.* (2001b). Correlates of initiation to cannabis use: a 5-year follow-up of 15–19 year old adolescents. *Drug and Alcohol Dependence,* **62**, 175–180.

Prescott-Clarke, P. and Primatesta, P. (1997). *Health Survey for England: The Health of Young People '95–97.* London: Department of Health. http://www.official–documents.co.uk/document/doh/survey97/hse95.htm.

Pudney, S. (2002). *The Road to Ruin? Sequences of Initiation into Drug Use and Offending by Young People in Britain.* London: Home Office Research, Development and Statistics Directorate.

Settertobulte, W., Jensen, B. B., & Hurrelmann, K. (2001). *Drinking Among Young Europeans.* Copenhagen: World Health Organization. http://www.euro.who.int/document/E71921.pdf.

Simon, R., Hoch, E., Hüllinghorst, R., Nöcker, G., & David-Spickermann, M. (2001). *Federal Report on the Drug Situation in Germany 2001.* Munich: German Reference Centre for the European Monitoring Centre for Drugs and Drug Addiction.

Steinhausen, H. C. & Metzke, C. W. (1998). Frequency and correlates of substance use among preadolescents and adolescents in a Swiss epidemiological study. *Journal of Child Psychology and Psychiatry,* **39**, 387–397.

Strauss, B. M. & Kaechele, H. (1998). The writing on the wall: comments on the current discussion about empirically validated treatments in Germany. *Psychotherapy Research,* **8**, 158–170.

Sullivan, T. & Farrell, A. D. (2002). Risk factors. In C. A. Essau (ed.), *Substance Abuse and Dependence in Adolescence* (pp. 87–118). London: Brunner-Routledge.

UK Drug Strategy Directorate (1998). *The Government's Ten Year Strategy for Tacking Drugs.* London: The stationery office. http://www.archive.official-documents.co.uk/document/cm39/3945/3945.htm.

von Sydow, K., Lieb, R., Pfister, H., Höfler, M., & Wittchen, H.-U. (2002). What predicts incident use of cannabis and progression to abuse and dependence? A four-year prospective examination of risk factors in a community sample of adolescent and young adults. *Drug and Alcohol Dependence,* **68**, 49–64.

Verhulst, F. C., van der Ende, J., Ferdinand, R. F., & Kasius, M. C. (1997). The prevalence of DSM-III-R diagnoses in a national sample of Dutch adolescents. *Archives of General Psychiatry,* **54**, 329–336.

Wennberg, P., Andersson, T., & Bohman, M. (2002). Psychosocial characteristics at age 10; differentiating between alcohol use pathways: a prospective longitudinal study. *Addictive Behaviors,* **27**, 115–130.

Wittchen, H.-U., Nelson, C. B., & Lachner, G. (1998). Prevalence of mental disorders and psychosocial impairments in adolescents and young adults. *Psychological Medicine,* **28**, 109–126.

Wittchen, H.-U. & Pfister, H. (1996). *DIA-X-Manual: Instrumentsmanual zur Durchführung von DIA-X-Interviews.* Frankfurt: Swets & Zeitlinger.

7

The Drug Abuse Treatment Outcomes Studies: outcomes with adolescent substance abusers

Christine Grella

Integrated Substance Abuse Programs, University of California at Los Angeles, Los Angeles, CA, USA

Large-scale studies of drug abuse treatment effectiveness provide benchmarks that can be used to gauge drug abuse treatment services at a given point in time, as well as over time. Such large-scale studies have inherent strengths and weaknesses: they provide a broad view of the nature of treatment services offered in community-based programs, yet, because of their breadth, they do not address the implementation or effectiveness of specific clinical treatment approaches. Consequently, national evaluation studies are best suited to examining global questions about the characteristics of individuals who utilize substance abuse treatment across a broad sample of settings and the outcomes associated with their treatment participation. Findings from these studies can help to advance the field by identifying gaps in existing treatment systems and, by informing the development of both clinical and policy approaches, to improve the quality of treatment provided.

Since the 1970s, three national treatment outcome studies sponsored by the NIDA have been conducted in the USA. The goals of these studies have been to examine the effectiveness of substance abuse treatment, to provide information for policy makers that can be used for developing national treatment plans and policies, and to obtain information that can be used to improve service delivery and clinical practices. In this chapter, we provide a brief review of the first two national treatment outcome studies (the Drug Abuse Reporting Program [DARP] and Treatment Outcome Perspectives Study [TOPS]) and examine in depth the last study (Drug Abuse Treatment Outcome Studies for Adolescents [DATOS-A]), which was the first to include a separate sample of adolescents who were treated in adolescent-oriented programs. We discuss the methodological features of these studies, within the historical contexts that they were undertaken; the major findings from these national treatment-outcome studies and the clinical and policy implications of these findings; and the future role of such studies, including research questions that remain to be addressed. Key aspects of the research designs and the characteristics of clients in these three studies are summarized in Table 7.1.

Adolescent Substance Abuse: Research and Clinical Advances, ed. Howard A. Liddle and Cynthia L. Rowe. Published by Cambridge University Press. © Cambridge University Press 2006.

Table 7.1 Characteristics of the youth sample in three national drug treatment outcome studies

	DARP	TOPS	DATOS-A
Sample recruitment	1969–1973	1979–1981	1993–1995
Intake sample size	6259	1042	3382
Treatment modality (%)			
Therapeutic community/residential	22.6	38.6	48.1
Outpatient drug-free	50.8	61.4	24.4
Outpatient methadone	11.4	NA	NA
Detox	15.2	NA	NA
Short-term inpatient	NA	NA	27.5
Follow-up sample size	587[a]	240[b]	1785[c]
Gender of intake sample (%)			
Male	66.0	67.0	73.8
Female	35.0	33.0	26.2
Ethnicity of intake sample (%)			
White	60.1	80.0	51.6
African-American	26.3	20.0	23.9
Hispanic	12.2	NA	20.5
Other	1.3	NA	4.0
Age range of intake sample (%)			
≤ 17 years	51.4	56.6	91.1
18–19 years	48.6	43.4	8.9
Substance use (%)			
Opiate[d]	66.8	15.8	4.8
Alcohol, heavy[e]	NA	40.8	33.8
Marijuana	46.8[d]	54.3[f]	80.4[f]
Prior drug treatment (%)	NA	21.5	30.2

NA, data not available.

[a] Interviewed at 4–6 years following admission; 87% location rate for total follow-up sample.

[b] Interviewed approximately 1 year after leaving treatment; interview rate is 57% for youth < 18 years and 73% for youth aged 18–19 years.

[c] Interviewed approximately 12 months after discharge; location and follow-up rates in Kristiansen & Hubbard (2001).

[d] Weekly or more frequent use.

[e] Defined as drinking five or more drinks in one sitting at least weekly.

[f] Daily use.

Drug Abuse Reporting Program

The first USA large-scale national drug abuse treatment outcome study conducted by NIDA (begun under the National Institute of Mental Health) was DARP. The intake sample consisted of approximately 44 000 admissions to 52 drug treatment facilities throughout the USA and Puerto Rico. Patients were sampled from four treatment modalities over three consecutive cohorts from 1969 to 1973: therapeutic community, outpatient drug-free (non-methadone) (ODF), outpatient methadone maintenance, and detoxification. The DARP study predated the widespread development of specialized substance abuse treatment programs for youth; therefore, youth sampled in DARP were treated in the same programs as adult patients. Most younger patients were admitted to residential programs or ODF programs; in the 1971–1972 DARP cohort, 47% of ODF admissions and 44% of therapeutic community admissions were of people younger than 21 years of age.

Characteristics of the youth admissions

Among the 6259 youth in the admission sample, one third were female; the sample was approximately equally divided between patients under 18 years of age and those aged 18 or 19; and ethnicity was 60% White, 26% African-American, 8.8% Puerto Rican, and 3.4% Mexican-American. The proportions of males relative to females, and African-Americans relative to Whites increased with age. Approximately half (51%) of the youth were treated in ODF programs, 23% were treated in therapeutic communities, 15% were in detoxification, and 11% received methadone maintenance treatment.

The subsample of White and African-American youth in DARP who were 19 years and younger (5405) was analyzed separately with regard to their characteristics at treatment admission, time in treatment, type of discharge from treatment, and post-treatment outcomes (Sells & Simpson, 1979).[1] Youth in DARP had distinctive patterns of drug use and treatment utilization by age and ethnicity. In general, African-American youth were older at the onset of first drug use and at treatment admission, and they were more likely to be daily opioid users. White youth were younger at the onset of drug use and more likely to be non-opioid users. Accordingly, African-American youth had higher rates of methadone treatment, whereas White youth had higher rates of treatment in ODF programs. Similarly, daily use of opioids was more common among older youth, since these youth were more likely to have been sampled from methadone treatment.

---

[1] The subsample was restricted to White and African-American youth in order to conduct analyses by ethnicity, age, and modality; Puerto Rican and Mexican American subjects were dropped from analyses because their number was too small.

Treatment retention and posttreatment outcomes

Time in treatment and discharge status were examined in DARP as key indicators of therapeutic progress. In general, younger clients in DARP remained in treatment longer than the total sample. The youth subsample stayed in therapeutic community treatment for a median of 96 days compared with 90 days for the total sample; the median days in ODF treatment for youth was 117 compared with 108 for the total sample. Conversely, youth treated in methadone programs had shorter lengths of stay than the total sample (median days of 267 versus 380, respectively); however, this was probably a function of age restrictions that precluded their participation in methadone treatment prior to the age of 18. African-American youth aged 18–19 years had longer retention in therapeutic community programs compared with White youth (63% and 56% over 60 days, respectively), but shorter retention in ODF programs (55% and 73% over 60 days, respectively). The youth subsample had higher rates of treatment completion than the total sample in methadone treatment (14% versus 7%) and ODF treatment (27% and 22%, respectively) however, drop-out rates for youth were relatively high, ranging from 67% in therapeutic community treatment to 48% in ODF programs.

Follow-up analyses were conducted with data collected 4–6 years after admission from 587 youth, of whom 38% were African-American and 62% were White. Comparisons at follow-up were made between the youth subsample and the total sample, as well as between older and younger youth ($<$ 18 years versus $\geq$ 18 years), and between White and African-American youth. Opioid use decreased following treatment from 93% to 33% among those in methadone treatment, from 76% to 9% among those in therapeutic community treatment, and from 49% to 15% among those in ODF treatment. Marijuana use remained about the same for White youth, but increased among African-Americans to a level equivalent to that of Whites: approximately 70% at follow-up. Alcohol use was relatively low in the youth sample overall (approximately 10%), slightly increased among those in methadone treatment, remained stable among those in therapeutic community treatment, and slightly decreased among those in ODF treatment at follow-up. Employment increased in all groups, but White youth in the older age group (18–19 years) had the largest increase. Similarly, this group had the greatest decrease in criminal activity. Overall, the White youth in the older age group had the most favorable outcomes, and African-American youth in the younger age group ($<$ 18 years) had the least favorable outcomes. Hence, these adult-oriented programs appeared to be most effective for older youth whose drug use patterns were more similar to those of adults. Younger adolescents, particularly African-Americans, fared less well in these mainstream treatment programs.

In sum, DARP provided the first USA national examination of the characteristics and outcomes of youth entering into non-specialized drug treatment programs in the early 1970s. Both the characteristics of these youth and the programs where they received treatment reflected this historical period, when heroin and other opioids were the predominant substances used among individuals entering drug treatment in the USA. Although this study showed that opioid use was reduced following treatment, there was little improvement in either alcohol or marijuana use among youth. These findings from DARP established the importance of addressing adolescent-specific treatment issues, as well as the need to examine differences in the characteristics and outcomes of youth by ethnicity, age group, and types of substance used. The lack of information specific to adolescent-treatment issues, such as developmental aspects of alcohol and drug use, the influence of family members and peers on the treatment process, and the prevalence of co-occurring disorders among young substance abusers, foreshadowed a growing need to develop adolescent-specific treatment approaches, which would become more commonplace in the ensuing decade.

Treatment Outcomes Prospective Study

The TOPS was the second of NIDA's national treatment outcome studies. Individuals were sampled from 1979 to 1981 in 10 cities from three types of treatment modalities: residential, ODF, and outpatient methadone. As with DARP, youth were intermingled with adults in the same treatment settings. Programs that were school based or designed specifically for adolescents were excluded from the study design (Hubbard *et al.*, 1985). Overall, 18% of the 1042 TOPS patients admitted to residential and outpatient programs were adolescents (less than 20 years of age); they constituted 14% of residential program admissions, and 22% of the ODF clients (Hubbard *et al.*, 1989).[2]

Youth characteristics

Approximately two thirds (67%) of the adolescent sample in TOPS were male and over 80% were White (Hubbard *et al.*, 1985). Most (61%) were treated in outpatient programs, with the remainder (39%) treated in residential programs. About 80% of the males and 65% of the females less than 18 years of age lived with their families; the remainder lived independently of their families of origin. About two thirds of youth in residential programs and close to 90% of those in outpatient programs had no prior treatment for drug abuse. As with adults in drug treatment, males reported higher rates of criminal activity than did females.

---

[2] Youth less than 21 years of age constituted 2.1% of subjects admitted to methadone maintenance treatment; however, given their small number, these youth were not included in analyses of the youth subsample.

Reflecting changes in the epidemiology of substance use from the 1970s to the 1980s, TOPS included clients who used a broader range of substances, especially cocaine, and who used multiple substances. Marijuana was the most frequently reported primary drug of abuse among youth, although the rates of use were higher among males than females and among patients in outpatient than in residential programs. Females in residential treatment who were 18–19 years old had the highest rates of cocaine, heroin, and amphetamines as their primary drugs of abuse. Males aged 18–19 years had the highest rates of heavy alcohol use (i.e., use of five or more drinks in one sitting at least weekly), and rates of heavy alcohol use were higher among patients in residential than in outpatient programs. Females had higher rates of depressive symptoms; three quarters reported at least one symptom of depression across age and modality groups, compared with about half of the males (varying by age and modality).

In-treatment services provided to youth

TOPS included measures of services received during the first 3 months of treatment (based on self-report) to enable examination of variation in service delivery by modality and patient characteristics. About three quarters of youth in residential programs and two thirds of those in ODF programs reported receiving two or more services while in treatment. Females received more types of service in both modalities. Psychological and family-related services were most frequently reported, although there was considerable variation across gender, age, and modality. Over half of the youth in ODF programs received family-related services, although the rates were lowest for males aged 18–19 years (30%). Youth in residential programs had higher rates of educational services, particularly those younger than 18 years old (over 75%). However, greater proportions of youth reported needs for services than actually received services in some areas. Unmet needs (i.e., youth who needed but did not receive services) were highest for employment services among youth in outpatient programs (22%), and for employment and financial services (about 50% unmet needs), family services (41%), and legal services (18%) among youth in residential programs.

Treatment retention and post-treatment outcomes

Rates of treatment retention were generally low among adolescents treated in TOPS. Only approximately one third remained in treatment for more than 3 months and over one third left treatment within 30 days in both types of treatment, although clients in ODF programs tended to drop out of treatment more rapidly. Comparisons made with DARP showed that retention rates were lower among participants in TOPS. Among youth treated in DARP, one in every eight admitted to residential treatment left within the first 30 days, as did about one quarter of youth in ODF programs, compared with approximately one third of the youth in both types of program in TOPS. Although the lack of comparable data on patient characteristics in DARP and TOPS prevents direct comparisons of patient severity, it is possible that these lower retention levels reflect greater problem severity among patients in TOPS than in DARP, as well as greater problems in integrating these younger patients in the TOPS programs.

Analyses were conducted with the subsample of 240 youth who received follow-up interviews at approximately 1-year after treatment (conducted from May 1980 to December 1982). The follow-up sample was stratified by modality and time in treatment to ensure sufficient representation for sub-group analyses on these variables. Among youth in residential programs, more positive behavioral changes were found in the first year after treatment for those who remained in treatment for 3 months or more. The results for adolescents treated in ODF programs were mixed, however, and generally were not as good as those for youth in residential programs. Daily marijuana use among youth in outpatient programs declined from approximately half of the sample to approximately one fourth. There was little change in the proportion of patients reporting heavy alcohol use, however, which remained at one third or more of the sample, depending on age and time in treatment. Weekly or more frequent use of drugs other than marijuana or alcohol declined from approximately one half of the sample prior to treatment to approximately one third of the sample in the year after treatment. Although the proportion of patients reporting drug-related problems decreased substantially, approximately half still reported a drug-related problem in the year after treatment. Suicidal thoughts or attempts were reported by approximately one fifth of the patients after treatment, compared with over half who reported such thoughts or attempts in the year prior to treatment.

Overall, TOPS established the complexity of problems among youth who were admitted into adult-oriented drug treatment programs in the late 1970s and early 1980s, including the interrelationships of drug use, criminality, family problems, and psychological distress. TOPS also furthered our understanding of how youth treatment outcomes differed by gender, age, and type of treatment received. Reflecting advances from research into the effectiveness of substance abuse treatment, TOPS assessed a broader range of indicators of psychosocial functioning compared with DARP, such as problems related to drug use across functional domains. Further, consistent with a growing emphasis on health-services-related research, TOPS assessed the types of service received while in treatment and the degree to which services received matched self-perceived needs.

TOPS provided evidence that positive behavioral changes occurred subsequent to treatment participation, especially for youth who stayed in treatment longer; however, the study also demonstrated that outcomes were not uniform across age groups or treatment modalities. Yet, given its focus on "adult" treatment programs, TOPS did not address more complex issues related to social, psychological, and developmental processes of adolescent substance abuse, and how treatment for youth should be designed to address these issues. At the time that TOPS was underway, studies in this area were making significant advances in conceptualizing and identifying the risk factors for and consequences of substance abuse among youth (Botvin & Botvin, 1992; Jessor & Jessor, 1977; Hawkins, Catalano, & Miller, 1992; Newcomb & Bentler, 1988) yet this emerging context had not yet been incorporated within national treatment outcome research on youth.

The Drug Abuse Treatment Outcome Studies

Findings from both DARP and TOPS underscored the need for distinctive treatment approaches for substance-abusing adolescents. Reflecting the increased recognition of this need, beginning in the 1970s, some programs began developing special treatment tracks for adolescents or separate programs specifically for youth (Kajdan & Senay, 1976). Specialized youth programs continued to increase in numbers throughout the 1980s, along with the development of treatment protocols specifically for youth (Dennis *et al.*, 2003). As a result, the third national treatment outcome evaluation study sponsored by NIDA was designed to include a separate cohort of adolescents sampled from youth-oriented treatment programs. The DATOS program included both adult and adolescent cohorts, the latter known as DATOS-A. Concurrent with the growth in specialized programs for adolescents, admissions of younger patients to drug treatment programs not specializing in adolescent treatment declined over this time. Only approximately 5% of DATOS admissions to residential or outpatient programs (in the "adult" sample) were less than 20 years of age, compared with approximately one quarter of those in DARP and one fifth of those in TOPS.

With some modifications to account for issues specific to adolescents (Kristiansen & Hubbard, 2001), the DATOS-A followed the general research design used in the adult DATOS study (Flynn *et al.*, 1997). The intake sample consisted of approximately 3000 admissions between 1993 and 1995 to 13 residential, nine short-term inpatient (STI), and 14 ODF programs specifically intended to treat adolescent drug abusers in six cities (Chicago, Miami, Minneapolis, New York, Pittsburgh, and Portland, OR). Subjects were not sampled from methadone maintenance treatment facilities, as in the adult DATOS and in the previous national studies, given the regulation that individuals admitted to methadone treatment be at least 18 years of age. Subjects received a comprehensive assessment at intake into treatment and were assessed (if still enrolled) after 1, 3, and 6 months in treatment with regard to services received and various treatment processes. A subset of the sample (1785) received a 12-month post-treatment follow-up interview. In addition, information on program characteristics and treatment services was collected from administrators of the participating programs (Fletcher & Grella, 2001).

Characteristics of programs in the youth study

Programs included in DATOS-A were recruited from six of the same cities where the adult DATOS study was conducted in order to utilize the existing research infrastructure that had been established for recruiting, interviewing, and tracking subjects for follow-up (Kristiansen & Hubbard, 2001). In those locations, adolescent-based programs were recruited for study participation if they had been in existence for at least 2–3 years and were judged by the study investigators to be typical community-based treatment providers. These programs were viewed as stable, ongoing providers that would remain viable throughout the study period. Moreover, the study programs were required to have a rate of patient admission of at least five patients per month. Lastly, all programs had to agree to participate in the research protocols for subject recruitment and assessment, including all human subjects requirements. No programs that were selected to participate refused study participation, although programs that were demonstration projects or primarily designed for research or for special populations other than adolescents were excluded from the sampling frame.

All programs in DATOS-A were either entirely adolescent based or had a separate program component for adolescents, and all primarily treated drug problems (including alcohol use), as opposed to providing primary alcohol treatment. Most had a mixture of funding from both public and private sources. They averaged 14 years in operation. Programs reflected a variety of treatment orientations, clinical interventions, and services. The treatment provided was not manual driven nor based on experimental or enhanced treatment protocols. Below is a brief description of the types of service provided within each treatment modality, based on the survey of program administrators.

Residential treatment programs

Residential programs were a mixture of milieu treatment and therapeutic communities. The programs provided residential living, education, counseling sessions, and interventions designed to resocialize patients. One half of the residential programs provided group sessions almost daily, and 88% provided individual counseling sessions at least once per week. One half of the programs provided had a "major" emphasis on family therapy (based on three-point scale, ranging from none to major). Planned or recommended duration of stay ranged from 3 to 12 months (median, 5 months). Many of the residential programs modified their approach to accommodate adolescents (e.g., shortening the duration of treatment, placing less emphasis on confrontation, and incorporating parents and family members in treatment).

Outpatient drug-free programs

The ODF programs included regular and intensive day treatment. Services included counseling sessions, education, and skills training. Approximately 78% of the programs provided group sessions three or more times per week; 56% of the programs had individual sessions once per week; and 22% of programs had individual sessions two to three times per week. All but one reported great emphasis on family therapy. Planned duration of treatment ranged from 1 to 6 months (median, 1.6 months).

Short-term inpatient programs

The STI programs provided services (e.g., counseling sessions and 12-step groups) within a medically controlled environment. A majority of the programs had daily group sessions and weekly individual sessions. All reported a strong emphasis on family therapy. Planned duration of stay ranged from 5 to 35 days (median, 18 days). Patients were typically referred for continued outpatient treatment at discharge.

Youth characteristics

The youth sampled in DATOS-A have a distinct profile from that of adults in treatment, which reflects their unique patterns of treatment referral and access, age-related developmental processes, and earlier stage of development of their drug use and treatment careers (Anglin *et al.*, 2001; Hser *et al.*, 1997). Further, adolescent patient profiles differed by modality (Rounds-Bryant, Kristiansen, & Hubbard, 1999). Generally, adolescents in ODF had lower levels of problem severity than those in STI or residential programs, with a somewhat lower percentage of patients meeting drug-dependence diagnoses and a higher percentage of referrals to treatment from family and friends. Patients in ODF programs were also slightly younger than patients in the other modalities and were more likely to be attending school at the time of treatment admission. The STI programs had a higher percentage of patients with mental health disorders and who had private insurance coverage. Patients in residential programs were more likely to be criminally involved, to be under legal supervision at the time of treatment admission, and to have been referred to treatment through the legal system (Hser *et al.*, 2001).

Demographic characteristics

Participants in DATOS-A were primarily aged 15–16 years (mean, 15.7; SD, 1.3). The majority of subjects were male (73.8%), with more males in residential treatment (82%) than in STI (60%) or ODF (62%) programs. Approximately half of the subjects were White, close to one quarter (24%) were African-American, and 21% were Hispanic, although there were more African-Americans in residential programs (28%) and more Whites in STI programs (79%).

Drug use

Because of their younger age, adolescents in drug treatment have generally used substances for shorter periods of time than adults in drug treatment and hence are less likely to have developed the problems typically associated with chronic drug usage. Nevertheless, youth who entered into treatment in DATOS-A often displayed symptoms of dependence and many met dependence criteria based on DSM-III-R (American Psychiatric Association, 1987). Close to two thirds of adolescents in DATOS-A (73%) met criteria for alcohol and/or drug dependence: 64% met dependence criteria for marijuana, 36% for alcohol, and 10% for cocaine. In contrast to adults in drug treatment and to youth in the previous national treatment outcomes studies, only a small percentage was dependent on opiates (approximately 3%). Approximately, 80% of the sample reported using marijuana at least weekly in the year prior to treatment entry, and nearly half (48%) reported use of other drugs (e.g., cocaine, heroin, stimulants, hallucinogens). One quarter of the sample reported having used three or more substances.

Mental disorders

Studies of adolescents in alcohol and drug abuse treatment have estimated that as many as 75% of drug-abusing adolescents have a comorbid mental disorder, with conduct disorder, affective disorders, and attention-deficit hyperactivity disorder (ADHD) being the most prevalent (Brown *et al.*, 1996; Crowley *et al.*, 1998; Greenbaum, Foster-Johnson, & Petrila, 1996). By the time DATOS-A was developed, major improvement had been made in the methods for obtaining psychiatric diagnoses with adolescents, including the use of manual-guided assessments based on standardized diagnostic criteria (Orvaschel, 1994). DATOS-A included assessments of several mental disorders based on DSM-III-R criteria.

The prevalence rates for comorbid disorders among youth in DATOS-A were fairly consistent with those found in other studies conducted with adolescents in substance abuse treatment, which are mostly derived from small-scale clinical trials or demonstration programs for youth. Among patients in DATOS-A, 63% had a comorbid mental disorder: 57% had conduct disorder, 15% had major depression, and 12% had ADHD (Grella *et al.*, 2001). Most of those with either depression or ADHD were also diagnosed with conduct disorder.

Youth with conduct disorder, depressive disorder, and/or ADHD had a more severe profile of substance use prior to treatment admission. Youth with comorbid problems had initiated alcohol and marijuana use at earlier ages; had higher rates of dependence on marijuana, alcohol, and cocaine; and had used more substances than the non-comorbid adolescents. They also reported more family, school, or legal-related problems at the time of treatment admission. Interestingly, youth with conduct disorder had higher levels of treatment motivation (i.e., problem recognition, desire for help, and treatment readiness) at the time of admission, which may be related to their higher levels of problem severity (Hser *et al.*, 2003).

Criminal involvement

The connection between criminal activity and substance use among adults who enter drug treatment is well established, but much less is known about the interrelationship of drug use and criminal behavior among youth, as well as the treatment outcomes among juvenile offenders. Approximately, two thirds of youth in DATOS-A were criminally active at the time of treatment admission (defined as being on probation or parole, awaiting trial or having a case pending, or reporting a period of weekly involvement in illegal activities during the past year), with the highest rate among patients in residential programs (89%) and the lowest rate among those in outpatient programs (47%). Over half were involved with the legal system at the time of treatment entry. The likelihood of being under legal supervision was higher for youth who were male, who were African-American or Hispanic, who were not attending school, who reported having family or friends who were involved in crime and/or drug use, who had conduct disorder, and who came from households that did not have two parents (Farabee *et al.*, 2001). There were no differences, however, between groups based on legal status with regard to frequency of alcohol and drug use at treatment admission.

Comparison of the Treatment Outcome Perspectives Study and the Drug Abuse Treatment Outcomes Studies

Changes in characteristics of adolescents in TOPS & DATOS-A

The use of similar instruments, common measures, and research designs allowed for comparative analyses over time, treatment sites, and study populations in TOPS (1979 to 1981) and DATOS-A (1993 to 1995) for residential and ODF modalities (STI programs were not included in TOPS) (Etheridge *et al.*, 2001). Patients in DATOS-A were younger than those in TOPS; approximately 60% of DATOS-A patients were 14 and 15 years of age compared with 27% in TOPS. The DATOS-A sample had significantly lower concentrations of Whites and higher concentrations of African-American and Hispanic youth. Moreover, there were more males in residential programs in DATOS-A than in TOPS. The rate of referral by the criminal justice system to residential treatment was higher in

DATOS-A than TOPS, reflecting the increased importance of the criminal justice system as a conduit to drug treatment for youth. A larger percentage of patients in DATOS-A had public insurance, whereas a smaller percentage had no insurance compared with TOPS.

In general, patients in DATOS-A appeared to have less-severe substance abuse problems than those in TOPS. They had lower rates of "weekly or greater" cocaine use in residential programs, lower rates of weekly or greater marijuana use in ODF programs, and lower rates of weekly or greater use of hallucinogens. Fewer DATOS-A patients in ODF were heavy alcohol users than TOPS outpatient adolescents. Similarly, use of hallucinogens among patients in residential programs was lower in DATOS-A than in TOPS. In both TOPS and DATOS-A, and in contrast with adults in these studies, heroin use was low (less than 5% across modalities). The more severe profile of youth in TOPS may have stemmed from more selective criteria for admitting youth into adult-oriented programs, such as those in TOPS. Further, the increased rate of referrals to treatment through the criminal justice system in DATOS-A, particularly to residential programs, may reflect a lower threshold for treatment admission among youth in the juvenile justice system.

Changes in treatment service profiles

Comparisons made between TOPS and DATOS-A demonstrated that there were differences in levels of service needs and in service delivery across the two studies. However, these comparisons must be framed by the context that youth in DATOS-A were treated in specialized programs for youth, whereas those in TOPS were not. In general, there were lower rates of self-reported needs for services among youth in treatment in DATOS than in TOPS (Etheridge *et al.*, 2001). Self-reported needs for medical, psychological, family, employment, and financial services were lower among patients in ODF programs in DATOS-A compared with those in TOPS. Patients in residential programs in DATOS-A had lower needs for medical, psychological, and financial services compared with residential patients in TOPS, but they had higher needs for legal and employment services. These lower rates of service needs most likely stem from differences between youth in adult-oriented programs, as in TOPS, and youth in specialized adolescent treatment programs, as in DATOS-A. As noted previously, adolescent patients in DATOS-A were generally younger and had lower levels of drug use severity.

Although the rate of self-reported service needs was lower among youth in DATOS-A than in TOPS, the rate of service delivery in DATOS-A was also lower and partially offset the lower levels of service needs. The percentage of patients in DATOS-A reporting that they had received any mental health services was less than half of that in TOPS. However, a significantly larger percentage of patients in

DATOS-A than in TOPS had unmet needs for psychological services in both residential and ODF programs. There were also higher rates of unmet needs among patients in DATOS-A for employment services, particularly in residential programs, and for family services, particularly in ODF programs. Further, there was a greater emphasis in DATOS-A on group counseling services rather than individual counseling, particularly in ODF programs, and shorter stays in treatment, particularly in residential programs. These patterns of decreased number and intensity of services provided and increased levels of unmet needs were also found in comparisons made between adults in TOPS and DATOS (Etheridge *et al.*, 1995). These reductions in the provision of services were probably driven by cost-containment efforts that broadly affected substance abuse treatment programs in the 1990s (Etheridge *et al.*, 2001).

Much less is known about the content of substance abuse treatment for adolescents than for adults, such as the types of service typically provided, the degree of involvement of family members in treatment, the characteristics and training of staff, and the structure and financing of programs. One study conducted with data obtained from program administrators in DATOS-A showed that there were distinct profiles of services provided by programs within each of the treatment modalities, and these service profiles were related both to organizational factors and to patient-problem profiles (Delany *et al.*, 2001). Among ODF programs, three clusters of service arrays were found, from minimal (i.e., psychiatric, family, after-care) to a fairly broad range (i.e., psychiatric, educational, vocational, legal, family, after-care). Accreditation was positively related to a broader range of service offerings in ODF programs, and there was a tendency for ODF programs with a greater diversity of patient needs and greater staff resources to offer a wider array of services. Among residential programs, the primary distinction in the availability of services was in whether programs provided financial or after-care services. Further, a higher level of professional training was related to more extensive service offerings.

Treatment processes

Given the relatively recent emergence of adolescent-oriented drug treatment programs, few studies have examined the relationships between treatment processes and treatment outcomes for adolescents (Blood & Cornwall, 1994; Dakof, Tejeda, & Liddle, 2001; Friedman & Glickman, 1986, 1987). Some studies have shown that, in addition to patient characteristics, several aspects of treatment are important predictors of positive outcomes, including treatment duration, treatment completion, and participation in after-care (Hawke, Jainchill, & De Leon, 2000; Jainchill *et al.*, 2000; Latimer *et al.*, 2000a,b; Winters *et al.*, 2000). Moreover, studies with adolescents in treatment have emphasized the role of developmental processes and the relationships between youth and their family and peers (Brown & D'Amico, 2001), and their effects upon treatment participation.

Motivation and engagement

There are few models of treatment engagement that specify how substance-abusing adolescents perceive and participate in drug treatment. One study attempted to replicate a model of treatment engagement originally developed for adults in DATOS with the DATOS-A sample (Broome, Joe, & Simpson, 2001). Although there was some variation between the models developed for patients in residential and ODF programs, in general, pretreatment social support and family/peer deviance (defined as illicit drug use, heavy alcohol use, history of arrests) were positively associated with readiness for treatment (measured by indicators of willingness to enter drug treatment as a means to addressing one's drug problem). Treatment readiness and social support, in turn, were associated with higher levels of therapeutic involvement, which was measured by indicators of confidence in treatment, commitment to treatment, and rapport with one's counselor. In contrast with models of treatment engagement developed for adults (Simpson, 2001), however, a greater degree of therapeutic engagement was not related to longer treatment retention among the adolescents in DATOS-A. Another study with DATOS-A showed that treatment compliance (defined as agreeing with treatment goals, meeting treatment expectations, and following staff instructions) was positively related to desire for help and negatively related to psychological maladjustment (Wong, Hser, & Grella, 2003).

Services received

Information on services received was obtained from youth while in treatment in DATOS-A using the seven problem areas of the Addiction Severity Index (McLellan et al., 1992). There were significant differences in the types of service and in service intensity received within the first month of treatment among youth treated in the different modalities (Grella, Joshi, & Hser, 2004). Youth treated in residential programs received more services overall, had higher rates of participation in 12-step groups, and participated in more group counseling sessions. Youth treated in STI programs had higher rates of family participation in treatment. Service matching (i.e., having received a service for which one identified a need) was least common among youth treated in ODF programs. However, the level of service delivery overall was very low. Approximately one fifth of participants (18%) received no services (other than drug treatment) during 1 month of treatment; 29% received only one other service, and 31% reported having received two additional services, although nearly all of the patients (95%) reported having two or more service needs at treatment entry. The lack of greater congruence between service needs and service delivery suggests that organizational and environmental factors, in addition to patient needs, influence access to needed services among adolescents in drug treatment (Delany *et al.*, 2001; Friedmann, Alexander, & D'Aunno, 1999). However, more research is needed to improve our understanding of the process of service delivery within adolescent-oriented treatment programs, as well as the relationships of the program with other service providers to youth. In particular, research on strategies for coordinating services across delivery systems (i.e., juvenile justice, mental health, child welfare, educational, health services) is needed to address the complex needs of youth who access treatment through these various service systems (Dembo, 1996; Nissen *et al.*, 1999; Terry *et al.*, 2000).

Retention

The adult DATOS study showed that minimum thresholds of time in treatment, specific for each modality, were associated with better post-treatment outcomes (Hubbard *et al.*, 1997; Simpson *et al.*, 1999). However, it has been unclear whether these same retention thresholds are applicable to adolescents in treatment. Overall, 58% of the patients in residential programs stayed in treatment for at least 90 days, as did 27% of the patients in ODF programs. Close to two thirds (64%) of the patients in STI programs stayed 21 or more days in treatment. One analysis demonstrated that youth who stayed in treatment for a minimum of 90 days in either residential or ODF programs, or 21 days in STI programs, had significantly better post-treatment outcomes in terms of lower rates of alcohol and drug use and of arrests compared with youth who stayed in treatment for shorter periods (Hser *et al.*, 2001).

Treatment outcomes among patients in the Drug Abuse Treatment Outcome Studies for Adolescents

The widespread development of adolescent-oriented treatment interventions and programs since the mid-1990s has yielded a body of research showing that treatment for substance-abusing youth is generally effective in reducing their drug use and other behavioral problems compared with no treatment (Williams & Chang, 2000). Although much of this research suffered from small sample sizes and methodological problems, the extant research has established the importance of examining outcomes across the domains of psychosocial functioning specific to adolescent developmental processes, including interpersonal, educational/occupational, and familial (Brown *et al.*, 1994, 2001). Several studies have shown that family dysfunction, including parental or sibling substance use (Jainchill *et al.*, 1999), social pressures to drink/use (Brown, Vik, & Creamer, 1989), and affiliation with deviant peer groups (Jainchill *et al.*, 2000) are related to treatment outcomes among substance-abusing youth. Moreover, the previous findings from DARP and TOPS showed the importance of comparing outcomes for youth treated in different types of modalities and across ethnic, gender, and age groups.

The outcome analyses from DATOS-A were restricted to the subsample of youth from four cities where follow-up rates exceeded 65% (administrative and logistical problems in the other two cities resulted in lower follow-up rates).

Drug use

In the DATOS-A study, weekly marijuana use fell from 80% in the year before treatment to 44% at the 1-year follow-up, and use of other illicit drugs fell from 48% to 42% (Hser *et al.*, 2001). Use of cocaine actually increased from 15% to 23% among youth treated in STI programs and from 9% to 17% among those in ODF programs, but it decreased from 23% to 17% among those in residential programs. Similarly, use of hallucinogens decreased among those in residential programs (31% to 19%) and stayed stable at approximately one third of that seen in the STI group and one quarter of that in the ODF programs. These findings suggest that, although marijuana is the most frequently used substance among youth in drug treatment, more attention and resources may be required to address effectively the treatment needs of the minority of adolescents who abuse drugs that are more commonly used by adults.

Alcohol use

Over half (55%) of the youth in DATOS-A either used alcohol at least weekly or had alcohol dependence. These heavy alcohol users were more likely to be female and White and had higher rates of comorbidity, other drug use, family drug use, and history of physical or sexual abuse. Overall, there were significant reductions in alcohol use from before to after treatment at the 12-month follow-up. The rate of no-use increased from 12% to 29%, and weekly or more frequent use decreased from 46% to 27%. Over half of the sample (54%) reported lower rates of alcohol use at follow-up; 22% reported an increased rate of use; 18% reported no change in the frequency of alcohol use; and 6% reported no-use at both time points (Chung *et al.*, 2003). Males were approximately one third less likely to reduce their alcohol use compared with females, and African-Americans and Hispanics were more likely to reduce their alcohol use compared with Whites.

Outcomes for youth with comorbid mental disorders

Youth in DATOS-A who had a comorbid mental disorder (i.e., conduct disorder, depressive disorder, and/or ADHD) significantly reduced their drug use and other problem behaviors following treatment (Grella *et al.*, 2001). However, consistent with other research, youth with comorbidity had poorer outcomes when compared with non-comorbid youth. They were one third more likely than non-comorbid youth to use marijuana weekly and over half as likely to use hallucinogens at the 12-month follow-up, after controlling for pretreatment levels of use. Youth with comorbid disorders were also more likely than other youth to report engaging in illegal acts and being arrested during the follow-up period. Youth with comorbid disorders had higher rates of retention, compared with non-comorbid youth, in residential programs, basically the same rates of retention in STI, but had lower rates of retention in ODF programs. These findings suggest that substance-abusing youth with co-occurring mental disorders may require more intensive treatment in order to address their more complex treatment needs.

Criminal activity

There was an overall reduction in the rate of illegal activity from 76% at treatment admission to 53% at follow-up; similarly the rates of arrest decreased from one half to one third from before to after treatment. Although the likelihood of committing a drug-related crime decreased following treatment, those adolescents under legal supervision accounted for the majority of positive change in this domain (Farabee *et al.*, 2001). Further, reductions in alcohol or marijuana use were independently associated with significant reductions in the likelihood of committing crimes following treatment.

Risk of infection with human immunodeficiency virus

Reflecting the high rates of transmission of human immunodeficiency virus (HIV) among drug users in the decade between the TOPS and DATOS-A studies, DATOS-A included assessments of attitudes and behaviors regarding HIV risk. Over half of the adolescents reported reductions in risky sex behavior (defined as having two or more sexual partners without always using a condom) after treatment, or remained at a low level of risk (Joshi *et al.*, 2001). Youth with conduct disorder, unmet physical and emotional needs, and a lower commitment to school were less likely to change their high-risk sexual behaviors. HIV risk reduction following treatment was also significantly associated with higher levels of abstinence, self-esteem, empathy, and school commitment. In contrast, higher levels of HIV risk following treatment were associated with more illegal activity, negative peer group influence, and hostility.

Differences by ethnicity

DARP and TOPS demonstrated differences in pretreatment profiles and treatment outcomes by ethnicity, as have other studies conducted with substance-abusing youth (Jainchill, De Leon, & Yagelka, 1997; Stewart, Brown, & Myers, 1998). Patients in DATOS-A were similar across ethnic groups with respect to gender, age, and type of primary drug use (Rounds-Bryant & Staab, 2001). However,

African-American and Hispanic youth were more likely than Whites to have been referred to treatment through the criminal justice system. White youth were more likely than others to meet criteria for alcohol dependence, whereas Hispanic youth had the highest rate of cocaine dependence. White youth also had higher rates of conduct disorder and depressive disorder compared with African-Americans. Approximately half of all subjects reported engaging in serious illegal activity prior to treatment, although the rate among African-Americans was significantly lower than that of Hispanics and Whites. Moreover, White youth were twice as likely as African-Americans to report criminal activity following treatment.

Differences by gender

Prior studies have established that there are gender differences among substance-abusing adolescents that have implications for treatment processes and outcomes (Latimer *et al.*, 2000b). In particular, substance-abusing girls have higher rates of internalizing symptoms and family dysfunction compared with boys (Dakof, 2000). In DATOS-A, boys had higher rates of illegal activity and involvement with the criminal justice system, whereas girls were younger and had higher rates of alcohol dependence (Rounds-Bryant *et al.*, 1998). As in studies of adults in drug treatment, females in DATOS-A were more likely to have a diagnosis of depressive disorders, higher rates of suicidal attempts, and higher rates of mental health treatment. Consistent with other studies of youth in treatment (Titus *et al.*, 2003), girls were more likely to report a history of sexual abuse, whereas boys had higher rates of physical abuse (Grella & Joshi, 2003). There were also gender differences in the rates of post-treatment outcomes and in the predictors of post-treatment abstinence (Y. I. Hser & C. E. Grella, unpublished data). For girls, criminal involvement during the follow-up period was associated with a lower likelihood of abstinence from marijuana; among boys, having a psychiatric disorder was associated with a lower likelihood of abstinence from marijuana and other illicit drugs. African-American and Hispanic males were also more likely to be abstinent from illicit drugs (other than marijuana), compared with White males, but there was no effect of ethnicity on post-treatment abstinence for girls.

Conclusions

The findings from DARP, TOPS, and DATOS-A illustrate the changes that have occurred in substance abuse treatment services provided to youth in the USA and the outcomes associated with their treatment participation over the latter part of the twentieth century. Although neither DARP nor TOPS was intended to study youth in particular, the separate analyses conducted with the youth subsamples in both of these studies provided a foundation for examining the cohort of youth sampled from specialized treatment providers in DATOS-A. Analyses conducted with DATOS-A reflected improvements in research methods that occurred subsequent to both DARP and TOPS, including the use of standardized diagnostic measures (e.g., DSM), expanded assessment domains (e.g., HIV risk, history of physical and/or sexual abuse, treatment motivation), the application of advanced statistical modeling (e.g., structural equation modeling), and the availability of data on program characteristics and in-treatment processes. These advances enabled more complex and multitiered analyses, which have expanded our understanding of treatment processes and outcomes among youth treated in youth-oriented treatment programs. Below we consider the contributions, limitations, and future directions of national drug treatment evaluation studies for youth.

In general, findings from DARP and TOPS showed that treatment outcomes for adolescents in "adult" programs were mixed at best, particularly for younger adolescents, and clearly established the importance of addressing adolescent-specific treatment issues. Moreover, the relatively low levels of treatment retention among youth in both of these studies showed the need to develop treatment practices that enhance treatment engagement and retention among youth. Findings from DATOS-A further elucidated differences between adults and adolescents who enter substance abuse treatment, particularly regarding the types of substance used, psychosocial problems associated with school and family, referral patterns and pathways to treatment, and differences by gender and ethnicity in pretreatment characteristics and treatment outcomes. DATOS-A showed that there were significant reductions in marijuana and alcohol use following treatment; however, use of other "harder" substances remained stable or even increased among a minority of the sample, suggesting that treatment was not as effective for youth who used substances other than these "entry-level" substances. Moreover, youth with multiple and more severe problems, including those with comorbid disorders, legal involvement, histories of abuse, and negative peer involvement, generally showed less-consistent behavioral improvement and pose a further challenge in requiring the development of treatment protocols that address their complex treatment needs.

Naturalistic studies, such as DATOS-A, lack comparisons with non-treatment control groups, as well as control over the treatment processes that occur within the participating programs. Consequently, attributions of causality, or "treatment effects," must be carefully qualified and conclusions about treatment effectiveness must be interpreted within the confines of these observational research designs. Moreover, as with any large-scale evaluation study, the breadth of the assessment protocol given to subjects means that data available in any one content area are typically of a more general nature and often lack the detailed assessment that is needed for more in-depth analyses. However, the relatively large sample size affords a high level of statistical power to detect group differences and enables comparisons across multiple subgroups. Although DATOS-A provided data on service delivery and treatment processes, information was not available on the nature of the clinical services delivered that would allow for assessment of the effectiveness of specific clinical or treatment protocols. Yet the strength of the research design used in DATOS-A is that it is based on patients and services in naturally occurring treatment settings, and thus has a high degree of external validity and generalizability of findings (Simpson *et al.*, 1999). Such studies are a rich source for contextual information on the "real world" diversity in settings, clinicians, and patients that characterizes the national treatment system; this is essential for developing strategies for transporting findings from clinical trials into community-based treatment settings (Carroll & Rounsaville, 2003).

The findings from DATOS-A raise important questions for future studies regarding substance abuse treatment services for adolescents in the USA. The study clearly demonstrated the complex nature of substance abuse and other associated problems among youth who enter substance abuse treatment, and their need for services across multiple sectors. Future national evaluation studies are needed to describe the systems-of-care available for substance-abusing adolescents, particularly as service delivery systems are rapidly changing in response to new pressures for cost containment and constantly shifting policy imperatives. Longer-term follow-up studies are also needed to determine if youth who successfully reduce or eliminate substance use following their initial treatment episode sustain these positive outcomes or relapse and reenter treatment, either as older adolescents or as adults, over time. Moreover, DATOS-A examined youth and adults in separate cohorts, but the transition from youth- to adult-oriented services is not well understood.

There is a growing consensus that substance abuse treatment for adolescents needs to incorporate empirically validated techniques (Dennis *et al.*, 2003; Kaminer, 2001). New program models (Stevens & Morral, 2003) and treatment protocols that have been developed specifically for treatment of substance-abusing youth, or have been adapted from protocols originally developed for adults (Wagner & Waldron, 2001), have the potential to improve significantly substance abuse treatment provided to youth in community-based programs. Moreover, the results of clinical trials of adolescent-specific treatment approaches have become the basis for developing standards of clinical practice with this population (Bukstein, 1997). As the field of substance abuse treatment has moved into a new era that emphasizes the transfer of empirically based knowledge into community-based treatment settings (Lamb, Greenlick, & McCarty, 1998), national treatment outcome studies can be used to assess the degree to which community-based programs for youth have incorporated these empirically validated treatment protocols. Such research is crucial to evaluating the degree of dissemination of treatment protocols throughout the substance abuse treatment system for adolescents, as well as the characteristics of programs and treatment processes that are associated with successful incorporation of these treatment techniques.

ACKNOWLEDGEMENTS

This work was supported by NIDA Grant U01-DA10378 as part of a Cooperative Agreement on the Drug Abuse Treatment Outcome Studies (DATOS). The project includes a coordinating DATOS research center (Robert L. Hubbard, Principal Investigator at National Development and Research Institutes, Inc.) and two collaborating research centers (M. Douglas Anglin, Principal Investigator at University of California at Los Angeles and D. Dwayne Simpson, Principal Investigator at Texas Christian University) to conduct treatment evaluation studies in connection with NIDA (Bennett W. Fletcher, Principal Investigator at NIDA). The interpretations and conclusions contained in this paper do not necessarily represent the positions of the other DATOS Research Centers, NIDA, or the US Department of Health and Human Services.

REFERENCES

American Psychiatric Association, (1987). *Diagnostic and statistical manual of mental disorders: DSM-III-R* (3rd ed.). Washington, DC: American Psychiatric Press.

Anglin, M. D., Hser, Y. I., Grella, C. E., Longshore, D., & Prendergast, M. L. (2001). Drug treatment careers: conceptual overview and clinical, research, and policy applications. In F. M. Tims, C. G. Leukefeld, & J. J. Platt (eds.), *Relapse and Recovery in Addictions* (pp. 18–39). New Haven, CT: Yale University Press.

Blood, L. & Cornwall, A. (1994). Pretreatment variables that predict completion of an adolescent substance abuse treatment program. *Journal of Nervous and Mental Disease, 182,* 14–19.

Botvin, G. J. & Botvin, E. M. (1992). Adolescent tobacco, alcohol, and drug abuse: prevention strategies, empirical findings, and assessment issues. *Developmental and Behavioral Pediatrics, 13,* 290–301.

Broome, K. M., Joe, G. W., & Simpson, D. D. (2001). Engagement models for adolescents in DATOS-A. *Journal of Adolescent Research, 16,* 608–623.

Brown, S. A. & D'Amico, E. J. (2001). Outcomes of alcohol treatment for adolescents. In M. Galanter (ed.), *Recent Developments in Alcoholism,* Vol. 15: *Services Research in the Era of Managed Care.* New York: Plenum Press.

Brown, S. A., Vik, P. W., & Creamer, V. A. (1989). Characteristics of relapse following adolescent substance abuse treatment. *Addictive Behaviors, 14,* 291–300.

Brown, S. A., Myers, M. G., Mott, M. A., & Vik, P. W. (1994). Correlates of success following treatment for adolescent substance abuse. *Applied and Preventive Psychology*, **3**, 61–73.

Brown, S. A., Gleghorn, A., Schuckit, M. A., Myers, M. G., & Mott, M. A. (1996). Conduct disorder among adolescent alcohol and drug abusers. *Journal of Studies on Alcohol*, **57**, 314–324.

Brown, S. A., D'Amico, E. J., McCarthy, D. M., & Tapert, S. F. (2001). Four-year outcomes from adolescent alcohol and drug treatment. *Journal of Studies on Alcohol*, **62**, 381–388.

Bukstein, O. (1997). Practice parameters for the assessment and treatment of children and adolescents with substance use disorders. *Journal of the American Academy of Child and Adolescent Psychiatry*, **36**, 140–156.

Carroll, K. M. & Rounsaville, B .J. (2003). Bridging the gap: a hybrid model to link efficacy and effectiveness research in substance abuse treatment. *Psychiatric Services*, **54**, 333–339.

Chung, T., Martin, C. S., Grella, C. E., *et al.* (2003). Course of alcohol problems in treated adolescents. *Alcoholism: Clinical and Experimental Research*, **27**, 253–261.

Crowley, T. J., Mikulich, S. K., MacDonald, M., Young, S. E., & Zerbe, G. O. (1998). Substance-dependent, conduct-disordered adolescent males: severity of diagnosis predicts 2-year outcome. *Drug and Alcohol Dependence*, **49**, 225–237.

Dakof, G. A. (2000). Understanding gender differences in adolescent drug abuse: issues of comorbidity and family functioning. *Journal of Psychoactive Drugs*, **32**, 25–32.

Dakof, G. A., Tejeda, M., & Liddle, H. A. (2001). Predictors of engagement in adolescent drug abuse treatment. *Journal of the American Academy of Child and Adolescent Psychiatry*, **40**, 274–281.

Delany, P. J., Broome, K. M., Flynn, P. M., & Fletcher, B. W. (2001). Treatment service patterns and organizational structures: an analysis of programs in DATOS-A. *Journal of Adolescent Research*, **16**, 590–607.

Dembo, R. (1996). Problems among youths entering the juvenile justice system, their service needs and innovative approaches to address them. *Substance Use and Misuse*, **31**, 81–94.

Dennis, M. L., Dawud-Noursi, S., Muck, R. D., & McDermeit, M. (2003). The need for developing and evaluating adolescent treatment models. In S. J. Stevens & A. R. Morral (eds.), *Adolescent Substance Abuse Treatment in the United States: Exemplary Models from a National Evaluation Study* (pp. 3–34). Binghamton, NY: Haworth Press.

Etheridge, R. M., Craddock, S. G., Dunteman, G. H., & Hubbard, R. L. (1995). Treatment services in two national studies of community-based drug abuse treatment programs. *Journal of Substance Abuse*, **7**, 9–26.

Etheridge, R. M., Smith, J. C., Rounds-Bryant, J. L., & Hubbard, R. L. (2001). Drug abuse treatment and comprehensive services for adolescents. *Journal of Adolescent Research*, **16**, 563–589.

Farabee, D., Shen, H., Hser, Y., Grella, C. E., & Anglin, M. D. (2001). The effect of drug treatment on criminal behavior among adolescents in DATOS-A. *Journal of Adolescent Research*, **16**, 679–696.

Fletcher, B. W. & Grella, C. E. (2001). Preface to the *JAR* special issue: the drug abuse treatment outcome studies for adolescents. *Journal of Adolescent Research*, **16**, 537–544.

Flynn, P. M., Craddock, S. G., Hubbard, R. L., Anderson, J., & Etheridge, R. M. (1997). Methodological overview and research design for the Drug Abuse Treatment Outcome Study (DATOS). *Psychology of Addictive Behaviors*, **11**, 230–243.

Friedman, A. S. & Glickman, N. W. (1986). Program characteristics for successful treatment of adolescent drug abuse. *Journal of Nervous and Mental Disease*, **174**, 669–679.

——— (1987). Effects of psychiatric symptomatology on treatment outcome for adolescent male drug abusers. *Journal of Nervous and Mental Disease*, **175**, 425–430.

Friedmann, P. D., Alexander, J. A., & D'Aunno., T. A (1999). Organizational correlates of access to primary care and mental health services in drug abuse treatment units. *Journal of Substance Abuse Treatment*, **16**, 71–80.

Greenbaum, P. E., Foster-Johnson, L., & Petrila, A. (1996). Co-occurring addictive and mental disorders among adolescents: prevalence research and future directions. *American Journal of Orthopsychiatry*, **66**, 52–60.

Grella, C. E. & Joshi, V. (2003). Treatment processes and outcomes among adolescents with a history of abuse who are in drug treatment. *Child Maltreatment*, **8**, 7–18.

Grella, C. E., Hser, Y. I., Joshi, V., & Rounds-Bryant, J. (2001). Drug treatment outcomes for adolescents with comorbid mental and substance use disorders. *Journal of Nervous and Mental Disease*, **189**, 384–392.

Grella, C. E., Joshi, V., & Hser, Y. I. (2004). Effects of comorbidity on treatment processes and outcomes among adolescents in drug treatment programs. *Journal of Child and Adolescent Substance Abuse*, **13**, 13–31.

Hawke, J. M., Jainchill, N., & De Leon, G. (2000). Adolescent amphetamine users in treatment: client profiles and treatment outcomes. *Journal of Psychoactive Drugs*, **32**, 95–105.

Hawkins, J. D., Catalano, R. F., & Miller, J. Y. (1992). Risk and protective factors for alcohol and other drug problems in adolescence and early adulthood: implications for substance abuse prevention. *Psychological Bulletin*, **112**, 64–105.

Hser, Y. I., Anglin, M. D., Grella, C. E., Longshore, D., & Prendergast, M. L. (1997). Drug treatment careers: a conceptual framework and existing research findings. *Journal of Substance Abuse Treatment*, **14**, 1–16.

Hser, Y. I., Grella, C. E., Hubbard, R. L., *et al.* (2001). An evaluation of drug treatments for adolescents in four US cities. *Archives of General Psychiatry*, **58**, 689–695.

Hser, Y. I., Grella, C. E., Collins, C., & Teruya, C. (2003). Drug use initiation and conduct disorder among adolescents in drug treatment. *Journal of Adolescence*, **26**, 331–345.

Hubbard, R. L., Cavanaugh, E. R., Craddock, S. G., & Rachal, J. V. (1985). Characteristics, behaviors and outcomes for youth in the TOPS. In A. S. Friedman & G. M. Beschner (eds.), *Treatment Services for Adolescent Substance Abusers* (pp. 49–65). Rockville, MD: National Institute on Drug Abuse.

Hubbard, R. L., Marsden, M. E., Rachal, J. V., *et al.* (1989). *Drug Abuse Treatment: A National Study of Effectiveness*. Chapel Hill, NC: University of North Carolina Press.

Hubbard, R. L., Craddock, S. G., Flynn, P. M., Anderson, J., & Etheridge, R. (1997). Overview of 1-year follow-up outcomes in the Drug Abuse Treatment Outcome Study (DATOS). *Psychology of Addictive Behaviors*, **11**, 261–278.

Jainchill, N., De Leon, G., & Yagelka, J. (1997). Ethnic differences in psychiatric disorders among adolescent substance abusers in treatment. *Journal of Psychopathology and Behavioral Assessment*, **19**, 133–148.

Jainchill, N., Yagelka, J., Hawke, J., & De Leon, G. (1999). Adolescent admissions to residential drug treatment: HIV risk behaviors pre and post-treatment. *Psychology of Addictive Behaviors*, **12**, 163–173.

Jainchill, N., Hawke, J., De Leon, G., & Yagelka, J. (2000). Adolescents in therapeutic communities: one-year post-treatment outcomes. *Journal of Psychoactive Drugs*, **32**, 81–94.

Jessor, R. & Jessor, S. L. (1977). *Problem Behavior and Psychosocial Development: A Longitudinal Study of Youth.* New York: Academic Press.

Joshi, V., Hser, Y. I., Grella, C. E., & Houlton, R. (2001). Sex-related HIV risk reduction behavior among adolescents in DATOS-A. *Journal of Adolescent Research*, **16**, 642–660.

Kajdan, R. A. & Senay, E. C. (1976). Modified therapeutic communities for youth. *Journal of Psychoactive Drugs*, **8**, 209–214.

Kaminer, Y. (2001). Adolescent substance abuse treatment: where do we go from here? *Psychiatric Services*, **52**, 147–149.

Kristiansen, P. L. & Hubbard, R. L. (2001). Methodological overview and research design for adolescents in the Drug Abuse Treatment Outcome Studies. *Journal of Adolescent Research*, **16**, 545–562.

Lamb, S., Greenlick, M. R., & McCarty, D. (eds.) (1998). *Bridging the Gap Between Practice and Research: Forging Partnerships with Community-based Drug and Alcohol Treatment.* Washington, DC: National Academy Press.

Latimer, W. W., Newcomb, M., Winters, K. C., & Stinchfield, R. D. (2000a). Adolescent substance abuse treatment outcome: the role of substance abuse problem severity, psychosocial, and treatment factors. *Journal of Consulting and Clinical Psychology*, **68**, 684–696.

Latimer, W. W., Winters, K. C., Stinchfield, R., & Traver, R. E. (2000b). Demographic, individual, and interpersonal predictors of adolescent alcohol and marijuana use following treatment. *Psychology of Addictive Behaviors*, **14**, 162–173.

McLellan, A. T., Cacciola, J., Kushner, H., et al. (1992). The fifth edition of the Addiction Severity Index: cautions, additions and normative data. *Journal of Substance Abuse Treatment*, **5**, 312–316.

Newcomb, M. D. & Bentler, P. M. (1988). *Consequences of Adolescent Drug Use: Impact on the Lives of Young Adults.* Newbury Park, CA: Sage.

Nissen, L. B., Vanderburg, J., Embree-Bever, J., & Manky, J. (1999). *Strategies for Integrating Substance Abuse Treatment in the Juvenile Justice System: A Practice Guide.* Washington, DC: Center for Substance Abuse Treatment.

Orvaschel, H., (1994). Psychiatric interviews suitable for use in research with children and adolescents. In J. E. Mezzich & M. R. Jorge (eds.), *Psychiatric Epidemiology: Assessment Concepts and Methods* (pp. 509–522). Baltimore, MD: Johns Hopkins University Press.

Rounds-Bryant, J. L. & Staab, J. (2001). Patient characteristics and treatment outcomes for African American, Hispanic, and White adolescents in DATOS-A. *Journal of Adolescent Research*, **16**, 624–641.

Rounds-Bryant, J. L., Kristiansen, P. L., Fairbank, J. A., & Hubbard, R. L. (1998). Substance use, mental disorders, abuse, and crime: gender comparisons among a national sample of adolescent drug treatment clients. *Journal of Child and Adolescent Substance Abuse* **7**, 19–34.

Rounds-Bryant, J. L., Kristiansen, P. L., & Hubbard, R. L. (1999). Drug abuse treatment outcome study of adolescents: a comparison of client characteristics and pretreatment behaviors in three treatment modalities. *American Journal of Drug and Alcohol Abuse* **25**, 573–591.

Sells, S. B. & Simpson, D. D. (1979). Evaluation of treatment outcome for youths in the Drug Abuse Reporting Program (DARP): a follow-up study. In G. M. Bescher & A. S. Friedman (eds.), *Youth Drug Abuse: Problems, Issues, and Treatment* (pp. 571–638). Lexington, MA: Lexington Books.

Simpson, D. D. (2001). Modeling treatment process and outcomes. *Addiction*, **96**, 207–211.

Simpson, D. D., Joe, G. W., Fletcher, B. W., Hubbard, R. L., & Anglin, M. D. (1999). A national evaluation of treatment outcomes for cocaine dependence. *Archives of General Psychiatry*, **56**, 507–514.

Stevens, S. J. & Morral, A. R. (eds.) (2003). *Adolescent Substance Abuse Treatment in the United States: Exemplary Models from a National Evaluation Study*. Binghamton, NY: Haworth Press.

Stewart, D. G., Brown, S. A., & Myers, M. G. (1998). Antisocial behavior and psychoactive substance involvement among Hispanic and non-Hispanic Caucasian adolescents in substance abuse treatment. *Journal of Child and Adolescent Substance Abuse*, **6**, 1–22.

Terry, Y. M., van der Waal, C. J., McBride, D. C., & van Buren, H. (2000). Provision of drug treatment services in the juvenile justice system: a system reform. *Journal of Behavioral Health Services and Research*, **27**, 194–214.

Titus, J. C., Dennis, M. L., White, W. L., Scott, C. K., & Funk, R. R. (2003). Gender differences in victimization severity and outcomes among adolescents treated for substance abuse. *Child Maltreatment*, **8**, 19–35.

Wagner, E. F. & Waldron, H. B. (eds.), (2001). *Innovations in Adolescent Substance Abuse Interventions*. New York: Pergamon.

Williams, R. J. & Chang, S. Y. (2000). A comprehensive and comparative review of adolescent substance abuse treatment outcome. *Clinical Psychology: Science and Practice*, **7**, 138–166.

Winters, K. C., Stinchfield, R. D., Opland, E., Weller, C., & Latimer, W. W. (2000). The effectiveness of the Minnesota model approach in the treatment of adolescent drug abusers. *Addiction*, **95**, 601–612.

Wong, M. M., Hser, Y. I., & Grella, C. E. (2003). Compliance among adolescents during drug treatment. *Journal of Child and Adolescent Substance Abuse*, **12**, 13–31.

8

Adolescent treatment services: the context of care

M. Katherine Kraft, Kristin Schubert, Anna Pond, and
Marliyn Aguirre-Molina

Robert Wood Johnson Foundation, Princeton, NJ, USA

As the problem of substance abuse grows among youth of many nations, ensuring that young people have access to the highest quality and most effective drug and alcohol treatment becomes an ever more pressing public health issue. Since the mid-1990s, there have been a number of scientific advancements that have led to new medications and therapies with promising potential for substance abuse treatment (McLellan, 2002). However, while great strides have been made in research and in laboratory, many of these findings are not being transported into active treatment settings (McLellan, 2002). The translation of research into practice is significantly hindered by a disconnect between the clinical development and testing of effective interventions and the existing substance abuse treatment practice settings and the policy dictates that govern them.

For decades, the social sciences have linked organizational structures and processes to worker productivity and product quality. From Fredrick Taylor's work, which demonstrated increased productivity of assembly line processes, to the human relations school, which linked worker satisfaction and happiness to greater productivity, researchers have tried to determine the impact of organizational structure and processes on worker ability and product quality. This understanding has informed health-services research efforts to identify the delivery characteristics associated with efficient and effective patient care and the organizational environments needed to support the practice of evidence-based medicine in hospitals. For substance abuse services, studies examining organizational and service delivery attributes and characteristics are increasing; however, these studies often lack links to clinical approaches and fail to examine the quality of treatment provided. Generally, clinical interventions for substance abuse are developed and tested in exemplary settings, making replication very difficult in most organizations. These difficulties are partly a result of the limited attention being given to the

Adolescent Substance Abuse: Research and Clinical Advances, ed. Howard A. Liddle and Cynthia L. Rowe.
Published by Cambridge University Press. © Cambridge University Press 2006.

context in which the care will be provided. As evidenced in health care, the context of care or practice setting can either facilitate or prevent quality care, but it is never a neutral influence.

This chapter will examine the context within which adolescent substance abuse treatment is provided and the impact service delivery systems, provider and workforce characteristics, and financing options have on translating new evidence-based interventions into practice. Ultimately, the structure and processes of organizational development and the realities of practice settings must be linked to the practices and patterns of clinical researchers to allow the delivery of well-designed interventions that are effective with adolescent drug abusers and their families.

Background

A recent adolescent treatment "renaissance" has successfully tested clinical approaches and created manual-guided care protocols. In fact, the number of formally evaluated programs for adolescents more than doubled between 1997 and 2001, and it promises to double again in the next 3 years (Dennis *et al.*, 2002). As discussed in several chapters in this volume, we now have proven interventions that are effective in reducing adolescent substance use, that successfully engage families in treatment, that can be provided in different settings, and that are appropriate to the developmental, cultural, and gender differences of substance-abusing youth.

These recent advances in adolescent treatment efficacy will be tempered if the challenges of moving these models into practice settings are not given adequate attention. Clinical researchers are not necessarily knowledgeable about the constraints of organizational development. Traditionally, issues of workforce development and financing have not been the focus of clinical research in psychology or counseling. Yet, contemporary researchers in these fields are increasingly facing the need to address these issues in applied research settings. Substantial effort to understand and modify the impact of these context characteristics needs to be considered.

To that end, CSAT and the Robert Wood Johnson Foundation convened an expert meeting in the winter of 2002 to examine the current evidence and to identify existing challenges in the service delivery of adolescent substance abuse treatment. The meeting reviewed the literature on the efficacy of systems of care development and implementation; it identified the workforce data gaps, the limited funding mechanisms, and the misunderstood processes of knowledge transfer. Information for this chapter was compiled from briefing papers and key informant interviews from that meeting, as well as a review of the literature on substance abuse treatment and technology transfer. While this analysis provides a wide scope of information, it nevertheless has its limitations. Although there is a wealth of recent literature on adolescent treatment, the discussion of service delivery, workforce, and standards of care is very limited. This analysis attempts to categorize the challenges being faced and to suggest strategies that researchers, policy makers and funders might pursue to address them. These strategies are not meant to be exhaustive but should be regarded more as a platform from which to launch continued discussion with experts in the field.

Systems of care: the existing system

The current adolescent treatment system (some question the use of the term "system") is a collection of public and private agencies and institutions that have, for the most part, grown out of the adult treatment arena. There are approximately 10 800 treatment facilities in the USA (SAMHSA, 1998); over 80% are private organizations that primarily provide outpatient treatment. Public funds finance almost two thirds of all the substance abuse treatment provided. While many of these provide treatment to adolescents, only 37% have specialty adolescent programs (SAMHSA, 2000). Likewise, over 75% of these treatment organizations treat fewer than 100 clients, and almost half treat fewer than 30 clients (Hargan & Levine, 1998). In reality, most treatment is provided in small, publicly financed community-based organizations. They provide outpatient treatment to fewer than 30 clients and do not offer ancillary or supportive services (i.e., general education development tests or academic supports). Most are unlikely to be part of any continuum of care and they may have few connections with other social service agencies.

While substance abuse treatment in general is a challenging field, working with adolescents and their families adds complex issues that must be addressed. Young people are using alcohol and other drugs at an earlier age, while this same population of users is becoming more diverse. The illegal drug market is constantly shifting as new drugs enter the market, old drugs reenter, potencies increase, and young people discover new uses. Most often, the use of alcohol is endemic, resulting in multidrug use. Only 10% of youth who need treatment for substance use disorders receive any care (CSAT, 2001; NIDA 2001). Of those who do, only 25% receive appropriate services to address the extent of their problems (CSAT, 2001; NIDA 2001). Over 80% of the adolescents entering outpatient treatment have three or more diagnoses or other major problems (e.g., victimization, violence, illegal activity), with even more problems being associated with higher severity of substance use (Dennis *et al.*, 2002). Treatment providers reported that their adolescent clients are younger, with more problems than they had previously, have much greater treatment needs, and increasingly come from families with multiple problems (O'Neill, 2001).

Youth who do access care are often in other systems (child welfare, juvenile justice, mental health) and have multiple issues. Consequently, the needs of each young person may be managed by multiple agencies (e.g., juvenile justice, child welfare, foster care, etc.), and providing quality treatment for adolescent substance abusers could require navigation across multiple service systems. The evidence indicates that effective treatment for adolescent drug abusers requires comprehensive services that span across multiple systems and include their families.

The optimal system

Unfortunately, service providers often operate independently from each other and are often fragmented and disconnected from each other and their constituents. Given the multiple systems in which youth drug abusers are involved and the usual fragmentation of services, finding mechanisms for effective coordination across systems of care (e.g., mental health, substance abuse, juvenile justice, schools, health) is critical. Systems-of-care strategies have been developed to deliver the multiple services that troubled youth and their families may need.

This type of collaboration must be built on common objectives, and resources must be shared and secured (Mattessich, Murray-Close, & Monsey, 2001). Developing systems of care requires building partnerships among separate systems and across traditional organizational boundaries.

These service delivery designs were first developed in the early 1980s for child welfare and children's mental health care. The term *systems of care* was developed to represent a cohesive network of entities from various service sectors working together to meet the total requirements of children with special needs and their families (Brannan *et al.*, 2002). Ideally, these systems would seek to prevent problems and cultivate health and well-being through an integrated, effective, and holistic approach (Chang & Bruner, 1998; Cross *et al.*, 1989).

The purpose of the systems-of-care framework is to increase interagency coordination in planning, developing, and delivering services to children and their families. The goals are to provide flexible, individualized services that are tailored to the unique needs of each family, while demonstrating cost-effectiveness (Stroul, McCormack, & Zaro, 1996). The process by which these systems can be developed is well documented (Pires, 2002), and research describing the impact of systems of care for children with emotional disturbances has been promising. Programs such as the Child and Adolescent Service System Program (1983), the Fort Bragg Child and Adolescent Mental Health Demonstration (1990), the Mental Health Services Program for Youth (1989), and the Comprehensive Community Mental Health Services for Children and Their Families Program (ongoing) have led to a better understanding of the impact systems of care can have on children with mental illness and their families. These efforts have identified several organizational and process challenges involved in developing such systems (for comprehensive reviews of these programs, see Pires [2002]). At a minimum, they require shared client information, mutual understand of terminology and labels, mechanisms for sharing costs, shared vision and belief in the possibilities, and effective leadership to address the challenges.

Parents of children receiving services in systems of care have appeared to be more satisfied with the services and with the support they receive. Children demonstrated improvements in overall functioning that included symptom reductions and decreases in negative behaviors. Movement away from expensive treatment and shifts in resource allocation led to a decrease in costs overall (Stroul *et al.*, 1996). However, the organizational stimulus and appropriate policies necessary for development and sustainability are less understood. How the system-of-care framework is implemented varies across communities and changes over time to fit an individual community's needs and development.

The emphasis on creating systems of care for adolescents with substance use disorders is a much more recent development. In the 1990s, CSAT initiated two federal programs to address the need for coordinated collaboration among substance abuse treatment system and other various health and human service systems: Targeted Cities and the Criminal/Juvenile Justice Treatment Networks (C/JJTN).

The C/JJTN began in 1995 to address the increasing prevalence of substance use disorders among youth involved in the juvenile justice system. It sought to improve the effectiveness, efficiency, and appropriateness of needed services by creating a new level of service integration for these youth and their families through redesigning patterns of service delivery (CSAT, 1995).

These integrated networks faced extraordinary challenges to reconfigure existing and disparate service delivery systems, including barriers to information sharing, professional cultures of exclusion, and resistance to pooled financing. However, the networks were successful in meeting the goals of developing a continuum of services for clients. Collaboration between agencies improved and clients had greater access to services. Referral patterns of youth among systems, the flow of information, and case management practices within and among systems improved (Caliber, 2001a–c). This project made a strong case that integrating service approaches is a promising approach to providing substance-abusing youthful offenders with the services they need (Caliber, 2001a–c).

Given the many interacting problems of substance-abusing youth, the lack of coordinated systems of care is particularly detrimental and hampers the delivery of proven multiservice treatment approaches. Most evidence suggests that coordinated care systems can effectively address youth issues and may be a method for providing holistic approaches. Despite empirical support for integrated services, community services remain fragmented and categorical in approach. Providers can be territorial with resources and client information. Policies that promote categorical funding and limited problem definitions force agencies to operate in a vacuum. Furthermore, the components of systems of care have been difficult to operationalize and their development and maintenance are time consuming; ultimately, they require changes and cooperation at all levels (policy, culture, practice, and mission) if they are to work. Policy makers and funders could support new generations of projects that build on the lessons learned from past projects, such as Robert Wood Johnson's Reclaiming Futures program, and test more thoroughly the efficacy of developing systems of care for this population. Research focusing on time-efficient strategies of implementation, more detailed understanding of the attributes of collaboration, and better documentation of the benefits of systems approaches could assist in improving adolescent treatment. Ultimately, research that fails to focus on the development and implementation challenges of comprehensive systems of care and service delivery will be significantly limited in its usefulness and understanding of the treatment experience.

Providers of care

Whether delivered within a system of care or in a stand-alone agency, treatment is provided by individual counselors, therapists, and direct line staff. Few studies have been conducted on the workforce involved in substance abuse treatment. Even fewer provide data specific to those serving adolescents. Various regional Addiction Technology Transfer Centers (ATTCs), as well as CSAT, are initiating surveys to improve the knowledge base on substance abuse treatment workforce characteristics, issues, and needs. The Northwest Frontier ATTC (NFATTC) (includes Alaska, Idaho, Oregon, and Washington) is one of the first to present its findings. Results of their survey, which assessed substance abuse treatment programs in four states, have important implications for the national substance abuse treatment workforce generally, including providers who work with adolescents. The key findings (NFATTC, 2000) are given below.

- The substance abuse treatment workforce, particularly those serving adolescents, includes a variety of service providers ranging from physicians and nurses to social workers and counselors.
- The workforce is predominantly White (84%), largely female (57%), and is aging, with an average age of 47 years.
- The average time in the field is 11 years, with managers staying longer (14 years) than direct service staff (8 years). On average, there is a 25% staff turnover each year.
- A little under half (47%) are in direct service positions, with the remaining (53%) in management.

- More than three quarters (76%) of direct service staff earn between $15 000 and $34 999, with only 17% earning $35 000 or greater. Nearly three quarters (73%) of management staff earns $35 000 or more.
- The substance abuse treatment counselors, particularly those serving adolescents, are often former users themselves and possess a diverse range of educational and training backgrounds. Most have a bachelor's degree or greater, particularly among those aged 20 to 30 years (81%). A comparable number (70%) have also completed some form of specific substance abuse treatment coursework, with about half (48%) completing coursework at a 2-year college (figures varied significantly across states, which could be the result of different state certification and managed care/third party payer requirements).
- More than three quarters (77%) have current or pending certification as substance abuse counselors, with direct service staff (70%) and management staff (69%) almost equally certified (no significant difference across states despite the range of certification requirements).

Staff who treat adolescents report a unique array of challenges, which range from the evolving needs of youth and their families to systems issues created by the current state of youth services, such as low funding levels and contract restrictions on care types and amounts. These challenges can be examined in terms of barriers at systems levels, organizational levels, and staffing levels.

The primary systems and policy issues include fragmentation of youth-serving systems, lack of uniform licensing and certification standards, limited availability and dissemination of education and training curricula on adolescent-specific treatment approaches, lack of a complete demographic profile of the workforce involved in adolescent treatment, and financing and regulatory challenges that prevent comprehensive service planning and create the context of care for substance-abusing youth.

Organizational issues that prevent translation of research into practice for high-quality care further complicate these challenges. Specifically, inadequate communication between organizational management and staff in adolescent treatment, the lack of capacity to assess and understand workforce needs, and an organizational culture or leadership that cultivates unsupportive work environments are all influences on the type and quality of treatment that is ultimately provided within adolescent treatment programs.

From the staffing perspective, the practice setting can be adversely influenced by poor compensation, diverse experiences and education of counselors and those applying to be counselors, limited understanding of the existing proficiencies and skills required of staff in adolescent treatment, the excessive amount of time required for administrative rather than treatment responsibilities, and the stigma associated with pursuing a career in substance abuse treatment.

Some even say that working in the field of substance abuse treatment is truly the "toughest job you'll ever love" (Gallon, Gabriel, & Knudsen, 2003). The hours are long, the pay is low, the pressure is high, and the recognition, particularly from those outside the field, is extremely limited. Much of the public regards substance abuse as a preventable condition and is unsympathetic to drug abusers and insensitive to their treatment needs. Government support for treatment varies according to each administration's level of priority, or lack thereof, for substance abuse in its political agenda. Under these circumstances and within this environment, recruiting and retaining workers in this field is becoming more difficult and is rapidly approaching a crisis stage.

These agency realities impact provider ability to recruit, retain, and train staff, further eroding the possibilities of providing high-quality evidence-based care. As one focus group respondent stated (NYSOASAS 2002):

Programs are typically understaffed; vacancies are difficult to fill, staff are stressed out, underpaid, and often performing duties for which they have not been adequately trained; staff turnover continues to climb; complying with regulatory staffing mandates is becoming more and more difficult; career advancement opportunities are limited or non-existent; and the work environment is typically unappealing, when compared to other career options. Why, one might ask, would anyone want to work in the addictions field?

The system, itself and its organization and staffing levels all present unique and complex challenges to providing quality services to youth. To date, our understanding of their influence on the treatment practice setting is limited, and research about which arrangements create the most effective setting is needed.

Financing mechanisms and funding streams

Many will argue that funding is the primary driver of what and how treatment gets delivered. Most substance abuse treatment programming for adolescents is funded by a variety of state and federal programs. These programs represent a patchwork of entitlements, funding streams, and coverage levels. They include the entitlement programs of Medicaid (Title 19); the Early and Periodic Screening, Diagnosis, and Treatment (EPSDT) mandate of Medicaid; and the State Children's Health Insurance Program (SCHIP) program (Title 21). Nationally, the largest source of funding for substance abuse treatment is the Substance Abuse Block Grant, administered by CSAT. In 1997, the total amount spent on treatment was 11.9 billion dollars for the care of almost 1 million people; only 8% of these were under 18 years of age. Of this spending, 64% came from public sources and the rest came from private insurers, philanthropy, or out of the pockets of clients or their families. The public sector's share of substance abuse expenditures increased from 53% in 1987 to 64% in 1997, greatly exceeding the portion of public spending on all other health conditions.

To insure that available funding streams are utilized fully and appropriately, it is necessary to know what they are, how to access them, and what barriers to their utilization exist. The majority of Substance Abuse Block Grant funding is directed towards adult treatment, and no set-aside portion is required for adolescent treatment as with other special populations (e.g., women). Consequently, providers who serve adolescents are more reliant on the public insurance programs than Block Grant funding.

Medicaid, the primary insurance program for low-income families and individuals, requires certain mandated health services (i.e., inpatient and outpatient hospital care, home health services, etc.) as part of a state's benefit package and supports 20% of substance abuse treatment expenditures (Coffey *et al.*, 2001). States can select to add additional mandates from a list of approved optional services; however, substance abuse treatment is not included on any list of mandated or optional services. States have, though, funded substance abuse treatment through other categories, such as rehabilitation services or case management. For instance, 29 states have used Section 1115 or Section 1915(b) waivers to cover substance abuse treatment services under Medicaid (National Governors Association Center for Best Practices, 2002). In 1999, 28 states offered Medicaid benefits that covered adolescent substance abuse treatment; eight states provided substance abuse treatment services for adolescents similar to those provided by health care sponsored by private employers; 14 states provided substance abuse treatment for adolescents with limited annual or lifetime benefits; and only one state provided no coverage for treatment (CSAT, 1999). Understanding the ways and means by which those decisions were made might be instructive to other states as they look for ways to maintain current Medicaid benefits.

Another Medicaid mechanism by which all states could fund substance abuse treatment services for adolescents is through EPSDT mandates. This provision of Medicaid is intended to identify problems at earlier stages and provide corrective interventions. These mandates cover prevention and treatment services for children and adolescents under the age of 22. Under EPSDT, states must screen and must furnish all appropriate medically necessary treatment to "correct or ameliorate defects and physical and mental illness and conditions discovered by the screening services" (42 US code 1396d(a)). Even though states can elect not to cover alcohol and drug treatment services for adults, EPSDT requires that all services "whether or not such services are covered under the State plan" (Social Security Act 1905r(5)) be made available.

Theoretically, EPSDT could be used to cover alcohol and drug treatment and prevention services for adolescents. Medicaid is required to provide medically necessary treatment regardless of the state Medicaid plan. Even the courts have interpreted the federal EPSDT mandate to require states to ensure that children receive early diagnosis and treatment before conditions become serious (Bazelon Center, 1998). Continuing to document the medical necessity of adolescent substance abuse treatment is necessary to secure more EPSDT treatment funding.

Unfortunately, low EPSTD screening rates, lack of behavioral health screening generally, and limited follow-up procedures have undermined the potential of this policy provision. Screening rates through EPSDT are very low. In most states, fewer than half of eligible children receive Medicaid health screenings, in some states even less (Selby-Harrington *et al.*, 1995). Screening for behavioral health issues is even lower as effective screening and referral protocols for adolescents with alcohol and drug problems have not been adopted (Office of Treatment Improvement, 1991). Current state policies and practices about EPSDT funding for alcohol and drug treatment services are not clear, with the last national review of these policies over 10 years old (Fox *et al.*, 1993). Fragmentation of youth service systems and continued disconnects between health providers and community services has limited the development of the critical referral networks for utilizing EPSDT funding for adolescent treatment. These undeveloped treatment referral networks, unclear procedures, and low screening rates have substantially limited the potential of this funding mechanism to increase the availability of quality adolescent treatment.

The SCHIP was created in 1997 in the wake of the Clinton health plan to help states to expand insurance coverage for uninsured, low-income children. It is a block grant with $24 billion in appropriations (fiscal years 1998–2002) allocated through a formula to states with USA Department of Health and Human Services-approved SCHIP plans. As of February 2000, 24 states and territories had chosen to expand Medicaid; 15 had chosen to operate a separate state program, and 17 had chosen a combination (National Conference of State Legislatures, 2000). As with Medicaid, states have the option of covering inpatient, outpatient, and residential alcohol and drug treatment services, but it is not a requirement. To date, SCHIP coverage has not substantially increased funding for adolescent substance abuse treatment, and it is unlikely to improve access to services in the coming years because of critical budget shortfalls in state budgets. Realizing this objective will be even more difficult in coming years as states are dealing with critical budget shortfalls.

There are several other governmental funding sources from education, justice and labor. Each offers a particular funding stream for limited adolescent treatment. The combination of all these sources still leaves large numbers of adolescents unable to get treatment, and many treatment providers striving to provide care with fewer resources. These funding challenges do not create a practice setting that is particularly able to retrain staff and incorporate the fundamental changes that translation strategies might require. Likewise, they do not provide the organizational stability, incentives, understanding, or time required to change intervention approaches. Research could help to document the complexities of these mechanisms, assist in developing efficient models that maximize existing funding opportunities, and inform policy makers about the barriers to using existing mechanisms.

Technology transfer and treatment quality

Many attributes and service realities of the practice setting prevent technology transfer and delivery of high-quality care. Funding parameters govern the availability of treatment. Policy barriers, such as licensure requirements and confidentiality laws, dominate service delivery and complicate the development of comprehensive systems of care. Workforce issues and funding are central to the practice of evidence-based interventions and the improvement of treatment quality. Despite substantial research on what adolescents need, evidence-based interventions are not widely practiced. Fragmented services, limited institutional resources (staff and other), and limited compatibility of research with agency realities present numerous operational barriers to technology transfer. Likewise, the realities of funding and regulatory challenges create an organizational culture that can be hostile to innovation and resentful of change. Inconsistent leadership and the marginal management skills often found in treatment agencies can further hamper efforts to improve quality and promote evidence-based approaches. Policies that affect funding, service collaboration, and worker recruitment, retention and credentials all impact the practice settings where treatment is conducted. They influence our ability to translate evidence-based models into actual practice and often dictate the quality, quantity, and kind of care available to youth and their families.

In addition to this complex array of policy, operational, and service-delivery barriers, technology transfer is impacted by political processes. Since it emerged as a priority of the National Institute of Mental Health (NIMH) in the 1970s, the transfer of substance abuse research into treatment settings has been influenced by each presidential administration's overall commitment to the drug abuse issue, the priority given to prevention versus treatment efforts, and the shifting views on the role of the federal government and its relationship to states (which, in turn, impacts the way in which funding is allocated) (Brown & Flynn, 2002). Since the 1970s, technology transfer for substance abuse treatment has been spearheaded by the federal government through the creation of multiple agencies specifically mandated to focus on substance abuse research (Brown & Flynn, 2002). Not surprisingly, technology transfer appears most prevalent in federally supported practice research projects (i.e., research-based interventions being tested in community settings; Ozechowski & Liddle, 2000). Such projects are only available in a limited number of communities.

These realities of service delivery can inhibit the process of innovation and frustrate attempts to transport empirically supported interventions for adolescent drug abuse into practice settings. To expand the ability of service systems to deliver effective treatment and improve the quality of care provided, funders, policy makers, researchers, and practitioners will need to find additional ways to operate; sound research that is grounded in service-delivery realities is a step in that direction. Understanding the constraints and working to remove policy barriers seems a necessary component of good clinical research.

Conclusions and recommendations

In summary, high-quality, evidence-based adolescent substance abuse treatment is characterized by complex interactions between service delivery, clinician competency, and program availability. Systems of care, the providers of care, and funding mechanisms are fundamental components of adolescent treatment that influence the practice setting. Each has a significant impact on the type and quality of treatment provided. Regardless of the evidence supporting coordinated systems of care and research-to-practice protocols, most treatment continues to be provided through fragmented service networks, in agencies that have limited connections to outside supports, and by inconsistently trained professionals. Numerous barriers and challenges experienced during the day-to-day operations of adolescent treatment providers, which include categorical funding streams, restrictive client confidentiality laws, narrow professional paradigms and exclusive professional cultures, and limited leadership, are in part responsible for the existing situation. Changing systems and transcending service-delivery inertia requires that policy makers, funders, researchers, and practitioners change. If they do not, they can further hinder the process of adopting and delivering evidence-based care. Saving money, training staff, and coordinating care do not always work together seamlessly. Closer ties between practice-setting realities and clinical research tools are necessary. Consumer involvement in decision making regarding substance abuse research and a broader policy agenda for clinical researchers that focuses on increasing funding and improving service collaboration, as well as clinical practice, could be helpful.

Researchers and practitioners need to collaborate on intervention design and testing. Research needs to document clearly the skills and personal characteristics necessary to work effectively with youth, and to create training programs and recruitment strategies that will deliver those skills. Policy makers and funders should find ways to reward clinicians for competently delivered interventions and make sure that incentives are in place for providing more comprehensive, coordinated care. Innovative support options should be encouraged and non-traditional supports (i.e., horse riding programs or physical activity programming) should be linked to rigorous testing opportunities. Policy makers should understand the administrative and eligibility requirements of existing funding mechanisms, and streamlined procedures should be developed.

Foundations and other private funders can provide more investment in creating service-delivery models and can focus on developing community capacity to deliver these services. Part of capacity building should include training opportunities to engage in cross-discipline work. Such funders can require non-traditional partners to come together to provide a range of supports for youth and provide quality, evidence-based treatment in organizations and settings that are family and youth oriented.

Policy makers can rethink funding requirements and focus more on comprehensive youth outcomes rather than targeted problems. Funding and budgets could be linked to youth performance on a range of developmental outcomes, not just reducing problem behaviors.

Researchers need to provide a better understanding of what it takes to implement comprehensive systems of care, and they should develop implementation manuals for administrators and practitioners similar to treatment manuals. Practitioners, direct line staff, supervisors, and management levels can learn to transcend professional boundaries and begin creating care teams that deliver high-quality, evidence-based treatment and necessary supportive services.

For evidence-based interventions to be delivered, viable treatment systems, competent providers, and available funding streams must be in place. The recent economic downturn has left states financially strapped as new public health issues and security concerns demand resources. These pressures are being played out in every social service system but are particularly difficult for adolescent treatment services, where only one in ten adolescents needing treatment can access services (Muck *et al.*, 2001). The increased financial constraints that substance abuse providers are facing is coupled with the maturing of requirements for measuring performance monitoring outcomes, and establishing credentials, each of which requires additional capital investments on the part of treatment organizations. The combination of increased demands and fewer resources will further diminish existing treatment capacity. Critical stakeholders must begin to work together now to prevent such diminution from happening.

REFERENCES

Bazelon Center (1998, April). *Protecting Consumer Rights in Public Systems' Managed Mental Health Care Policy* (p. 6). Washington, DC: Judge David L. Bazelon Center for Mental Health Law.

Brannan, A., Baughman, L., Reed, E., & Katz-Leavy, J. (2002). System-of-care assessment: cross-site comparison of findings. *Children's Services: Social Policy, Research, and Practice*, **5**, 4–5.

Brown, B. S. & Flynn, P. M. (2002). The federal role in drug abuse technology transfer: a history and perspective. *Journal of Substance Abuse Treatment*, **22**, 245–257.

Caliber (2001a). *Denver Juvenile Justice Integrated Treatment Network Systems-level Report*. Fairfax, VA: Caliber & Associates.

(2001b). *Lane County Youth Intervention Network Systems-level Report*. Fairfax, VA: Caliber & Associates.

(2001c). *Travis County's Juvenile Offender Substance Abuse Treatment Services Systems-level Report*. Fairfax, VA: Caliber & Associates.

CSAT (Center for Substance Abuse Treatment) (1995). *Demonstration Cooperative Agreements for Development and Implementation of Criminal Justice Treatment Networks*. [*Guidelines for Applicants*, TI 95–04] Rockville, MD: US Department of Health and Human Services.

(1999). *Contracting for Managed Substance Abuse and Mental Health Services: A Guide for Public Purchasers*. Rockville, MD: Substance Abuse and Mental Health Services Administration Department of Health and Social Services. Retrieved September 20, 1999 from http:www.samhsa.ove/oas/tap22.1/chapteriii-bbav-15.htm.

(2001). *Treatment Episode Data Set*. Washington, DC: Substance Abuse and Mental Health Services Administration Department of Health and Human Services. Available www.icpsr.umich.edu/SAMHDA/das.html.

Chang, H. & Bruner, C. (1998). *A Matter of Commitment Community Collaboration Series*, guidebook 3: *Valuing Diversity and Practicing Inclusion: Core Aspects of Collaborative Work*. Des Moines, IA: National Center for Service Integration.

Coffey, R., Mark, T., King, E., et al. (2001). *National Estimates of Expenditures for Substance Abuse Treatment, 1997*. [Publication No. SMA–01–3511] Rockville, MD: Center for Substance Abuse Treatment and Center for Mental Health Services.

Cross, T., Bazron, B. R., Dennis, K. W., & Isaacs, M. R. (1989). *Toward a Culturally Competent System of Care: A Monograph on Effective Services for Minority Children who are Severely Emotionally Disturbed*. Washington, DC: Georgetown University Child Development Center.

Dennis, M. L., Dawud-Noursi, S., Muck, R. D., & McDermitt, M. (2002). The need for developing and evaluating adolescent treatment models. In S. J. Stevens & A. R. Morral (eds.), *Adolescent Substance Abuse Treatment in the United States: Exemplary Models from a National Evaluation Study* (pp. 3–56). Binghamton, NY: Haworth Press.

Fox, H. B., Wicks, L. N., McManus, M. A., & Kelly, R. W. (1993). *Medicaid Financing for Mental Health and Substance Abuse Services for Children and Adolescents*. Rockville, MD: US Department of Health and Human Services.

Gallon, S. L., Gabriel, R. M., & Knudsen, J. R. W. (2003). The toughest job you'll ever love: a Pacific Northwest Treatment Workforce survey. *Journal of Substance Abuse Treatment*, **24**, 183–196.

Hargan, C. M. & Levine, H. J. (1998). The substance abuse treatment system: what does it look like and whom does it serve? In S. Lamb, M. R, Greenlick, & D. McCarty (eds.), *Bridging the*

Gap between Practice and Research: Forging Partnerships with Community-based Drug and Alchohol Treament (pp. 186–197). Washington, DC: National Academy of Sciences.

Mattessich, P. W., Murray-Close, M., & Monsey, B. R. (2001). *Collaboration: What Makes it Work – A Review of Research Literature on Factors Influencing Successful Collaboration.* St. Paul, MN: Amherst H. Wilder Foundation.

McLellan, A. T. (2002). Technology transfer and the treatment of addiction: what can research offer practice? *Journal of Substance Abuse Treatment,* **22,** 169–170.

Muck, R., Zempolich, K. A., Titus, J. C., *et al.* (2001). An overview of the effectiveness of adolescent substance abuse treatment models. *Youth and Society,* **33,** 143–168.

National Conference of State Legislatures (2000). *State Children's Health Insurance Program (SCHIP): State Action Snapshot.* Washington, DC: National Conference of State Legislatures. www.ncsl.org.

National Governors Association Center for Best Practices (2002). *Medicaid Grants and Waivers.* Washington, DC: NGA. www.nga.org/center/ (accessed 25 September 2004).

NFATTC (Northwest Frontier Addiction Technology Transfer Center) (2000). *Substance Abuse Treatment Workforce Survey: A Regional Needs Assessment.* Salem, OR: RMC Research.

NIDA (National Institute for Drug Abuse) (2001). *Monitoring the Future.* Rockville, MD: National Institutes of Health. Available at www.icpst.umich.edu/SAMHDA/das.html.

NYSOASAS (New York State Office of Alcoholism and Substance Abuse Services) (2002). *The Addictions Profession: A Workforce in Crisis: A Compilation of the Results of the 2001 Regional Workforce Development Focus Groups.* New York: New York State Office of Alcoholism and Substance Abuse Services.

Office of Treatment Improvement (1991). *Medicaid Financing for Mental Health and Substance Abuse Services for Children and Adolescents (TAP 2).* Washington, DC: Office of Treatment Improvement.

O'Neill, C. (2001). *Adolescent Treatment Programs in the 21st Century.* Unpublished manuscript; copy available from the chapter authors.

Ozechowski, T. J. & Liddle, H. A. (2000). Family-based therapy for adolescent drug abuse: knowns and unknowns. *Clinical Child and Family Psychology Review,* **3,** 269–298.

Pires, S. A. (2002). *National Technical Asistance Center for Children's Mental Health.* Washington, DC: Center for Child Health and Mental Health Policy, Georgetown University Child Development Center.

SAMHSA (Substance Abuse and Mental Health Services Administration) (1998). *National Expenditures for Mental Health, Alcohol, and Other Drug Abuse Treatment, 1996.* Rockville, MD: Substance Abuse and Mental Health Services Administration.

(2000). *National Survey of Substance Abuse Treatment Services, 2000.* Rockville, MD: Substance Abuse and Mental Health Services Office of Applied Sciences.

Selby-Harrington, M., Sorensen, J. R., Quade, D., *et al.* (1995). Increasing Medicaid child health screenings: the effectiveness of mailed pamphlets, phone calls, and home visits. *American Journal of Public Health,* **85,** 1412–1417.

Stroul, B., McCormack, M., & Zaro, S. M. (1996). Measuring outcomes in systems of care. In B. Stroul (ed.), *Children's Mental Health: Creating Systems of Care in a Changing Society* (pp. 313–336). Baltimore, MD: Paul H. Brookes.

9

The principles of service organization and practice in England

Paul McArdle and Eilish Gilvarry

Fleming Nuffield Unit, Newcastle upon Tyne, UK
Centre for Alcohol and Drug Studies, Newcastle upon Tyne, UK

This chapter describes the common legal and policy context and the pattern of resources that frame and determine how services in England respond to young people in difficulty. It also aims to conceptualize how apparently different organizations can knit together to provide integrated services for young people with complex difficulties. In doing so, it draws on a recent report (Gilvarry *et al.*, 2001) and focuses particularly on those young people who abuse substances and who may attend clinical services. Also, while legislators and designers of policy did not necessarily have youth drug abuse uppermost in mind, the structures and processes they create are clearly relevant to the needs of this vulnerable group.

The legal framework in England

Professionals working with children require familiarity with the relevant legislation. This includes the criminal law, including laws regulating access to drugs and alcohol, and the rights of children and young people, for example to education (United Nations, 1989). In England and Wales, it also includes the Children Act 1989, the pre-eminent law regarding the welfare of children and young people of 16 years of age and younger. This describes a number of key principles.

- The welfare of the child is paramount.
- The child's wishes and views must be considered: it is important to note that the wishes and the interests of the child or young person may not be identical.
- The welfare of the child or young person is the parents' responsibility until the child is 18 years of age. This may lead to difficulty if a young person refuses to involve parents; experienced clinicians will usually find means both to respect these wishes and to involve parents in a way in keeping with the welfare of the young person (Kaplan & McArdle, 2004). Also, in UK law, young people under 16 years are generally regarded as unable to consent to treatment in their own

Adolescent Substance Abuse: Research and Clinical Advances, ed. Howard A. Liddle and Cynthia L. Rowe.
Published by Cambridge University Press. © Cambridge University Press 2006.

right. However, it is possible for a person under 16 years to give consent to treatment without parental permission if he or she can be judged to have reached "sufficient understanding" or competence. There are recommended criteria with which to judge the latter (Dale-Perera & Hamilton, 1997). However, it is doubtful if many younger adolescent drug users are competent to give consent without parental permission.

- There is a duty to safeguard and promote the welfare of the child: this may mean that the welfare of the child or young person requires breaking confidentiality regarding, for instance, circumstances potentially harmful to the child.
- Agencies working with children and young people should cooperate in the best interests of the child: this will often mean that, in complex clinical circumstances, good practice requires interagency and interprofessional cooperation. It would be unusual for one agency to contain all the resources required to meet the needs of children or young people with complex needs.

Recent policy initiatives

Over recent years there have been significant policy developments aiming to maximize the inclusion of vulnerable youth in mainstream services, drawing out in a sense some of the implications of the Children Act 1989. There has been a strong emphasis on cooperation across government departments, as well as across services, to fulfil the demand of Prime Minister Tony Blair for "joined-up solutions to joined-up problems." Think-tank organizations leading the search for such solutions include the Children and Young People's Unit, responsible for an "overarching strategy for all services for children and young people." However, although many of the policy developments are meant to be the product of cross-departmental initiatives, they tend to address one or other aspect of child and youth vulnerability and so appear as quite separate and apparently unlinked initiatives. It is an important task of the clinician to be aware of and take advantage of these initiatives in order to create integrated solutions for young people and their families.

The Quality Protects (http://www.doh.gov.uk/qualityprotects/) program is an important example of a government initiative. It aims to provide more effective protection, access to relevant services, and greater equity for children and young people in the care of local authorities (local democratic organizations comprising elected councillors and permanent officials with responsibility for a range of local services). Specific objectives include prompt allocation of social workers to vulnerable children, increasing stability of foster placements, reducing time to adoption for children in the care system, and enhancing staff training, an area traditionally neglected. Broader goals relate to reduction of truancy and criminality. While these policy ideas aim to embrace vulnerable children and young people in a range of situations, they offer the opportunity for those young people with substance-related problems to benefit, either directly or indirectly.

Local authorities are charged too with the early reintegration back into mainstream education of pupils (under 16 years) who have been expelled from school. They can facilitate this process by offering additional funding (or "dowries"). For those for whom reintegration is not feasible, local authorities now have to provide alternative full-time education. In these pupil referral centers, educational programs can be more tailored to needs. For instance, "for those whose behaviour problems stem from a lack of basic skills … " there should be additional focus on literacy and numeracy, as well as, for all pupils, some creative activity and physical education.

However, excluded pupils represent a minority of those not attending school, most of whom are truants. The government Department for Education and Skills has developed a set of principles in the form of a checklist to enable local authorities to address truancy. This includes setting attendance targets with schools, analysis of local data, liaison with police, support for families in difficulties, and meeting the needs of children with "special educational needs," amounting to the development of local strategic thinking about truancy.

The 1996 Education Act (law in England and Wales) regulates how the needs of children with " … disabilities [in] learning … in thinking and understanding … emotional and behavioural difficulties … or [in] how they relate to and behave with other people … " should be met (www.dfes.gov.uk/sen/documents/ACF5DF.pdf). If a parent considers that measures within the school are not meeting the child's needs, they can request "a statutory assessment" of needs, usually coordinated by an educational psychologist. This will incorporate advice from other services, such as health and social services, and will lead to a "Statement" of special educational needs. This document (against which parents have a right of appeal) potentially acts to reframe a child's difficulties (e.g., from bad to in need) and so offers a measure of protection and understanding. It may also facilitate release of significant funds and additional support, or sometimes special schooling.

It is important to note that these systems do not always work smoothly; they do not, for instance, dispense scarce funds without a strong case. Informed by their knowledge of the young person and local resources, clinicians find themselves arguing for the most appropriate response from local resources. Indeed, liaison and advocacy form a large part of the work of most UK health-based clinicians working with complex young people.

The Children's National Service Framework (http://www.doh.gov.uk/nsf/children.htm) aims to improve standards and reduce national variations in health and social services. While so far not directly addressing substance abuse, it is likely that its work on vulnerable young people will encompass those who misuse substances and have other related problems. Key issues are likely to be the setting of standards, protection of children, comprehensive assessments, competence in the work force, and effective cooperative working between service providers and evidence-based interventions.

However, because of the perception that drug use and crime are linked, "lead responsibility for driving forward delivery of the drug strategy" (for the reduction of drug use and abuse in England) now lies with the Home Office "responsible for internal affairs (and) ... security of the public ... in England and Wales." The Home Office refers to an "updated strategy" (http://www.drugs.gov.uk/ NationalStrategy/YoungPeople) that aims to engage services in "driving down" drug use. In this relatively new role, the Home Office (with its rather authoritarian style) has instructed local organizations, the "drug action teams," to meet a list of targets in relation to young people (e.g., 100% of schools will have drug education programs; 100% of certain high-risk groups will receive targeted interventions). It is attempting to stretch the criminal justice system to address the needs of young people with substance abuse problems, for instance by employment of a professional in all community-based youth-offending teams and through development of a range of treatment interventions in custodial institutions.

The Home Office and Department of Health have now handed over responsibility for aspects of promoting effective control of drug abuse to the National Treatment Agency (http://www.nta.nhs.uk). This is "a special health authority created by the Government in 2001 to improve the availability, capacity and effectiveness of treatment for drug misuse in England. In other words, to ensure that there is more treatment, better treatment and fairer treatment available to all those who need it." It defines treatment as "a range of interventions which are intended to remedy an identified drug-related problem or condition relating to a person's physical, psychological or social (including legal) well-being ... structured drug treatment follows assessment and is delivered according to a care plan, with clear goals, which is regularly reviewed with the client." It is taking an active role in shaping services for adults but has a section interested in young people and is likely, in time, to assert its role also in relation to young people.

The Youth Justice Board for England and Wales also has roots in the Home Office. It describes itself as "an executive non-departmental public body" (http:// www.youth-justice-board.gov.uk). Within the Home Office, it is responsible for the youth justice system, which comprises "Youth offending teams (YOT), the police, youth courts and the institutions in which young people are held in custody." Its stated aims are "to prevent offending by children and young people ... by ... preventing crime and the fear of crime; identifying and dealing with young offenders; reducing re-offending." It aims to achieve this by targeting resources "on young people at high risk of offending ...; [using] ... robust community penalties ... as alternatives to short custodial sentences; custody as a last resort; partnership (with families ... communities ... and all other services)." The Home Office and linked agencies also fund research in order to inform policy. The Youth Justice Board website links, for example, to a literature review focused on prevention of crime written from a UK perspective.

None of this legal and government-endorsed guidance and provision can be ignored by clinicians. Moreover, it is clear that there are practice benchmarks based in law (that have generally emerged from long consultation informed by evidence and practice) and important legally sanctioned rights and resources, and sometimes coercive measures, available to or that impinge on young people. These resources are scattered through different agencies with overlapping but non-identical goals, who may view young drug abusers differently. Hence, a key goal of clinical practice is not only to assess a young person's needs correctly but also to respond lawfully, and often through networking and advocacy, to extract the best management plan for the young person. This case-management approach has been a mainstay of child and adolescent mental health services (CAMHS: multi-disciplinary teams and agencies encompassing child and adolescent psychiatry, clinical psychology, social work, specialist teachers, occupational therapists, nurses and others). However, neither CAMHS nor any child or youth service has traditionally addressed the needs of substance abusers, partly because substance abuse by children and younger adolescents is a relatively new phenomenon. Also, those services that have attempted to do so have often, sometimes inappropriately, introduced adult models of assessment and intervention to the area of youth substance abuse.

The Health Advisory Service

In order to address these deficiencies, the UK Department of Health and the Home Office commissioned the Health Advisory Service (HAS) to present an updated blue print for drug and alcohol services in relation to children and young people services (Gilvarry et al., 2001). The HAS is a semi-autonomous body designed to formulate strategic advice on selected health-related matters. The issue of youth substance abuse was addressed as part of two earlier HAS reports addressing CAMHS (Williams et al., 1995) and substance abuse (Williams et al., 1996).

The most recent report (Gilvarry et al., 2001) was commissioned by a cross-departmental group of senior personnel from the government departments of Health, Education and the Home Office. It was intended as an update following the change in UK Government to Labour in 1997; this party had introduced or modified a range of policies for young people and had taken a renewed interest in youth substance misuse. It was particularly intended to provide a current rationale and methodology to engage health professionals in the problem of youth substance misuse.

The working party was chaired by a consultant addiction psychiatrist with an interest in young people. It consisted of a range of co-editors and contributors with special interests in aspects of substance abuse, for example from child and adolescent mental health, education, criminal justice, social services, and the voluntary sector. These individuals provided written or oral submissions. In addition, a wide range of senior individuals (e.g., directors of social services) and representatives of important organizations (e.g., Royal College of Psychiatrists, Royal College of Nursing) were consulted and asked for views. Hence, the report represented the distilled views of a broad spectrum of informed opinion.

Aims, objectives and principles of the *Substance of Young Needs 2001 Review*

The HAS reports are not primarily scientific documents. They are designed to incorporate the lessons and the realities of clinical experience and of service capabilities, while interpreting and rendering accessible the scientific evidence base. All aim to describe good practice in the light and of relevant UK policy and law. The HAS reports are not quite the same as guidelines or practice parameters: they have a broader audience than practitioners and are "advisory." However, they do aim to conceptualize services in a way that enables them to be viewed strategically by purchasers and providers.

Gilvarry *et al.* (2001) described the widespread effect of substance abuse on development, educational achievement, physical and mental health, the family, and the general public. Their report emphasized that children and younger adolescents are developing, dependent, require care and protection from, and reduction of, harm, and that they have rights, for instance to family life and education. Also, services should be centered on the child or young person, but respectful of parental responsibility, as well as lawful, equitable, competent, and responsible. They should espouse good practice, be accountable, holistic, efficient, effective, and targeted.

A Strategic Framework

The relationships between clinicians, disciplines, and agencies can appear competitive, overlapping, and complex. In order to clarify roles and to emphasize cooperation, Williams *et al.* (1995) proposed a four-tier strategic framework, which was adopted throughout CAMHS. The report by Williams *et al.* (1996) adapted this framework to services for young people abusing substances and Gilvarry *et al.* (2001) further adapted this framework.

The tiered concept emphasizes functions rather than professions, and promotes integration between sectors, agencies, and disciplines. It has enabled clinicians to formulate integrated, multidisciplinary and multiagency, comprehensive assessment and intervention plans for the child and family, and for stakeholders in general, to think strategically about services. There are four tiers: (1) universal primary-level services; (2) youth-oriented services; (3) service provided by teams that specialize in treating young people who misuse substances; and (4) very specialized and highly intensive services for young people who misuse substances.

The advantages to commissioners (those who are charged with purchasing services) include a clear framework for identification of current provision and gaps in provision, and a better understanding of organizational relationships for planning and investing in comprehensive services. The advantages to providers are clarity of roles and responsibilities, avoidance of fragmentation and duplication, delivery of seamless and multicomponent responses, facilitation of skill transfer between services, matching young people to the most appropriate services and interventions, and a sense of common enterprise across professions and agencies.

Tier 1

The first tier is the frontline of service delivery to which all young people and their families have direct access and which generally provides the first response. It involves those who may have specialized skills, but not necessarily skills in addressing substance abuse specifically. These include, for example, teachers, primary-care physicians and nurses, police, some workers within the criminal justice system, and many social workers. The essence of this tier is to provide universal access and continuity of care, to identify and screen those with vulnerability, and to embed identification, accurate information, and advice into mainstream services.

The role of tier 1 is to identify unmet needs, if any (health, learning, etc.), and to dispense accurate information and advice. A service at this level should pay attention to parental involvement and family difficulties. It may advise to aid individuation but will also ensure parental help and support for the young person, one of the hallmarks of a service attuned to the needs of young people. Screening for drug and alcohol use should be central to any meaningful assessment of the health and well-being of young people, with referral of those with more complex problems. However, a tier 1 service would often not be sufficient to understand or respond to complex problems associated with substance misuse. This tier may be involved also in the delivery of universal prevention programs and in the formulation of situation-related policy and procedures, such as drug-intoxication policies, handling of illicit drugs, and emergency procedures in particular settings (e.g., schools, children's homes).

All tier 1 and primary-care workers should acquire, and have access to training in, basic skills in recognition and provision of initial interventions, such as support, accurate information, and advice concerning substance abuse. They should be familiar with child-protection (against abuse) policies (every local authority is charged with developing such procedures) and be sufficiently familiar with the law and guidelines in relation to parental involvement and consent. When in doubt, they should have ready access to support from tier 2 workers. Contact between tier 1 workers and their colleagues in other tiers, often around particular clinical problems, should facilitate continued professional development and in-service training. The goal should be to achieve a degree of standardization of training of all practitioners.

Tier 2

Tier 2 is the frontline of specialist services. Its practitioners have in common expertise in the developmental needs of young people and in links between substance abuse and normal and abnormal development and environment, and an ability to discern good and lawful practice in even complex circumstances. Practitioners will include child and adolescent psychiatrists and clinical psychologists based in CAMHS, specialized voluntary youth services (e.g., counseling services), pediatric and psychology staff, some specialist primary-care and social workers, and some staff working in the youth justice system. It also includes providers of universal young people's services, who also have specific specialist skills (e.g., special-needs teachers, some primary-care physicians with a special interest, school or other community nurses with mental health training). Although they may also be attached to teams, tier 2 is characterized by individual practitioners networking around the needs of individual young people. The key aims are the reduction of risks and vulnerabilities and the reintegration or maintenance of young people in mainstream services (e.g., return to school).

Tier 2 is designed for all young people but in particular for those with more problematic use (Zoccolillo, Vitaro, & Tremblay, 1999) and substance use disorders: often combined with other vulnerabilities. Practitioners in this tier should identify and actively attempt to engage vulnerable young people. Assessment should identify the various developmental, educational, family conflict, or physical problems and predicaments of these young people, and to clarify the degree and significance of substance use and misuse.

Tier 2 will offer more elaborate responses such as school liaison, identifying and negotiating responses to special educational needs, or diversionary activities for those engaged in delinquent activity – and, of course, detection of and responses to poor care or indeed abuse. It will have a capacity for family support, for counseling (e.g., using problem-solving approaches and motivational techniques), for psychotherapeutic or other interventions with the young person, and for non-addiction-related pharmacological therapies, as in stimulant medication for attention-deficit hyperactivity disorder. It will ensure parental involvement as far as possible. This may require specific attention to allow individuation of adolescents while seeking to ensure parental help and support for the young person, often using family therapy techniques.

Some young people who abuse substances, and who often have multiple difficulties, are reluctant to attend services. Effective management of pre-engaged young people (e.g., persistent truants, runaways, and homeless youth with complex needs) hinges on recognition, outreach, and continuous care to enable negotiation of referral pathways and other barriers to treatment (Kipke *et al.*, 1997). This may require active engagement that may take many contacts and the development of a relationship with a professional to retain the adolescents in services, itself linked to reduced harm (Hser *et al.*, 2001). Outreach services may be a function of tier 2, leading and cooperating with tier 1 services. This is particularly evident for those young people who have multiple problems and are disaffected or excluded from mainstream provision (Kipke *et al.*, 1997). For similar reasons, services need to be flexible and provided in several settings (including the young person's home) to encourage engagement and nurture young people into services. These settings must be appropriate and appealing to children and their parents and carers, as well as adolescents. These assertive outreach principles are not dissimilar to those articulated in relation to adults with persistent mental health problems (Wright *et al.*, 2003).

Tier 3

Tier 3 comprises a team of professionals able to demonstrate a threshold of aggregate expertise and competence and who are capable of comprehensive assessment and formulation of care plans for those young people with substance abuse/dependence and multiple complex problems. Like all the tiers, it is concerned with outcomes across all domains of functioning, not substance abuse alone. The team includes professionals with specialist knowledge of addictions, practitioners in child and adolescent mental health, specialist teachers, psychologists, social workers, and other therapists. Although in small centers, practitioners in this team may also work at tier 2: the aggregation of specialists forming tier 3 leads to enhanced skills and capacities. The cornerstone of such a team is likely to be a permanent collaboration between those with skills in addictions and those with skills in child health and mental health.

This team is capable of comprehensive assessments of complex presentations, such as young pregnant users and comorbid conditions, including conduct disorder, attention-deficit hyperactivity disorder, or perhaps psychosis, and substance abuse/dependence. It has skills in engagement, assessment of, and intervention with complex young people and families. It will have skills in family and individual psychotherapeutic interventions, interprofessional and intersectoral liaison, as well as in pharmacological interventions such as detoxification and substitution therapy. It will link with other tiers, enhancing their capabilities and capitalizing on existing relationships; where necessary, and in partnership with others, it will mobilize multicomponent, multiagency interventions. Much of the clinical research conducted in the field might be generated at this level.

Tier 4

Tier 4 is the most resource intensive and so should be a last-resource tier, adjunctive to tier 3. In the health context, it might consist of inpatient adolescent psychiatric or forensic services, medicine or obstetric (e.g., for young pregnant users) units complemented by specialist young people's addiction services for complicated detoxifications, specialized crisis placements, highly intensive interventions with a residential component, or perhaps unusually intensive outpatient therapies. For younger adolescents, it may be more likely that the host service would be education (specialist boarding schools), voluntary organizations (therapeutic communities for young people), or social services (specialist children's homes), rather than health. However, as with the other tiers, there is likely to be interagency cooperation in designing and maintaining the management plan. The aims are to reduce substance abuse by providing specialist intervention(s) and settings; sometimes providing crisis assessment and management for a limited time, or containment and care; and providing education and treatment for a highly disturbed child over a longer period.

The current UK reality is that services in tier 4 explicitly designed for youth drug abuse are few. However, residential facilities for other purposes, such as specialist children's homes, may provide, in effect, the same function, albeit appropriately focused on underlying difficulties rather than substance abuse itself. Also, the HAS report recommended there should not be an explicitly substance-abuse-focused tier 4 service unless the other tiers are in place. Otherwise, existing resources are not effectively mobilized; too few will receive intervention, and those that do may not receive an intervention geared to their needs. Hence, consideration should be given to augmenting already available units, such as local authority children's homes and inpatient and day-patient adolescent and forensic psychiatric services. This would require specific additional training.

Links between tiers

Although described separately, the tiers of service should be closely linked. For instance, a social worker or nurse who initially recognizes a set of problems at tier 1 might follow their client or patient through the tiers; perhaps temporarily participating as a tier 3 member in relation to a particular young person. In this way, their initial engagement and knowledge of the young person is not lost to other tiers; there is continuity of care and sharing of skills (in this way it is also possible to avoid the potentially corrosive notion of an explicit hierarchy). Indeed, young people should never be referred from service to service with the case closed behind them. As often the point of first contact, and in cooperation with other tiers, tier 1 may be in some cases the key to the outreach and engagement capabilities that specialists lack, particularly for hard-to-reach young people.

Example of tiers of service

Table 9.1 shows an example of the tiers of service for a 14-year-old boy who is a heavy cannabis user, smokes and drinks regularly, and may also be offending and truanting. Social services would be involved with the family as he is at risk and beyond parental control. The table shows a possible set of interventions at various levels.

Links of the framework with evidence

Law, policy, and the pattern of resources in England provide a framework for practice. This practice in the tiered framework reflects a hierarchy of needs (and rights) determining, in effect, clinical priorities: safety from harm, family life, education, healthy activities, normalizing of peer affiliation, and cooperation between agencies. The tiers system also relies on mobilizing what may be significant latent capacity in the health-care and other systems in the pursuit of these clinical priorities. Indeed, the UK model of multidimensional assessment, emphasis on the role of parents (while respecting appropriately the autonomy of the young person), and multidimensional/multisystems intervention appears consistent and sympathetic with the USA family therapy interventions that have been experimentally developed and formally evaluated (Henggeler *et al.*, 2002; Liddle *et al.*, 2001).

However, while serious attempts have been made to evaluate health-care systems, services for youth engaged in substance misuse are too limited in scale to evaluate as an entire system using national data (World Health Organization: www.who.int/whr2001/2001/archives/2000/en/index.htm). Indeed the scale and distribution of services for youth substance abuse probably bear more resemblance to general health provisions 100 years ago in the developed world than to current general health provisions. Also, despite progressive language, the disorders suffered by young people in Western countries are not taken seriously by health planners, who are often wedded to definitions linked to physical health and are only able to evaluate if routinely gathered statistics are available; the latter are often

Table 9.1 The four-tier strategic framework as it might be utilized for an adolescent with a drug-abuse problem

Tier	Components	Professional involvement
1	Accurate information within the educational curriculum concerning tobacco, alcohol, and drugs	Teachers; school health or general practitioner
	Educational assessment and support to maintain in school	
	General medical services including routine advice on health issues, parental support and advice, hepatitis B vaccination, appropriate referral	
2	Assessment of risk and child care/protection issues	Social services
	Programme of activities to address offending	Youth offender teams
	Counseling addressing lifestyle issues	Youth counseling services
	Interventions regarding parenting and family communication	Mental health services
	Institution of educational rehabilitation measures and regular attendance	Education services
3	Specialist assessment, augmenting and coordinating that already activated in tiers 1 and 2	Specialist, young-person drug and alcohol services (collaboration between the child and adolescent mental health services and adult drug services)
	Interagency planning and communication	
	Specialist substance-specific interventions e.g., cognitive–behavioral therapy	
	Assessment and intervention for mental disorder	
	Family assessment and therapy	Specialist educational provision
	Intensive liaison with education	
4	Short-period accommodation by social services or specialist health facility	Forensic child and adolescent psychiatry; social services
	In/day patient psychiatric or secure unit to assist detoxification, if required	Substance misuse services
	Continued tier 1, 2, and 3	Mutiagency involvement

overtly health or economy related. Even large-scale evaluations of existing services (e.g., Hser *et al.*, 2001) almost certainly do not include the majority of young people with relevant problems in their catchments. Hence, although statistics are available (e.g., from NIDA [http://www.nida.nih.gov/Newsroom/02/NR12-16.html] or the European Monitoring Centre for Drugs and Drug Abuse [http://www.emcdda.org/]), these have not been linked to services. Nevertheless, it would be theoretically possible to evaluate the tiered approach, for instance in terms of access (the estimated proportion of the affected population involved in a meaningful way with an identifiable tier of service) and engagement, youth and carer satisfaction, degrees to which professionals feel that they are part of a coherent delivery system, and outcome according to a range of dimensions. Data such as these could be obtained continuously for a district attempting to develop in this way, linking where possible with relevant databases, such as truancy or crime statistics. This might require a new breadth of vision for funders. However, new UK organizations, such as Children's Trusts (http://www.doh.gov.uk/childrenstrusts/), might be a vehicle for such an investment.

Achievements

The HAS reports as a whole have succeeded dramatically in conceptualizing in a widely acceptable way a complex service provision. They have enabled strategic thinking by both providers and purchasers of services. This has reduced "in-fighting" between providers in particular (e.g., community pediatrics and child psychiatry). The 2001 report has drawn attention to the complex needs of users and the appropriateness, in particular, of including services for users within the broader CAMHS provision. Without the HAS report, it is possible that, as with adult services, an attempt at separate provision or provision by unmodified adult services would have gathered pace.

Nevertheless, the 2001 report has not had the impact yet that it deserves. This is in part a function of the Home Office's focus on crime reduction as the inspiration behind its interest in drug policy, and its use of non-health funding and planning mechanisms to develop interventions for offenders. Also, the Department of Health has invested in much wider reviews of child health services. It is a function, too, of long-standing provision of services (in the absence of mainstream provision) by voluntary organizations with their own cultures and generally adult-oriented training. Furthermore, CAMHS services are hugely overstretched with conventional responsibilities and resist taking on what they have perceived as yet further burdens. Additionally, while the HAS 1995 report on CAMHS described and creatively conceptualized what was already in existence, the 1996 and 2001 reports aimed to describe at least in part what should be: a much more ambitious task.

The enthusiastic official sanction that the HAS report required to progress to actual services has had to wait on the National Treatment Agency, the youth component of which is generating guidance for commissioners of services that is likely to refer to and paraphrase the HAS report. This agency has also sponsored training for pediatricians and other professionals based on the principles outlined in Gilvarry *et al.* (2001). It is anticipated that this will result in accredited training though the Royal College of Paediatrics and Child Health and the Royal College of Psychiatrists. The Royal College of General Practitioners already accredits a course for family practitioners, but this is aimed mainly at the needs of adult users.

Conclusions

There have been developments in the UK system of response to substance abuse and in provision of treatment since the turn of the century. However, the challenge now is to incorporate substance misuse services within existing children's services. The HAS reported that substance abuse services for children and young people should be led by children's systems rather than by commissioners for drug services alone (who may tend to adapt an adult model). The key conclusion is that services should strive to respond to all the problems presented by young drug abusers by an integrated and evidence-based approach. The National Treatment Agency has adopted the HAS report as the basis for its work guiding treatment services for young people.

REFERENCES

Dale-Perera, A. & Hamilton, C. (1997). *An Outline of Some of the Key Issues Raised during the Development of National Policy Guidelines on Working with Young Drug Users.* London: Children's Legal Centre.

Gilvarry, E., Christian, J., Crome, I., *et al.* (2001). *The Substance of Young Needs 2001 Review.* London: Health Advisory Service.

Henggeler, S., Clingempeel, W., Brondino, M., & Pickrel, S. (2002). Four-year follow-up of multisystemic therapy with substance-abusing and substance-dependent juvenile offenders. *Journal of the American Academy of Child and Adolescent Psychiatry.* **41**, 868–74.

Hser, Y., Grella, C., Hubbard, R., *et al.* (2001). An evaluation of drug treatments for adolescents in four US cities. *Archives of General Psychiatry* **58**, 689–695.

Kaplan, C. & McArdle, P. (2004). Ethical and legal principles. In I. Crome, H. Ghodse, E. Gilvarry, & P. McArdle (eds.), *Young People and Substance Misuse* (pp. 184–198). London: Gaskell.

Kipke, M., Unger, J., O'Connor, S., Palmer, R., & LaFrance, S. (1997). Street youth, their peer group affiliation and differences according to residential status, subsistence patterns, and use of services. *Adolescence* **32**, 655–669.

Liddle, H., Dakof, G., Parker, K., *et al.* (2001). Multidimensional family therapy for adolescent drug abuse: results of a randomized clinical trial. *American Journal of Drug and Alcohol Abuse*, **27**, 651–688.

United Nations (1989). *Convention on the Rights of the Child*. New York: United Nations Publications.

Williams, R., Richardson, G., Bates, P., *et al.* (1995). *Together We Stand: Child and Adolescent Mental Health Services*. London: Health Advisory Service.

Williams, R., Christian, J., Gay, M., & Gilvarry, E. (1996). *The Substance of Young Needs. Commissioning and Providing Services for Children and Young People who Use and Misuse Substances*. London: Health Advisory Service.

Wright, C., Burns, T., James, P., *et al.* (2003). Assertive outreach teams in London: models of operation. Pan-London Assertive Outreach Study Part 1. *British Journal of Psychiatry*, **183**, 132–138.

Zoccolillo, M., Vitaro, F., & Tremblay, R. (1999). Problem drug and alcohol use in a community sample of adolescents. *Journal of the American Academy of Child and Adolescent Psychiatry*. **38**, 900–907.

10

Health services with drug-abusing adolescents: the next frontier of research

Jerry P. Flanzer

National Institute on Drug Abuse, Bethesda, MD, USA

The public health care needs of the USA have been steadily shifting from acute, episodic care to treatment for chronic conditions. Chronic conditions are now the leading causes of illness, disability, and death, affecting almost half of the USA population and accounting for the majority of health-care expenditures (Hoffman, Rice, & Sung, 1996). Today, few clinical programs have the infrastructure required to provide the full complement of services needed by people with common chronic conditions (Wagner, Austin, & Korff, 1996). The fact that more than 40% of people with chronic conditions have more than one condition argues for a more sophisticated mechanism to communicate and coordinate care (Robert Wood Johnson Foundation, 1996; Institute of Medicine, 2001).

The treatment of drug abuse, one of the most pervasive chronic conditions and one that often coexists with mental illness and other health problems, similarly lacks the support of an adequate infrastructure for service delivery. The services infrastructure and access to and availability of such services for adolescent drug abusers are even more limited than those for their adult counterparts. Indeed, the actual number of treatment programs serving adolescents with drug abuse problems (mental health as well) has been shrinking in the last few decades (Etheridge *et al.*, 2001). The majority of the programs that do exist are oriented to treat short acute episodes, not taking into account the need to have treatment protocols that follow the treatment career of adolescents and deal with the chronic nature of the disease.

This is the case despite the fact that a number of efficacious treatments for drug-abusing adolescents have been developed and validated. In fact, treatment research for adolescent drug abuse has matured to the point that it now addresses nuanced questions such as focusing on interventions that increase treatment engagement and retention, target different subpopulations, and produce a range of positive outcomes in addition to reducing drug use. Health-services research has matured

Adolescent Substance Abuse: Research and Clinical Advances, ed. Howard A. Liddle and Cynthia L. Rowe.
Published by Cambridge University Press. © Cambridge University Press 2006.

as well, to encompass not only research on the effectiveness of a treatment for an individual (adolescent) patient (Aday *et al.*, 1994), which predominated in the 1960s and 1970s, but also research on treatment economics, organization, and technology transfer (AcademyHealth, 2000). Yet much still remains to be done. The focus of inquiry now must move beyond treatment development and innovation to studies of which treatments are most effective and cost-effective, depending on the specific developmental needs of the adolescents and the progression of their substance abuse and related problems. These real world issues of how interventions can be best tailored and implemented in practice and within the scope of available resources are the domain of health-services research.

Another way of looking at health-services research is that it is "the business approach to health care": the field that focuses on ways to make health-care delivery better (by providing quality services within a range of organizational structures and with improved outcomes), cheaper (by providing services in the most cost-efficient manner possible) and faster (by increasing access to and utilization of services and minimizing barriers so that the most people can benefit from them).

Stated in a more formal way, the 2004 NIDA Blue Ribbon Task Force on Health Services Research offered the following definition of health-services (Weisner & McLellan, 2004, p. 2):

Health services research is a multidiscipline field of inquiry, both basic and applied, that examines how social factors, financing systems, organizational structures and processes, health technologies and personal beliefs and behaviors impact access to and utilization of health care, the quality and cost of health care, and in the end our health and well-being. Ultimately the goals of health services research are to identify the most effective ways to organize, manage, finance and deliver high quality care.

This chapter aims to present some key findings and highlight the gaps and next directions for future health-services research with drug-abusing adolescents. To this end, the chapter is organized around the key care components of health-services research based on the following principles for ideal treatment services (Institute of Medicine, 2001).

<u>Effective</u> – providing services to all who could benefit from them and refraining from providing services to those not likely to benefit, all based on scientific knowledge and affirmative *technology transfer*.

<u>Patient centered</u> – providing care that is respectful and responsive to individual patient preferences, needs and values, and ensuring that patient values guide all clinical decisions.

<u>Timely</u> – reducing wasteful and sometimes harmful delays in delivering care and responding appropriately to phases of the patient's treatment career.

<u>Efficient</u> – avoiding waste, of equipment, supplies, ideas and energy, and ensuring that services are cost-effective and cost-beneficial.

Equitable – providing care that does not vary in quality because of personal characteristics such as gender, ethnicity, geographic location and socio-economic status.

Redesigned – organized around the creation of new structures that support the delivery of evidence based practices and improve care.

Effective

Until the early 1980s, the bulk of health services research focused on measuring the effectiveness of various treatments for individual patients. The typical research question was, "Does drug abuse treatment really work?" That is, does the patient's addictive behavior change in response to treatment implemented in "real world" settings? To answer this question, NIDA funded three large-scale national treatment evaluations covering three decades: the 1970s, 1980s, and 1990s. Collectively, these naturalistic studies, known, respectively, as the Drug Abuse Reporting Program, the Treatment Outcome Prospective Study, and the Drug Abuse Treatment Outcome Study, supported the importance of an adequate length of stay as the cornerstone of effective treatment (http://www.ibr.tcu.edu/resources/rc-natlevals.html; Fletcher, Tims, & Brown, 1997; Simpson, Joe, & Brown, 1997; Simpson, Joe, & Broome, 2002). However, they did not deal exclusively or even primarily with adolescent drug abusers. Grella (Ch. 7) provides findings from these studies specific to adolescent drug abusers.

More recently, Williams and Chang (2000) reviewed 53 treatment studies to determine the effectiveness of treatment for drug-abusing adolescents. Virtually all of those studies, whether inpatient, outpatient, therapeutic community, or outward-bound programs, reported a decline in the amount and frequency of adolescent drug use after treatment. However, the results were far from overwhelming in that, on average, only 38% of the adolescents reported abstinence at 6 months after treatment in these studies, and fewer than half of the discharged adolescents followed through with after-care. Moreover, adolescents diagnosed with comorbid disorders relapsed more often and were less likely to stay in after-care programs than adolescent drug abusers without additional diagnoses, pointing to the need for services better tailored to the multiple problems experienced by many drug-abusing teenagers. An important conclusion of the Williams and Chang (2000) review was that, while little difference was found among different treatment approaches, family-based interventions consistently emerge as superior to alternative interventions.

Other research has shown tailored services to be effective in bringing about behavioral and psychological improvements, including decreases in drug use, criminal activity, family problems, and other risky behaviors, as well as improvements in school and job functioning (Azrin *et al.*, 2001; Hser *et al.*, 2001; Jainchill *et al.*, 2000). For instance, the recently completed randomized multisite Cannabis Youth Treatment study has shown that there are several effective treatments for adolescent marijuana abusers (see Ch. 5). The interventions that are used most commonly and that show the most efficacy with substance-abusing adolescents include family-based and multisystemic therapies, cognitive–behavioral therapy, pharmacotherapy, 12-step treatments, and therapeutic communities (Crome, 1999; Deas and Thomas, 2001; Dennis, 2002). However, effective interventions are not readily available in practice settings (Dennis, 2002). Many drug-abusing adolescents also suffer from mental illness and/or infectious diseases, such as human immunodeficiency virus or hepatitis C. Integrated programs that deal with these co-occurring diseases require greater resources and targeted treatments than do programs for drug abuse alone. In this era of limited resources, communities tend to focus on acute needs, often providing services only for the most problematic cases and sacrificing support for those evidence-based services that address prevention and early intervention needs or offer a continuum of care (Cavanaugh, 2002; Perry, 2002).

Part of the effectiveness equation involves treatment accessibility. That is, does the treatment structure facilitate service delivery? Answering this question requires attention to the sociopolitical environment, organization, management, economic (cost), and financial systems (private or public, insurance or government payers) that affect drug abuse prevention and treatment delivery systems. Financial barriers and disincentives exist in the USA that impede the treatment delivery process. For instance, payment for early assessment and intervention for adolescents who are in the experimentation phase of drug abuse is rare. Such early assessments may lead to a myriad of service costs that third-party payers, worried about the bottom-line, seek to avoid. Fear of stigmatizing the adolescent also plays a role in resistance to the identification of early substance abuse. Professionals working in primary care and other medical settings, schools, and other potential points of contact for screening and assessing adolescent drug users rarely have the organizational capacity, knowledge, or incentive to identify and assess these youths or intervene on their behalf (Petrila, Foster-Johnson, & Greenbaum, 1996).

The USA government has launched several efforts geared toward overcoming organizational barriers and increasing the application of scientific advances in adolescent drug abuse treatment into the field. These efforts include the work of the Addiction Technology Transfer Centers and the Practice Improvement Collaboratives, both supported by CSAT, a division of SAMHSA, as well as the Clinical Trials Network, funded by NIDA. Similarly, some technology transfer efforts by states and local agencies are also under way (Pond, Aguirre-Molina, & Orleans, 2002). Most promising, Join Together On-Line (www.jointogether.com), an umbrella organization of stakeholder intervention groups for substance abuse, has used the internet and email as a way of closing some of the gaps between research and practice. However, very little has been done to assess the impact of these efforts on treatment practices and outcomes.

The federal drug abuse research institute, NIDA, and the federal treatment services funding agency, SAMHSA, recognizing the need to move evidence-based practice into the practice community, have launched a strong new science-to-practice policy effort supporting joint activities to remove these barriers. The operation of this effort can be seen in the new publication *NIDA Science & Practice Perspectives* and in SAMHSA's *National Registry of Evidence-based Programs and Practices*. Still, government efforts in this regard have been handicapped by the dearth of research on the best means of achieving technology transfer. Liddle *et al.* (2002) have directly addressed the challenges of technology adaptation and transfer with drug-abusing adolescents in treatment. In implementing multidimensional family therapy (Liddle, 2002) within an intensive day-treatment program, Liddle's group described (a) the conceptual and empirical basis for these technology-transfer efforts, (b) the technology being adapted and transferred, and (c) the critical events and processes that shaped the transfer effort. Similar empirical studies of adoption and transfer of treatment for substance-abusing adolescents are sorely needed.

Patient Centered

Providing patient-centered care to adolescents is made difficult by the fact that a large portion of adolescents receiving drug abuse treatment are coerced into treatment and do not seek it voluntarily. Treatment utilization and engagement is strongly related to several individual-level factors: the adolescents stage of change readiness, pressure to remain in treatment, the degree of support from family and friends, and presence of co-occurring disorders. Other program-level factors influence treatment participation including establishing a positive, therapeutic relationship between the adolescent and treatment provider; developing a comprehensive treatment plan; linking the adolescent with indicated medical, psychiatric, and social services; and providing appropriate after-care that takes account of and can counter negative social influences in the adolescent's everyday life.

Association with drug-abusing peers has been found to be the most common psychosocial trigger of relapse among young people, followed by difficulties coping with negative feelings, interpersonal conflict, and lack of social supports (Shoemaker & Sherry, 1991). Approximately half of drug-abusing adolescents are in and out of recovery once or more following treatment; even when they are on probation or parole, they often have few supports to help them to sustain their recovery or make it back from a relapse (Dennis *et al.*, 2002a). This is not surprising, given the chronicity of the disease. In fact, compared with other chronic diseases, these relapse rates are not remarkably high (McLellan *et al.*, 2000). A reintegration component is typically part of the treatment plan for teenagers in residential programs, but, surprisingly, ongoing after-care for teens in non-residential outpatient programs is not often considered or funded. Linkages to continuing care services are often non-existent or poorly coordinated (Godley *et al.*, 2002).

Current studies of relapse, retention, and reintegration all point to a need for effective continuity-of-care models that address each adolescent's unique needs. Future research must focus on factors affecting reintegration of the drug-abusing adolescent into the community from residential programs and juvenile justice facilities, including engagement and motivation to seek continued treatment, mental health issues, social skills, peer relationships, and linkages with community agencies. Innovative studies of reentry strategies utilizing evidence-based family-focused interventions are currently being funded through NIDA's Criminal Justice Drug Abuse Treatment Studies (NIDA, 2002). In addition, the Community Reinforcement Approach is a continuity-of-care treatment model that relies upon financial and other incentives to reward the adolescent and the community agencies for maintaining ongoing reciprocal contact. However, it is one of the only comprehensive care models to be empirically tested (Azrin *et al.*, 1982; Meyers & Smith, 1995).

Timing

Timing is an important and understudied component of seeking care and of the treatment process itself. Wait-list delays and poorly coordinated care of different treatment components are concrete examples of case timing mismanagement that affect treatment costs, as well as youths' motivation, engagement, and adherence (Tucker & Davidson, 2000). Providing appropriate care at the appropriate time, in a manner that is matched to the patient's level of abuse and/or phase in his/her treatment career, is no easy task. A comprehensive array of services and a community continuity-of-care model needs to be in place to fulfill this diagnostic/assessment–treatment match (Etheridge *et al.*, 2001). In fact, drug-abusing adolescents tend to receive the same treatment intervention, the one that is the specialty of an addiction program/agency, no matter where the adolescent is in the addiction cycle or in their treatment career (Aarons *et al.*, 2001). This further reflects the gap between evidence-based research findings and everyday practice.

Efficient

Achieving efficiencies in treatment delivery and avoiding wasteful expenditures of time, money, treatment resources, and energy requires attention to organization-level issues. Drug abuse treatment services are generally separated from traditional health-care settings and are provided by a range of institutions, including free-standing addiction programs, dual diagnosis addiction programs, criminal justice systems, and human service/social welfare agencies. Issues related to the workforce employed at these varying sites have only recently been studied. The available research points to a wide gap between the demographic profiles of treatment providers and the adolescents they treat (Northwest Frontier Addiction Technology Transfer Center, 2000). For instance, the workforce is predominantly composed of white middle-aged women (average age 47 years) with a history of drug abuse themselves. By contrast, the treatment population of adolescent substance abusers is predominantly male, is growing more racially and ethnically diverse, and is initiating drug use at an increasingly younger age. Studies exploring the impact of differences between the adolescents in treatment and the providers who treat them has yet to be conducted. Clearly, the lack of providers who are sufficiently trained to deal with the issues specific to treating adolescent substance abusers is reflected in the dearth of licensing requirements for counselors working with this age group (Pollio, 2003). The questionable competence of many providers working with adolescent drug abusers naturally compromises the ability to transfer proven technologies and practices into the field.

Lower staff-to-patient ratios facilitate attention to individually targeted patient needs. Staff members who experience peer and supervisory support are more likely to maintain treatment fidelity (Knudsen, Johnson, & Roman, 2003). Negative experiences in supervision may adversely influence patient care, as the counselor's confidence in treating patients erodes (Ramos-Sanchez *et al.*, 2002). Maintenance of treatment fidelity can be expected to suffer accordingly. By contrast, training, supervision, and a supportive environment increase the likelihood that the professionals will have access to, and be more likely to use faithfully, the latest treatment technologies – with resultant cost benefits (French *et al.*, 2002). Management principles of supervisory support and training have been shown to enhance service efficiency in business and health-care fields outside the substance abuse arena (Mael, 1991). Workers who have feelings of low personal power in an organization are less likely to report feelings of service effectiveness and accomplishment with their clients, as well as greater emotional exhaustion and a greater intent to leave their jobs in the near future. As worker power increases, self-reported service also tends to increase, and clients mirror the workers' perception of the worker's power and effectiveness (Bargal & Guterman, 1996). Yet these principles are seldom taken into account in planning and implementing drug abuse treatment programs, and certainly very infrequently in the adolescent specialty.

Issues related to turnover of staff in service delivery for drug abuse also have not been examined, even though turnover is estimated to cost an organization 100% of the departing employee's salary and benefits (Gering & Conner, 2002). This translates into a turnover cost of approximately $35 000 per counselor (Roman, Blum, & Johnson, 2002). It also has significant clinical consequences, as client recovery is known to be associated with a continuous treatment provider (Alverson, Alverson, & Drake, 2000). In fact, staff turnover is one of the most frequently reported obstacles to recovery for patients diagnosed with two comorbid disorders (Bargal & Guterman, 1996).

Who owns the service agency can and often does affect the organization of services and the quality of care provided. Yet health-services research has yet to explore adequately the issue of ownership. Ownership differences are evident in service funding (amount and priorities), and referrals and selection of client groups to receive substance abuse services. Several surveys have shown that the assessment and provision of services in the for-profit and not-for-profit agencies are similar. Contrary to pervasive beliefs, for-profit agencies are not more efficient in their delivery of services, even though they charge more for similar services than non-profit agencies. However, there are important differences in service delivery between the two agency types. For-profit agencies are networked into a different array of services than the not-for-profit programs; their clients are also more affluent, less disabled, less vulnerable, less likely to be incarcerated, and less likely to leave treatment involuntarily. Market specialization is also more pronounced among for-profit agencies (Wheeler & Nahra, 2000).

In terms of costs of services, only recently have the actual costs, cost-effectiveness, and cost–benefits of adolescent drug abuse treatments been examined. Three major studies, plus a smaller pilot study, have shed some light on this issue by actually comparing the costs of treatment for adolescent drug abusers: the Fort Bragg Demonstration (King *et al.*, 2000), the Washington State study (Barnowski & Aos, 2004), and the Cannabis Youth Treatment study (French *et al.*, 2002). In the Fort Bragg study, estimates of the average treatment costs for adolescents with comorbid drug abuse and psychiatric disorders were more than twice the costs for adolescents with only one of these disorders (King *et al.*, 2000). The Washington State study was the first state-wide experiment adopting evidenced-based treatment programs for adolescents involved in the juvenile justice system (functional family therapy, aggression replacement therapy, coordination of services, and multisystemic therapy). The effectiveness of each approach was compared between a center with good training and one with a limited training and no quality assurance. The multisystemic therapy component failed to yield interpretable results because of problems in implementation and training; among the other treatments, the higher adherence programs all showed strong decreases in recidivism and drug abuse rates. By contrast, in lower adherence programs, the accompanying quality assurance, recidivism, and cost rates actually increased (Barnowski & Aos, 2004), implicating better outcomes and lower costs associated with careful adherence and monitoring to evidence-based models. In the third study, French and colleagues (2002) adapted the Drug Abuse Treatment Cost Analysis Program, a standardized measure of service utilization and costs, to analyze the cost data from the Cannabis Youth Treatment study (Dennis *et al.*, 2002b). Costs generally reflected intensity, duration, and number of services provided. Unlike Barnowski and Aos (2004), French *et al.* did not find significant cost differences between types of treatment. Finally, in a small experimental pilot study, Robertson, Grimes, & Rogers (2001) demonstrated that intensive out-patient counseling with cognitive–behavioral therapy imposed significantly fewer costs on the juvenile justice system than did an alternative, intensive probation supervision and monitoring program.

These studies illustrate the feasibility of studying service costs and their potential benefits to policy decision makers. However, further cost estimates and standardization of measurement across studies will be needed as an essential step towards responsible decisions regarding resource allocation based on rigorous cost–benefit analyses. Public health stakeholders who set policies and make decisions on budgeting and resource allocation need to know the optimal configurations of staffing treatment services and the related costs. The full costs of the delivery of treatment services must be evaluated (Cartwright, 1998; French *et al.*, 2002).

The enormous advances in research on adolescent drug abuse treatment will be for naught if the means to pay for proven interventions are not provided. Two thirds of all children in the USA have private insurance, mainly through their parents' employers or through family purchased plans (Kaiser Commission on Medicaid and the Uninsured, 2002). Yet in terms of drug abuse treatment, their care is limited (Fox, McManus, & Reichman, 2002). For instance, the number of outpatient therapy visits allowed for drug abuse in insurance plans is generally quite limited and not sufficient to cover ongoing treatment of this chronic disorder. Part of the problem is that drug abuse treatment is not regarded as being on par with general medical care in the USA. As a result, the benefit limits and patient/family cost-sharing requirements for drug abuse services generally exceed those for general medical care (American Academy of Pediatrics, 2001).

Funding for services also varies by geographic location, partly because public funding for drug abuse treatment is primarily controlled by state governments. States, in turn, vary in their allocation of funds, as well as in the amount and distribution of treatment services offered and the settings in which they are delivered to adolescents (within the mental health system, free-standing substance abuse programs, or as attachments to juvenile justice programs; Perry, 2002). Under federal policy, funds from Medicaid and from comprehensive health-care plans, and smaller amounts from a host of other federal projects (Flanzer, 2005), may be used to cover emergency services for substance abuse and outpatient treatment services, but the states have wide latitude in the type, amount, and intensity of adolescent substance abuse services that they provide under Medicaid (Geshan, 1999; Johnson, 1999). Furthermore, reimbursement rates and the supply of providers in some geographic areas are low (Pringle & Flanzer, 2004).

Federal support for treating adolescent substance abuse comes primarily through the Substance Abuse Prevention and Treatment Performance Partnership Block Grant, administered by SAMHSA. States support over half of all treatment services in substance abuse with these dollars. In many states, however, the block grant funds for youth are spent primarily on prevention services, with little money targeted for treatment (Cavanaugh, 2002). Primary-care providers and other medical specialists provide little treatment for substance abusers, and their avoidance of the diagnosis of substance abuse reflects the billing disincentives prevalent in the USA health-care system. Annual access to Medicaid-paid substance abuse treatment services remains low for adolescents in all states (Heflinger, Renfrew, & Saunders, 2003). Although the Medicaid funds for drug abuse treatment services are set aside by these states, they are not frequently accessed because of low reimbursement rates, administrative hassles, and potential referrers' lack of knowledge of the existence of Medicaid money available for treatment (Heflinger *et al.*, 2003). Research that could shed light on new funding and resource allocation structures and gradually change these unfortunate circumstances is sorely needed.

Equitable

There is clearly an inequitable distribution of services for adolescent drug abusers in the USA. Urban areas offer more services than rural areas. Whites continue to enjoy disproportional access to services compared with African-American, American-Indian, and Hispanic youth. African-American youth are significantly more likely to be processed in the juvenile justice system and access treatment through the courts. As mentioned above, the staff of most adolescent substance abuse treatment programs is not representative of the racial and ethnic groups the programs serve. While case management approaches (Siegal *et al.*, 1997) can increase access and reduce barriers to treatment, particularly for disadvantaged and disenfranchised groups, financing issues and issues of social capital continue to block much progress toward equitable delivery of services to the economically disadvantaged and politically powerless.

Dwayne Simpson and colleagues at Texas Christian University and Thomas McLellan and his colleagues at the University of Pennsylvania and the Treatment Research Institute have demonstrated that core drug abuse treatment components must be accompanied by comprehensive adjunctive services in order for treatment gains to be fully realized (McLellan *et al.*, 2000; Simpson *et al.*, 1997). Simpson's group has shown that treatment programs are integrally linked to their affiliated agency systems and the social capital of their surrounding environment. Ultimately, it is the local neighborhoods' social capital (that is, the strength of their network of support services, their attitude toward treatment programs situated in their "backyard," the availability of jobs, and the community's intolerance of drug dealing) that creates an equitable treatment-friendly environment. Disadvantaged populations tend not to be proportionately represented in social capital efforts. Therefore, for meaningful research to develop and for effective technology transfer to take place, all "community" stakeholders need to be involved. Research is sorely needed on how to increase the involvement of stakeholders and on the effect of social capital for all groups within and among the adolescent drug-abusing population.

Redesign

In review, recently developed treatments for drug-abusing adolescents offer promise, but research illustrating how to implement them in the most effective, cost-effective manner must now take priority. The time has come to build upon efficacy studies with research investigating the optimal utilization of resources and integrative models of treatment.

There are many challenges ahead. Key challenges for the redesign of health-care organizations include organizing and financing services in ways that make sense to patients and clinicians and that foster coordination of care, collaborative work, technology transfer, and educating the workforce. Agency structures and ownership should be considered in ways that involve all stakeholders. All of this work should be based on sound design principles and make use of information technologies that can integrate data for multiple uses and answer the many remaining questions about organizational adaptation and adoption of treatment services. The research cited above points to the need for coordinated care across patient conditions, services, and settings over time, and that incorporate performance and outcome measures for improvement and accountability relevant to consumers, regulators, health professionals, and educational institutions.

Government and private funding, and related organizational changes, is needed to create an environment that fosters and rewards improvements in care by building an infrastructure to support evidence-based practice, facilitating the use of information technology, aligning payment policies and incentives with quality improvements, and preparing the workforce to serve patients better in a world of expanding knowledge and rapid change. More in-depth research is needed on the economics and financing of treatment services.

Health-services researchers also need to involve the stakeholders, the policy makers, and the administrators more fully in the research process in order to guarantee the adoption and maintenance of evidence-based, patient-centered treatments in practice settings. Health-services research is witnessing an ongoing transition from patient-focused treatment applications to organizational-level systems research. This is leading to increased interest in, and cooperation from, numerous federal, state, and treatment-provider stakeholders. As evidenced by NIH's roadmap effort (NIH website) and by the NIDA-SAMHSA-AHRQ service-to-practice collaborative initiatives, efforts have been undertaken to:

- explore new models of continuous training, treatment adherence, and staff development and their effects on service-delivery outcomes
- explore the effect of social capital on access to and development of adolescent drug abuse prevention and treatment services
- acknowledge and test resource allocation, social and fiscal costs, and financing streams as key variables in the implementation of adolescent drug abuse treatment services.

With major initiatives now underway and further commitment from funders to invest in health-services research and implementation efforts, the adolescent drug abuse treatment field is in a solid position to make remarkable advances in the years to come.

NOTE

The views expressed in this paper are the views of the author and should not be necessarily construed as the views of the National Institute on Drug Abuse.

REFERENCES

Aarons, G. A., Brown, S., Hough, R. L., Garland, A. F., & Wood, P. A. (2001). Prevalence of adolescent substance use disorders across five sectors of care. *Journal of the American Academy of Child and Adolescent Psychiatry*, **40**, 419–426.

AcademyHealth (2000). *Definition of the Field of Health Services Research*. Washington, DC: AcademyHealth. Retrieved July 2002 from http://www.academyhealth.org/hsrproj/hsr.htm.

Aday, L. A., Youssef, A., Liu, S. W., Chao, W. H., & Zhang, C. (1994). Estimating the risks and prevalence of hypertension in a suburban area of Beijing. *Journal of Community Health*, **19**, 331–341.

Alverson, H., Alverson, M., & Drake, R. (2000). An ethnographic study of the longitudinal course of substance abuse among people with severe mental illness. *Community Mental Health Journal*, **36**, 557–569.

American Academy of Pediatrics (2001). Improving substance abuse prevention, assessment, and treatment financing for children and adolescents. *Pediatrics*, **108**, 1025–1029.

Azrin, N. H., Sisson, W., Meyers, R., & Godley, M. (1982). Alcoholism treatment by disulfram and community reinforcement therapy. *Journal of Behavior Therapy and Experimental Psychiatry*, **13**, 105–112.

Azrin, N. H., Donohue, B., Teichner, G. A., *et al.* (2001). A controlled evaluation and description of individual cognitive problem solving and family-behavior therapies in dually diagnosed conduct-disordered and substance-dependent youth. *Journal of Child and Adolescent Substance Abuse*, **11**, 1–43.

Bargal, D. & Guterman, N. (1996) Perception of job satisfaction, service effectiveness and burnout among social workers in Israel. *[In Hebrew] Society and Welfare [Hevrah U'revaha]*, **16**: 541–565.

Barnowski, R. & Aos, S. (2004). *Outcome Evaluation of Washington State's Research-based Programs for Juvenile Offenders*. Seattle, WA: Washington Institute for Public Policy. http://www.wsipp.wa.gov.

Cartwright, W. S. (1998). Cost–benefit and cost-effectiveness analysis of drug abuse treatment services, *Evaluation Review*, **2**, 609–636.

Cavanaugh, D. A. (2002). Financing a system of care for adolescents with substance use disorders: Opportunities and challenges. In *Proceedings of the Center for Substance Abuse Treatment/Robert Wood Johnson Foundation Adolescent Treatment Systems and Support Summit*, Rockville, MD, September.

Crome, I. B. (1999). Treatment interventions: looking toward the millennium. *Drug and Alcohol Dependence*, **55**, 247–263.

Deas, D. & Thomas, S. E. (2001). An overview of controlled studies of adolescent substance abuse treatment. *American Journal of Addictions*, **10**, 178–189.

Dennis, M. (2002). Treatment research on adolescent drug and alcohol abuse: despite progress, many challenges remain. In AcademyHealth (ed.), *Connection* (pp. 1–2, 7). Washington, DC: AcademyHealth. http://www.academyhealth.org/publications/connection/may02.pdf.

Dennis, M. L., Dawud-Noursi, S., Muck, R., & McDermott, M. (2002a). The need for developing and evaluating adolescent treatment models. In S. J. Stevens & A. R. Morral (eds.), *Adolescent Substance Abuse Treatment in the United States: Exemplary Models from a National Evaluation Study*. Binghampton, NY: Haworth Press.

Dennis, M. L., Titus, J. C., Diamond, G., *et al.* and the CYT Steering Committee. (2002b). The Cannabis Youth Treatment (CYT) experiment: rationale, study design and analysis plans. *Addiction*, **97**(Suppl. 1), 16–34.

Etheridge, R. M., Smith, J. C., Rounds-Bryant, J. L., & Hubbard, R. L. (2001). Drug abuse treatment and comprehensive services for adolescents. *Journal of Adolescent Research*, **16**, 563–589.

Flanzer, J. (2005). The status of health services research on adjudicated drug-abusing juveniles: selected findings and remaining questions. *Substance Use and Misuse*, **40**, 887–911.

Fletcher, B. W., Tims, F. M., & Brown, B. S. (1997). The Drug Abuse Treatment Outcome Study (DATOS): treatment evaluation research in the United States. *Psychology of Addictive Behaviors*, **11**, 216–229.

Fox, H. B., McManus, M. A., & Reichman, M. B. (2002). *Private Health Insurance for Adolescents: Is It Adequate?* Washington, DC: Maternal and Child Health Policy Research Center.

French, M., Roebuck, M. C., Dennis, M., *et al.* (2002). The economic cost of outpatient marijuana treatment for adolescents: findings from a multisite field experiment. *Addiction,* **97**(Suppl. 1), 84–97.

Gering, J. & Conner, J. (2002). A strategic approach to employee retention. *Healthcare Financial Management,* **56**, 40–44.

Geshan, S. (1999). *TIE Communique: Substance Abuse Benefits in State Children's Health Insurance Program* (pp. 25–27). Rockville, MD: Center for Substance Abuse Treatment.

Godley, M. D., Godley, S. H., Dennis, M. L., Funk, R., & Passetti, L. L. (2002). Preliminary outcomes from the assertive continuing care experiment for adolescents discharged from residential treatment. *Journal of Substance Abuse Treatment,* **23**, 21–32.

Heflinger, C. A., Renfrew, J. W., & Saunders, R. C. (2003, March). Medicaid non-specialty services to adolescents to adolescents with drug and alcohol diagnoses. In *Proceeding of the NIMHDAA Conference Beyond the Clinic Walls: Expanding Mental Health, Drug and Alcohol Services Research Outside the Specialty Care System.* Washington, DC: National Institutes on Mental Health, Drug Abuse, and Alcoholism.

Hoffman, C., Rice, D. P., & Sung, H. (1996). Persons with chronic conditions: their prevalence and costs. *Journal of the American Medical Association,* **276**, 1473–1479.

Hser, Y., Grella, C. E., Hubbard, R. L., *et al.* (2001). An evaluation of drug treatments for adolescents in four US cities. *Archives of General Psychiatry,* **58**, 689–695.

Institute of Medicine (2001). *Crossing the Quality Chasm: A New Health System for the 21st Century.* Washington, DC: National Academy Press for the Institute of Medicine, Committee on Quality of Health Care in America.

Jainchill, N., Hawke, J., DeLeon, G., & Yagelka, J. (2000). Adolescents in therapeutic communities: one year post treatment outcomes. *Journal of Psychoactive Drugs,* **32**, 81–94.

Johnson, P. (1999). *Substance Abuse Treatment Coverage in State Medicaid Programs.* Washington, DC: National Conference of State Legislatures.

Kaiser Commission on Medicaid and the Uninsured (2002). *Health Coverage for Low Income Children* [*Fact Sheet*] Washington, DC: Kaiser Commission. http://www.kff.org.

King, R. D., Gaines, L. S., Lambert, E. W., Summerfelt, W. T., & Bickman, L. (2000). The co-occurrence of psychiatric and substance use diagnoses in adolescents in different service systems: frequency, recognition, cost, and outcomes. *Journal of Behavioral Health Services and Research,* **27**, 417–430.

Knudsen, H. K., Johnson, J. A., & Roman, P. M. (2003). Retaining counseling staff at substance abuse treatment centers: effects of management practices. *Journal of Substance Abuse Treatment,* **24**, 1–7.

Liddle, H. A. (2002). *Cannabis Youth Treatment (CYT) Manual Series,* Vol. 5: *Multidimensional Family Therapy for Adolescent Cannabis Users.* Rockville, MD, Center for Substance Abuse Treatment, Substance Abuse and Mental Health Services Administration. Retrieved from http://www.samhsa.gov.csat.csat.htm.

Liddle, H. A., Rowe, C. L., Quille, T. J., *et al.* (2002). Transporting a research-based adolescent drug treatment into practice. *Journal of Substance Abuse Treatment,* **22**, 231–243.

Mael, F. (1991). Desire for career mobility and workplace adaptation. *International Journal of Career Management*, **3**, 10–16.

McLellan, A. T., Lewis, D. C., O'Brien, C. P., & Kleber, H. D. (2000). Drug dependence, a chronic medical illness: implications for treatment, insurance, and outcome evaluation. *Journal of the American Medical Association*, **284**, 1689–1695.

Meyers, R. J. & Smith, J. E. (1995) *Clinical Guide to Alcohol Treatment: The Community Reinforcement Approach*. New York: Guilford Press.

NIDA (National Institute on Drug Abuse) (2002). *National Criminal Justice Drug Abuse Treatment Services Research System*. [Report RFA-DA-02-011] Rockville, MD: National Institutes of Health. Retrieved May 15, 2004 from http://grants2.nih.gov/grants/guide/rfa-files/RFA-DA-02-011.html.

NFATTC (Northwest Frontier Addiction Technology Transfer Center) (2000). *Advancing the Current State of Addiction Treatment: A Regional Needs Assessment of Substance Abuse Treatment Professionals in the Pacific Northwest*. Portland, OR: RMC Research.

Perry, P. D. (2002). Fragmented funding: friend or foe? A multi-state case study of publicly supported adolescent alcohol and substance abuse treatment. In *Proceedings of the Center for Substance Abuse Treatment/Robert Wood Johnson Foundation Adolescent Treatment Systems and Support Summit*, Rockville, MD, September.

Petrila, A. T., Foster-Johnson, L., & Greenbaum, P. E. (1996). Serving youth with mental health and substance abuse problems. In B. A. Stroul (ed.), *Children's Mental Health: Creating Systems of Care in a Changing Society* (pp. 493–511). Baltimore, MD: Brookes.

Pollio, D. E. (2003). States need to ensure expertise of adolescent providers through training and certification. In AcademyHealth (ed.), *Connection* (pp. 4–8). Washington, DC: AcademyHealth.

Pond, A. S., Aguirre-Molina, M., & Orleans, J. (2002). *Technology Transfer in Adolescent Substance Abuse Treatment: Status, Challenges, and Strategies to Improve the Transfer Process*. Princeton, NJ: Robert Wood Johnson Foundation.

Pringle, B. & Flanzer, J. (2004). Treatment services for adolescent substance abuse. In Steele, R. G. & Roberts, M. C. (eds.)., *Handbook of Mental Health Services for Children, Adolescents, and Families* (pp. 181–200). New York: Kluwer/Plenum.

Ramos-Sanchez, L., Esnil, E., Goodwin, A., *et al.* (2002). Negative supervisory effects: effects on supervision satisfaction and supervisory alliance. *Professional Psychology: Research and Practice*, **33**, 197–202.

Robert Wood Johnson Foundation (1996). *Chronic Care in America: A 21st Century Challenge*. Princeton, NJ: Robert Wood Johnson Foundation. www.rwjf.org/library/chrcare.

Robertson, A., Grimes, P., & Rogers, K. (2001). A short-run cost–benefit analysis of community-based interventions for juvenile offenders. *Crime and Delinquency*, **47**, 265–284.

Roman, P., Blum, T. C., & Johnson, J. A. (2002). *National Treatment Center Study*. [*Summary Report No. 5, Third Wave On-Site Results*.] Atlanta, EA: University of Georgia, Institute for Behavioral Research.

Shoemaker, R. H. & Sherry, P. (1991). Posttreatment factors influencing outcome of adolescent chemical dependency treatment. *Journal of Adolescent Chemical Dependency*, **2**, 89–106.

Siegal, H. A., Rapp R. C., Li, L., Saha, P., & Kirk, K. (1997). The role of case management in retaining clients in substance abuse treatment: an exploratory analysis. *Journal of Drug Issues*, **27**, 821–831.

Simpson, D. D., Joe, G. W., & Brown, B. S. (1997). Treatment retention and follow-up outcomes in the Drug Abuse Treatment Outcome Study (DATOS). *Psychology of Addictive Behaviors*, **11**, 294–307.

Simpson, D. D., Joe, G. W., & Broome, K. M. (2002). A national 5-year follow-up of treatment outcomes for cocaine dependence. *Archives of General Psychiatry*, **59**, 538–544.

Tucker, J. & Davidson, J. (2000). Waiting to see the doctor: the role of time constraints in the utilization of health and behavioral health services. In W. Bikel & R. Vuchinich (eds.), *Reframing Health Behavior Change with Behavioral Economics*. Hillsdale, NJ: Lawrence Elbaum.

Wagner, E. H., Austin, B. T., & Korff, M. V. (1996). Organizing care for patients with chronic illness. *Milbank Quarterly*, **74**: 511–42.

Williams, R. J. & Chang, S. Y. (2000). A comprehensive and comparative review of adolescent substance abuse treatment outcome. *Clinical Psychology: Science and Practice*, **7**, 138–166.

Weisner, C. & McLellan, A. T. (2004) *The Blue Ribbon Task Force on Health Services Research at the National Institute on Drug Abuse*. Rockville, MD: National Institute of Drug Abuse. Retrieved February 20 2004 from http://www.drugabuse.gov/about/organization/nacda/HSRReport.pdf.

Wheeler, J. & Nahra, T. (2000). Private and public ownership in outpatient substance abuse treatment: do we have a two-tiered system? *Administration Policy of Mental Health*, **27**, 197–209.

Part III

Comprehensive assessment and integrative treatment planning with adolescent substance abusers

11

Clinical perspectives on the assessment of adolescent drug abuse

Kenneth C. Winters

University of Minnesota, Minneapolis, MN, USA

The purpose of this chapter is to provide an overview of clinical best practices for assessing adolescent drug abuse. To achieve this purpose, a multidimensional model of screening and assessment is proposed. This model provides a theoretical framework sufficiently broad as to be applicable to most research and treatment assessment challenges (Winters, 1999) and to be relevant for problem identification, referral, and treatment. In addition, the chapter highlights clinical challenges and approaches when applying the model.

Assessment model

For the purposes of this chapter, the central task of the assessment process is to characterize the client's drug use behaviors, as well as a range of personal and environmental risks and strengths. This process has three basic components – method, content, and source – and each component intersects as a function of assessment level (brief screening, screening, and comprehensive). Table 11.1 offers an overview of how these components can form an assessment model. Three broad types of assessment are characterized: brief screening, screening, and comprehensive assessment. Domains associated with content, methods, and sources are associated with each type. The two screening processes focus on drug use behaviors based on the client's self-report. The assessment goal of these two processes is to determine if the client should receive a comprehensive assessment. "Positive" cases would receive an in-depth evaluation of the pattern and extent of problems in order to address decisions related to referral and treatment planning.

The availability of several information resources greatly facilitates the task of locating and judging the adequacy of appropriate measures for screening and in-depth assessment. The measure's published validity is paramount in this evaluation. Validity evidence provides the basis for the scientific utility of the instrument, that is, "how well

Adolescent Substance Abuse: Research and Clinical Advances, ed. Howard A. Liddle and Cynthia L. Rowe.
Published by Cambridge University Press. © Cambridge University Press 2006.

Table 11.1 Assessment model

Evaluation	Methods	Sources	Content
Brief screening (5–10 min)	Short questionaire	Client	Drug use severity
Screening (30–60 min)	Short questionaire; brief interview; urinalysis	Client; parent	Drug use severity; biopsychosocial
Comprehensive (2–4 h)	Comprehensive questionaire; detailed interview; observation; archival records	Client; parent	Drug use severity; biopsychosocial; comorbidity; problem recognition; response distortion

it measures what it purports to measure" (Nunnally & Bernstein, 1994). Given that the field of adolescent drug abuse assessment has seen considerable growth in the development of sound instruments – ranging from very brief screens, to multiple domain questionnaires, to detailed interviews – it is no longer necessary for treatment programs to use in-house, untested assessment instruments. Provided below is a summary of several resources for selecting measures in this field.

Print resources

Several print sources provide information on instruments for the assessment of substance use disorders and related constructs. Reviews of psychometric instruments have been reported in peer-reviewed literature (e.g., Lecesse & Waldron, 1994), and others are sponsored by several federal agencies, including CSAT, NIDA, and NIAAA. Three particularly relevant and useful sources are contained in Winters (1999), CSAT (1999), and Allen & Columbus (2004). The first provides information on screening and assessment instruments for evaluating adolescents for substance use disorders. In addition to measures focused exclusively on substance use and related disorders, other relevant dimensions are also considered, including measures of mental disorders, family functioning, school achievement, and health. The CSAT guide (1999) to risk factor and outcome instruments provides a similar instrument index. The NIAAA's updated edition of their assessment handbook (Allen & Columbus, 2004) includes several chapters from experts in the field that address various assessment topics (e.g., screening, biological assessment, diagnosis), as well as summaries of over 100 instruments and measures. Instrument selection required, among other criteria, that it be specific to alcohol and other drug abuse treatment, that it yield a quantitative score, and that its psychometric properties be published in at least one source. The guide also presents copies of the instruments and information on how to obtain a copy. The second edition contains an expanded section on adolescent measures.

Among more general print resources, the *Mental Measurements Yearbook*, published since 1938, annually provides reviews of new and revised measures. A companion volume, *Test in Print*, provides a comprehensive list of measures described in all volumes of *Mental Measurements Yearbook*.

Public access internet sites

Public access internet sites provide ready access to information about test instruments and, in some instances, links to the instruments themselves. In some cases, these electronic resources provide more extensive information than would be practical in the print format. Of note are the websites for the CSAT *Treatment Improvement Protocols Series* (www.text.nim.nih.gov), the *ERIC/AE Test Locator* (www.ericae.net/testcol.html), and the *Buros Institute of Mental Measurements* (www.unl.edu/buros/).

Developmental considerations

The effective application of the assessment model in Table 11.1 requires an appreciation by the assessor of several developmental characteristics of adolescent drug involvement. A developmentally informed assessment approach is critically important to the clinician and researcher given that drug use behaviors, and the risk and protective factors that underlie drug involvement, unfold across qualitatively distinct stages of emotional and behavioral growth (Achenbach, 1995). A developmental perspective of drug use should emphasize the contrast between normal and atypical development, qualitative change over time, and mediator and moderator variables, which vary in effects according to developmental stages (Cicchetti & Cohen, 1995). Without these considerations, treatment referral decisions and conclusions from research investigations may be invalid.

Consequently, a paramount challenge of the assessment process is to provide an objective foundation for accurate and time-relevant data necessary for clinical and research decisions. Fortunately, progress has been made in constructing developmental conceptualizations of the onset of drug use and substance use disorders (Tarter *et al.*, 1999; Zucker, Fitzgerald, & Moses, 1995), and these conceptualizations have been translated into useful assessment strategies and instruments (Winters, 1999). For example, state of the art assessment tools recognize that the development of drug use problems during adolescence has multiple facets, including the identification of relevant substances, determination of consumption histories, and description of substance-specific and substance-general problems. Also, in contrast to the more traditional approach, which is focused on a given point without historical referents, many extant assessment tools depict changes in drug involvement over time in order to distinguish infrequent use versus frequent use (Clark & Winters, 2002).

Finally, many well-developed instruments include standardized norms that distinguish normative developmental roles played by drug use in this age group from roles that reflect clinical problems. As described in the classic research by Kandel and colleagues (Kandel, 1975; Yagamuchi & Kandel, 1984), adolescents experiment with drugs typically in a social context that involves the use of so-called gateway substances, such as alcohol and cigarettes. This pattern makes it difficult to determine when adolescent drug use has negative long-term implications versus short-term effects and social payoff. Whereas the best available epidemiological data suggest that relatively small percentages of adolescents advance to later and more serious levels of drug use, such as the development of a substance dependence disorder (Kandel, 1975; Martin & Winters, 1998), some youth continue heavy drug use into young adulthood (Shedler & Block, 1990). A developmentally sensitive assessment tool should include content coverage for the following drug use behaviors: age of drug-specific onset, which drugs are used on a weekly or more frequent basis during the prior year, how often binge drinking occurs during the prior year, and to what extent polydrug use occurs.

In this chapter's next sections, the three key components of the assessment process, method (collection of data from the client), source (collection of data from other sources), and content (factors affecting level of risk or motivation), will be discussed. Following each section, clinical implications will be discussed.

Method

Client self-report

The main method for collecting assessment data is gathering it from the client's self-report. Common types of self-report formats are reviewed below, and the validity of these formats is also discussed.

Diagnostic interviews

Generally speaking, it is advisable to use diagnostic interviews to assess drug use behaviors and related problems. Such interviews, in which clients are asked a set of predetermined questions, are considered by many researchers and clinicians to be the preferred method. For example, with the introduction of definable diagnostic criteria for substance use disorders, diagnostic interviews can quite precisely and reliably elicit the information needed to make a diagnosis. Variability in responses is minimized by the use of standardized symptom definitions and question formats. The use of follow-up questions provides important information that cannot always be obtained through the more rigid format of a paper–pencil questionnaire.

Most current interviews address several psychosocial domains, as well as a wide range of drug use behaviors, including drug use consumption history, the quantity and frequency of use over defined time periods, and substance use duration. For alcohol, tobacco, and licit drugs (i.e., prescription medications), quantity is more readily determined than is the case for most illicit substances.

Timeline follow-back

Given the pitfalls of collecting detailed retrospective data on drug use, the systematic timeline follow-back interview procedure developed by Sobell and Sobell (1992) has been widely adopted. It was originally created to collect retrospective data on daily alcohol consumption. There is an extensive literature demonstrating the reliability and accuracy of collecting retrospective alcohol consumption data for up to 1 year prior to the interview from clinical and non-clinical subjects aged 18 years and over (Sobell & Sobell, 1992). The use of timeline follow-back in adolescent drug-abusing subjects has also been researched (Winters, 2003). As already discussed, the relevance of drug use history assessments should be considered in the context that consumption variables do not play a major role in diagnosing substance use disorders.

Self-report questionnaires

The value of diagnostic interviews does not minimize the importance of self-report questionnaires. Indeed, there are an array of such questionnaires to assess the adolescent client's psychosocial risk and protective factors. Several of these multi-scale instruments have had norms established for both community and clinical adolescent samples, permitting comparisons of a client's score to relevant reference points. Also, many questionnaires have very favorable test-retest reliability, which accommodate their use for pre-post treatment analyses.

Validity of self-report

The validity of self-report of drug use behavior is a topic of considerable interest in research and clinical areas. Data from the Drug Use Forecasting study suggest that nearly half of all adolescents who are arrested deny or minimize illicit use of drugs (Harrison, 1995; Magura & Kang, 1997). Some investigators have reported that adolescents will report greater past use and related problems at treatment completion compared with their reports at treatment intake (Stinchfield, 1997). Nevertheless, the literature provides several lines of evidence for the validity of adolescent self-reports of alcohol and other drug problems: a large proportion of youth in drug treatment settings admit to use of alcohol and other drugs and associated problems; few treatment-seeking adolescents endorse questions that indicate blatant faking of responses (e.g., admit to the use of a fictitious drug); and the information provided by adolescents is usually in general agreement with other knowledgeable sources (e.g., parents and peers) (Johnston & O'Malley, 1997; Maisto, Connors, & Allen, 1995; Winters *et al.*, 1991, 2000).

Several factors and approaches contribute to the validity of self-report. Among instrumentation factors, questionnaires that contain measures of response distortion provide an opportunity for the assessor to detect faking tendencies and to respond (e.g., instructing the client to retake the questionnaire). Computer-administered and audio assessments using a cognitive abilities screening instrument have shown some promise in contributing to greater disclosure by youth of their problems, including drug use (Winters, 2003). Several assessor considerations are noteworthy as well. Valid self-report is likely to be enhanced if the assessor can legitimately ensure confidentiality of self-report and engage the client in a non-confrontational style. And it is prudent to keep in mind that an invalid self-report does not always stem from a client's conscious attempt to engage in self-management tactics. Other sources of invalidity include inattention and poor comprehension.

Data other than client self-report

One form of data that is not self-report is direct observation. This can be an objective view of the client's appearance and behavior during the interview assessment (e.g., smell of alcohol or marijuana; slurred, incoherent or too rapid speech).

Another conventional method of collecting data that does not rely on the self-report is laboratory testing. Laboratory tests can be used to detect drugs in body fluid samples of blood and urine. Given its convenience related to collection and its low cost, urinalysis is the preferred laboratory procedure. Several factors determine whether a urinalysis is positive or negative: dose, frequency of use, time from drug use to sample collection, and test sensitivity. However, because most drug detection periods are relatively short, little can be inferred from a positive result. Also, several factors may contribute to a negative result. Nonetheless, urine testing is appropriate when the detection of recent drug use is highly important, such as in juvenile justice settings or when the adolescent has denied recent drug use.

Clinical implications of data sources

Self-report data provide the optimal vehicle for gathering information pertaining to an individual's drug use behaviors and related psychosocial consequences.

Despite valid concerns about the adequacy of self-report, the adolescent is typically the best source for obtaining the most detailed and accurate information during the assessment process. Within the self-report domain, it is preferable to use several methods. Naturally, time and resource constraints may require the use of only one approach. In many instances, the use of well-researched, comprehensive semi-structured or structured interviews may be the preferred method. Semi-structured interviews require more training than structured ones, but they allow considerable latitude in adapting questions to suit the respondent. With a skilled interviewer, this format can produce comprehensive information without sacrificing reliability.

Source

Several information sources may be relevant when evaluating an individual's drug abuse problems. This chapter's earlier discussion of self-report, laboratory testing, and direct observation addressed methods for obtaining information from the client. Three other main sources of information relevant to adolescent drug abuse assessment are parents, peers, and archival records.

Parents

It goes without saying that the parents of an adolescent client play an important role in providing information during screening and comprehensive assessment. In addition to inquiring about relevant clinical information, the assessor must determine who has legal custody, whom the adolescent defines as family members, and which family member is likely to be the best informant. Generally speaking, parents will not be able to provide detailed information about the child's drug use, but they may be useful in establishing obvious warning signs. It is advisable to focus parent assessments largely on the client's psychological and social functioning and on family issues. There is one parent psychometrically evaluated questionnaire in the literature that was designed for use in assessing adolescent drug abuse: the Personal Experience Inventory–Parent Version (Winters et al., 2000). It contains one set of scales that asks the parent to rate their child's problem with drugs and their psychosocial functioning, and another set of scales asks the parent to rate family life and personal drug involvement.

Peers

It is probably too idealistic to assume that a client's peers will prove to be a valuable source of information, particularly if they are using drugs themselves. The most logical opportunity for a peer to serve as a valid assessment source is when he or she is a non-drug-using friend or a person in recovery who may be able to describe the client's recent behavioral changes, or provide information about the possible presence of drug abuse warning signs.

Archival records

Archival records can supply relatively inexpensive and unobtrusive information about school performance, social or behavioral problems at school, legal status (history of delinquency, for example), and mental and physical health status. It is important to keep in mind that archival data may not include information relevant to the assessment, may not always be recorded or collected systematically, may contain errors, and may not be accessible if the agency is unwilling to make the records available or the client has not granted consent.

Clinical implications of data from other sources

Both research literature and clinical experience provide a converging view that parent and peer informants have, at best, a limited role in the assessment process. Parents are probably not aware of many of the key behaviors of interest. Peers may be a good source of information about a client, but it is unlikely that knowledge-able peers will willingly discuss the problems of their friend. Certain situations or conditions may encourage disclosure from a peer, but there is no formal research on this topic. As for archival data, the aforementioned limitations are important reminders that this method should be used cautiously. Perhaps the greatest value with archival data may be that it can be used to corroborate personal consequences that would most certainly be recorded in official documents (e.g., school suspension, contact with the court system). Nonetheless, even in the best situation in which parents, peers, and archival data provide valuable inform-ation, it is incumbent on the assessor to seek reliable and detailed information from the client.

Content

The interrelated core variables of content are drug use behaviors and the range of risk factors that may contribute to the initiation, maintenance, and desistance of drug use behaviors.

Drug use history

Drug use history refers to several variables, including whether the drug has ever been used, how old the person was when he/she first used the drug, and how many times in the recent past (e.g., last 12 months, last 1 month) the drug has been used. For alcohol and tobacco use, it is appropriate to inquire about quantity. It is common on national surveys and clinical instruments to inquire how many

12-ounce cans or bottles of alcohol the person drinks and how many cigarettes, cigars, or pipes the person smokes on a typical day. These questions allow the calculation of average consumption. However, there is a growing consensus among experts that consumption variables have minimal relevance to determining the presence of a substance use disorder, and they only moderately correlate with drug use problems. Indeed, the criteria for substance use disorders in DSM-IV (American Psychiatric Association, 1994) do not include any specific criteria directly linked to drug use, frequency, and quantity. Despite this caveat, drug use history is still important in a clinical setting because yearly national norms are available concerning drug use characteristics for high school students (e.g., Johnston, O'Malley, & Bachman, 1999), thus permitting comparison of a client's usage frequency against national norms that are updated yearly. For researchers, drug use history is vital in order to accommodate comparison of baseline and follow-up data.

Abuse and dependence diagnostic symptoms

Several adolescent-specific instruments measure formal diagnostic criteria for substance use disorders. Abusive-like symptoms of drug use include negative consequences related to role impairment, use when it is physically hazardous, recurrent drug-related legal problems, and drug-related social and interpersonal difficulties. These symptoms are expected to be associated with clinically signi-ficant impairment or distress but are meant to fall short of true physical depen-dence or a pattern of compulsive use. Whereas abuse reflects use related to negative consequences, dependence refers to continued and compulsive-like use in the face of these negative consequences. The constellation of symptoms for dependence reflects this notion of compulsive and pathological patterns of drug use, as well as symptoms related to physical dependence.

Are these symptoms relevant for adolescents? Only to some degree (Martin & Winters, 1998). The diagnostic utility of some criteria are limited in that they have a very low prevalence rate, even in clinical samples (e.g., withdrawal and drug-related medical problems). An important criteria for dependence, tolerance, appears to have low specificity because the development of tolerance for drugs is likely a normal developmental phenomenon that happens to most adolescents; this is particularly the case for alcohol. Also, the criteria for DSM-IV substance abuse produce a great deal of heterogeneity because these symptoms cover a broad range of problems, and only one symptom is required to meet the criteria. In addition, there is evidence that symptoms of abuse do not always precede symptoms of dependence, contrary to the notion that abuse should be a pro-dromal category with respect to dependence (Martin et al., 1996). Finally, there is the finding in the adolescent and adult literature that some individuals "fall through the cracks" of the DSM-IV system. That is, some individuals reveal one or two dependent symptoms, and no abuse symptoms, and, therefore, do not qualify for any diagnosis (Hasin & Paykin, 1998). These "diagnostic orphans" have been found to range from 10 to 30% among adolescent drug users (Harrison, Fulkerson, & Beebe, 1998; Lewinsohn, Rohde, & Seeley, 1996).

Family functioning and parenting practices

The literature on drug abuse provides several examples, including prospective data, that point to poor parent management as a significant risk of youth drug involvement, including poor monitoring of the whereabouts of the child (August et al., 1996; Chassin et al., 1993), inconsistent disciplining (Kandel, Kessler, & Marguiles, 1978; Lerner & Vicary, 1984), lack of nurturance and attachment (Baumrind & Moselle, 1985; Brook et al., 1990), and parental conflict, including physical or sexual abuse (Gutierres, Molof, & Ungerleider, 1994). Also, parent and sibling drug use and attitudes about drug use have been identified as significant risk factors of adolescent drug use (Hawkins, Catalano, & Miller, 1992; Kaminer, 1990; McGue, Sharma, & Benson, 1996; Sher, 1991). Naturally, the association between the presence of these family variables and drug use in a child could reflect etiological influences from both genetic and experiential factors. Moreover, such risk variables may serve to frustrate favorable treatment outcome. Family functioning scales are common in several multidimensional instruments (e.g., the Comprehensive Addiction Severity Index for Adolescents: Meyers et al., 1995), and other well-researched instruments exist that focus on this domain (e.g., the Family Assessment Measure: Skinner, Steinhauer, & Santa-Barbara, 1983).

For assessing family variables, the multiplicity of family constellations and differences in perception of relationships among family members complicate interpretation of family interaction measures. For example, mother and adolescent perceptions of general family functioning, dyadic relationships, and parenting practices systematically differ (Clark et al., 1998). If neither the mother nor the father participates in the care of the adolescent, it is advisable to have the adolescents rate their attachment relationship with their primary caregiver. Direct observation of family interaction is considered by many investigators to be the "gold standard" of family-functioning assessment and serves to provide inter-actional process data (Alexander et al., 1995). While observational measures may be optimal for some purposes, the resources necessary to implement and score such measures are prohibitive for many clinical and research settings.

Peer drug involvement

The construct of peer drug use has been emphasized repeatedly in the adolescent drug abuse literature as a key precipitating factor (Newcomb & Bentler, 1989;

Oetting & Beauvais, 1986) and potential moderator of escalation of use (Winters *et al.*, 1999a). Accordingly, many assessment scales for adolescent drug abuse measure peer drug use and drug-seeking behaviors. The assumption that personal drug use is influenced by peer involvement is based on the consistent finding that adolescents who report having drug-using friends also indicate higher levels of personal drug use compared with young people who do not report such friends (Farrell & Danish, 1993; Oetting & Beauvais, 1986). Other peer-related factors empirically linked to youth drug abuse include peer attitudes about substance use and the increased orientation of youth to their peers (Hawkins *et al.*, 1992; Patterson *et al.*, 1998). The influence of peers on drug use is likely complex, and its importance may be overstated (Bauman & Emmett, 1994). Peer and personal drug use may be associated as a result of underlying socialization and environmental influences, such as cohesive peer groups making drugs available to each other, drug use being modeled by friends within the group, peer group support and norms favoring drug use, and the role of drug use in friendship selection (i.e., already drug-using individuals may tend to select friends with similar habits) (Bauman & Emmett, 1994; Oetting & Beauvais, 1986).

Educational status

Academic failure, low academic aspirations, and poor progress in high school and post-high school have been noted as strong premorbid factors of youth drug use (Jessor, 1976; Robins, 1980). Furthermore, adolescents with a substance use disorder are more likely to drop out of high school, repeat grades, not seek post-high school education, and suffer from learning disabilities (Hawkins *et al.*, 1992). Instruments in the field have addressed this construct directly (by inquiring about school status, and level of engagement and interest in school work) and more broadly in the context of measuring the adolescent's future aspirations of graduating from high school.

Coexisting psychopathology

The forms of psychopathology most likely to be relevant in the etiology and treatment of drug abuse may be conceptualized as forms of dysregulation. Deficits in regulation are hypothesized to result in psychopathology when the demands and expectations of the social environment exceed the individual's adaptive capacities (Tarter *et al.*, 1999). *Behavioral* dysregulation is manifested as antisocial behavior, including the diagnostic categories of conduct disorder and oppositional defiant disorder; *emotional* dysregulation is manifested as anxiety and depression, including anxiety disorders and major depression; and *cognitive* dysregulation is manifested as attentional problems and impulsivity, including attention-deficit hyperactivity disorder (ADHD). The relevance of these dysregulations for understanding adolescent drug use behaviors is reinforced by cross-sectional observations of elevated rates of these disorders in drug-abusing samples (Clark & Bukstein, 1998). Further support is given by prospective research showing that conduct disorder and oppositional deficient disorder predict later substance involvement (Boyle *et al.*, 1992; Clark, Parker, & Lynch, 1999), and ADHD may predict substance use and related problems, although this relationship may be mediated by the presence of conduct disorder (B. Molina *et al.*, unpublished data).

Fortunately, several measures have been developed for comorbid psychiatric disorder in adolescent assessments. These measures include comprehensive, stand-alone diagnostic interviews (e.g., the Diagnostic Interview Schedule for Children: Fisher *et al.*, 1993), modules contained within drug abuse interviews (e.g., the Adolescent Diagnostic Interview: Winters & Henly, 1993), and general scales of psychological distress as part of standardized questionnaires (e.g., Adolescent Self-Assessment Profile: Wanberg, 1992). One of the biggest hurdles in gathering accurate and clinically useful data on disorders comorbid to the drug use behaviors is the challenge of assessing the relative independence/dependence of the psychiatric disorders and the substance use disorder. Relevant here are the issues of which came first, and is one disorder a consequence of the other or are they etiologically independent yet one exacerbates the other (Clark & Bukstein, 1998). The diagnostic interview provides the optimal source for gathering complex data such as these. Also, there is the issue of child versus parent as informant. Parent informants improve validity in the assessment of some psychiatric disorders in children and adolescents (Herjanic & Reich, 1982). With preadolescent children or retrospective assessment of early development, mothers tend to report more symptoms of ADHD and oppositional deficient disorder, whereas children report more symptoms of mood and anxiety disorders. Also, behaviors associated with conduct disorder are typically concealed from the parent; therefore, here the adolescent is typically the best source for such information.

Clinical implications of content factors

These content areas represent a core list of factors that are vital to the assessment process, and there are other highly relevant factors that also deserve consideration (e.g., motivational variables, such as readiness for change; exposure to childhood maltreatment and other adverse life events; use of leisure and recreation time). It can be difficult to assess all core content areas adequately, let alone additional factors. For example, a comprehensive historical assessment of coexisting disorders using a semi-structured or structured interview can easily take 2 hours.

A careful review of an adolescent's drug use behaviors, including use history and signs and symptoms of abuse and dependence, can easily add another hour to the assessment. Realistically, it is best to use a mix of interview and self-administered questionnaires during the intake assessment. It is our clinical (and research) experience that for content areas such as drug use behaviors and coexisting psychopathology, in which temporal characteristics are important (e.g., age of onset and offset of behaviors), a semi-structured or structured interview is preferred. With respect to psychosocial risk and protective factors that are presumed to be relatively stable over time (e.g., self-esteem, delinquency, conventionality), a well-developed self-administered questionnaire is preferred.

Bridging assessment and referral decisions

Clinically, assessment information provides the framework for treatment referral decisions. Table 11.2 represents a general model for matching level of treatment and severity of drug use and related psychosocial problems. For the sake of parsimony, three levels of treatment are considered: brief intervention, non-intensive drug treatment, and intensive drug treatment. In general, specialized treatments, such as intensive and non-intensive treatment, are appropriate referrals for youth with severe drug use problems, such as a substance dependence disorder, and for whom abstinence is the treatment goal. Brief interventions are appropriate responses for adolescents with a substance abuse disorder; such approaches often broaden treatment goals to include harm and risk reduction (Bien, Miller, & Tonigan, 1993). Naturally, the referral model becomes more

Table 11.2 Guidelines for substance abuse treatment placement along a continuum of care

Level of intervention or treatment	Suggested characteristics
Brief intervention (2–4 sessions)	Mild-to-moderate drug use: absence of substance dependence disorder; absence of poly-drug use pattern; absence of acute coexisting psychiatric disorder; relatively supportive and stable home life
Low-intensive treatment (e.g., 7–20 days or sessions)	Substance abuse disorder(s), or a single substance dependence disorder with recent onset; if coexisting disorder present, then mild symptoms; relatively supportive and stable home life
Intensive treatment (e.g., 21 or more days or sessions)	Substance dependence disorder; severe coexisting disorder present; relatively unsupportive and unstable home life

complex as more client characteristics are included in the decision-making process.

Conclusions and future directions

Considerable maturity in the assessment field has transpired since the mid-1980s. Numerous tools have been developed and psychometrically evaluated. Of particular note is the large group of well-researched comprehensive instruments that obtain information from typically the best source of information: the adolescent respondent. An appropriate mix of self-administered measures and a detailed structured or semi-structured interview should serve to provide reliable and detailed information without overextending the assessment process. When time and resource constraints impinge on the assessment, more reliance on semi-structured or structured interviews is advisable.

Nonetheless, much work needs to be done in adolescent drug abuse assessment in order to address the myriad health-service delivery challenges. There is far less psychometric research on screening tools compared with the larger instruments. The clinical arena would benefit from the development of very brief and accurate drug abuse screens for use in settings such as health clinics, juvenile courts, and school health clinics. An example of excellent progress in this area is CRAFFT, a brief screen that has been validated in pediatric clinics (Knight *et al.*, 2002).

There is also a significant lack of empirical evidence as to how assessment profiles can translate to predictions in order to improve the efficiency and effectiveness of treatment referral decisions. Some assessment tools in the field provide guidelines for treatment referrals, but such instruments usually offer very general suggestions based on narrow criteria (Winters, Latimer, & Stinchfield, 1999b). Treatment-matching research has the potential to clarify with precision the extent to which the severity and nature of a problem complex can lead to treatment–client matching models. Many matching research questions come to mind, including the following: How severe should a drug problem be to benefit optimally from intensive treatment? How heterogeneous is an appropriate group of mild-to-moderate drug-abusing teenagers for referral to a brief intervention? Are there indications when the intensity of family therapy can be minimal in the treatment regimen and when its intensity should be maximized? What configuration of risk and protective factors contributes to optimal treatment matching?

Despite these needs for further growth and sophistication, clinicians and researchers have many resources and strategies from which to choose when faced with challenges of problem identification, referral, and treatment for adolescents suspected of drug abuse.

ACKNOWLEDGEMENT

Partial support for this chapter was provided by NIDA grant DA05104.

REFERENCES

Achenbach, T. M. (1995). Developmental issues in assessment, taxonomy, and diagnosis of child and adolescent psychopathology. In D. Cicchetti & D. J. Cohen (eds.), *Developmental psychopathology*, Vol. 1: *Theory and Methods* (pp. 57–80). New York: John Wiley.

Alexander, J. F., Newell, R. M., Robbins, M. S., & Turner, C. W. (1995). Observational coding in family therapy process research. *Journal of Family Therapy*, **9**, 355–365.

Allen, J. P. & Columbus, M. (eds.) (2004). *Assessing Alcohol Problems: A Guide for Clinicians and Researchers*, 2nd edn. Bethesda, MD: National Institute on Alcohol Abuse and Alcoholism.

American Psychiatric Association (1994). *The Diagnostic and Statistical Manual*, 4th edn (*DSM-IV*). Washington, DC: American Psychiatric Association.

August, G. J., Realmuto, G. M., MacDonald, A., Nugent, S. M., & Crosby, R. D. (1996). Prevalence of ADHD and comorbid disorders among elementary school children screened for disruptive behavior. *Journal of Abnormal Child Psychology*, **24**, 571–595.

Bauman, K. E. & Emmett, S. T. (1994). Peer influences on adolescent drug use. *American Psychologist*, **49**, 820–822.

Baumrind, D. & Moselle, K. A. (1985). A developmental perspective on adolescent drug abuse. *Advances in Alcohol and Substance Abuse*, **4**, 41–67.

Bien, T. H., Miller, W. R., & Tonigan, J. S. (1993). Brief interventions for alcohol problems: a review. *Addiction*, **88**, 315–336.

Boyle, M. H., Offord, D. R., Racine, Y. A., *et al.* (1992). Predicting substance use in late adolescence: results of the Ontario Child Health Study Follow-up. *American Journal of Psychiatry*, **149**, 761–767.

Brook, J. S., Brook, D. W., Gordon, A. S., Whiteman, M., & Cohen, A. (1990). The psychosocial etiology of adolescent drug use: a family interactional approach. *Genetic, Social, and General Psychology Monograph*, **116**, 111–267.

Chassin, L., Pillow, D. R., Curran, P. J., Molina, B. S. G., & Barrera, M., Jr. (1993). Relation of parental alcoholism to early adolescent substance use: a test of three mediating mechanisms. *Journal of Abnormal Psychology*, **102**, 3–19.

Cicchetti, D. & Cohen, D. J. (1995). Perspectives on developmental psychopathology. In D. Cicchetti & D. J. Cohen (eds.), *Developmental Psychopathology: Theory and Methods* (pp. 3–20). New York: John Wiley.

Clark, D. B. & Bukstein, O. G. (1998). Psychopathology in adolescent alcohol abuse and dependence. *Alcohol Health Research World*, **22**, 117–121.

Clark, D. B. & Winters. K. C. (2002). Measuring risks and outcomes in substance use disorders prevention research. *Journal of Consulting and Clinical Psychology*, **70**, 1207–1223.

Clark, D. B., Neighbors, B. D., Lesnick, L. A., & Donovan, J. E. (1998). Family functioning and adolescent alcohol use disorders. *Journal of Family Psychology*, **12**, 81–92.

Clark, D. B., Parker, A., & Lynch, K. (1999). Psychopathology and substance-related problems during early adolescence: a survival analysis. *Journal of Clinical Child Psychology*, **28**, 333–341.

CSAT (Center for Substance Abuse Prevention) (1999). *Guide to Risk Factor and Outcome Instruments for Youth Substance Abuse Prevention Program Evaluation*. [DHHS No. 99–3279] Rockville, MD: Substance Abuse Mental Health Services Administration.

Farrell, A. D. & Danish, S. J. (1993). Peer drug associations and emotional restraint: causes and consequences of adolescents' drug use? *Journal of Consulting and Clinical Psychology*, **61**, 327–334.

Fisher, P., Shaffer, D., Piacentini, J. C., et al. (1993). Sensitivity of the Diagnostic Interview Schedule for Children, 2nd edition (DISC-2.1) for specific diagnoses of children and adolescents. *Journal of the American Academy of Child and Adolescent Psychiatry*, **32**, 666–673.

Gutierres, S. E., Molof, M., & Ungerleider, S. (1994). Relationship of "risk" factors to teen substance use: a comparison of abstainers, infrequent users, and frequent users. *International Journal of Addictions*, **29**, 1559–1579.

Harrison, L. D. (1995). The validity of self-reported data on drug use. *Journal of Drug Issues*, **25**, 91–111.

Harrison, P. A., Fulkerson, J. A., & Beebe, T. J. (1998). DSM-IV substance use disorder criteria for adolescents: a critical examination based on a statewide school survey. *American Journal of Psychiatry*, **155**, 486–492.

Hasin, D. & Paykin, A. (1998). Dependence symptoms but no diagnosis: diagnostic orphans in a community sample. *Drug and Alcohol Dependence*, **50**, 19–26.

Hawkins, J. D., Catalano, R. F., & Miller, J. Y. (1992). Risk and protective factors for alcohol and other drug problems in adolescence and early adulthood: implications for substance abuse prevention. *Psychological Bulletin*, **112**, 64–105.

Herjanic, B. & Reich, W. (1982). Development of a structured psychiatric interview for children: agreement between child and parent on individual symptoms. *Journal of Abnormal Child Psychology*, **10**, 307–324.

Jessor, R. (1976). Predicting time of onset of marijuana use: a developmental study of high school youth. *Journal of Consulting and Clinical Psychology*, **44**, 125–134.

Johnston, L. D. & O'Malley, P. M. (1997). The recanting of earlier reported drug use by young adults. In L. Harrison & A. Hughes (eds.), *Research Monograph*, No. 167: *The Validity of Self-reported Drug Use: Improving the Accuracy of Survey Estimates* (pp. 59–80). Rockville, MD: National Institute on Drug Abuse.

Johnston, L. D., O'Malley, P. M., & Bachman, J. G. (1999). *National Survey Results on Drug Use from the Monitoring the Future Study 1975–1998*. Rockville, MD: National Institute on Drug Abuse.

Kaminer, Y. (1990). *Adolescent Substance Abuse: A Comprehensive Guide to Theory and Practice*. New York: Plenum Press.

Kandel, D. B. (1975). Stages in adolescent involvement in drug use. *Science*, **90**, 912–914.

Kandel, D. B., Kessler, R. C., & Marguiles, R. Z. (1978). Antecedents of adolescent initiation into stages of drug use: a developmental analysis. In D. B. Kandel (ed.), *Longitudinal Research on Drug Use: Empirical Findings and Methodological Issues* (pp. 73–99). Washington, DC: Hemisphere (Halstead-Wiley).

Knight, J. R., Sherritt, L., Shrier, L. A., Harris, S. K., & Chang, G. (2002). Validity of the CRAFFT substance abuse screening test among general adolescent clinic patients. *Archives of Pediatric Adolescent Medicine*, **156**, 607–614.

Lecesse, M. & Waldron, H. B. (1994). Assessing adolescent substance use: a critique of current measurement instruments. *Journal of Substance Abuse Treatment*, **11**, 553–563.

Lerner, J. V. & Vicary, J. R. (1984). Difficult temperament and drug use. *Journal of Drug Education*, **14**, 1–8.

Lewinsohn, P. M., Rohde, P., & Seeley, J. R. (1996). Alcohol consumption in high school adolescents: frequency of use and dimensional structure of associated problems. *Addiction*, **91**, 375–390.

Magura, S. & Kang, S. Y. (1997). The validity of self-reported cocaine use in two high-risk populations. In L. Harrison & A. Hughes (eds.), *Research Monograph*, No. 167: *The Validity of Self-reported Drug Use: Improving the Accuracy of Survey Estimates*, (pp. 227–246). Rockville, MD: National Institute on Drug Abuse.

Maisto, S. A., Connors, G. J., & Allen, J. P. (1995). Contrasting self-report screens for alcohol problems: a review. *Alcoholism: Clinical and Experimental Research*, **19**, 1510–1516.

Martin, C. S. & Winters, K. C. (1998). Diagnosis and assessment of alcohol use disorders among adolescents. *Alcohol Health and Research World*, **22**, 95–105.

Martin, C. S., Kaczynski, N. A., Maisto, S. A., & Tarter, R. E. (1996). Polydrug use in adolescent drinkers with and without DSM-IV alcohol abuse and dependence. *Alcoholism: Clinical and Experimental Research*, **20**, 1099–1108.

McGue, M., Sharma, A., & Benson, P. (1996). Parent and sibling influences on adolescent alcohol use and misuse: evidence from a US adoption cohort. *Journal of Studies on Alcohol*, **57**, 8–18.

Meyers, K., McLellan, A. T., Jaeger, J. L., & Pettinati, H. M. (1995). The development of the Comprehensive Addiction Severity Index for Adolescents (CASI-A): an interview for assessing multiple problems of adolescents. *Journal of Substance Abuse Treatment*, **12**, 181–193.

Newcomb, M. D. & Bentler, P. M. (1989). Substance use and abuse among children and teenagers. *American Psychologist*, **44**, 242–248.

Nunnally, J. C. & Bernstein, I. H. (1994). *Psychometric Theory*, 3rd edn. New York: McGraw-Hill.

Oetting, E. R. & Beauvais, F. (1986). Peer cluster theory: drugs and the adolescent. *Journal of Counseling and Development*, **65**, 17–22.

Patterson, G. R., Forgatch, M. S., Yoerger, K. L., & Stoolmiller, M. (1998). Variables that initiate and maintain an early-onset trajectory for juvenile offending. *Development and Psychopathology*, **10**, 531–548.

Robins, L. N. (1980). The natural history of drug abuse. *Acta Psychiatrica Scandinavia*, **62**(Suppl. 384), 7–20.

Shedler, J. & Block, J. (1990). Adolescent drug use and psychological health. *American Psychologist*, **45**, 612–630.

Sher, K. J. (1991). *Children of alcoholics*. Chicago, IL: University of Chicago Press.

Skinner, H. A., Steinhauer, P. D., & Santa-Barbara, J. (1983). The Family Assessment Measure. *Canadian Journal of Community Mental Health*, **2**, 91–105.

Sobell, L. C. & Sobell, M. B. (1992). Time-line follow-back: a technique for assessing self-reported alcohol consumption. In R. Z. Litten & J. P. Allen (eds.), *Measuring Alcohol Consumption* (pp. 73–98). Totowa, NJ: Humana Press.

Stinchfield, R. D. (1997). Reliability of adolescent self-reported pretreatment alcohol and other drug use. *Substance Use and Misuse*, **32**, 63–76.

Tarter, R., Vanyukov, M., Giancola, P., *et al.* (1999). Epigenetic model of substance use disorder etiology. *Development and Psychopathology*, **11**, 657–683.

Wanberg, K. W. (1992). *Adolescent Self-Assessment Profile*. Arvada, CO: Center for Alcohol/Drug Abuse Research and Evaluation.

Winters, K. C. (ed.) (1999). *Screening and Assessing Adolescents for Substance Use Disorders. [Treatment Improvement Protocol Series, No. 31.]* Rockville, MD: Substance Abuse and Mental Health Services Administration.

Winters, K. C. (2003). Screening and assessing youth for drug involvement. In J. Allen & M. Colombus (eds.), *NIAAA Handbook on Assessment Instruments for Alcohol Researchers*, 2nd edn. Rockville, MD: National Institute on Alcohol Abuse and Alcoholism.

Winters, K. C. & Henly, G. A. (1993). *Adolescent Diagnostic Interview Schedule and Manual*. Los Angeles, CA: Western Psychological Services.

Winters, K. C., Stinchfield, R. D., Henly, G. A., & Schwartz, R. H. (1991). Validity of adolescent self-report of alcohol and other drug involvement. *International Journal of Addictions*, **25**, 1379–1395.

Winters, K. C., Latimer, W. W., Stinchfield, R. D., & Henly, G. A. (1999a). Examining psycho-social correlates of drug involvement among drug clinic-referred youth. *Journal of Child and Adolescent Substance Abuse*, **9**, 1–18.

Winters, K. C., Latimer, W. W., & Stinchfield, R. D. (1999b). Clinical and research uses of the PEI in assessing adolescent drug abuse. In M. Maruish (ed.), *The Use of Psychological Testing for Treatment Planning and Outcomes Assessment*, 2nd edn (pp. 599–630). Hillsdale, NJ: Lawrence Erlbaum.

Winters, K. C., Anderson, N., Bengston, P., Stinchfield, R. D., & Latimer, W. W. (2000). Development of a parent questionnaire for the assessment of adolescent drug abuse. *Journal of Psychoactive Drugs*, **32**, 3–13.

Yagamuchi, K. & Kandel, D. B. (1984). Patterns of drug use from adolescence to young adulthood: III. Patterns of progression. *American Journal of Public Health*, **74**, 673–681.

Zucker, R. A., Fitzgerald, H. E., & Moses, H. D. (1995). Emergence of alcohol problems and the several alcoholisms: a developmental perspective on etiologic theory and life course trajectory. In D. Cicchetti & D. J. Cohen (eds.), *Developmental Psychopathology*, Vol. 2: *Risk, Disorder and Adaptation* (pp. 677–711). New York: John Wiley.

12

Psychopharmacology of adolescents with substance use disorders: using diagnostic-specific treatments

Oscar G. Bukstein and Jack Cornelius

Presbyterian University Hospital, Pittsburgh, PA, USA

Treatments for adolescent substance use disorders (SUDs) in the community use a variety of modalities and settings and almost always reflect a psychosocial approach. In recent years, the use of medications (pharmacotherapy) has increased. This chapter will explore the current situation for pharmacotherapy as a treatment for adolescents with SUDs, particularly the rationale and empirical basis for pharmacological treatment in this population. The goal is to understand the limited scope of the current literature, and the broad potential for empirically based pharmacological therapies to assume a more prominent role in the treatment of adolescents with SUDs.

Current status of pharmacotherapy

Pharmacotherapy can be used to target the symptoms or behaviors directly or indirectly related to SUDs. Unlike psychosocial treatments, which may target a host of different individual and family processes underlying adolescent SUDs, pharmacological treatments usually focus on a more specific target, such as comorbid psychiatric disorders or neurophysiological processes underlying addictive behavior (e.g., the reinforcing properties of substances of abuse on the brain). The ample evidence pointing to the role of neuropsychiatric factors in the etiology and development of SUDs in adolescents supports serious consideration of pharmacological strategies in SUD treatment (Bukstein & Tarter, 1998). The dependence liability of psychoactive compounds is indicated by the propensity of laboratory animals to self-administer the substance (Brady & Lucas, 1984). Drug reinforcement involves activation of the dopaminergic system subserving reward centers of the brain (Gardner, 1992; Wise & Rompre, 1989). Different substances may have different mechanisms of activating or influencing dopaminergic

Adolescent Substance Abuse: Research and Clinical Advances, ed. Howard A. Liddle and Cynthia L. Rowe. Published by Cambridge University Press. © Cambridge University Press 2006.

systems. Complicating the picture, neurotransmitter systems, such as the seroto-nergic, adrenergic, and gamma-aminobutyric acid-utilizing pathways, are involved in regulating motivated behavior and, consequently, are also linked to the reinforcement effects of drugs (Jaffe, 1990).

Despite the substantial pharmacological treatment literature for adults, the empirical basis for the pharmacological treatment of adolescents is sparse and underdeveloped (Bukstein & Kithas, 2002; Solhkhah & Wilens, 1998). While this situation mirrors the paucity of empirically based psychosocial treatments for adolescents versus the many interventions tested and established for adults, there are many reasons for research and the development of adolescent SUD treatments to lag behind that for adults. First, there is a general trend for novel treatments to be initially tested in adults and then, later, to be adapted and tested in adolescent populations. Second, similar to the initial reluctance to use medications for adults with SUDs, there may be a greater reluctance to do so for adolescents. Parents and clinicians worry about replacing one drug with another, the potential effects of medications on the physical and mental development of youth, other potential adverse effects of medications, the potential for abuse or overdose of medications, and/or the fact that medications cannot provide adolescents with the behavioral skills that they will need for their recovery from SUDs. Third, the general denial by parents of the presence or severity of SUDs in their offspring may limit their enthusiasm for a seemingly intrusive intervention, such as medication. Fourth, the frequent denial and poor compliance of the adolescents themselves may limit valid tests of the efficacy of specific medications. Poor compliance limits tests of efficacy as patients need to be compliant for weeks to months for the medications of this type to work. Resulting high attrition rates and biased samples in studies could limit generalization of study findings to active treatment. Fifth, the number of well-trained investigators interested in conducting such trials is limited. Finally, the field of adolescent psychopharmacology is generally a nascent area. Few empirically based pharmacological treatments exist for adolescents with non-comorbid disorders, such as major depressive disorder (MDD), bipolar disorder, anxiety disorders, and even attention-deficit hyperactivity disorder (ADHD). Despite the common occurrence of psychiatric comorbidities in clinical popula-tions of adolescents, there is a reluctance to test pharmacotherapies in comorbid populations prior to more definitive work with adolescents having single disor-ders, such as MDD.

Lessons from the adult literature

The limited research literature on the use of pharmacotherapies with adolescents necessitates some guidance from the adult literature to assist the clinician in identifying the most supported potential approaches for adolescents. Common pharmacotherapeutic strategies in adults consist of treating withdrawal symptoms, substitution therapy (e.g., replacing heroin with methadone), craving reduction plus blocking strategies (e.g., using naltrexone for treatment of alcoholism), and aversive therapy (i.e., using disulfiram to maintain alcohol abstinence) (Solhkhah & Wilens, 1998). This list of potential strategies can be further expanded to include treating comorbid psychiatric conditions that lead to early use or contribute to continued use. Overall, the focus of pharmacotherapy for SUDs in youth has been directed toward the treatment of comorbid psychiatric disorders. The adult literature on the treatment of withdrawal symptoms, and the use of agents for substitution therapy, craving reduction, and aversive therapy is extensive, and even a summary of this literature is beyond the scope of this chapter.

There are several well-controlled studies of the treatment of comorbid psychiatric disorders in the adult literature. The treatment of depression in adults with alcohol dependence has received much attention in the literature. In the first double-blind, placebo-controlled study of a selective serotonin reuptake inhibitor (SSRI) antidepressant (fluoxetine) in adult depressed alcoholics, Cornelius et al. (1997) reported efficacy for fluoxetine versus placebo in treating both the depression and the drinking in adult alcoholics with comorbid MDD. Studies using SSRIs in mostly non-depressed adults have had more equivocal results (Kranzler et al., 1995), suggesting that treating the comorbid psychiatric disorder or problem may be the mechanism for improvement, rather than the action of the agent on the SUD per se. Other controlled studies of depressed alcoholics show the efficacy of sertraline (Pettinati et al., 2001; Roy, 1998), nezafazadone (Roy-Byrne et al., 2000), and tricyclic antidepressants (Mason et al., 1996; McGrath et al., 1996; Nunes et al., 1998). Controlled trials of cocaine- and opiate-dependent individuals with depression have also been carried out but results have been more mixed. Some using imipramine have been positive (Nunes et al., 1998), while others using fluoxetine have found no medication–placebo differences (Petrakis et al., 1998; Schmitz et al., 2001). Despite the prevalence of marijuana use, no controlled trials of medications for marijuana abuse have been published. Given the potential importance of depressive symptoms in the maintenance of relapse of substance use behavior in adolescents, implementing similar studies for adolescents will be critical.

Despite the substantial impact of bipolar disorder on the course of SUDs, there are a limited number of controlled trials of comorbid bipolar disorder and SUDs in adults (Salloum & Thase, 2002). In a 24-week, double-blind, placebo-controlled, randomized parallel-group trial of valproate, Salloum and coworkers (2005) reported that the valproate group had a significantly lower proportion of heavy drinking days, fewer drinks per heavy drinking day, and fewer drinks per drinking day when medication adherence was added as covariate. Based on several controlled trials, lithium appears to have at most limited efficacy in adult alcoholics without mood disorders. The efficacy of lithium in alcoholics with bipolar disorder has yet to be firmly established. Anticonvulsants, among the mainstays of the pharmacological treatment of bipolar disorder, have shown much potential in the treatment of acute alcohol withdrawal (Myrick, Brady, & Robert, 2001). Recent studies of anticonvulsants, including controlled trials of carbamazepine (Mueller *et al.*, 1997) and case studies of gabapentin (Karam-Hage & Bower, 2000), show lower relapse rates in alcoholics taking these medications. A double-blind, placebo-controlled pilot study of divalproex reported a significantly smaller percentage of patients relapsed to heavy drinking in the medication group, although there were no group differences in other alcohol-related outcomes (Brady *et al.*, 2002). Divalproex also had a modest impact on the reduction of irritability in this sample. In summary, medication studies using mood stabilizers or antidepressants in adults with SUDs show positive effects on both mood and reductions in substance use, but only in adults with mood disorders. However, even in studies where treating the depression improved substance use outcomes, rates of sustained abstinence have been low, and both placebo response rates and medication effect sizes have been highly variable.

The literature on the use of pharmacotherapy for comorbid anxiety disorders and SUDs is limited even in adults. Four studies examining the anxiolytic drug buspirone in the treatment of patients with anxiety and alcoholism had different outcomes. In an 8-week trial with patients suffering mild-to-moderate alcohol abuse and mild-to-moderate anxiety, buspirone reduced alcohol craving, depression, anxiety, and global psychopathology (Bruno, 1989). In an open trial, Kranzler and Meyer (1989) reported that buspirone diminished anxiety symptoms, as well as craving for alcohol in anxious alcoholics. In a controlled 12-week trial with similar patients, Kranzler *et al.* (1994) found that those treated with buspirone delayed return to heavy drinking and engaged in drinking on fewer days during both treatment and the 6-month post treatment follow-up than did placebo controls. Tollefson, Montague-Clouse, and Tollefson (1992) also reported positive effects of buspirone in abstaining alcoholics with generalized anxiety disorder. The use of buspirone for 24 weeks resulted in lower anxiety, greater global reduction of drinking, and better retention in treatment than did placebo. Unlike these previous studies, Malcom and colleagues (1992) failed to confirm effects of buspirone on either anxiety or alcohol consumption in alcohol-dependent but abstinent participants with a comorbid generalized anxiety disorder. Surprisingly, there are no controlled studies of SSRIs and anxiety disorders in adults. Unfortunately, the reality of the frequent comorbidity of anxiety disorders with other psychiatric disorders, especially depression, serves to confuse further a definable phenomenology or target for medication trials.

Despite the presumed importance of ADHD in children and adolescents, few studies have examined pharmacological treatment of ADHD in adults. Case reports and other open studies have suggested the efficacy of stimulant medications in adults with SUDs (Castaneda *et al.*, 2000; Levin *et al.*, 1998; Schubiner *et al.*, 1995; Turnquist *et al.*, 1983). In a 12-week double-blind placebo-controlled trial of methylphenidate in 48 cocaine-dependent adults with ADHD, Schubiner *et al.* (2002) reported greater symptom relief in the methylphenidate group (versus placebo), but no differences in self-reported cocaine use, urinalysis results, or cocaine craving. Non-stimulants with a low abuse potential such as bupropion (Spencer *et al.*, 1996) and atomoxetine (Wilens *et al.*, 2001), a noradrenergic agent recently approved by the US Food and Drug Administration (FDA), have also been shown to be effective in adults, children, and adolescents with ADHD, thus suggesting their potential usefulness in patients with SUDs.

In summary, although the adult medication research is more extensive and developed than the pharmacological treatment literature for adolescents, it is inconsistent and has many gaps, especially in providing large, controlled studies for patients with bipolar or anxiety disorders. Not all of these therapies work or work well. For example, Haney *et al.* (2001) have found evidence that bupropion actually worsens mood (increases irritability and depressive symptoms) during marijuana withdrawal. Rates of sustained abstinence have been low, and both placebo response rates and medication effect sizes have been highly variable. The high placebo response rates in adult studies (up to 45%) portend potential problems in studies of adolescents, where pharmacological studies have demonstrated high placebo response. The literature for adults would also benefit from longer follow-up periods (i.e., over 1 year) to determine long-term effects and treatment utilization for those with treated comorbid disorders, and a more consistent paradigm across studies regarding the time at which a given comorbid disorder is diagnosed (e.g., during an enforced or prolonged period of abstinence or prior to the onset of the SUD) and the diagnostic or symptom criteria used to select study samples. Nevertheless, existing adult studies do provide useful methodological models for adolescent studies, although the latter will require developmentally appropriate assessment variables, instruments, and procedures.

Pharmacological treatment studies in adolescents

Common adult pharmacotherapeutic strategies for addiction, such as treating withdrawal symptoms and reducing craving, and the use of blocking, substitution, and aversive agents, have not been tested in adolescents. While approaches such as nicotine replacement have been used in adolescents, placebo-controlled studies are the exception rather than the rule. Although many of these therapies hold promise in adolescents, as with adults, it is necessary to combine these pharmacological approaches with psychosocial or behavioral interventions in order to improve compliance and to target environmental issues not addressed by medications.

Withdrawal treatment

The existing literature (Martin *et al.*, 1995; Vingilis & Smart, 1981) suggests that adolescents experience considerably fewer symptoms of physiological withdrawal than adults, who usually have a more extensive history of alcohol or other substance abuse in terms of quantity, duration, and frequency of use. No controlled studies of alcohol and drug withdrawal in the adolescent population are available, and this perceived or real lack in the severity of withdrawal or frequency of symptoms may be one of the reasons for the paucity of studies. Currently, adolescents experiencing clinically significant withdrawal symptoms are generally treated using adult guidelines, and the reader is referred to several guidelines and reviews for a detailed examination of the clinical management of substance withdrawal (APA, 1995; Claassen & Adinoff, 1999; NIH, 1998).

In order to develop intervention strategies for withdrawal, a better description and understanding of the phenomenology and course of withdrawal from specific or multiple substances in adolescents is needed. Even the publication of a small series of cases with common assessment techniques would be valuable. Investigators also need to focus on points of entry, such as emergency room and detention centers, for addicted adolescents who may be in withdrawal. With improved access to these adolescents, researchers can begin to test and refine in adolescents the withdrawal interventions developed for adults.

Substitution therapy

The purpose of substitution therapy is to replace an addictive harmful substance with another substance that prevents symptoms of withdrawal along with functional impairment. Substitution therapy is a common yet controversial strategy for treating adults with opiate addiction. Such treatment consists of either methadone or levo-α-acetylmethadyl, a longer acting opiate. The goals of treatment are to prevent withdrawal, eliminate drug craving, and to block the euphoric effects of illicit opiate use (Kaminer, 1994). Adolescent opiate abusers can be admitted to methadone maintenance treatment programs only if state or local laws or regulations allow, and an adult provides written consent. Additional guidelines for adolescents include at least two failed attempts at short-term detoxification or drug-free treatment (Bukstein & Kithas, 2002; Kaminer, 1994). Given the obstacles above, other substitution treatments are being sought. One promising drug is the recently FDA-approved opiate agonist/antagonist buprenorphine, which can be prescribed in the outpatient office. It has showed efficacy in the treatment of opiate dependence in adults (NIDA, 2000; Ling, Huber, & Rawson, 2001). However, there are no published controlled trials or case studies for the use of buprenorphine in adolescents.

Craving reduction and blocking strategies

Various strategies have been employed to decrease craving, which is the urge or desire to use a particular drug, or to block the positive reinforcing qualities of a drug. Similar to adults, many adolescents with SUDs experience cravings for drugs (Deas *et al.*, 2002). For adolescents, there are few controlled trials of these strategies, although case reports suggest their potential usefulness and the necessity of clinical trials. The pharmacotherapy of cocaine craving has been addressed in the adolescent literature in three case reports on the use of desipramine by Kaminer (1994). Naltrexone, the most prominent example of an anticraving agent, reduces the positive reinforcing pleasurable effects of alcohol, as well as its craving (Swift, 1999). As a result, alcohol consumption can be reduced and abstinence prolonged. Although case reports support the potential use of naltrexone in reducing alcohol craving in adolescents (Lifrak *et al.*, 1997; Wold & Kaminer, 1997), there are no controlled trials using naltrexone for either opiate or alcohol dependence in adolescents. Naltrexone is also used in opiate addiction to lessen craving and prolong recovery periods; however, the adolescent literature is without case studies or controlled trials of its use with opiate dependence. Opiate and cocaine craving have also been treated by pharmacotherapeutic interventions. In the adult literature, buprenorphine, an opiate agonist/antagonist, has been successful in treating opiate dependence (NIDA, 2000; Ling *et al.*, 2001). Recent reviews have stated that buprenorphine carries less risk of overdose given its agonist/antagonist mechanism of action (Ling *et al.*, 2001). Currently, the NIDA Clinical Trials Network is conducting a study (the Buprenorphine/Naloxone-facilitated Rehabilitation for Heroin Addicted Adolescents/Young Adults) that compares two 3-month treatments for adolescents/young adults who are addicted to heroin: either buprenorphine/naloxone combined with psychosocial therapy and "treatment as usual," or a 7–14 day detoxification with buprenorphine and 3 weeks of psychosocial therapy ("treatment as usual"). In a double-blind, placebo-controlled study of acamprosate in 26 adolescents, aged 16–19 years, with alcohol dependence, Niederhofer and Staffen (2003) reported that the cumulative abstinence duration was significantly greater in the acamprosate group than in the placebo group.

The increased prevalence of opiate dependence among adolescents necessitates testing and possible expansion of proven strategies for adults. At this time, naltrexone and buprenorphine appear to be the best candidates for controlled studies in adolescents.

Aversive therapy

Aversive interventions refer to treatments that aim to reduce or eliminate the craving or desire for alcohol or other drugs by presenting a noxious consequence immediately following substance use or psychosocial cues related to use (Bukstein, 1995). One of the most common and controversial forms of aversive therapy is disulfiram (Antabuse). Despite its wide use and promising effects with adult alcoholics, there are no published controlled trials, and limited case reports have yielded mixed results (Myers, Donahue, & Goldstein, 1995). Aversive agents are potentially problematic with adolescents, given the potential harmful physical effects if alcohol is taken, and common adolescent issues of non-compliance, impulsiveness, and questionable motivation. Adolescents must be supervised in taking disulfiram and similar agents and must also be medically healthy, intellectually competent, insightful about their drug use, and highly motivated for recovery (Solhkhah & Wilens, 1998). Given the presence of other less potentially dangerous pharmacological options for treatment, the development and testing of adverse agents for adolescents is a very low priority for investigators.

Tobacco cessation

The pharmacological treatment of tobacco cessation largely involves substitution therapy or nicotine replacement. Tobacco-dependent adolescents manifest similar types and severity of withdrawal symptoms as those reported by adults (Moolchan, Ernst, & Henningfield, 2000; Rojas *et al.*, 1998). In studies of adult smokers, nicotine replacement therapy has been shown to increase cessation rates over placebo (Hughes *et al.*, 1999). In the single published adolescent study (an 8-week open-label trial of nicotine replacement therapy using a patch), Smith, House, and Croghan (1996) reported that only 1 of 22 adolescents remained abstinent after 6 months. Nicotine substitution is *not* contraindicated in adolescents, and given the significant health risk from smoking, additional studies are needed. Buproprion, an atypical antidepressant, also shows significant promise when treating nicotine addiction since it doubles quit rates (Hughes, 2000). The success of bupropion in smokers is not linked to treatment of depression in this population, as it has proved efficacious in people without any current or past symptoms of depression (Hughes, 2000). Buproprion is commonly used in adolescent patients for treatment of depression and ADHD, but no guide-lines are available for buproprion dosage in adolescents who desire to quit smoking.

The most salient issue of using tobacco substitution therapies with adolescents involves motivation, as adolescents often do not recognize their use patterns as problematic. For tobacco smoking, motivational interviewing techniques have demonstrated preliminary success in affecting smoking cessation among adolescents (Colby *et al.*, 1998). Nicotine cessation trials should eventually combine medication with psychosocial interventions, such as psychoeducation, motivational enhance-ment, or cognitive–behavioral therapy (Moolchan *et al.*, 2000).

The pharmacological treatment of comorbid disorders in adolescents

Importance of comorbidity in adolescents

Significant rates of adolescents with coexisting SUDs and psychiatric disorders (disruptive behavior disorders, mood disorders, and anxiety disorders) are reported in both clinical and general populations (Grella *et al.*, 2001; Lewinsohn *et al.*, 1993; Wilens *et al.*, 1997). Furthermore, the comorbidity of psychiatric disorders, particularly conduct disorder and, to a lesser extent, MDD, may have an effect on the alcohol and substance use and related problems both at baseline and at follow-up, and they may impair an adolescent's ability to engage effectively in treatment (Riggs & Whitmore, 1999).

Disruptive behavior disorders are the most common psychiatric disorders diagnosed in adolescents with SUDs (Huizinga & Elliot, 1981; Loeber, 1988; Milan *et al.*, 1991). Clinical populations of adolescents with SUDs manifest rates of conduct disorder ranging from 50% to almost 80%, and also commonly display aggressive behavior (Bukstein, 1994) and often have ADHD (Kaminer, 1994; Wilens *et al.*, 1994).

Mood disorders, particularly depression, frequently have onsets both preceding and consequent to the onset of substance use and SUDs in adolescents (Bukstein, Glancy, & Kaminer, 1992; Deykin, Buka, & Zeena, 1992). The prevalence of depressive disorders in these studies of clinical populations ranged from 24% to more than 50%. The occurrence of SUDs among adolescents are also a risk factor for suicidal behaviors, including ideation, suicide attempts, and completed suicide (Crumley, 1990; Lewinsohn, Rohde, & Seeley, 1996). Evidence suggests that depression increases the rate and rapidity of relapse (Cornelius *et al.*, 2004; Maisto *et al.*, 2001).

A number of studies of clinical populations show high rates of anxiety disorders among youth with SUDs, ranging from 7% to over 40% (Clark *et al.*, 1995; Grella *et al.*, 2001). Adolescents with SUDs often have a past history or current manifestation of post-traumatic stress disorder (Clark *et al.*, 1995; van Hasselt *et al.*, 1992), and SUDs are very common among individuals, especially young and chronically impaired, who are diagnosed with schizophrenia (Kutcher *et al.*, 1992).

The heterogeneity of substance use and mental disorders among adolescents suggests that adolescents with different subtypes of comorbidity may respond differently to substance abuse treatment (Bennett & McCrady, 1993; Bukstein, Brent, & Kaminer, 1989; Estroff, Schwartz, & Hoffman, 1989), yet drug treatment providers focus treatment on the mental health needs of these youth or develop diagnosis-specific treatment modalities, such as pharmacotherapy (Crowley & Riggs, 1995).

Although evidence is accumulating regarding the effectiveness of specific psychosocial or non-pharmacological interventions for adolescents with SUDs (e.g., family therapy, cognitive–behavioral therapy), it is not yet established whether or how effective substance abuse treatment is for adolescents with comorbid mental disorders. Some initial studies have suggested that psychopathology is associated with poorer treatment outcomes among substance-abusing adolescents (Brown *et al.*, 1994, Crowley *et al.*, 1998a; Kennedy & Minami, 1993). The DATOS-A study and other studies have reported that comorbidity is associated with more severe substance use (Crowley *et al.*, 1998b; Grella *et al.*, 2001; Wilens *et al.*, 1997), as indicated by youth with comorbid disorders having higher rates of drug and alcohol dependence, having ever used a greater number of substances, and initiating alcohol and marijuana use at earlier ages than the adolescents without comorbidity. Severity of drug use has been identified as a precursor of earlier treatment initiation, repeated treatment utilization, and generally poorer treatment outcomes over the course of an addiction/treatment career (Anglin, Hser, & Grella, 1997; Hser *et al.*, 1999). These findings indicate the importance of intervention for adolescents with comorbid psychiatric disorders. The persistence of depressive symptoms after drug treatment was partially, although not wholly, explained by their continued drug and alcohol use. This finding is consistent with other studies showing the persistence of depressive symptoms after drug treatment and short-term abstinence for adolescents (Bukstein *et al.*, 1992; Riggs *et al.*, 1995) and emphasizes the need for concurrent psychiatric treatment for these adolescents, both during and after drug treatment (Riggs & Davies, 2002).

There is an emerging but still nascent research literature on the pharmacotherapy of comorbid disorders in adolescents with SUDs. The following will examine existing medication studies in the areas of mood disorders and ADHD. Unfortunately, there are no controlled trials or even reported series of cases examining medication approaches in adolescents with SUDs and anxiety disorders. Similar to the adult literature, such patients often suffer from the common adolescent problem of multiple psychiatric comorbidities (e.g., anxiety disorder plus mood disorder plus disruptive behavior disorder), thus limiting an investigator's ability to control for medication effects on concurrent, but not explicitly targeted, problems.

Mood disorders

Similar to the adult literature, pharmacological studies of depressive disorders are represented by several open and controlled studies of adolescents. For MDD, three published studies have evaluated the efficacy of fluoxetine or any other SSRI antidepressant in adolescents with substance dependence. Riggs *et al.* (1997) conducted an open label trial involving eight male adolescent subjects with a diagnosis of either cannabis abuse or cannabis dependence and conduct disorder in addition to an alcohol use disorder and MDD; the adolescents were treated with a 20 mg daily dose of fluoxetine for 7 weeks. Seven subjects demonstrated marked improvement in depressive symptoms on the Clinical Global Impression scale, as well as on observer-rated and self-rated measures of depressive symptoms. As the study was conducted in the controlled environment of a residential treatment center, the efficacy of fluoxetine for reducing alcohol or substance use could not be assessed. Cornelius *et al.* (2000) conducted a 12-week open-label study of fluoxetine in an outpatient setting with 13 adolescents diagnosed with comorbid alcohol use disorder and MDD. The study found a significant within-group decrease (improvement) for both depressive symptoms and drinking. Deas *et al.* (2000) conducted a 12-week, double-blind placebo-controlled trial of sertraline plus cognitive–behavioral group therapy in 10 adolescents with a depressive disorder and comorbid alcohol use disorder. Both groups showed significant reductions in drinking variables and depression scores, although there were no group differences.

In perhaps the only published double-blind placebo-controlled trial in adolescents with SUDs and bipolar disorder, Geller and colleagues (1998) conducted a 6-week study of 25 adolescents, aged 12–18 years, who were randomly assigned to receive either placebo or lithium carbonate. Using both intent-to-treat and completer analyses, there were significant differences on continuous and categorical measures between the lithium and the placebo groups for both psychopathology measures and weekly random urine drug screens.

Attention-deficit hyperactivity disorder

Psychostimulant medications, which include methylphenidate, dextroamphetamine (dexamfetamine), and pemoline, have been consistently shown to be effective in treatment of ADHD (Barkley *et al.*, 1990). While there are many studies of treatment for children with ADHD, there are only a few dozen published studies of stimulant treatment with adolescents, and very few controlled studies. Although these studies show improvement in ADHD symptoms, stimulants appear to be less effective in adolescents than in children (Klorman, Coons, & Borgstadt, 1987; Pelham *et al.*, 1991; Smith *et al.*, 1998). Controversy remains regarding their use among adolescents with problems related to substance use. Methylphenidate and amphetamines are classified as Schedule II by the Drug Enforcement Administration (DEA), thus indicating a high potential for abuse (DEA, 1995; Jaffe, 1991; Riggs, 1998). The use of stimulant medication as a secondary prevention modality for children and adolescents with ADHD is supported by at least two studies reporting an association between decreased SUD and use of stimulant medication for adolescents with ADHD (Barkley *et al.*, 2003; Biederman *et al.*, 1999). However, a recent study by Pelham *et al.* (2003) reported that stimulant use is unrelated to substance use in adolescents but, in young adults with ADHD there is a consistent, positive prediction from lifetime stimulant treatment to heavy use of alcohol, marijuana, and cigarettes. Therefore, concerns still remain about the appropriate use or possible misuse of stimulant medication by adolescents with conjoint substance abuse and ADHD problems.

Despite the behavioral pharmacological profile of methylphenidate, it is generally accepted that the rates of methylphenidate abuse are minimal compared with those of cocaine or even dextroamphetamine (NIDA Community Epidemiology Work Group, 1995). Although the case reports in the literature suggest that some individuals develop problems with methylphenidate use (Jaffe, 1991), much of the popular press and anecdotal information regarding non-medical use of the drug centers on its use as a more mild stimulant for recreational use. The prevalence of stimulant abuse or dependence among adolescents or young adults with a history of ADHD and therapeutic stimulant use is very low. The reinforcing properties of drugs of abuse suggest that the rapidity of drug delivery to the brain affects the reinforcing properties of drugs. The shorter the interval between intake and the perceived effects of the drug, the greater the addictive potential of the drug. Research on the influence of rate of onset of effects and stimulant use support that the abuse potential of immediate-release methylphenidate may be greater than that of the sustained-release formulation (Kollins *et al.*, 1998; Volkow *et al.*, 1995). These findings suggest that the longer-acting stimulants such as those in Oros controlled delivery formulations or once-a-day formulations of methylphenidate (Concerta) or the extended-release formulation of mixed amphetamine salts (Adderall XR) may have a lower abuse potential than immediate-release preparations of psychostimulants. Similarly, there may be differential abuse or dependence liabilities between methylphenidate and amphetamines.

Pemoline, another central nervous system stimulant and a schedule IV medication, has a lower abuse potential, as indicated by animal and human studies (Langer *et al.*, 1986; Riggs *et al.*, 1996). Riggs and colleagues (1996) conducted a 1-month open trial of pemoline in 13 adolescents aged 14 to 18 years with SUD, ADHD, and conduct disorder who were being treated in a residential drug and alcohol treatment center. After 1 month of pemoline treatment, scores of mean Conners Hyperactivity Index scores and physical activity decreased from baseline. In a 12-week randomized double-blind placebo trial of pemoline, Riggs, Mikulich, and Hall (2001) found that the 35 subjects in the pemoline group had significantly lower Parent Conners Hyperactivity scores but no differences in substance use from the 34 subjects in the placebo group.

Bupropion is a noradrenergic and dopamine reuptake blocker that is in current use as an antidepressant (Davidson & Conner, 1998). It has a low side effect profile and low cardiotoxicity (Ferris, Cooper, & Maxwell, 1983). A newer sustained-release preparation is an attractive candidate agent for the treatment of comorbid ADHD. Bupropion appears to have a low abuse potential on physiological measures compared with dextroamphetamine (Griffith *et al.*, 1983). The approval by the US FDA for the use of bupropion for smoking cessation and its efficacy in controlled clinical trials (Hurt *et al.*, 1997; Goldstein, 1998) suggests the potential value of this agent for addictive disorders. Similarly, the noradrenergic medication atomoxitine may hold promise as a medication with efficacy for ADHD and with low abuse potential. Clinical trials using atomoxetine in adolescents or adults with ADHD and SUDs are expected in the near future.

The current status of pharamacotherapy in adolescents with substance use disorders

Despite past and continuing concerns about using any type of medications in adolescents with SUDs, the use of pharmacotherapy is increasing rapidly, not only in adolescents with SUDs but for all adolescents (Safer & Zito, 2002). As little as a decade ago, the use of pharmacotherapy was discouraged by addiction professionals. Today, the use of medications for adolescents with SUDs, particularly those with comorbid psychiatric disorders, appears to be widespread, although few data exist on the full extent of its use among this adolescent population. Unfortunately, the database from existing pharmacotherapy studies often provides little positive support for such widespread use. The "off label" (i.e., not having an indication by the FDA for a particular use) use of medications approved for use by adults is the rule rather than the exception in adolescents, despite there being inadequate data on efficacy, safety, and appropriate dosing. In the area of SUDs, data are inadequate even in the adult literature in such areas as the pharmacological treatment of SUDs when comorbid with bipolar disorder or anxiety disorders. Currently, there is insufficient evidence for the use of any pharmacological agent for any specific disorder related to SUDs in adolescents.

As adolescents with SUDs are often considered a difficult population to assess and treat, such treatment often falls to adult addiction specialists with little understanding of the relevant developmental and psychopathological differences present in adolescents, or to child and adolescent psychiatrists who often have little understanding of SUDs and have little connection or inadequate communication with SUD treatment programs. The need for more training for child and adolescent psychiatrists in understanding how to assess and treat adolescents with SUDs within a multimodal context is as critical as the need for more research into pharmacotherapy.

Future directions in research

The success of pharmacotherapies in adults with SUDs and the presumed importance of medication treatment of psychiatric disorders suggest a vigorous research agenda for studying pharmacotherapies in various adolescent populations.

Training of investigators

The number of investigators with adequate research and clinical training to conduct such studies is limited. The NIDA, the NIAAA, and the American Academy of Child and Adolescent Psychiatry have supported increased training of physicians and psychologists interested in developing careers in treatment aspects of pharmacotherapy research. This support must extend to the major research departments of psychiatry and/or psychology, as well as to the major addiction research centers.

Extension of the adult literature on agents for withdrawal, substitution, craving, or blocking

While studies on agents for withdrawal, craving, or blocking should be reserved for adolescents with severe, persistent substance dependence, these adolescents represent the core of those who will continue with severe problems well into adulthood, and they should have access to these medications if they are proven to be safe and effective for youth.

Studies of adolescents with specific comorbid psychiatric disorders, using specific agents

Almost every agent currently in use for adolescents with specific psychiatric disorders, such as depression, bipolar disorder, anxiety disorder and ADHD, needs to be empirically tested in controlled studies. These studies need to be large enough to establish the primary aim of efficacy, but also potentially large enough to examine mediators and moderators of treatment.

The use of multicenter trials

The difficulty of recruiting and retaining sufficient numbers of youth with SUDs within a reasonable time period will require multisite trials using the cooperation of centers with experience and expertise. Such efforts as NIDA's Clinical Trials Network provide examples of cooperative efforts that are encouraged and supported by the federal government and that utilize both adult and adolescent addiction expertise. The advantage of larger, multisite studies is the ability to do subgroup and other secondary analyses, and to examine mediators and moderators of treatment response.

The use of common, salient variables among studies

Treatment research will advance more rapidly if some basic conventions are adopted. In order to achieve some level of uniformity, a set of core variables should be developed that is relatively consistent, or at least comparable, across studies. Within two major types of variable, baseline and outcome, are core variables that represent critical content domains. Core variables are those that should be measured in every treatment study. Examples include DSM-IV psychiatric diagnoses as a baseline variable(s) and occasions of specific substance use in the past month as outcome variables. Adoption of a "gold standard" of core variables and the resulting uniformity should allow cross-study comparison and ease in meta-analyses of adolescent SUD pharmacotherapy studies.

Studies of safety, abuse, and diversion

Common objections to pharmacotherapy in adolescents with SUDs are the potential for interactions between the therapeutic agent and drugs of abuse, abuse of the therapeutic agent, and diversion of the agent to others who are not prescribed the agent. Unfortunately, there is no literature to provide guidance for the clinician. Measurement of potential adverse effects of medication, therapeutic–illicit drug interactions, abuse, and diversion will require creative research strategies and methods.

Studies of compliance and the development of motivational strategies to improve compliance

Adolescents with SUDs seldom seek help. Poor compliance with pharmacotherapy may have a role in treatment response or relapse. Future studies need to develop valid and reliable measures of compliance and strategies to improve compliance.

Multimodal studies using a combination of pharmacotherapy and psychosocial intervention modalities

Several recent studies suggest that medications may have a limited role in targeting substance use behavior, and perhaps, overall levels of psychosocial functioning. Therefore, as in the adult research literature, multimodal studies, especially involving adolescents with comorbid disorders, may offer an advantage over single modality interventions. The combination of these modalities may improve outcomes over single modality strategies. Behavioral intervention (including family, individual, or group therapies) strategies may be needed, even more with adolescents than adults, in order to implement a trial of medication successfully in the first place, and to get adolescents to take the medications long enough and consistently enough to see if they work.

Even quasi-experimental models where adolescents are allowed to receive medication treatment(s) through established a-priori algorithms as an adjunct to controlled, randomized trials of psychosocial modalities may help to answer some questions about the relative value of medication treatment. Similar to the Cannabis Youth Treatment study, adding on additional modalities, such as medication, to a core empirically proven treatment, such as a specific type of family therapy, is another potential methodology. Such combination approaches for adolescents with SUDs are starting (Riggs & Davies, 2002).

Pharmacotherapy is a potentially fertile area for the discovery and development of efficacious treatments for adolescents with SUDs. To contribute to the field of treatment research, agencies and institutions need to support and develop researchers with expertise in pharmacotherapy clinical trials and promote multi-center efforts, and multimodal projects.

ACKNOWLEDGEMENT

The work in this chapter was supported by grants AA000301 and AA013370-01.

REFERENCES

American Psychiatric Association (1995). Practice guidelines for the treatment of patients with substance use disorders: alcohol, cocaine, opioids. *American J Psychiatry*, **152**(Suppl.), 1–59.

Anglin, M. D., Hser, Y. I., & Grella, C. E. (1997). Drug addiction and treatment careers among clients in the drug abuse treatment outcome study. *Psychology of Addictive Behaviors*, **11**, 308–323.

Barkley, R. A., Fischer, M., Edelbrock, C. S., & Smallish, L. (1990). The adolescent outcome of hyperactive children diagnosed by research criteria, I: An 8-year prospective follow-up study. *Journal of the American Academy of Child and Adolescent Psychiatry*, **29**, 546–557.

Barkley, R. A., Fischer, M., Smallish, L., & Fletcher, K. (2003). Does the treatment of attention-deficit/hyperactivity disorder with stimulants contribute to drug use/abuse? A 13-year prospective study. *Pediatrics*, **11**, 97–109.

Bennett, M. E. & McCrady, B. S. (1993). Subtype by comorbidity in young adult substance abusers. *Journal of Substance Abuse Treatment*, **5**, 365–378.

Biederman, J., Wilens, T., Mick, E., Spencer, T., & Farone, S. V. (1999). Pharmacotherapy of attention-deficit hyperactivity disorder reduces risk for substance use disorder. *Pediatrics*, **104**, e20.

Brady, J. V. & Lucas, S. E. (1984). *Testing Drugs for Physical Dependence Potential and Abuse Liability*. [*NIDA Research Monograph Series*, No. 52.] Rockville, MD: National Institute on Drug Abuse.

Brady, K. T., Sonne, S. C., Malcom, R., *et al.* (2002). Carbamazepine in the treatment of cocaine dependence: subtyping by affective disorder. *Experimental and Clinical Pharmacology*, **10**, 276–285.

Brown, S. A., Myers, M. G., Mott, M. A., & Vik, P. W. (1994). Correlates of success following treatment for adolescent substance abuse. *Applied and Preventive Psychology*, **3**, 61–73.

Bruno, F. (1989). Buspirone in the treatment of alcoholic patients. *Psychopathology*, **22**, 49–59.

Bukstein, O. G. (1994). Substance abuse. In M. Herson, R. T. Ammerman, & L. A. Sisson (eds.), *Handbook of Aggressive and Destructive Behavior in Psychiatric Patients* (pp. 445–468). New York: Plenum Press.

(1995). *Adolescent Substance Abuse: Assessment, Prevention and Treatment*. New York: John Wiley.

Bukstein, O. G. & Kithas, J. (2002). Adolescent substance use disorders. In D. Rosenberg, P. A. Davanzo, & S. Gershon (eds.), *Child and Adolescent Psychopharmacology* (pp. 346–373). New York: Maecel-Dekker.

Bukstein, O. G. & Tarter, R. E. (1998). Substance use disorders in children and adolescents. In E. Coffey (ed.), *Textbook of Pediatric Neuropsychiatry* (pp. 595–616). New York: American Psychiatric Press.

Bukstein O. G., Brent D. A., & Kaminer, Y. (1989). Comorbidity of substance abuse and other psychiatric disorders in adolescents. *American Journal of Psychiatry*, **146**, 1131–1141.

Bukstein O., Glancy, L. J., & Kaminer, Y. (1992). Patterns of affective comorbidity in a clinical population of dually diagnosed substance abusers. *Journal of the American Academy of Child and Adolescent Psychiatry*, **31**, 1041–1045.

Castaneda, R., Levy, R., Hardy, M., & Trujillo, M. (2000). Long-acting stimulants for the treatment of attention-deficit disorder in cocaine-dependent adults. *Psychiatric Services*, **51**, 169–171.

Claassen, C. A. & Adinoff, B. (1999). Alcohol withdrawal syndrome: guidelines for management. *CNS Drugs*, **12**, 279–291.

Clark, D. B., Bukstein, O. G., Smith, M. G., *et al.* (1995). Identifying anxiety disorders in adolescents hospitalized for alcohol abuse or dependence. *Psychiatric Services*, **46**, 618–620.

Colby, S. M., Monti, P., Barnett, N., *et al.* (1998). Brief motivational interviewing in a hospital setting for adolescent smoking: a preliminary study. *Journal of Consulting and Clinical Psychology*, **66**, 574–578.

Cornelius, J. R., Salloum, I. M., Ehler, J. G., *et al.* (1997). A double-blind, placebo-controlled study of fluoxetine in depressed alcoholics. *Archives of General Psychiatry*, **54**, 700–705.

Cornelius, J. R., Bukstein, O. G., Birmaher, B., *et al.* (2000). Fluoxetine in adolescents with major depression and an alcohol use disorder: an open label trial. *Addictive Behaviors*, **25**, 1–6.

Cornelius, J. R., Maisto, S. A., Martin, C. S., *et al.* (2004). Major depression associated with earlier alcohol relapse in treated teens with AUD. *Addictive Behaviors*, **29**, 1035–1038.

Crowley, T. J. & Riggs, P. D. (1995). Adolescent substance use disorder with conduct disorder and comorbid conditions. In E. Rahdert & D. Czechowicz (eds.), *Adolescent Drug Abuse: Clinical Assessment and Therapeutic Interventions* (pp. 49–111). Rockville, MD: National Institute on Drug Abuse.

Crowley, T. J., Macdonald, M. J., Whitmore, E. A., & Mikulick, S. K. (1998a). Cannabis dependence, withdrawal and reinforcing effects among adolescents with conduct symptoms and substance use disorders. *Drug and Alcohol Dependence*, **50**, 27–37.

Crowley, T. J., Mikulich, S. K., MacDonald, M. J., Young, S. E., & Zerbe, G. O. (1998b). Substance-dependent, conduct-disordered adolescent males: severity of diagnosis predicts 2-year outcome. *Drug and Alcohol Dependence*, **49**, 225–237.

Crumley, F. E. (1990). Substance abuse and adolescent suicidal behavior. *Journal of the American Medical Association*, **263**, 3051–3056.

Davidson, J. T. & Connor, K. M. (1998). Bupropion sustained release: a therapeutic overview. *Journal of Clinical Psychiatry*, **58**(Suppl. 4), 25–31.

DEA (Drug Enforcement Administration (1995). *Methylphenidate Review Document.* Washington, DC: DEA Office of Diversion Control, Drug and Chemical Evaluation Section.

Deas, D., Randall, C. L., Roberts, J. S., & Anton, R. F. (2000). A double-blind, placebo-controlled trial of sertraline in depressed adolescent alcoholics: a pilot study. *Human Psychopharmacology*, **15**, 461–469.

Deas, D., Roberts, J. S., Randall, C. L., & Anton, R. F. (2002). Confirmatory analysis of the Adolescent Obsessive Compulsive Drinking Scale (A-OCDS): a measure of 'craving' and problem drinking in adolescents/young adults. *Journal of the National Medical Association*, **94**, 879–887.

Deykin, E. Y., Buka, S. L., & Zeena, T. H. (1992). Depressive illness among chemically dependent adolescents. *American Journal of Psychiatry*, **149**, 1341–1347.

Estroff, T. W., Schwartz, R. H., & Hoffmann, N. G. (1989). Adolescent cocaine abuse: addictive potential, behavioral and psychiatric effects. *Clinical Pediatrics*, **28**, 550–555.

Ferris, R. M., Cooper, B. R., & Maxwell, R. A. (1983). Studies of bupropion's mechanism of antidepressant activity. *Journal of Clinical Psychiatry*, **44**, 74–78.

Gardner, E. L. (1992). Brain reward mechanisms. In J. H. Lowinson, P. Ruiz, & R. B. Millman (eds.), *Substance Abuse: A Comprehensive Text book* (pp. 70–99). Baltimore, MD: Williams & Williams.

Geller, B., Cooper, T. B., Sun, K., *et al.* (1998). Double-blind and placebo-controlled study of lithium for adolescent bipolar disorders with secondary substance dependency. *Journal of the American Academy of Child and Adolescent Psychiatry*, **37**, 171–178.

Goldstein, M. G. (1998). Bupropion sustained release and smoking cessation. *Journal of Clinical Psychiatry*, **59**, 66–72.

Grella, C. E., Hser, Y., Joshi, V., & Rounds-Bryant, J. (2001). Drug treatment outcomes for adolescents with comorbid mental and substance use disorders. *Journal of Nervous and Mental Disorders*, **9**, 384–392.

Griffith, J. D., Carranza, J., Griffith, C., & Miller, L. I. (1983). Bupropion: clinical assay for amphetamine-like potential. *Journal of Clinical Psychiatry*, **44**, 206–208.

Haney, M., Ward, A. S., Comer, S. D., Hart, C. L., Foltin, R. W., & Fischman, M. W. (2001). Bupropion SR worsens mood during marijuana withdrawal in humans. *Psychopharmacology*, **155**, 171–179.

Hser, Y., Joshi, V., Anglin, M. D., & Fletcher, B. (1999). Predicting post-treatment cocaine abstinence for first-time admissions and treatment repeaters. *American Journal of Public Health*, **89**, 666–671.

Hughes, J. R. (2000). New treatments of smoking cessation. *CA: A Cancer Journal for Clinicians*, **50**, 143–151.

Hughes, J. R., Goldstein, M. C., Hurt, R. D., & Shiffman, S. (1999). Recent advances in the pharmcotherapy of smoking. *Journal of the American Medical Association*, **281**, 72–76.

Huizinga, D. & Elliot, D. S. (1981). *A Longitudinal Study of Drug Use and Delinquency in a National Sample of Youth: An Assessment of Causal Order.* [Project Report No. 16, A National Youth Study.] Boulder, CO: Behavioral Research Institute.

Hurt, R. D., Sachs, P. P. L., Glover, E. D., et al. (1997). A comparison of sustained-release bupropion and placebo for smoking cessation. *New England Journal of Medicine*, **337**, 1195–1202.

Jaffe, J. (1990). Drug addiction and drug abuse. In G. A. Goodman (ed.), *The Pharmacological Basis of Therapeutics* (pp. 522–573). New York: MacMillan.

Jaffe, S. L. (1991). Intranasal abuse of prescribed methylphenidate by an alcohol and drug abusing adolescent with ADHD. *Journal of the American Academy of Child and Adolescent Psychiatry*, **30**, 773–775.

Kaminer, Y. (1994). Cocaine craving. *Journal of the American Academy of Child and Adolescent Psychiatry*, **33**, 592.

Karam-Hage, M. & Bower, K. (2000). Gabapentin treatment for insomnia associated with alcohol dependence. *American Journal of Psychiatry*, **157**, 151.

Kennedy, B. P. & Minami, M. (1993). The Beech Hill Hospital/outward bound adolescent chemical dependency treatment program. *Journal of Substance Abuse Treatment*, **10**, 395–406.

Klorman, R., Coons H. W., & Borgstadt, A. D. (1987). Effects of methylphenidate on adolescents with a childhood history of attention-deficit disorder. I: Clinical findings. *Journal of the American Academy of Child and Adolescent Psychiatry*, **26**, 363–367.

Kollins, S. H., Rush, C. R., Pazzaglia, P. J., & Ali, J. A. (1998). Comparison of acute behavioral effects of sustained-release and immediate-release methylphenidate. *Experimental and Clinical Psychopharmacology*, **6**, 367–374.

Kranzler, H. R. & Meyer, R. E. (1989). An open trial of buspirone in alcoholics. *Journal of Clinical Psychopharmacology*, **9**, 379–380.

Kranzler, H. R., Burleson, J. A., Del Boca, F. K., et al. (1994). Buspirone treatment of anxious alcoholics: a placebo-controlled trial. *Archives of General Psychiatry*, **51**, 720–731.

Kranzler, H. R., Burleson, J. A., Korner, P., et al. (1995). Placebo-controlled trial of fluoxetine as an adjunct to relapse prevention in alcoholics. *American Journal of Psychiatry*, **152**, 391–397.

Kutcher, S., Kachur, E., Marton, P., & Szalai, J. (1992). Substance abuse among adolescents with chronic mental illnesses: a pilot study of descriptive and differentiating features. *Canadian Journal of Psychiatry*, **37**, 428–431.

Langer, D. H., Sweeney, K. P., Bartenbach, D. E., Davis, P. M., & Menander, K. B. (1986). Evidence of lack of abuse or dependence following pemoline treatment: results of a retrospective survey. *Drug and Alcohol Dependence*, **17**, 213–227.

Levin, F. R., Evans, S. M., McDowell, D. M., & Kleber, H. D. (1998). Methylphenidate treatment for cocaine abusers with adult attention-deficit/hyperactivity disorder: a pilot study. *Journal of Clinical Psychiatry*, **59**, 300–305.

Lewinsohn, P. M., Hops, H., Roberts, R. E., & Seeley, J. R. (1993). Adolescent psychopathology: I. Prevalence and incidence of depression and other DSM-III – R disorders in high school students. *Journal of Abnormal Psychology*, **102**, 133–144.

Lewinsohn, P. M., Rohde, P., & Seeley, J. R. (1996). Alcohol consumption in high school adolescents: frequency of use and dimensional structure of associated problems. *Addiction*, **91**, 375–390.

Lifrak, P. D., Alterman A. I., O'Brien, C. P., & Volpicelli, J. R. (1997). Naltrexone for alcoholic adolescents. *American Journal of Psychiatry*, **154**, 439–440.

Ling, W., Huber, A., & Rawson, R. A. (2001). New trends in opiate pharmacotherapy. *Drug and Alcohol Review*, **20**, 79–94.

Loeber, R. (1988). Natural histories of conduct problems, delinquency and associated substance use. In B. B. Lahey & A. E. Kazdin (eds.), *Advances in Clinical Child Psychology* (pp. 73–124). New York: Plenum Press.

Maisto, S. A., Pollock, N. K., Lynch, K. G., Martin, C. S., & Ammerman, R. (2001). Course of functioning in adolescents 1 year after alcohol and other drug treatment. *Psychology of Addictive Behavior*, **15**, 68–76.

Malcolm, R., Anton, R. F., Randall, C. L., *et al.* (1992). A placebo-controlled trial of buspirone in anxious inpatient alcoholics. *Alcoholism, Clinical and Experimental Research*, **16**, 1007–13.

Martin, C. S., Kaczynski, N. A., Maisto S. A., Bukstein O. G., & Moss, H. B. (1995). Patterns of alcohol abuse and dependence symptoms in adolescent drinkers. *Journal of Studies in Alcohol*, **56**, 672–680.

Mason, B. J., Kocis, J. H., Ritvo, E. C., Cutler, R. B. (1996). A double blind, placebo-controlled trial of desipramine for primary alcohol dependence stratified on the presence or absence of major depression. *Journal of the American Medical Association*, **275**, 761–767.

McGrath, P. J., Nunes, E. V., Stewart, J. W., *et al.* (1996). Imipramine treatment of alcoholics with primary depression: a placebo-controlled clinical trial. *Archives of General Psychiatry*, **53**, 232–240.

Milan, R., Halikas, J. A., Meller, J. E., & Morse, C. (1991). Psychopathology among substance abusing juvenile offenders. *Journal of the American Academy of Child and Adolescent Psychiatry*, **30**, 569–574.

Moolchan, E. T., Ernst, M., & Henningfield, J. E. (2000). A review of tobacco smoking in adolescents: treatment implications. *Journal of the American Academy of Child and Adolescent Psychiatry*, **39**, 682–693.

Mueller, T. I., Stout, R. L., Rudden, S., *et al.* (1997). A double-blind, placebo controlled pilot study of carbamazepine for the treatment of alcohol dependence. *Alcoholism, Clinical and Experimental Research*, **21**, 86–92.

Myers, W. C., Donahue, J. E., & Goldstein, M. R. (1995). Disulfiram for alcohol use disorders in adolescents. *Journal of the American Academy of Child and Adolescent Psychiatry*, **34**, 2–4.

Myrick, H., Brady, K. T., & Robert, R. (2001). New developments in the psychopharmacology of alcohol dependence. *American Journal of Addictions*, **10**, 3–15.

NIDA (National Institute on Drug Abuse) Community Epidemiology Work Group (1995). *Epidemiologic Trends in Drug Abuse*. Washington, DC: National Institutes of Health.

NIDA (National Institute on Drug Abuse 2000). *Buprenorphine update: Questions and Answers*. Rockville, MD: National Institute on Drug Abuse. Retrieved from, http://www.nida.nih.gov/bupupdate.html.

Niederhofer, H. & Staffen, W. (2003). Acamprosate and its efficacy in treating alcohol-dependent adolescents. *European Child and Adolescent Psychiatry*, **12**, 144–148.

NIH (National Institute of Health 1998). Effective medical treatment of opiate addiction. *Journal of the American Medical Association*, **280**, 1936–1943.

Nunes, E. V., Quitkin, F. M., Donovan, S. J., *et al.* (1998). Imipramine treatment of opiate dependant patients with depressive disorders: a placebo-controlled trial. *Archives of General Psychiatry*, **55**, 153–160.

Pelham, W. E., Vodde-Hamilton, M., Murphy, D. A., Greenstein, J., & Vallano, G. (1991). The effects of methylphenidate on ADHD adolescents in recreational, peer group and classroom settings. *Journal of Clinical and Child Psychology*, **20**, 293–300.

Pelham, W. E., Molina, B. S., Meichenbaum, D., Gnagy, E., & Greenhouse, J. (2003, May). *Stimulant effects on long term outcomes in ADHD individuals*. In *Proceedings of the 43rd Annual New Clinical Drug Evaluation Unit Meeting*, Boca Raton, FL [poster].

Petrakis, I., Carroll, K. M., Nich, C., Gordon, L., Kosten, T., & Rounsaville, B. (1998). Fluoxetine treatment of depressive disorders in methadone-maintained opioid addicts. *Drug and Alcohol Dependence*, **50**, 221–226.

Pettinati, H. M., Volpicelli, J. R., Luck, G., *et al.* (2001). Double-blind clinical trial of sertraline treatment for alcohol dependence. *Journal of Clinical Psychopharmacology*, **21**, 143–153.

Riggs, P. D. (1998). Clinical approach to treatment of ADHD in adolescents with substance use disorders and conduct disorder. *Journal of the American Academy of Child and Adolescent Psychiatry*, **37**, 331–332.

Riggs, P. D. & Davies, R. D. (2002). A clinical approach to integrating treatment for adolescent depression and substance abuse. *Journal of the American Academy of Child and Adolescent Psychiatry*, **41**, 1253–1255.

Riggs, P. D. & Whitmore, E. A. (1999). Substance use disorders and disruptive behavior disorders. In R. L. Hendren (ed.), *Disruptive Behavior Disorders in Children and Adolescents. Review of Psychiatry Series* (pp. 133–173). Washington, DC: American Psychiatric Press.

Riggs, P. D., Baker, S., Mikulich, S. K., Young, S. E., & Crowley, T. J. (1995). Depression in substance-dependent delinquents. *Journal of the American Academy of Child and Adolescent Psychiatry*, **34**, 764–771.

Riggs, P. D., Thompson, L. L., Mikulich, S. K., Whitmore, E. A., & Crowley, T. J. (1996). An open trial of pemoline in drug-dependent delinquents with attention-deficit hyperactivity disorder. *Journal of the American Academy of Child and Adolescent Psychiatry*, **35**, 1018–1024.

Riggs, P. D., Mikovich, S. K., Coffman, L. M., & Crowley, T. J. (1997). Fluoexetine in drug-dependant delinquents with major depression: an open trial. *Journal of Child and Adolescent Psychopharmacology*, **7**, 87–95.

Riggs, P. D., Mikulich, S. K., & Hall, S. (2001). Effects of pemoline on ADHD, antisocial behaviors, and substance use in adolescents with conduct disorder and substance use disorder. In *Proceedings of the 63rd Annual Scientific Meeting of the College on Problems of Drug Dependence*, Scottsdale, AZ.

Rojas, N., Killen, J., Haydel, K., & Robinson, T. (1998). Nicotine dependence among adolescent smokers. *Archives of Pediatric Adolescent Medicine*, **152**, 151–156.

Roy, A. (1998). Placebo-controlled study of sertraline in depressed recently abstinent alcoholics. *Biological Psychiatry*, **44**, 633–637.

Roy-Byrne, P. P., Pages, K. P., Russo, J. E., *et al.* (2000). Nefazodone treatment of major depression in alcohol-dependent patients: a double-blind, placebo-controlled trial. *Journal of Clinical Psychopharmacology*, **20**, 129–136.

Safer, D. & Zito, J. M. (2002). Adolescent stimulant use. *Canadian Medical Association Journal*, **167**, 15.

Salloum, I. M. & Thase, M. E. (2002). Impact of substance abuse on the course and treatment of bipolar disorder. *Bipolar Disorders*, **2**, 269–280.

Salloum, I. M., Cornelius, J. R., Daley, D. C., *et al.* (2005). Efficacy of valproate maintenance in patients with bipolar disorder and alcoholism. *Archives of General Psychiatry*, **62**, 37–45.

Schmitz, J. M., Averill, P., Stotts, A. L., *et al.* (2001). Fluoxetine treatment of cocaine-dependent patients with major depressive disorder. *Drug and Alcohol Dependence*, **63**, 207–214.

Schubiner, H., Tzelepis, A., Isaacson, J. H., & Warbasse, L. H. (1995). The dual diagnosis of attention-deficit/hyperactivity disorder and substance abuse: case reports and literature review. *Journal of Clinical Psychiatry*, **56**, 146–150.

Schubiner, H., Downer, K. K., Arfken, C. L., *et al.* (2002). Double-blind placebo-controlled trial of methylphenidate in the treatment of adult ADHD patients with comorbid cocaine dependence. *Experimental and Clinical Psychopharmacology*, **10**, 286–294.

Smith, B. H., Pelham, W. E., Gnagy, E., & Yudell, R. S. (1998). Equivalent effects of stimulant treatment for attention-deficit hyperactivity disorder during childhood and adolescence. *Journal of the American Academy of Child and Adolescent Psychiatry*, **37**, 314–321.

Smith, T. A., House, R. F., & Croghan, I. T. (1996). Nicotine patch therapy in adolescent smokers. *Pediatrics*, **98**, 659–667.

Solhkhah, R. & Wilens, T. E. (1998). Pharmacotherapy of adolescent AOD use disorders. *Alcohol Health and Research World*, **22**, 122–126.

Spencer, T., Biederman, J., Wilens, T., *et al.* (1996). Pharmacotherapy of attention-deficit hyperactivity disorder across the life cycle. *Journal of the American Academy of Child and Adolescent Psychiatry*, **24**, 325–347.

Swift, R. M. (1999). Drug therapy: drug therapy for alcohol dependence. *New England Journal of Medicine*, **340**, 1482–1490.

Tollefson, G. D., Montague-Clouse, J., & Tollefson, S. L. (1992). Treatment of comorbid generalized anxiety in a recently detoxified alcoholic population with a selective serotonergic drug (buspirone). *Journal of Clinical Psychopharmacology*, **22**, 19–26.

Turnquist, K., Frances, R., Rosenfeld, W., & Mobarak, A. (1983). Pemoline in attention deficit disorder and alcoholism: a case study. *American Journal of Psychiatry*, **140**, 622–624.

van Hasselt, V. B., Ammerman, R. T., Glancy, L. J., & Buksein, O. G. (1992). Maltreatment in psychiatrically hospitalized dually diagnosed adolescent substance abusers. *Journal of the American Academy of Child and Adolescent Psychiatry*, **31**, 868–874.

Vingilis, E. & Smart, R. G. (1981). Physical dependence on alcohol in youth. In Y. Israel, F. B. Gleser, & H. Kalant (eds.), *Research Advances in Alcohol and Drug Problems* (pp. 197–215). New York: Plenum Press.

Volkow, N. D., Ding, Y., Fowler, J. S., *et al.* (1995). Is methylphenidate like cocaine? Studies on their pharmacokinetics and distribution in the human brain. *Archives of General Psychiatry*, **52**, 456–463.

Wilens, T. E., Biederman, J., Spencer, T. J., & Frances, R. J. (1994). Comorbidity of attention-deficit disorder and psychoactive substance use disorders. *Hospital and Community Psychiatry*, **45**, 421–435.

Wilens, T. E., Biederman, J., Abrantes, A. M., & Spencer, T. J. (1997). Clinical characteristics of psychiatrically referred adolescent outpatients with substance use disorder. *Journal of the American Academy of Child and Adolescent Psychiatry*, **36**, 941–947.

Wilens, T. E., Spencer, T. J., Biederman, J., *et al.* (2001). A controlled clinical trial of bupropion for attention deficit hyperactivity disorder in adults. *American Journal of Psychiatry*, **158**, 282–288.

Wise, R. A. & Rompre, P. P. (1989). Brain dopamine and reward. *Annual Review of Psychology*, **40**, 191–225.

Wold, M. & Kaminer, Y. (1997). Naltrexone for alcohol abuse. *Journal of the American Academy of Child and Adolescent Psychiatry*, **36**, 6–7.

13

Developmentally informed diagnostic and treatment considerations in comorbid conditions

Elizabeth A. Whitmore and Paula D. Riggs

University of Colorado School of Medicine, Denver, CO, USA

A burgeoning of research into child and adolescent substance use in the 1990s has significantly advanced our understanding of adolescent substance use disorders (SUDs) and of effective treatment approaches (Muck *et al.*, 2001; Drug Strategies, 2003). Developmental research has demonstrated that adolescents who present for drug treatment have a broad range of behavioral problems, skills deficits, academic difficulties, and family and mental health problems, which have generally been shaped by a series of environmental adversities and biological vulnerabilities from early childhood (Dawes *et al.*, 2000; Hops *et al.*, 2000; Tarter, 2002; Tims *et al.*, 2002). Developmental research has also supported the development of a number of manual-guided, behavioral, cognitive–behavioral, and family-based modalities that integrate treatment across multiple problem domains (Deas & Thomas, 2001; Muck *et al.*, 2001; Riggs & Whitmore, 1999). A growing research and clinical consensus indicates that substance treatment is most effective when it attends to the multiple psychosocial problems and medical and mental health needs of adolescents in addition to their drug abuse. Such multimodal treatment, including the concurrent assessment and treatment of psychiatric comorbidity, is recommended by the leading research and clinical professional organizations in the field (AACAP, 1997; Drug Strategies, 2003; NIDA, 1999). Despite these recommendations, implementation of integrated treatment of comorbidity in substance treatment programs has lagged behind the integration of other treatment services owing to a number of barriers, including a lack of research evaluating the safety and efficacy of psychotropic medications in adolescents with SUD (Sohlkhah & Wilens, 1998). The lack of research, in turn, has impeded the development of empirically grounded integrated practice guidelines.

Fortunately, recent advances have begun to address this research gap and can now shed light on several of the most vexing clinical questions and treatment

Adolescent Substance Abuse: Research and Clinical Advances, ed. Howard A. Liddle and Cynthia L. Rowe. Published by Cambridge University Press. © Cambridge University Press 2006.

conundrums posed by comorbidity in adolescents across assessment, treatment, development, research, funding, and policy domains. There are a number of key questions. What is the general sequence of onset of the various common comorbid disorders and SUDs? What are the clinical implications, if any, of the order of onset? Do childhood psychiatric disorders increase the risk of developing adolescent SUD and does treatment of those disorders decrease the risk? Is there a difference in treatment outcome if psychiatric disorders are treated before or after SUD has developed? Is it safe and effective to use medications to treat psychiatric comorbidity in non-abstinent adolescents? Is the abuse potential of medications an important clinical concern? Does our scientific knowledge support sequential or integrated treatment models? Has our science advanced sufficiently that integrated treatment principles can be empirically derived?

These questions will be addressed in the context of achieving the primary goals of this chapter: (a) to understand the clinical impact and treatment implications of comorbidity in adolescents with SUD; (b) to understand the current state of the science in treating psychiatric disorders comorbid with SUD; (c) to derive an empirically grounded treatment algorithm for integrating the treatment of both SUD and comorbid psychiatric disorders in adolescents.

Developmental context and bidirectional impact of substance use and comorbid psychiatric disorders

A relatively large body of developmental research has led to a greater understanding of the interactions of biopsychosocial risk factors that increase a child's vulnerability to develop SUD. These risk factors include "difficult temperament" in early childhood, often characterized as behavioral and affective dysregulation, impulsivity, hyperactivity, aggression, poor persistence, and poor frustration tolerance (Tarter, 2002). Family risk factors, such as attachment problems, ineffective parental monitoring, parental or sibling substance abuse, and physical or sexual abuse, are also important (Dawes *et al.*, 2000; Hops *et al.*, 2000; Riggs & Whitmore, 1999; Tarter, 2002). When such children enter school, they often have few experiences of success or mastery, given their high rates of attention-deficit hyperactivity disorder (ADHD) and learning disorders, which are often coupled with immature social skills, ongoing behavioral dysregulation, and family problems. These problems can often lead to their removal from mainstream classes and placement into separate classes for the emotionally and behaviorally disturbed, thereby increasing their association with peers who may also be at increased risk for school failure and deviant social development (Dishion *et al.*, 1991; Riggs & Whitmore, 1999; Tarter, 2002).

In late childhood and early adolescence, the interplay of these biobehavioral risk factors together with the hormonal changes associated with puberty may further exacerbate preexisting dysregulation. These then influence gene expression, the hypothalamic–pituitary–adrenal and hypophyseal–pituitary–gonadal axes, and the developing brain (including the prefrontal cortex, extended amygdala and "brain reward system"); these, in turn, influence motivation and reactivity to environmental stressors. Common comorbid psychiatric disorders such as ADHD, learning disabilities, oppositional defiant disorder, conduct disorder, affective disorders, and anxiety disorders are often present and may also contribute to greater vulnerability and risk of developing SUD.

Although more than 85% of youths in US culture experiment with substances of abuse before graduating from high school, those who are most vulnerable to progression from experimentation to SUD are those who have been on an "at risk" developmental trajectory from an early age (Dawes *et al.*, 2000; Hops *et al.*, 2000; Tarter, 2002). Development is then further arrested by regular substance abuse, which interferes with the achievement of many of the normal developmental tasks of adolescence, including individuation, consolidation of identity, moral development, development of coping skills, and conceptualization of future educational, vocational, and family goals (Grella *et al.*, 2001; Grilo *et al.*, 1995; Tims *et al.*, 2002). Drug abuse also contributes to what is often already poor school performance and truancy, which may lead to increasing amounts of time spent with deviant peers involved in activities associated with using or obtaining drugs, resulting in further social marginalization (Riggs & Whitmore, 1999).

The role of psychiatric comorbidity

The high prevalence of the dual diagnosis of psychiatric and SUD disorders is becoming increasingly recognized and documented in the literature concerning both adolescents and adults (Crowley *et al.*, 1998; Kandel *et al.*, 1997; Whitmore *et al.*, 1997). Two large population-based studies have reported on adolescents who have both psychiatric disorders and SUD. Lewinsohn *et al.* (1993) reported on a large sample of 14–18-year-old adolescents with SUD and found the lifetime prevalence of any psychiatric disorder to be 60%. In addition, 49% had unipolar depression, 25% had a disruptive disorder, and 16% had an anxiety disorder. Similarly, the Methods for the Epidemiology of Child and Adolescent Mental Disorders (MECA) study found the prevalences over the past 6 months for comorbid psychiatric disorders with an adolescent SUD sample to be 76% for any comorbid disorder, 68% for any disruptive behavior disorder, 32% for any mood disorder, and 20% for any anxiety disorder (Kandel *et al.*, 1997). In addition, Rohde, Lewinsohn, & Seeley (1996) found that disruptive behavior disorders were 10 times more prevalent among adolescents with alcohol abuse/dependence than among non-drinkers.

In sum, comorbidity is the rule, rather than the exception, among adolescents in treatment for SUD. The poorer treatment outcomes, higher costs, recidivism, and relapse rates associated with comorbidity may be related to poorer access to both medical and psychiatric services in comorbid youth, as evidenced by the fact that the majority of such youth in substance treatment do not receive psychiatric treatment (Grella *et al.*, 2001; Whitmore *et al.*, 1997; Wise, Cuffe, & Fischer, 2001). An important barrier that has impeded integration of psychiatric services with treatment for drug abuse has been the lack of research in this field. The following section examines what is known about the relationships between psychiatric disorders and adolescent SUD and the clinical implications from a developmental perspective, highlighting recent advances that address this significant research gap.

Disruptive behavior disorders

The most common comorbid disorders associated with adolescent SUD are the disruptive behavior disorders (i.e., oppositional defiant disorder, conduct disorder, ADHD), with conduct disorder being the most common (60–80%). Once conduct disorder develops, it becomes one of the most robust predictors of progression from "experimentation" with drugs and alcohol to the development of a SUD (Crowley & Riggs, 1995). Most children and adolescents who meet diagnostic criteria for conduct disorder previously met diagnostic criteria for oppositional defiant disorder when they were younger. However, only about 50% of children with oppositional defiant disorder progress to conduct disorder, and the former often does not share the same severe correlates and outcomes (Biederman *et al.*, 1996). Both disorders generally precede the onset of SUD, and if identified early, there is an opportunity for early intervention. Evidence-based treatment interventions have been shown to improve family functioning and reduce the risk of progression to more severe behavior problems and development of adolescent SUD. Such treatments include parent and family management training, generally with individual skills training for the child (Kazdin, Siegel, & Bass, 1992); family behavior therapy (Donohue & Azrin, 2001); motivational enhancement therapy/cognitive–behavioral therapy (Muck *et al.*, 2001); school- and community-based interventions (Wagner *et al.*, 1999), and multidimensional approaches (Henggeler *et al.*, 1999; Liddle & Hogue, 2001). Because of the high rates of co-occurrence of conduct disorder with SUD in adolescents, most substance treatment programs have developed programming that addresses both disorders.

The onset of ADHD is prior to age 7; consequently, it also precedes the development of SUD (American Psychiatric Association, 1994). Most studies indicate that ADHD alone does not impart a significant increase in the risk for developing SUD in adolescence unless associated with conduct disorder (Barkley *et al.*, 1990; Mannuzza *et al.*, 1993). However if both ADHD and conduct disorder co-occur, the risk of developing SUD in adolescence rises dramatically. As many as 30–50% of adolescents with SUD have both ADHD and conduct disorder, which not only increases the risk of adolescent SUD but is also associated with greater impulsivity, neuropsychological deficits, more severe substance abuse and behavior problems, worse treatment outcomes, and worse prognosis compared with either disorder alone (Crowley & Riggs, 1995; Forehand *et al.*, 1991; Gittelman *et al.*, 1985; Mannuzza *et al.*, 1993).

A recent meta-analysis of the existing studies demonstrated an approximate two-fold *reduction* in the risk for developing SUD in adolescence or adulthood if ADHD was treated with pharmacotherapy (generally psychostimulants) in childhood compared with children who were not treated for their ADHD (Wilens *et al.*, 2003). Moreover, these studies also indicated that treatment of ADHD with psychostimulants in childhood did not increase the risk of developing SUD, as this had been a concern for some investigators. Although treatment of ADHD in childhood may decrease the risk of developing an adolescent SUD, recent research in both adolescents and adults indicate that once a SUD develops, treatment of ADHD alone does not decrease substance abuse in the absence of specific substance treatment (Riggs, Mikulich, & Hall, 2001).

Internalizing disorders

Depressive disorders (major depression, dysthymia) occur in approximately 5–10% of school-age children and adolescents without SUD, with prevalence rates rising to 15–30% in adolescents with SUD. These disorders may impact the severity and patterns of their substance involvement (Barkley *et al.*, 1990; Chiles, Miller, & Cox, 1980; Gittelman *et al.*, 1985). Unlike some adults with chronic alcohol or drug dependence, depression in adolescents appears to be less likely to be substance induced and, therefore, is less likely to remit with abstinence (Bukstein, Glancy, & Kaminer, *et al.*, 1992; Riggs *et al.*, 1995).

In both epidemiological samples and clinically referred samples, approximately half report that depression started prior to SUD and about half report that depression had onset either concurrently or after onset of SUD (Lewinsohn *et al.*, 2002; Riggs *et al.*, 1995; Swendsen & Merikangas, 2000). Although there is some evidence that depression that arises in childhood increases the risk of developing adolescent SUD somewhat, it is not yet known whether treatment of depression in childhood and adolescence reduces the risk of later developing SUD. Standard clinical management of pediatric depression without SUD generally calls for combined psychotherapy and pharmacotherapy. The efficacy of interpersonal psychotherapy (Mufson *et al.*, 1999) and cognitive–behavioral therapy for depression have been demonstrated in both children and adolescents without SUD (Brent *et al.*, 1997), but they have not yet been evaluated in controlled trials in substance-involved adolescents. Selective serotonin reuptake inhibitors (SSRIs) are recommended as the first-line antidepressants for the treatment of depression in adolescents without SUD. Studies in adults also indicate that antidepressants may be safe and effective for comorbid depression in substance-dependent adults, but they do not effectively reduce substance use in the absence of specific behavioral treatment for SUD (NIDA, 1999; Riggs, 1998; Riggs & Davies 2002; Wilens *et al.*, 2003).

Although less is known about the prevalence of bipolar disorder among adolescents with SUD, it is most likely greater than the 1% prevalence found in the general population, with prevalence estimates ranging from 3 to 15% among adolescents with SUD (Wilens *et al.*, 1999; Wise *et al.*, 2001). There is some evidence that bipolar disorder in childhood may increase the risk of developing adolescent SUD, and that treatment may reduce this risk (Wilens *et al.*, 1999). Adolescent-onset bipolar disorder, however, dramatically increases the risk of developing a SUD (greater than eight times the risk compared with childhood onset, Wilens *et al.*, 1999). Treatment of mania or hypomania with lithium in adolescents with bipolar disorder and SUD has been shown to be relatively safe and effective in stabilizing mood even without abstinence, but it was not effective in "treating" substance abuse in the absence of specific treatment for SUD (Geller *et al.*, 1998).

Anxiety disorders also have a higher prevalence in adolescents with SUD than found in the general pediatric population, and they may increase the risk of developing SUD (e.g., generalized anxiety disorder, social anxiety disorder, post-traumatic stress disorder; Breslau *et al.*, 1997; Davies *et al.*, 2002; Lewinsohn *et al.*, 2002; Rohde *et al.*, 1996). Although there are data indicating that the onset of anxiety disorders may increase the risk of developing adolescent SUD (e.g., social anxiety disorder, post-traumatic stress disorder), there is not sufficient research currently to indicate whether treatment of anxiety disorders in childhood decreases this risk. Similarly, there is a lack of controlled psychotherapy or pharmacotherapy trials evaluating the impact of treating anxiety disorders in adolescents with SUD.

Taken together, the current body of research indicates that, in general, childhood psychiatric disorders appear to increase the risk of SUD, and treatment may decrease the risk they impart (Kaminer *et al.*, 1992; Lohman *et al.*, 2002). However, once SUD develops, current evidence-based practice guidelines have emphasized the importance of treating both comorbidity and SUD, as neither remits with treatment of the other alone (NIDA, 1999; Riggs *et al.*, 2001). Until recently, the lack of research in this area has been a significant barrier to implementing integrated treatment. Recent advances, with the completion of the first placebo-controlled medication trials in dually diagnosed adolescents, now provide some empirical data to help to guide clinical practice. These trials have demonstrated that pharmacotherapy for comorbidity may be both safe and effective, even in adolescents who may not yet be abstinent from substances of abuse, but that such treatment should be provided only in the context of concurrent substance treatment that enables close monitoring of urine drug screens, treatment motivation and compliance, psychosocial functioning, and monitoring of target symptom response and adverse side effects (Geller *et al.*, 1998; Lohman *et al.*, 2002; Riggs *et al.*, 2001). Although research into comorbidity is still quite limited, what currently exists provides sufficient data to advance the development of empirically grounded approaches to implementing the integrated treatment discussed below, until further research can guide modification and refinement of these principles.

Integrated clinical assessment of adolescent substance abuse and comorbidity

Performing a comprehensive individual and family assessment is the foundation for developing an integrated treatment plan. Clinicians may begin with this assessment in order to understand the sequential history of presenting problems from multiple perspectives, as well as to obtain relevant developmental history across the lifespan. Whenever possible, parents or guardians should be present at a patient's initial clinical interview. Their presence enables the counselor to establish the rules of confidentiality, including conditions under which confidentiality must be broken (e.g., reports of abuse, neglect, threats of harm to self or others, etc.). Subsequently, a private interview with the adolescent serves the purpose of establishing a strong treatment alliance and eliciting candid information about substance abuse and behavior problems that the patient may not be comfortable disclosing with parents present. Clinicians should use an empathic, non-judgmental, encouraging, and supportive interview style with adolescent patients.

Issues in the screening and assessment of adolescent substance use and disorders are covered elsewhere in this volume. There are, however, some clinical techniques derived from developmental research that may be particularly useful in evaluating the relationship between substance use and co-occurring psychiatric disorders. To organize the assessment information, it is useful for the clinician to construct a lifetime timeline (birth to present) onto which can be mapped important developmental and family history (e.g., risk factors such as family disruptions, divorce, trauma, major losses, abuse and neglect, association with deviant peers, school failure, etc.), as well as the onset and progression of psychiatric symptoms and substance use (Riggs, 1998; Riggs & Davies, 2002). This technique enables clinicians to conceptualize more clearly the developmental events that impact the patient's clinical presentation and to integrate these longitudinally. Utilization of the timeline also enables clinicians to establish psychiatric and SUD diagnoses as opposed to merely identifying symptom clusters that may confound diagnostic formulations. For example, many substance-involved adolescents may present with symptoms of irritability, impulsivity, aggression, dysphoria, and sleep disturbance. This symptom constellation may be present in a number of conditions including major depression, bipolar disorder, post-traumatic stress disorder, traumatic brain injury, ADHD, anxiety disorders, acute grief reactions, current abuse or neglect, conduct disorder, and drug intoxication or withdrawal states, all of which have different treatment approaches. For some of these conditions, pharmacotherapy would be first line (e.g., ADHD, bipolar); behavioral interventions would be indicated for others (e.g., conduct disorder, grief reaction); and a combined pharmacotherapy/psychotherapy approach would be indicated for other comorbid disorders (e.g., depression, anxiety disorders).

In teasing apart the relationships between SUD and co-occurring psychiatric illness, it is useful to obtain a history of the onset of psychiatric disorders in relationship to the onset of SUD, including the presence of psychiatric symptoms during periods of abstinence, intoxication, and withdrawal from specific substances of abuse. For example, if an adolescent reports transient symptoms of depression only during the month after abrupt discontinuation of regular cocaine abuse, and not at other times, then post-cocaine depression (which does remit with abstinence) is a more likely diagnosis than major depressive disorder. If, however, an adolescent reports the onset of depression at about the same time as the onset of regular marijuana use 8 months ago, subsequent to his parents' divorce and moving to a different state in the middle of seventh grade, both major depression and cannabis dependence should be specifically targeted in treatment because neither is likely to remit with treatment of the other disorder alone. Using the lifetime timeline enables clinicians to organize and conceptualize complex, multidimensional histories from multiple informants in order to establish meaningful clinical and diagnostic formulations to guide treatment.

A clinical approach to integrating treatment of substance abuse and comorbidity

The sequential organization of the assessment information anchored to a lifetime timeline provides the foundation for developing an integrated treatment plan. If the adolescent has a comorbid disorder for which medication is being considered, the following empirically grounded treatment algorithm can be used to guide medication initiation and management of a psychiatric disorder in the context of substance treatment. This general clinical algorithm can be modified as appropriate based on individual case details and consideration of available family, clinical, and community resources:

1. Initiating treatment
2. Assessing suitability for pharmacotherapy
3. Pharmacotherapy principles
4. Choosing specific medications for comorbidity
5. Evaluating improvement
6. Dealing with relapse.

1. Initiating treatment

In initiating treatment, it is helpful for clinicians to utilize motivational enhance-ment techniques (e.g., motivational enhancement therapy) and maintain an empathic stance throughout evaluation and treatment in comorbid adolescents in order to establish a strong treatment alliance and elicit patient-generated treatment goals (Monti *et al.*, 2001). The use of motivational interviewing techniques is particularly important in adolescents as they are generally resistant to more directive, confrontational approaches and are often ambivalent and relatively unmotivated for treatment (Drug Strategies, 2003; NIDA, 1999). In addition, it is important to be mindful of the impact that symptoms of psychiatric comor-bidity may have on initial clinical presentation and treatment motivation (e.g., cognitive distortions, tearfulness, irritability, poor concentration). Initiating substance treatment includes eliciting a detailed "functional analysis" of substance use (as specified in many treatment manuals for evidence-based treatment modalities [e.g., Godley *et al.*, 2001]) and establishing patient-elicited goals for treatment. Although abstinence is ideal, many adolescents do not begin treatment with a goal of abstinence but may develop this goal as they progress in treatment. Principles of motivational enhancement therapy can be effectively used in conjunction with another of the empirically supported treatment modalities, such as individual (e.g., cognitive–behavioral therapy) and/or family-based treatment (Muck *et al.*, 2001; Wagner *et al.*, 1999; Waldron *et al.*, 2001). A good example of an empirically supported, brief treat-ment that combines motivational enhancement therapy and cognitive–behavioral therapy has been published (Sampl & Kadden, 2001). Adolescents may also derive benefit from participating in (but not mandated to) 12-step programs as another component of multidimensional, multimodal treatment (Deas & Thomas, 2001). In addition, there is now considerable evidence demonstrating the effectiveness of family-based engagement strategies for motivating youth and families to initiate and engage in treatment (Coatsworth *et al.*, 2001; Henggeler *et al.*, 1996; Szapocznik *et al.*, 1988). Engaging parents or other caregivers in the treatment process increases the likelihood that an adolescent will participate and remain in treatment and that treatment gains will be sustained after the treatment ends (Drug Strategies, 2003). Intensive family-based treatments also have been shown to reduce both conduct problems and internalizing symptoms (Henggeler *et al.*, 1991, 2002; Liddle *et al.*, 2001), which can also help with engagement and may even mitigate the need for pharmacological treatment in some cases.

2. Assessing suitability for pharmacotherapy

Once the adolescent is effectively engaged in substance treatment, and if both urine drug screening and self-reports indicate either abstinence or significant reduction in substance use has been achieved, then carefully monitored pharmacotherapy may be initiated, if needed, to treat comorbid disorders for which pharmaco-therapy is indicated (e.g., ADHD, significant major depression) (AACAP, 1997; Lohman *et al.*, 2002; Riggs *et al.*, 2001). Although abstinence is ideal before initiating medication for comorbidity, it is often not a realistic initial goal for adolescent patients. Clinicians must weigh the risk of potential drug–medication interactions against the risk that the untreated psychiatric illness will thwart treatment engagement and precipitate early drop-out. It is important to provide patient psychoeducation, emphasizing the importance of discontinuing or main-taining significant reductions in drug and alcohol use in order to enhance the safety and effectiveness of medications. The empirically supported treatments for substance abuse mentioned above can often produce sufficient motivation and reduction in substance use in the first 2–3 weeks of treatment such that pharmaco-therapy may be initiated if patients are also compliant with at least weekly therapy sessions, urine drug screening, and clinical monitoring of adverse effects and target symptom response (Lohman *et al.*, 2002).

Ideally, a single clinician or treatment program would provide treatment for both SUD and any co-occurring disorders to achieve seamless integration of treatment. However, the current shortage of clinicians with dual training and the limited availability of truly integrated systems of care and provider networks often necessitates clinicians integrating treatment between two or more treatment providers (e.g., physician-monitored pharmacotherapy for a comorbid disorder with a different clinician providing individual and/or family therapy for SUD). In such cases, treatment may still be effectively coordinated by regular commun-ication among the treating clinicians or treatment teams. In addition, it is helpful for family members or caretakers to be involved in adolescent treatment and educated about the appropriate application of behavioral principles at home, as well as family dynamics and behaviors that diminish drug use and enhance support of abstinence (e.g., appropriate behavioral modeling; rewarding behaviors and activities incompatible with drug use; withholding reward or instituting negative consequences for ongoing drug use; monitoring medication compliance, substance use and target symptoms).

3. Pharmacotherapy principles

The following principles may be useful when pharmacotherapy for a comorbid disorder is a component of multidimensional treatment: (a) initiate pharmacotherapy for a comorbid psychiatric disorder within the context of concurrent treatment for SUD that includes mechanisms for monitoring medication compliance, regular therapy attendance (generally at least weekly individual and/ or family counseling), adverse effects, target symptom response, and ongoing substance use (by both self-report and urine drug screens); (b) choose medications with a good safety profile, low abuse liability, and, when possible, once per day dosing; (c) use a single medication (monotherapy) if possible; and (d) provide the patient and family with education about the potential for adverse interactions of medications with substances of abuse; the importance of maintaining abstinence or reduced substance use for reasons of safety and efficacy; the importance of compliance with regular appointments for medication monitoring and evaluation of side effects; and the importance of establishing mental health and substance treatment continuing care and regular follow-up visits, given the chronic, relapsing nature of SUD and many psychiatric disorders.

4. Choosing specific medications for comorbidity

Another chapter in this volume addresses issues related to the choice of pharmacotherapies for treating specific comorbid psychiatric and SUDs (see Ch. 12). Therefore, only key points related to medication choice will be highlighted here. The SSRIs are considered by many psychiatrists to be the first-line pharmacotherapy for depression *in adolescents*, both with and without SUD (Cornelius *et al.*, 1997; Emslie *et al.*, 1997; Riggs *et al.*, 1997). Fluoxetine (an SSRI) currently has the most empirical safety and efficacy data for adolescent depression, both with and without SUD (Emslie *et al.*, 1997; Lohman *et al.*, 2002; Riggs *et al.*, 1997). Tricyclic antidepressants are not recommended in substance-involved adolescents because of their overall questionable efficacy, significant anticholinergic and cardiac side effects, greater potential for adverse interactions with substances of abuse, and high lethality in overdose (Wilens *et al.*, 1997).

When both depression and ADHD are comorbid with SUD, bupropion may be considered as first-line pharmacotherapy, given the empirical support for its efficacy in treating both disorders in both adults and adolescents without SUD and preliminary safety and efficacy data in individuals with SUD (Riggs *et al.*,

1998; Wilens *et al.*, 2001). Schedule II psychostimulants (e.g., methylphenidate) are considered the first-line medications for ADHD in children and adolescents without comorbid substance use. The efficacy of psychostimulants is generally superior to non-psychostimulant medications (e.g., bupropion or atomoxetine) for ADHD (Spencer and Beiderman, 2002). However, careful consideration should be given to the use of scheduled medications in substance-involved adolescents because of their well-known potential for abuse and diversion, as noted in several reports (Garland, 1998; Jaffe, 2002). Clinicians also need to be mindful of the potential for psychostimulant abuse by peers, siblings, and parents, as well as the risk they may pose to counselors who are in recovery. If a Schedule II psychostimulant is used in this population, newer long-acting formulations should be considered over shorter-acting formulations. The former are likely to have a lower abuse liability than short-acting preparations, although this has not yet been systematically evaluated.

5. Evaluating improvement

If substance abuse and/or target symptoms do not significantly improve (or if there is evidence of escalation of drug abuse or clinical deterioration) within the first 2 months of treatment, the efficacy of the medication and the need for a change in medication should be considered, as well as reevaluation of the diagnosis (e.g., bipolar versus unipolar depression). In addition, a more intensive level of treatment (e.g., day treatment, residential, multisystemic/multidimensional therapy) or treatment frequency may need to be considered.

6. Dealing with relapse

The potential for relapse after achieving abstinence should be openly discussed and anticipated. A detailed and feasible plan for managing relapse and for mental health follow-up should be jointly developed by the patient, clinician, and caretakers. It is important that clinicians emphasize that relapse is common, given the chronic relapsing nature of both addictive disorders and most psychiatric disorders. Patients must be educated that relapse of either disorder increases the risk of destabilization of the other disorder. Relapse should be framed as neither a personal failure nor a treatment failure, but rather as an indication of the need to increase the intensity and frequency of treatment to restabilize illness rapidly to prevent further functional decline. This treatment model is similar to the medical management practice standards for many chronic medical illnesses (e.g., diabetes, hypertension) (McLellan *et al.*, 1993).

Conclusions

Despite the empirical support for the integration of co-occurring adolescent substance and psychiatric treatment, until recently there was little research to guide how this should be implemented. Recent advances have begun to address some of the barriers to implementation. Adolescents with SUD are now beginning to be included in placebo-controlled trials evaluating the safety and efficacy of medications for psychiatric disorders. As a result, there is now information (albeit still limited) that pharmacotherapy for comorbidity may be both safe and effective, provided there is careful monitoring and therapy is initiated in the context of concurrent substance treatment. Clinicians can utilize these new safety and efficacy data to support implementation of earlier and more comprehensive treatment of comorbid psychiatric disorders in adolescents in substance treatment programs, which may improve their poor treatment engagement and outcomes. In addition, the use of motivational enhancement, cognitive–behavioral therapy, skills training, family-based treatments, and an empathic, supportive approach may improve treatment of both comorbidity and SUD by increasing motivation, engagement, and retention in treatment.

As in other fields of medicine, large gaps exist between research and actual clinical practice. Overcoming these barriers to widespread adoption of evidence-based practice will require development of cooperative partnerships and integrated treatment networks that include primary medical care, substance treatment, and mental health services. Very few such collaborations or dual training programs currently exist, however. This has contributed to a critical shortage of both researchers and clinicians with expertise in mental health, addictions, and developmental psychopathology. Enhanced training needs to include not only professional training and certification programs but also the development and implementation of practical cross-discipline "in-service training" within existing treatment settings. For example, training in substance treatment programs might include brief training in the assessment of common psychiatric disorders comorbid with SUD, as well as the most frequently employed psychotherapy and pharmacotherapy approaches. Similarly, training for mental health professionals needs to include detailed information about substance abuse, treatment principles, urine monitoring, and intoxication and withdrawal symptoms that can mimic or be mimicked by psychiatric conditions. Training in motivational interviewing and learning to perform a thorough substance history and functional analysis of drug use behaviors would be invaluable to all mental health professionals.

Given that our systems of care are not well integrated, one of the greatest challenges in this field is how to provide comprehensive care for the individual diagnosed with more than one disorder. It is unreasonable to ask the individuals and families with the greatest burden of illness to be responsible for the integration of these systems of care. Until it becomes a public policy priority to move towards the routine availability of comprehensive, integrated medical and substance services, however, treatment programs and providers need to develop efficient communication mechanisms to be able to relay important relevant information back and forth among programs, systems of care, or diverse providers within a treatment program.

To broaden the implementation of integrated psychiatric services in community substance treatment programs further, much more research is needed in multiple areas. This includes systematic evaluation of a number of factors.

1. The neurobiological similarities and differences between psychiatric disorders and drug addiction, and the vulnerabilities that may be common to both.
2. The separate and combined efficacy of both pharmacotherapies and psychotherapeutic interventions in targeting addictions and comorbid psychiatric disorders.
3. The safety and efficacy of a broader range of medications for comorbid disorders and the abuse liability of these medications.
4. The impact of medications and drugs of abuse on the developing adolescent brain.
5. The potential for interactions between prescribed medications and substances of abuse.
6. The "active ingredients" of all types of treatment.
7. The feasibility and sustainability of implementing evidence-based integrated practices in community treatment settings with diverse populations.

Furthermore, in evaluating research outcomes, both medical/psychiatric (e.g., target symptoms, adverse effects, mechanisms of action and biological markers of response to treatment) and substance outcomes (e.g., cravings, impact on drug use behaviors) should be considered.

Finally, since few adolescents have economic resources of their own, the cost of providing both pharmacological and psychotherapeutic treatment to adolescents is an important concern. If adolescents wish to seek treatment without their families' knowledge, or if their families do not provide funding for treatment, it is usually difficult for an adolescent to find the resources needed to obtain treatment. Cost–benefit analyses of providing free or reduced treatment to adolescents are needed to assess the public health impact of providing concurrent treatment for psychiatric disorders and SUDs in adolescents versus the costs of recidivism; incarceration; loss of future productivity; suicide; higher-level, longer-term, and/or more expensive, separate SUD and mental health treatment; and the societal costs of chronic drug abuse and mental health needs.

In summary, the body of current adolescent research indicates that the developmental trajectories of children who are at risk for developing SUD in adolescence often begin early and are embedded in a complex matrix of biobehavioral, family, and psychosocial risks and vulnerabilities, leading to higher rates of problem behavior and comorbid psychiatric illness in addition to SUD. Comorbidity (often multiple comorbidities) is now recognized as the rule rather than the exception, yet routine screening and identification of these disorders in adolescents with SUD has not yet become mainstream, and not enough of these adolescents are receiving the integrated treatment they need. We know, however, that the adolescents with comorbid psychiatric disorders in addition to their SUD have worse prognosis and outcome than those without. Recent research advances have helped to overcome some of the former barriers to integrated treatment of comorbidity and SUD. Current research now clearly supports the integrated treatment of comorbidity and SUD rather than sequential treatment, given that neither disorder remits with treatment of the other alone, and that treatment of one disorder is less likely to be successful without co-occurring treatment of the other.

ACKNOWLEDGEMENTS

The preparation of this chapter was supported by the National Institute on Drug Abuse (R01-DA13176, 5U10-DA13716–03, R01–DA12845, 5R37–DA09842, and 5P60–DA11015) and the US Department of Health and Human Services, Substance Abuse Mental Health Services Administration/Center for Substance Abuse Treatment (H79-TI14188).

REFERENCES

AACAP (American Academy of Child and Adolescent Psychiatry) (1997). Practice parameters for the assessment and treatment of children and adolescents with substance use disorders. *Journal of the American Academy of Child and Adolescent Psychiatry*, **36** (Suppl. 10), 140S–156S.

American Psychiatric Association (1994). *Diagnostic and Statistical Manual of Mental Disorders* (DSM-IV), 4th edn. Washington, DC: American Psychiatric Press.

Barkley, R. A., Fischer, M., Edelbrock, C. S., & Smallish, L. (1990). The adolescent outcome of hyperactive children diagnosed by research criteria: I. An 8-year prospective follow-up study. *Journal of the American Academy of Child and Adolescent Psychiatry*, **29**, 546–557.

Biederman, J., Faraone, S. V., Milberger, S., *et al.* (1996). Is childhood oppositional defiant disorder a precursor to adolescent conduct disorder? Findings from a four-year follow-up of children with ADHD. *Journal of the American Academy of Child and Adolescent Psychiatry*, **35**, 1193–1204.

Brent, D. A., Holder, D., Kolko, D., *et al.* (1997). A clinical psychotherapy trial for adolescent depression comparing cognitive, family, and supportive therapy. *Archives of General Psychiatry*, **54**, 877–885.

Breslau, N., Davis, G. C., Andreski, P., Peterson, E. L., & Schultz, L. R. (1997). Psychiatric sequelae of posttraumatic stress disorder in women. *Archives of General Psychiatry*, **54**, 81–87.

Bukstein, O. G., Glancy, L. J., & Kaminer, Y. (1992). Patterns of affective comorbidity in a clinical population of dually diagnosed adolescent substance abusers. *Journal of the American Academy of Child and Adolescent Psychiatry*, **31**, 1041–1045.

Chiles, J. A., Miller, M. L., & Cox G. B. (1980). Depression in an adolescent delinquent population. *Archives of General Psychiatry*, **37**, 1179–1184.

Coatsworth, J. D., Santisteban, D. A., McBride, C. K., & Szapocznik, J. (2001): Brief strategic family therapy versus community control: engagement, retention, and an exploration of the moderating role of adolescent symptom severity. *Family Process*, **40**, 313–332.

Cornelius, J. R., Salloum, I. M., Ehler, J. G., *et al.* (1997). Fluoxetine in depressed alcoholics: a double-blind placebo-controlled trial. *Archives of General Psychiatry*, **54**, 700–705.

Crowley, T. J. & Riggs, P. D. (1995). Adolescent substance use disorder with conduct disorder and comorbid conditions. In E. Rahdert & Czechowicz (eds.), *NIDA Research Monograph*, Vol. 156: *Adolescent Drug Abuse: Clinical Assessment and Therapeutic Interventions* (pp. 49–111). Rockville, MD: National Institute on Drug Abuse.

Crowley, T. J., Mikulich, S. K., MacDonald, M., Young, S. E., & Zerbe, G. O. (1998). Substance-dependent, conduct-disordered adolescent males: severity of diagnosis predicts 2-year outcome. *Drug and Alcohol Dependence*, **49**, 225–237.

Davies, R. D., Chapman, M. C., Hall, S. K., Mikulich, S. K., & Riggs, P. D. (2002). Correlates of social phobia in depressed adolescents with conduct disorder and substance dependence. *Drug and Alcohol Dependence*, **66**: S41.

Dawes, M. A., Antelman, S. M., Vanyukov, M. M., *et al.* (2000). Developmental sources of variation in liability to adolescent substance use disorders. *Drug and Alcohol Dependence*, **61**, 3–14.

Deas, D. & Thomas, S. E. (2001). An overview of controlled studies of adolescent substance abuse treatment. *American Journal on Addictions*, **10**, 178–189.

Dishion, T. J., Patterson, G. R., Stoolmiller, M. & Skinner, M. L. (1991). Family, school, and behavioral antecedents to early adolescent involvement with antisocial peers. *Developmental Psychology*, **27**, 172–180.

Donohue, B. & Azrin, N. (2001). Family behavior therapy. In E. F. Wagner & H. B. Waldron (eds.), *Innovations in Adolescent Substance Abuse Interventions* (pp. 205–227). Oxford, UK: Elsevier Science.

Drug Strategies (2003). *Treating Teens: A Guide to Adolescent Drug Programs*. Washington, DC: Drug Strategies.

Emslie, G. J., Rush, A. J., Weinberg, W. A., *et al.* (1997). A double-blind, randomized, placebo-controlled trial of fluoxetine in children and adolescents with depression. *Archives of General Psychiatry*, **54**, 1031–1037.

Forehand, R., Wierson, M., Frame, C., Kempston, T., & Armistead, L. (1991). Juvenile delinquency entry and persistence: do attention problems contribute to conduct problems? *Journal of Behavioral and Experimental Psychiatry*, **22**, 261–264.

Garland, E. J. (1998). Intranasal abuse of prescribed methylphenidate. *Journal of the American Academy of Child and Adolescent Psychiatry*, **37**, 573–574.

Geller, B., Cooper, T. B., Sun, K., *et al.* (1998). Double-blind and placebo-controlled study of lithium for adolescent bipolar disorders with secondary substance dependency. *Journal of the American Academy of Child and Adolescent Psychiatry*, **37**, 171–178.

Gittelman, R. S., Mannuzza, R. S., Shenker, R., & Bonagura, N. (1985). Hyperactive boys almost grown up: I. Psychiatric status. *Archives of General Psychiatry*, **42**, 937–947.

Grella, C. E., Hser, Y., Joshi, V., & Rounds-Bryant, J. (2001). Drug treatment outcomes for adolescents with comorbid mental and substance use disorders *Journal of Nervous and Mental Diseases*, **189**, 384–392.

Grilo, C. M., Becker, D. F., Walker, M. L., *et al.* (1995). Psychiatric comorbidity in adolescent inpatients with substance use disorders. *Journal of the American Academy of Child and Adolescent Psychiatry*, **34**, 1085–1091.

Godley, S. H., Meyers, R. J., Smith, J. E., *et al.* (2001). *Cannabis Youth Treatment Series*, Vol. 4: *The Adolescent Community Reinforcement Approach for Adolescent Cannabis Users*. Rockville, MD: Center for Substance Abuse Treatment.

Henggeler, S., Borduin, C., Melton, G., *et al.* (1991). Effects of multisystemic therapy on drug use and abuse in serious juvenile offenders: a progress report from two outcome studies. *Family Dynamics of Addiction Quarterly*, **1**, 40–51.

Henggeler, S. W., Pickrel, S. G., Brondino, M. J. (1996). Eliminating (almost) treatment dropout of substance abusing or dependent delinquents through home-based multisystemic therapy. *American Journal of Psychiatry*, **153**, 427–428.

(1999). Multisystemic treatment of substance abusing and dependent delinquents: outcomes, treatment fidelity, and transportability. *Mental Health Services Research*, **1**, 171–184.

Henggeler, S., Schoenwald, S. K., Rowland, M. D., & Cunningham, P. B. (2002). *Serious Emotional Disturbance in Children and Adolescents: Multisystemic Therapy*. New York: Guilford Press.

Hops, H., Andrews, J. A., Duncan, S. C., Duncan, T. E., & Tildesley, E. (2000). Adolescent drug use development: a social interactional and contextual perspective. In A. J. Sameroff, M. Lewis, & S. M. Miller (eds.), *Handbook of Developmental Psychopathology*, 2nd edn (pp. 589–605). New York: Plenum Press.

Jaffe, S. L. (2002). Failed attempts at intranasal abuse of Concerta. *Journal of the American Academy of Child and Adolescent Psychiatry*, **41**, 5.

Kaminer, Y., Tarter, R. E., Bukstein, O. G., & Kabene, M. (1992). Comparison between treatment completers and noncompleters among dually diagnosed, substance-abusing adolescents. *Journal of the Amercian Academy of Child and Adolescent Psychiatry*, **38**, 693–699.

Kandel, D. B., Johnson, J. G., Bird, H. G., *et al.* (1997). Psychiatric disorders associated with substance use among children and adolescents: findings from the methods for the epidemiology of child and adolescent mental disorders (MECA) study. *Journal of Abnormal Child Psychology*, **25**, 121–132.

Kazdin, A. E., Siegel, T. C., & Bass, D. (1992). Cognitive problem-solving skills training and parent management training in the treatment of antisocial behavior in children. *Journal of Consulting and Clinical Psychology*, **60**, 733–747.

Lewinsohn, P. M., Hops, H., Roberts, R. E., Seeley, J. R., & Andrews, J. A. (1993). Adolescent psychopathology, I. prevalence and incidence of depression and other DSM-III-R disorders in high school students. *Journal of Abnormal Psychology*, **102**, 133–144. [Erratum in *Journal of Abnormal Psychology, 102*, 517.]

Lewinsohn, P. M., Rohde, P., Seeley, J. R., & Klein, D. N. (2002). Comorbidity between depression and substance abuse. In *Proceedings of the 2002 Annual Meeting of the American Academy of Child and Adolescent Psychiatry*, San Francisco, CA.

Liddle, H. A. & Hogue, A. (2001). Multidimensional family therapy for adolescent substance abuse. In E. F. Wagner & H. B. Waldron (eds.), *Innovations in Adolescent Substance Abuse Interventions* (pp. 229–261). Oxford: Elsevier Science.

Liddle, H. A., Dakof, G. A., Parker, K., *et al.* (2001). Multidimensional family therapy for adolescent drug abuse: results of a randomized clinical trial. *American Journal of Drug and Alcohol Abuse*, **27**, 651–688.

Lohman, M., Riggs, P., Hall, S. K., Mikulich, S. K., & Klein, C. A. (2002). Perceived motivations for treatment in depressed, substance-dependent adolescents with conduct disorder. In *Proceedings of the 64th Annual Meeting of the College on Problems of Drug Dependence*, Quebec City, Canada.

Mannuzza, S., Klein, R. G., Bessler, A., Malloy, P., & LaPadula, M. (1993). Adult outcome of hyperactive boys: educational achievement, occupational rank, and psychiatric status. *Archives in General Psychiatry* **50**, 565–576.

McLellan, A. T., Arndt, I. O., Metzger, D. S., Woody, G. E., & O'Brien, C. P. (1993). The effects of psychosocial services in substance abuse treatment. *Journal of the American Medical Association*, **269**, 1953–1959.

Monti, P. M., Barnett, N. P., O'Leary, T. A., & Colby, S. M. (2001). Motivational enhancement for alcohol-involved adolescents. In P. M. Monti & S. M. Colby (eds.), *Adolescents, Alcohol, and Substance Abuse: Reaching Teens through Brief Interventions* (pp. 145–182), New York: Guilford Press.

Muck, R., Zempolich, K. A., Titus, J. C., *et al.* (2001). An overview of the effectiveness of adolescent substance abuse treatment models. *Youth and Society*, **33**, 143–168.

Mufson, L., Weissman, M. M., Moreau, D., & Garfinkel, R. (1999). Efficacy of interpersonal psychotherapy for depressed adolescents. *Archives of General Psychiatry*, **56**, 573–579.

NIDA (National Institute on Drug Abuse) (1999). *Principles of Drug Addiction Treatment: A Research-based Guide.* [NIDA Publication No. 99–4180.] Rockville, MD: National Institute on Drug Abuse.

Riggs, P. D. (1998). Clinical approach to treatment of ADHD in adolescents with substance use disorders and conduct disorder. *Journal of the American Academy of Child and Adolescent Psychiatry*, **37**, 331–332.

Riggs, P. D. & Davies, R. D. (2002). A clinical approach to integrating treatment for adolescent depression and substance abuse. *Journal of the American Academy of Child and Adolescent Psychiatry*, **41**, 10.

Riggs, P. D. & Whitmore, E. A. (1999). Substance use disorders and disruptive behavior disorders. In R. L. Hendren (ed.), *Review of Psychiatry*, Vol. 18: *Disruptive Behavior Disorders in Children and Adolescents* (pp. 33–174). Washington, DC: American Psychiatric Press.

Riggs, P. D, Baker, S., Mikulich, S. K., Young, S. E., & Crowley, T. J. (1995). Depression in substance-dependent delinquents. *Journal of the American Academy of Child and Adolescent Psychiatry*, **34**, 764–771.

Riggs, P. D., Mikulich, S. K., Coffman, L. M., & Crowley, T. J. (1997). Fluoxetine in drug-dependent delinquents with major depression: an open trial. *Journal of Child and Adolescent Psychopharmacology*, **7**, 87–95.

Riggs, P. D., Leon, S. L., Mikulich, S. K., & Coffman, L. M. (1998). An open trial of bupropion for ADHD in adolescents with substance use disorders and conduct disorder. *Journal of the American Academy of Child and Adolescent Psychiatry*, **37**, 1271–1278.

Riggs, P. D., Mikulich, S. K., & Hall, S. (2001). Effects of pemoline on ADHD, antisocial behaviors, and substance use in adolescents with conduct disorder and substance use disorder. In *Proceedings of the 63rd Annual Meeting of the College of Problems of Drug Dependence*, Scottsdale.

Rohde, P., Lewinsohn, P. M., & Seeley, J. R. (1996). Psychiatric comorbidity with problematic alcohol use in high school students. *Journal of the American Academy of Child and Adolescent Psychiatry*, **35**, 101–109.

Sampl, S. & Kadden, R. (2001). *Motivational Enhancement Therapy and Cognitive Behavioral Therapy for Adolescent Cannabis Users: 5 sessions (DHHS Publication No. 01-3486)*. Rockville, MD: Center for Substance Abuse Treatment.

Sohlkhah, R. & Wilens, T. E. (1998). Pharmacotherapy of adolescent alcohol and other drug use disorders. *Alcohol Health and Research World*, **22**, 122–125.

Spencer, T. & Biederman, J. (2002). Non-stimulant treatment for attention-deficit hyperactivity disorder. *Journal of Attention Disorders*, **6**(suppl. 1), S101–S107.

Swendsen, J. D. & Merikangas, K. R. (2000). The comorbidity of depression and substance use disorders. *Clinical Psychology Review*, **20**, 173–189.

Szapocznik, J., Perez-Vidal, A., Brickman, A. L., et al. (1988). Engaging adolescent drug abusers and their families in treatment: a strategic structural systems approach. *Journal of Consulting and Clinical Psychology*, **56**, 552–557.

Tarter, R. E. (2002). Etiology of adolescent substance abuse: a developmental perspective. *American Journal on Addictions*, **11**: 171–191.

Tims, F. M., Dennis, M. L., Hamilton, N., et al. (2002). Characteristics and problems of 600 adolescent cannabis abusers in outpatient treatment. *Addiction*, **97**(Suppl. 1): 46–57.

Wagner, E. F., Brown, S. A., Monti, P. M., Myers, M. G., & Waldron, H. B. (1999). Innovations in adolescent substance abuse intervention. *Alcoholism: Clinical and Experimental Research*, **23**: 236–249.

Waldron, H. B., Slesnick, N., Brody, J., Turner, C., & Peterson, T. (2001). Treatment outcomes for adolescent substance abuse at 4- and 7-month assessments. *Journal of Consulting and Clinical Psychology*, **69**: 802–813.

Whitmore, E. A., Mikulich, S. K., Thompson, L. L., *et al.* (1997). Influences on adolescent substance dependence: conduct disorder, depression, attention deficit hyperactivity disorder, and gender. *Drug and Alcohol Dependence*, **87**, 97–107.

Wilens, T. E., Biederman, J., & Spencer, T. J. (1997). Case study: adverse effects of smoking marijuana while receiving tricyclic antidepressants. *Journal of the American Academy of Child and Adolescent Psychiatry*, **23**, 45–48.

Wilens, T. E., Biederman, J., Millstein, R. B., *et al.* (1999). Risk for substance use disorders in youths with child- and adolescent-onset bipolar disorder. *Journal of the American Academy of Child and Adolescent Psychiatry*, **38**, 680–685.

Wilens, T. E., Spencer, T. J., Biederman, J., *et al.* (2001). A controlled clinical trial of bupropion for attentional deficit hyperactivity disorder in adults. *American Journal of Psychiatry*, **158**, 282–288.

Wilens, T., Faraone, S., Biederman, J., & Gunawardene, S. (2003). Does the stimulant pharmacotherapy of ADHD beget later substance abuse? A meta-analysis of the literature. *Pediatrics*, **111**, 179–185.

Wise, B. K., Cuffe, S. P., & Fischer, T. (2001). Dual diagnosis and successful participation of adolescents in substance abuse treatment. *Journal of Substance Abuse Treatment*, **21**, 161–165.

14

Prevention of infection with human immunodeficiency virus in adolescent substance abusers

Robert M. Malow, Rhonda Rosenberg, and Jessy Dévieux

Florida International University, Miami, Florida

Despite considerable progress in the design, implementation and refinement of interventions, infection with the human immunodeficiency virus (HIV) and subsequent acquired immunodeficiency syndrome (AIDS) has only become a more entrenched pandemic, reaching into populations originally not deemed to be at risk. Adolescents are one such population. While the overall incidence of HIV has been declining in the USA, the opposite pattern has been true for adolescents, particularly those who abuse alcohol and other drugs (AOD).

Individuals between the ages of 10 and 24 years make up approximately one third of the world's population and 80% of these young people reside in developing countries where the burden from sexually transmitted diseases (STDs), including HIV, is greatest (Aggleton, 2000). Globally, it has been estimated that approximately half those who acquired HIV do so before age 25 (UNICEF, 2002). Similar estimates are provided by the Strategic Plan of the Center for Disease Control & Prevention (CDC, 2003), in which at least half of all new HIV seroconversions in the USA occur among adolescents or young adults under the age of 25. Between 1993 and 1999, the number of adolescents with HIV dramatically increased by 34% (Jemmott & Jemmott, 2000; Kirby, 2000; Rotheram-Borus, 2000; Rotheram-Borus et al., 2000). Moreover, the CDC reported in 2002 that the prevalence of AOD use "before last intercourse" among adolescents had increased 18% in the previous decade (CDC, 2002). The high prevalence rates of HIV/AIDS and other STDs, combined with AOD abuse, high rates of unprotected sex, and an increasingly earlier onset of sexual activity have increased focus on the development of well-targeted, effective HIV prevention interventions for adolescents (D'Angelo & DiClemente, 1996; Kirby, 2000; Rotheram-Borus, 2000).

The HIV/AIDS prevention community, however, faces a set of strategic and unique barriers in working with this population that are important to identify.

Adolescent Substance Abuse: Research and Clinical Advances, ed. Howard A. Liddle and Cynthia L. Rowe. Published by Cambridge University Press. © Cambridge University Press 2006.

- Adolescence is a developmental period, characterized by intense exploration, including sexual activity (Tapert *et al.*, 2001), often leading to episodic and risky experimentation.

- Risk calculations by adolescents are stereotypically characterized by invulnerability, particularly toward death and fatal disease (Trad, 1994), creating the tendency for adolescents to ignore health warnings (Palmquist, 1992) and underestimate personal risk for HIV/AIDS (Walter, Vaughan, & Cohall, 1991). Consequently, high prevalence rates of HIV risk behaviors are observed even among adolescents who have knowledge of the facts of transmission and prevention (Deas-Nesmith *et al.*, 1999).

- Adolescents often lack sufficient knowledge, motivation, and/or skills to implement safer sex behaviors (DiClemente *et al.*, 1991; Gardner & Herman, 1990).

- Distinctive filters (e.g., cognitive immaturity, undefined sexual identity, peer influences, autonomy struggles, physical development, emotional vulnerability, and cultural identity) influence how HIV/AIDS prevention information and skills will be assimilated and utilized by adolescents (Brown, DiClemente, & Reynolds, 1991; Fortenberry, 1995); in particular, the adolescent's "first theories" of sexuality from childhood may influence this process in ways still largely unstudied (Fraiberg, 1987).

- Adolescent sexual risk behavior is closely associated with AOD experimentation, which can escalate to clinical severity (Tapert *et al.*, 2001). Particular subgroups of substance abusers such as juvenile offenders are at increased risk because they tend to initiate sexual relations earlier than their peers (Gillmore *et al.*, 1994; Malow *et al.*, 1997, 2001) and are less likely to use condoms (D'Angelo & DiClemente, 1996).

- Depressive disorders and symptoms have been shown to be highly prevalent during adolescence, especially among AOD-abusing adolescents (Bukstein, Glancy, & Kaminer, 1992). Depressed adolescents represent an understudied subgroup at risk for HIV but may be one important key to deciphering observed paradoxes, such as how adolescents seem to "lose" or misplace what they know, perceive, or feel and proceed with risky sexual and substance abuse behavior (Lucenko *et al.*, 2003).

It is considered almost a truism today to reference the developmental nature of adolescence; yet it is a useful reminder of how HIV has exposed the gaps in our understanding of developmental origins and vulnerabilities, which all too often translate into adulthood. Basic research is substantiating this point even where alcohol and drug abuse is concerned. According to emerging neuroscience research, addiction itself may best be conceived as a developmental disorder during adolescence: as an exploiter of changes in cognitive functioning that mark the transition to adulthood (Chambers, Taylor, & Potenza, 2003). Though typically not identified as a direct causal agent, substance use and dependency are nevertheless repeatedly associated with high-risk sexual behavior, and this correlation may be said to signal a developmental deficit that follows these adolescents into adulthood. At the very least, the evidence is strong that the transition to adulthood for those with continuing substance use problems is decidedly marked by an increased vulnerability that includes risk behavior for HIV transmission (Tapert *et al.*, 2001).

The most pointed commentary, however, on the "stickiness" of developmental origins and the influence of formative experience on HIV transmission risk in adulthood is the increasingly sharpened focus on childhood sexual and physical abuse by the HIV/AIDS prevention community (Purcell *et al.*, 2005). Childhood sexual abuse, in particular, has been identified as an important predictor of sexual risk behavior in the Urban Men's Health Study (Paul *et al.*, 2001). For women in treatment for drug abuse, a history of child sexual abuse is common (up to 70% of some samples; NIDA, 1996). The influence is complex and the prevailing message from this research is that childhood abuse must be examined as a context-specific factor in which the type of abuse is delineated (physical, sexual, and emotional) and buffering factors, such as culture-specific social support and communal resources, are taken into account (Hobfoll *et al.*, 2002).

Structure and message of the chapter

The purpose of this chapter is to describe the empirical links between adolescent AOD abuse and HIV/AIDS and to highlight promising interventions at the individual, group, and community levels. First, the relationship between adolescent AOD abuse and HIV/AIDS will be presented, followed by examples of different levels of intervention, in which the emphasis will be on the potential for integration into AOD treatment programs, schools, and community settings. Finally, limitations of this research and areas of improvement are reviewed, with recommendations for future directions for advancing the field.

The "press release" opening of this chapter is common in publications addressing special population characteristics of the HIV/AIDS epidemic. Disconcerting seroprevalence rates among adolescents have become the rule rather than the exception. Surprise and dire prediction have become the norm, as yet another permutation of risk seemingly announces itself. For example, recent press releases point to the internet as the new vector for HIV in what were thought to be stabilized risk populations (CDC, 2003). Despite the lessons taught in the early years of the epidemic when prevention interventionists realized how little they knew about homosexual culture or how to affect the sexual and relational dimensions of people in general, the histories and structures of emergent risk populations are still not being recognized and integrated into intervention models. We are only beginning to understand how to operationalize the influence of developmental origins, communal and network situations, and supportive and affective resources at the individual, family, and group levels. All of this has come to be known in the HIV/AIDS prevention field as the *search for contextual predictors*.

Whether the intervention is at the individual, group, or community level, or a cognitively based behavioral skills or condom training framework, the major message of this chapter is that there is a contextual search that can be pursued. Condom use, for example, may appear to be an outcome measure, yet it is also a contextual vehicle, in which we may learn how it is an indicator of communication styles, dyadic intimacy, depression and aversion to loss, network and social norms, and survival stress. Where AOD is concerned, it is not enough merely to measure the association between condom use and the presence or quantity of the abused substance – or to throw in measures of use proximal to sex and call it contextual. Context is not a coinciding behavior or pathology. Context is the *holding environment* of an individual or a group of individuals, and in HIV/AIDS prevention, *context is the container of sexuality*, which, at the most fundamental level, begins with a dyad – both the real one and the one perceived by the individual.

In spite of the barriers noted above, adolescent HIV/AIDS prevention offers a distinct advantage in forcing our attention on context. For adolescents perhaps more than any other age group, an understanding of behavior requires reference to context, most importantly the family, neighborhood, geographic, educational, and political situations. There can be little question that adolescence is associated with sexuality. Even when absent or latent, the relational and sexual dimensions of adolescence are waiting for our attention as researchers.

Co-occurring patterns of HIV risk and substance use in adolescents

The relationship between adolescent AOD abuse and HIV risk behavior has been well documented. Numerous studies have found that AOD-abusing adolescents are at high risk of transmitting HIV (e.g., Brown *et al.*, 1997; DiClemente *et al.*, 1991; Gillmore *et al.*, 1994; Jemmott & Jemmott, 2000; Malow *et al.*, 1997, 2001). Moreover, this co-occurrence of sexual risk taking and the use of alcohol, marijuana, cocaine, or other illicit drugs has emerged repeatedly in samples across the full range of the adolescent population, as well as in the usual high-risk subgroups of runaway and homeless youth, those in drug treatment or the juvenile criminal justice system, those with severe mental illness, and, of course, inner-city ethnic minority young people and homosexual and bisexual youth. In fact, AOD-abusing adolescents can be expected to report more sexual risk taking than these other high-risk subgroups (St. Lawrence, Crosby, & O'Bannon, 1999). For those who receive treatment, the simple goal of cessation may not be enough to prevent an associated pattern of high-risk sexual behavior from continuing as they enter adulthood (Tapert *et al.*, 2001).

In a national survey performed by the CDC, almost 25% of USA high school students reported AOD use prior to sex (CDC, 1999). In a study of incarcerated youth, 24.8% of adolescent males reported AOD use before engaging in sexual activity, and 46.3% reported that alcohol was available the majority of the time at social gatherings (Rolf *et al.*, 1990). The mere drinking of alcohol has been found to increase youths' likelihood of engaging in sex by approximately 50% (Sikkema, Winett, & Lombard, 1995; Strunin & Hingson, 1992). Furthermore, a series of studies have all shown a relationship between alcohol use and the early initiation of sexual activity (Leigh, 1990; Tapert *et al.*, 2001), including an increased likelihood of intercourse on the first date (Cooper & Orcutt, 1997). Sizable and growing research indicates, however, that it is likely that unobserved variables, probably of a contextual nature, are driving this relationship, as investigators consider behavioral conundrums such as the observation that adolescents who use condoms when sober tend to use them when drunk (Leigh, 2002; Weinhardt & Carey, 2000).

The co-occurrence of AOD abuse and sexual risk behavior is frequent among adolescents despite the serious consequences that accompany such combined risk activities. A random dial telephone survey of 1773 adolescents aged 16–19 years revealed that those adolescents who consumed more than five drinks a day were 2.8 times less likely to use condoms than abstaining adolescents (Hingson *et al.*, 1990). For AOD-abusing adolescents, greater HIV risk behavior has been related to less-frequent use of condoms during sex and more sexual partners (Tapert *et al.*, 2001); more STDs (D'Angelo & DiClemente, 1996); less HIV-related knowledge and lower perceived susceptibility to HIV infection (Deas-Nesmith *et al.*, 1999); lower self-efficacy and perceived peer norms regarding safer sex practices and psychopathology (e.g., conduct disorder, impulsivity, affect lability, impaired attention, and judgment) (Malow *et al.*, 1997; Jemmott & Jemmott, 2000); varying patterns of HIV risk factors including prostitution for money, drugs, food, and shelter (DiClemente *et al.*, 1991); and more permissive attitudes toward sex (Canterbury *et al.*, 1995; D'Angelo & DiClemente, 1996; Gillmore *et al.*, 1994). Further, patterns of risky sexual behavior that emerge in adolescence appear to persist into young adulthood, particularly if AOD abuse continues to be in evidence (Tapert *et al.*, 2001). There is evidence that initiating interventions early before the onset of sexual activity is the most effective strategy of prevention (Kirby, 2001a).

Levels of intervention

Because of the developmental nature of adolescence, the integration of HIV/AIDS prevention and AOD treatment carries a dual burden: to reduce the adverse consequences of sexual behavior and to support the capacity for sexual intimacy and healthy relationships. In fact, relationship health at all levels – sexual partner, family, peer, and social – may be key to reducing HIV risk behavior (Giordano, 2003; Neighbors & O'Leary, 2003; Simoni, 2000). Two decades into the epidemic, we still do not have a compendium of relational indicators linked to risk behaviors per subpopulation.

Interventions that have been developed to reduce HIV risk among adolescents typically anchor their design at the *level* of intervention and so may be classified according to individual, small group, or community-based approaches. Individual-level approaches are advantageous in allowing more precise tailoring of activities and components to fit the separate needs of participants. The most common example of this type of intervention is HIV risk-reduction counseling in conjunction with HIV antibody testing, as well as one-on-one counseling outside of testing contexts. The small-group type of intervention is based on participation in collective activities to alter HIV-related attitudes and instil protective knowledge and skills. Small groups have been implemented within schools and also have incorporated family-based approaches. Community level interventions are also known as structural approaches and are characterized by outreach efforts, social network intervention, media campaigns, and social marketing.

Individual-level interventions: prevention counseling

Individualized one-on-one counseling has achieved success in areas as diverse as smoking cessation, cardiovascular risk reduction, and weight loss. However, there is little empirical research that has tested its effects within HIV risk-reduction efforts, particularly apart from HIV antibody testing and with adolescent target populations. A number of published case reports, however, have suggested that one-on-one counseling may be effective, especially motivational interviewing approaches. Unfortunately, these have been applied primarily in adult populations (e.g., Belcher *et al.*, 1998; Kalichman *et al.*, 2002).

Project RESPECT is a notable exception and is the largest HIV risk-reduction study of the client-centered interactive counseling model that also has included adolescents in its sample (Kamb *et al.*, 1998). The study randomly assigned almost 6000 patients aged 14 years and over (median age of 25 years) attending an STD clinic to one of three individual counseling models offered in conjunction with STD testing (chlamydia, syphilis, gonorrhea, and HIV): (a) a standard care, didactic, risk education-only control condition; (b) a brief counseling intervention of two sessions that focused on risk behavior change through personal goal setting; and (c) an enhanced four-session intervention based on the theory of reasoned action and social-cognitive theory. The enhanced intervention sessions used counseling procedures chosen to alter self-efficacy, attitudes, and perceived norms concerning condom use, along with behavior-change goal setting between sessions. Laboratory tests confirmed that the incidence of new STDs was 30% lower at the 6-month follow-up among those receiving the brief and enhanced counseling sessions relative to controls, although this effect diminished to 20% at 12 months. Subgroup analyses suggested that the client-centered model could have particular impact on those at higher (or unknown) risk, such as adolescents (age 20 or younger), those diagnosed at enrollment with an STD, or those who had never been tested for HIV.

Unfortunately, Project RESPECT could not comment on direct HIV risk-reduction effects from this model, though its primary message about HIV prevention appears to have been reinforced by other studies and literature reviews focused on this type of intervention. The first part of this message is that, however brief, counseling can still achieve an effect if something more than information is provided: namely, components that enhance motivation and behavioral skills, which are the other pillars of the intentions–motivation–behavioral skills theoretical model developed by Fisher and Fisher (1992). The second part of the message is that sustained risk reduction will most likely require yet additional components, the most likely candidates being some incorporation of social support and a pointed integration of condom skills training within any larger behavioral and role-playing framework. While knowing how to use and ask for a condom should perhaps not be the sole end of an HIV prevention intervention, what is becoming evident is that it is a prevention activity in which failure often signals deeper deficits in communication, intimacy, and relational dynamics, as well as social institutional deficiencies, all of which compromise safe sex intentions (O'Leary, 2002).

Prevention case management

With its point of delivery typically in a public health setting (e.g., STD clinic and HIV testing center; Purcell, DeGroff, & Wolitski, 1998), prevention case management is an individual-level intervention strategy, widely acknowledged in its applicability to a range of social ills. However, there has been little research examining the effect of case management on HIV risk behavior, particularly among at-risk youth such as AOD-abusing adolescents. The most notable study (Purcell *et al.*, 1998) covered 25 CDC-funded community-based organizations but was still confined to the practice and program implementation levels. A literature review by Murphy *et al.* (2003a) showed that there has been no progress in evaluation work beyond refinement of process outcome measures.

Because an intervention providing one-on-one support over time is potentially very costly, prevention case management was designed for people who have, or who are likely to have, "difficulty initiating and sustaining safer behavior" (CDC, 1995, p. 32). Consequently, it appears best suited for AOD-abusing adolescents whose lives are complicated by multiple, competing stressors such as mental illness, homelessness, and poverty. Unfortunately, a major stumbling block identified by Purcell *et al.* (1998) is that those high-risk subpopulations defined as most in need of this type of intervention very often do not self-identify as such and leave core services under-utilized. Something more is needed beyond standard outreach and marketing, and there are indications from the study that a few community-based organizations may have found a solution to this problem with small group adaptations of prevention core management that may facilitate self-identification through peer support and interaction. This adaptation is ripe for future efficacy studies.

Small-group interventions

Numerous studies have supported cognitive–behavioral skills training (CBST) within a small-group format in targeting HIV risk reduction among adolescents. Positive outcomes have been identified using these interventions with runaway street youth, teens in substance abuse treatment, and high school students in terms of increasing condom use among the sexually active and delaying sexual intercourse among the sexually inexperienced. In a review of 21 studies that evaluated this approach in community settings, Jemmott and Jemmott (2000) found significant reductions in the number of sexual partners and the frequency of unprotected intercourse and increases in condom use and acquisition: an outcome pattern that held across a variety of adolescent populations, including males and females, and African-American and White adolescents.

Though ecological validity has still not been firmly established, researchers have increasingly focused on adapting CBST group interventions to "real life" conditions and delivery points, and the NIH has made such studies a priority (Malow *et al.*, 2002). Card *et al.* (2001) have recently identified 23 such interventions that are effective and ready to be implemented in communities, schools, STD and family planning clinics, mental health centers, and AOD abuse rehabilitation programs. *Be A Responsible Teen (BART)* and *Be Proud–Be Responsible* are just two of the many CBST HIV risk-reduction interventions that have been packaged for mass dissemination. BART has been demonstrated by St. Lawrence *et al.* (1995) to be effective in reducing HIV risk among adolescents in community mental health centers. Jemmott and Jemmott have developed *Be Proud–Be Responsible* as a brief CBST group curriculum, which they have shown to be effective in schools, community centers, and other similar settings.

The adaptation of this design to AOD treatment has been a particular focus, and there is promise that interventions shown to be effective in schools may be generalizable to AOD rehabilitation settings. Kirby (2001b) identified a number of characteristics that may assist in integrating small-group CBST HIV prevention approaches within adolescent AOD abuse rehabilitation settings. The most promising may be interventions that incorporate (a) a few, specific behavior targets; (b) self-efficacy through skills-building activities; (c) rehearsal and feedback to model new behaviors (based in social cognitive theory); (d) personalization of information and multiple teaching methods; (e) small-group formats with at least 14 hours of contact; (f) basic risk information with strategies for resisting peer pressure; (g) components that reinforce social norms consistent with behavioral change targets; and (h) extensive training of interventionists. Promising models incorporating these features include Walter and Vaughan's (1993) six-session intervention delivered in health education classes in New York City, and a skills-building intervention tested in the Netherlands (Schaalma, Kok, & Paulussen, 1996).

The most effective and comprehensive school-based HIV prevention programs have supplemented the group intervention model with a multicomponent, multilevel design comprised of curriculum-based instruction that includes skills building, institution-wide peer-led programming, and health-promotion activities aimed at social norms. This is well illustrated by the *Safer Choices Program*, which seeks to reduce risks for STDs, HIV infection, and teen pregnancy (Coyle *et al.*, 1996, 1999, 2001) and has been designated by the CDC as one of few HIV risk "Programs that Work." The program reduced the frequency of unprotected intercourse and the number of sexual partners with whom students had intercourse without a condom at 3-month follow-up. Another study evaluating the school-wide effects of *Safer Choices* (Basen-Engquist *et al.*, 1997, 2001) found that the program decreased the frequency of sex without a condom 19 months after the intervention. At 31 months, when students in schools using *Safer Choices* reported unprotected sexual intercourse, they also reported this behavior with fewer partners. Consequently, this multicomponent, multilevel intervention not only had a positive effect on psychosocial variables and school climate for HIV/STD and pregnancy prevention; it also showed sustained effects that have been rare in HIV prevention interventions for adolescents.

Similarly, O'Hara *et al.* (1996) developed an intervention that utilized peer counselors and educators to deliver prevention activities at multiple levels in schools. Fisher *et al.* (2002) have recently developed another multicomponent school-based intervention, using a quasi-experimental controlled trial to compare it with two other theory-grounded HIV prevention programs. At 12 months, the classroom-based intervention resulted in sustained changes in condom use. These results point to the need of future development, replication, and evaluation of such an approach within adolescent AOD abuse treatment facilities.

Accounting for the effectiveness of group interventions

By the very fact that HIV transmission is largely preventable through behavioral change, the attention of the intervention community has been primarily anchored in developing testable theories of HIV risk behavior and securing prevention trials that produce reliable predictors and replicable designs. The result has been a prevailing tendency toward small-group behavioral interventions with multiple sessions and intensive interaction as the general format. Adherents of the public health approach, including those dissatisfied with the rapid decay of treatment effects and the largely unexplained variance of such models, increasingly have criticized group interventions for being too rooted in the individual, rational decision-making framework and not sufficiently structured to capture the social and institutional context of health and human behavior (Moatti & Souteyrand, 2000). Rotheram-Borus (2000) has pointed to the shallow treatment effects of such interventions, such as condom adherence increases of only 30% for perhaps as much as a year and little integration of substance abuse prevention. Nonetheless, Rapkin and Dumont (2000) argued that group interventions allow for the investigation of important contextual factors and the influence of the social, peer, and institutional norm dimensions. The basic message is that current research has not yet fully investigated the contextual factors of the group process and that future research must pay closer attention to these designs as micro-experiments in contextual influences.

As Benotsch and Kalichman (2002) have noted, the effectiveness of the small-group HIV intervention approach has been affirmed by more than one national review panel, with the scientific appeal of standardized manuals that can be adapted to new populations and allow the tailoring of components while remaining grounded in testable theory. The growing recognition of health disparities, in particular, has highlighted the need to identify and differentiate the most effective and predictive components for addressing the populations hardest hit by HIV/AIDS, as well as a confluence of preventable health problems. It is clear that group HIV prevention interventions have been able to affect the aggregate index of sexual behavior outcomes, including specific targets such as condom use, frequency of unprotected sexual intercourse, and number of sexual partners: all behaviors with recognized links to STI risk among adolescents (Jemmott & Jemmott, 2000).

This approach also has had ameliorative effects on many of the predictors and correlates of risk behavior, including self-efficacy, intentions, and attitudes. Studies of mediators have identified characteristics at the intervention and participant levels that may influence the magnitude and direction of effects. Jemmott and Jemmott (2000) found that group interventions that result in larger changes in theoretical mediator variables also have greater effects on risk behavior. For example, in a study of a single-session group intervention to promote STD protection among college students, Bryan, Aiken, and West (1996) showed that changes in the perceived benefits of condom use, acceptance of sexuality, sexual control, attitudes toward condoms, and self-efficacy in condom use were linked to behavioral intentions to use condoms. In analyses performed by Sanderson and Jemmott (1996), intentions to use condoms appeared to mediate the effects of group HIV interventions on condom use among college students. The evidence for other likely mediators, such as the sexual experience of participants, has been inconclusive (Jemmott & Jemmott, 2000). Attention has increasingly focused on indicators of the sexual dyad or partnership, and relationship status has been identified as a mediator of condom use (Plichta *et al.*, 1992; Sanderson & Jemmott, 1996). The analysis of mediators has allowed researchers to conclude that affective attitudes are a key mechanism of change in group interventions, specifically affective attitudes toward condoms and condom users, as well as self-efficacy in condom use.

It also appears conclusive that theory-based interventions have a definite advantage over atheoretical ones in producing desired effects. A comprehensive review of 40 HIV risk-reduction group interventions (Kim *et al.*, 1997) showed that those investigations that cited a culturally sensitive, theoretical framework were the ones most likely to demonstrate target effects among adolescents. Further, evaluations of school-based AOD abuse prevention programs have pointed to the intense, interactive framework that characterizes small-group interventions as an important medium for producing change. The sustenance of change still remains an issue, however, and change is often modest, suggesting that a goodness-of-fit with the context of high-risk adolescents – both as individuals and as members of a group – is still not in evidence (Masterman & Kelly, 2003).

Limitations of group interventions

Aside from the expected disincentive that groups may pose to certain individuals uncomfortable with this format, as well as the logistics involved for interventionists in scheduling and organizing group sessions, perhaps the most formidable limitation may be that those at greatest risk may be the least likely to participate or the most likely to drop out compared with other populations (Hoff *et al.*, 1997; Kalichman, Rompa, & Coley, 1997). To the degree that such individuals are compromised by multiple sources of survival stress (e.g., inadequate income and housing or family support, criminal record, addiction), the more likely they will be to succumb to the logistic and emotional challenges that any such participation poses. Research-based interventions invariably pay people to participate in studies, and alternative incentives such as meeting people, altruism, fun, and food may boost the willingness of such adolescents to participate. Nevertheless, attrition has remained high for this type of intervention, particularly in community settings. This has shifted attention to more formalized settings, such as adolescent AOD abuse treatment facilities or court-mandated juvenile rehabilitation programs. Paradoxically, the small-group format may be ideal for exceedingly risky individuals, such as AOD abusers if the intervention can be taken to them, as it can be in a treatment setting or could be in a community location when designed for "ground zero," that is, where risky behavior is initiated. Gains have been made with the help of sophisticated statistical techniques in delineating the mediators and moderators of behavioral change that will permit more tailored small-group formats for subpopulations; however, these factors are all too often at the level of individual characteristics, with few linkages to the dynamics and structural components of the group process that is purposely created by these interventions (Rapkin & Dumont, 2000).

Intervening at the family level

An important subset of structural support strategies is family-based intervention. Family approaches often focus on increasing the resource knowledge of parents and caregivers, and expanding the repertoire of communication and engagement with their children, particularly in relation to how to talk about HIV/AIDS, substance abuse, and other risky behavior. The National Association of Social Workers and other HIV-related providers have identified such elements as important training issues, especially how to adapt HIV/AIDS prevention strategies to the cultural context and communicative styles of families (Beauford, 2002).

In addition to education about HIV/AIDS, family programs have typically aimed at developing parental competencies that can influence adolescent behavior. Recent work has focused on understanding how family-related risk factors may mediate outcomes (Pequegnat & Szapocznik, 2000). For instance, parental monitoring of adolescent activities has been shown to delay initiation of sexual behavior (DiClemente *et al.*, 2002).

Given the critical role that parents can play in influencing the sexual behavior of their children, particularly as it relates to HIV risk, NIH has recently funded the evaluation of a number of parent-oriented HIV risk reduction interventions. Several excellent examples of these are detailed in a recent volume by Pequegnat and Szapocznik (2000) and provide a menu for those in search of effective components to adapt to HIV prevention programs involving AOD-abusing adolescents. An illustration is the prevention program developed by Krauss *et al.* (2000) aimed at mothers and fathers and their preadolescent children. This model, which consisted of parents participating in group training along with parent–child sessions, could be useful in structuring family involvement in the sexual health of AOD-abusing adolescents, including delay of sexual intercourse and performance of HIV risk reduction behaviors.

Another approach, developed by McKay *et al.* (2000), utilizes parent-only and child-only groups in combination with multiple-family groups, with the aim of fully recognizing parents as the fundamental social context of child development, as elaborated by Bronfenbrenner's (1986) social ecological theory. Others have created models that could be particularly helpful in acknowledging the special role that mothers play in the family structure of certain communities, such as the Dilorio *et al.* (2000) prevention program for mothers and their AOD-abusing adolescents. Interventions with mothers may be critical in reducing the HIV risk-associated sexual behaviors of AOD-abusing, African-American male adolescents. Jemmott and her colleagues (2000) have developed an intervention to help mothers to teach their sons about sex to reduce risky behavior. This program provides HIV prevention information and assists mothers in examining their personal values related to sexuality.

While the design and evaluation of family-based HIV prevention approaches is just beginning, it is unlikely that either group or family-level interventions alone will produce sustained behavioral changes for AOD-abusing adolescents at risk for HIV. What is most instructive from the research reviewed above is the importance of multiple levels and components of intervention in the maintenance of change (Ethier & St. Lawrence, 2002; Lonczak *et al.*, 2002). Such a framework recognizes the force of a *mix* of contextual influences and seeks to bring rigor to the analysis of context at the individual, group, family, and community levels. Future research will increasingly focus on the development of "smart" interventions, in which different components can be applied according to population profiles that include, but are not limited to, individual-level risks and mediators.

Community-level interventions

In contrast to intensive face-to-face interventions for individuals and small groups, community-level approaches are directed toward populations or specific population segments. These interventions seek to reduce the prevalence of high-risk behavior practices in communities by bringing about population-level changes in risk awareness; social norms concerning safer sex, condom-use attitudes or intentions; and collective self-efficacy for the enactment of behavior change.

Controlled trials of community-level HIV prevention interventions have been conducted with multiple hard-to-reach subgroups within communities (CDC, 1999), and they have differed in their approaches. Kelly *et al.* (1997) used principles derived from diffusion of innovation theory (Rogers, 2002), which postulates that new behavioral trends in a population can be initiated when a sufficient number of natural, popular opinion leaders are observed to model innovative behaviors. Applied to the issue of HIV prevention, interventions based on this model have identified, trained, and then engaged groups of popular opinion leaders to systematically disseminate risk-reduction messages endorsing condom use and safer sex during everyday discussions with members of their own social networks. The strategy is to create an intervention that is responsive to the network effect of peer norms, with the expectation that changes produced in social groups may extend to reductions in the sexual risk behavior of the target population (Kelly *et al.*, 1997; Sikkema *et al.*, 2000). This type of intervention also may be beneficial within AOD rehabilitation settings, as well as in communities with high prevalence rates of adolescent AOD abuse.

Another exemplary large-scale trial of a community-level HIV prevention was reported by the CDC AIDS Community Demonstration Projects Research Group (CDC, 1999). The project was implemented in five cities and targeted a variety of different groups, including high-risk youth. The intervention consisted of outreach contacts made by nearly 1000 volunteers and staff to target population members in community venues. Outreach consisted of "role-model stories," presented verbally and through picture books, portraying how persons similar to the target-population members were making behavior changes to reduce risk. In addition, small media materials were used to deliver similar role-model stories targeted to each population, and condoms and bleach kits were widely distributed. Cross-sectional interview waves of data collection took place with members of each target population over a 3-year period in both intervention and matched comparison communities. There was evidence of increased condom use with main and non-main partners, as well as greater rates of condom carrying in the intervention communities. Consistent condom use for at least 6 months increased from 9 to 17% with main partners and 25 to 33% with non-main partners.

On the international level, LoveLife is the largest community-level intervention ever launched in South Africa to change adolescent sexual behavior. This project aims to reduce the rate of HIV infection among 15–20 year olds by 50%, to reduce other STDs, and to reduce the incidence of teenage pregnancy (Stadler & Hlongwa, 2002). The design of LoveLife combines high-powered media awareness and education, development of adolescent-friendly reproductive health services, and outreach and support programs. A 5-year research and evaluation plan of the project includes a comprehensive observational study over several years, tracking change in a range of behavioral indicators and in sexual health outcomes. In its first 2 years, the project has reached more than 4 million adolescents and their families.

As evidenced in these studies, an effective or promising community-level intervention must take the popular culture of its target population seriously, as well as the more academically studied dimensions of ethnic and social context. Rotheram-Borus (2000) has encouraged researchers to reach beyond the randomized controlled trial design and to expand theoretical models to include interdisciplinary approaches. Operationally, this would include the use of diverse modalities (e.g., computers, videotapes, television, telephone groups, computerized telephones) and sites (e.g., parents' workplaces, religious organizations, self-help networks, primary health-care clinics), and the linkage of program components with key milestones in life.

Community-level interventions need not be complex to be effective. In developing countries and among at-risk adolescent populations in the USA without easy access to condoms, the distribution and social marketing of inexpensive or free condoms can constitute a significant intervention, particularly since risk-reduction objectives cannot be achieved under conditions in which condoms are not available. Further, given that STDs are HIV transmission-risk cofactors, more effective STD treatment (in high STD prevalent populations) may serve to reduce rates of sexually transmitted HIV. Research has shown that the transmission of HIV between heterosexual partners may become less biologically efficient if "traditional" STDs can be removed from the risk equation (Wasserheit, 1992). However, outcomes from STD treatment programs have been mixed in African countries, with reductions in heterosexual HIV transmission observed in some studies (Grosskurth *et al.*, 1995), but not in others (Wawer *et al.*, 1999). Therefore, like many other intervention components, STD treatment is merely one piece of a prevention strategy that must rest on some mechanism of revision and learning by researchers and those in the field. As HIV/AIDS has become chronic in communities characterized by other health disparities, structural interventions have come to serve such a purpose, and ways to differentiate effects and fine tune designs have come from the resulting focus on contextual factors.

Future as context: research to advance prevention of HIV infection and substance abuse in adolescents

The research outlined in this chapter indicates that significant progress has accompanied the design of high-quality evaluations and the application of theory-based interventions (Jemmott & Jemmott, 2000; Shoveller & Pietersma, 2002). A recent review of HIV/AIDS risk-reduction interventions in North America (Shoveller & Pietersma, 2002) suggested that more rigorous study approaches are being pursued in the evaluation of prevention interventions for adolescents. However, several important caveats exist in considering the progress to date in addressing HIV/AIDS prevention within adolescent AOD abuse treatment. Most notably is the tendency for effects to diminish over time even with interventions that have produced significant short-term (e.g., 30–90 days) effects (D'Angelo & DiClemente, 1996; Jemmott & Jemmott, 2000; Rotheram-Borus, 2000; Rotheram-Borus *et al.*, 2000). Challenges to recruiting and retaining large samples of adolescents (e.g., parental consent) to fulfill probability requirements often have prompted the use of small convenience samples and interfered with the design of long-term follow-up periods (Shoveller & Pietersma, 2002). While significant methodological issues remain, guidelines and innovations are gradually emerging, particularly in how to recruit the large samples needed for probability estimates, how to curb study attrition, and how to achieve consistent and standardized measurement of behavioral outcomes (Shoveller & Pietersma, 2002).

Increasingly, researchers have focused on the need to study the relationship between AOD use, sexual activity, and condom use within specific subgroups of adolescents. Those within AOD abuse treatment are of particular concern, since they are relatively unstudied and are at exceptionally high risk of HIV transmission, with features distinctly different from other subgroups that have been investigated (Dévieux *et al.*, 2002; Malow *et al.*, 2001). For example, using the Millon Adolescent Clinical Inventory in a study of ethnic minority adolescents who were court mandated into AOD treatment, our research identified the following as key predictors of sexual risk behavior in this subgroup: impulsivity, submissiveness, alcohol and marijuana use, and safer sex intentions. High impulsivity, low submissiveness to social norms, more frequent alcohol use, and less favorable intentions to engage in safer sex each characterized the substance-abusing adolescents who reported risky sexual behavior, with less frequent marijuana use distinguishing those reporting abstinence. This research also identified a striking heterogeneity within this recognized subgroup, emphasizing the importance of delineating risk variation within, as well as across, groups.

A primary theme is that contextual factors, ranging from individual to situational variables, may be complicating the interpretation of results of HIV prevention studies. Gender and age have been noted as significantly associated with HIV risk behavior (Jemmott & Jemmott, 2000; Newman & Zimmerman, 2000), as well as underlying characterological causal factors, such as impulsivity, sensation seeking, or some general psychopath deviancy factor (Dévieux *et al.*, 2002; Malow *et al.*, 2001). However, the literature on the nature and magnitude of the relationship between AOD use and sexual behavior has varied across diverse populations, with complex relationships being documented among characterological, situational, and behavioral factors (Leigh, 2002). This has occurred even with the use of similar methodologies to study this relationship, such as using event-related or situation covariation methodology. Therefore, while research has confirmed the complexities introduced by contextual factors, we are just at the beginning of understanding how to respond to them.

A key contextual variable now receiving priority in research with AOD-abusing adolescents is gender (Kalichman *et al.*, 2002). Female adolescent AOD abusers may be more susceptible to relational power dynamics, particularly when trading sex for drugs, a circumstance in which they have little power or control. Such gender–power relations have been shown to be important in explaining risk and protective behaviors in adolescents, as well as in adults (Wingood & DiClemente, 2000). According to the CDC (2002), adolescent girls are primarily infected through heterosexual contact, especially in the context of exchanging sex for survival needs or in relationships in which condom negotiation is compromised (Jemmott & Jemmott, 2000), and secondarily by injection drug use. Adolescent boys seem to be at greater risk from injection drug use, homosexual sex, and purchasing sex. These differences illustrate the need for more tailored research questions and prevention programming for AOD-abusing adolescent boys and girls (Smith, 2001).

Although data suggest that gender may influence the efficacy of HIV prevention interventions, only one study provides a rigorous model for evaluating the moderating effect of gender on the adoption and maintenance of protective behavior by adolescents. Joffe and Radius (1993) found that perceived ability to discuss safer sex and condom use with a partner was a significant predictor of intent to use condoms for adolescent males. However, among females, 29.8% of the variance for intent to use condoms was explained by their perceived ability to enjoy sex with a condom. Research from our group, however, does not support the role of gender or even expected personality factors, such as impulsivity or psychopathy, in moderating risk behavior outcomes. By far the most significant factor was alcohol abuse severity, coinciding with higher rates of sexual activity, unprotected sex, and intoxication proximate to sex, underscoring the importance of integrating alcohol screening and treatment referral with HIV prevention efforts for such subgroups.

By far the most significant vehicle of advance in the field has been the prioritization of *translational* research in an effort to reach groups at disproportionate risk for HIV/AIDS and substance abuse. Recent funding initiatives by various federal entities (e.g., CDC, NIAAA, NIDA, the National Institute on Child Health and Development, and the Office of Behavioral and Social Science Research) call for effective interventions to be "translated" to other groups, not only in terms of language and cultural realities but also according to contextual factors at issue for different subgroups. More than ever, there is the recognition that the traditional, rational decision-making model of risk behavior must be expanded and refined to embody the specificities of gender, culture, sexuality, and intimacy. Thus, the focus is shifting from individuals to relationships, from risk factors to contextual factors, from the individual as patient to the individual as a member of a family, peer group, or ethnic and cultural community. The result is that the model of human agency that has motivated many of our interventions to date – that is, the human capital model (education and training) – is being supplemented with the concept that assets or capacities for change go beyond the individual and must incorporate the social and physical environment. Consequently, organizations like the World Bank have found a new footing in various prevention efforts by expanding their concept of investment to include social and natural capital (wealth from social and ecological structures). What this has meant for high-risk adolescents is still developing.

The clearest move toward preparing the ground for designing intervention-based research on social capital and HIV/AIDS is the recent substudy by Crosby *et al.* (2002), in which the contextual factor of membership and activity in social organizations was built into and measured as part of an HIV prevention trial and then examined for predictive value in a target population's HIV and STD protective behavior. They found preliminary support for this hypothesis in their study population of African-American female adolescents. The implication of such research is that it may be possible to test an intervention that encourages and structures such participation and, in consequence, improves the social capital of a group or community, and thus their protective behavior.

Social network analysis has long been the route to tracing the social environmental influence on risk behavior, particularly in the field of substance abuse prevention. Exposure to high-risk networks has been identified as an individual risk factor for both substance abuse and sexual risk behavior. Moreover, association with high-risk peers may be predictive of relapse behavior; in fact, the power of such social contexts may be the single most determining factor in the decay function of risk-reduction interventions. As Moos (2003) makes clear, interventionists must face the fact that social contexts will limit (as well as sometimes enhance) the capacity to meet prevalence and incidence targets.

As noted repeatedly in this chapter, the foremost step forward in HIV prevention has been an increasingly concentrated search for contextual predictors, delineated according to mediators and moderators of intervention effects, as tied to subpopulations. However, more rigorous epidemiological studies of HIV seroprevalence among AOD-abusing youth are still needed to refine our understanding of differences in ethnicity, geographic region, socioeconomic status, and other contextual variables, all of which have been found to be especially salient for adolescents (e.g., Kalichman *et al.*, 2002).

Even if HIV primary prevention efforts are maximized with adolescents, we must face the prospect that the nature of prevention will increasingly focus on the transmission behavior of HIV-positive individuals, particularly those who are AOD abusers. Many identify this shift with the CDC policy announcement in the *MMWR Weekly* of April 18, 2003. However, it became something to be reckoned with as soon as effective antiretroviral treatment became available and, most importantly, became less intrusive in terms of regimen and cost. Those who were seropositive could then be offered proactive rather than reactive medical care. At the same time, this has meant that those living with HIV and also engaging in transmission risk behavior pose a more complex public health risk: not only that of spreading the virus but also that of increasing the probability of multiple and resistant strains, not to mention the possibility of reinfection for the individual.

The advent of a rapid and simple HIV test made this shift inevitable, especially in light of epidemiological trends indicating incidence may be increasing and that the initial positive impact of antiretroviral drugs on morbidity and mortality may be over. In a compelling way, the shift to transmission prevention crystallizes what is often amorphous in the attempts to achieve prevention intervention with the most vulnerable populations. To articulate the risks for adolescents in terms of how many fail to use condoms, how many do not know their serostatus or have never been tested, and how many are non-adherent to treatment is to underscore how little the current prevention messages have been digested by many in the adolescent population.

While condom use increased during the 1990s, there has been a leveling effect since 1999, with inconsistent or suboptimal use still occurring in one-third to one-half of adolescents, and more pessimistic indicators suggesting in 80–90% (CDC, 2002; Rotheram-Borus, 2000). Less than one-fifth of the HIV-positive adolescent population may know their serostatus and it may be as little as 7% (Rotheram-Borus, 2000; Rotheram-Borus et al., 2000). Among the more widely recognized at-risk group of men who have sex with men, at least 80% of those young men aged 15–22 years who are seropositive may not know they are infected (Valleroy et al., 2000). Further, less than one-third of HIV-positive adolescents may be adherent to antiretroviral regimens (Murphy et al., 2003b).

Adherence research will be key because of the need for complete compliance and mounting evidence of psychological factors as mediators of adherence and transmission risk behavior. Yet, even a highly individualized activity such as taking pills has a relational and social context. Transmission risk behavior and adherence by HIV-positive adolescents are the issues that will concentrate the attention of prevention interventionists on extending the frontier of contextual interventions. Even now, more researchers are focusing on how family and peer interventions improve not only adherence but also other health behaviors in adolescents, the family group approach by Lyon et al. (2003) being a good example. The effect on other health behaviors was unexpected in their study, which also found a positive impact on referral to substance abuse and mental health treatment.

Until there is a vaccine or cure for HIV, the role of context in the future of HIV-positive individuals – and ours – can be expected to go beyond formal institutions, such as supportive medical care, to include the degree of social involvement and trust existing in a community as a whole, as predicted by the social capital hypothesis. The physical environment is the concrete representation of that trust, and the micro-interactions in a neighborhood are as real as those that have come to be measured in the new science of mother–infant behavior. All such structural and contextual research, as reviewed in this chapter, expands our chances of reversing the pandemic trends of HIV/AIDS and the chronic devastation that usually follows for the populations affected, including the dreams that are destroyed for individuals at the beginning of life.

REFERENCES

Aggleton, R. K. (2000). Adolescent sexuality. [UNAIDS BP Digest Document 1999.] *AIDS* 2000 Jun; 14 Suppl 1:S33–40.

Basen-Engquist, K., Parcel, G. S., Harnst, R., *et al.* (1997). The Safer Choices Project: methodological issues in school-based health promotion intervention research. *Journal of School Health*, **67**, 365–371.

Basen-Engquist, K., Coyle, K. K., Parcel, G. S., *et al.* (2001). Schoolwide effects of a multi-component HIV, STD, and pregnancy prevention program for high school students. *Health Education and Behavior*, **28**, 166–185.

Beauford, C. (2002). *A Factsheet for Practitioners working with HIV/AIDS and Adolescents and Young Adults.* [National Association of Social Workers Fact Sheet.] Washington, DC: NASW Press. http://www.socialworkers.org/practice/hiv_aids/hiv_factsheet.asp.

Belcher, L., Kalichman, S., Topping, M., *et al.* (1998). A randomized trial of a brief HIV risk reduction counseling intervention for women. *Journal of Consulting and Clinical Psychology*, **66**, 856–861.

Benotsch, E. & Kalichman, S. (2002). Preventing HIV and AIDS. In L. A. Jason & D. S. Glenwick, (eds.), *Innovative Strategies for Promoting Health and Mental Health across the Life Span*, (pp. 205–226). New York: Springer.

Bronfenbrenner, U. (1986). Ecology of the family as a context for human development. *American Psychologist*, **32**, 513–531.

Brown, L. K., DiClemente, R. J., & Reynolds, L. A. (1991). HIV prevention for adolescents: utility of the health belief model. *AIDS Education and Prevention*, **3**, 50–59.

Brown, L. K., Danovsky, M. B., Lourie, K. J., DiClemente, R. J., & Ponton, L. E. (1997). Adolescents with psychiatric disorders and the risk of HIV. *Journal of the American Academy of Child and Adolescent Psychiatry*, **36**, 1609–1617.

Bryan, A. D., Aiken, L. S., & West, S. G. (1996). Increasing condom use: evaluation of a theory-based intervention to prevent sexually transmitted diseases in young women. *Health Psychology*, **15**, 371–382.

Bukstein, O. G., Glancy, L. J., & Kaminer, U. (1992). Patterns of affective comorbidity in a clinical population of dually diagnosed adolescent substance abusers. *Journal of the American Academy of Child and Adolescent Psychiatry*, **31**, 1041–1045.

Canterbury, R. J., McGarvey, E. L., Sheldon-Keller, A. E., *et al.* (1995). Prevalence of HIV-related risk behaviors and STDs among incarcerated adolescents. *Journal Adolescent Health*, **17**, 173–177.

Card, J. J., Benner, T., Shields, J. P., & Feinstein, N. (2001). The HIV/AIDS Prevention Program Archive (HAPPA): a collection of promising prevention programs in a box. *AIDS Education and Prevention*, **13**, 1–28.

CDC (Centers for Disease Control and Prevention) (1995). HIV prevention case management. In *Guidelines for Health Education and Risk Reduction* Activities (pp. 32–35). Atlanta, GA: Centers for Disease Control and Prevention.

——— (1999). The CDC AIDS Community Demonstration Projects: a multi-site community-level intervention to promote HIV risk reduction. *American Journal of Public Health*, **89**, 336–345.

——— (2002). *HIV/AIDS Surveillance Report*. Atlanta, GA: Centers for Disease Control and Prevention.

——— (2003). *The Strategic Plan of the Center for Disease Control and Prevention*. Atlanta, GA: Centers for Disease Control & Prevention. National Center for HIV, STD, and TB Prevention. Accessed on 9/12/2003 at http://www.cdc.gov/hiv/partners/psp.htm.

Chambers, R. A., Taylor, J. R., & Potenza, M. N. (2003). Developmental neurocircuitry of motivation in adolescence: a critical period of addiction vulnerability. *American Journal of Psychiatry*, **160**, 1041–1052.

Cooper, M. L. & Orcutt, H. K. (1997). Drinking and sexual experience on first dates among adolescents. *Journal of Abnormal Psychology*, **106**, 191–202.

Coyle, K., Kirby, D., Parcel, G., *et al.* (1996). Safer Choices: a multicomponent school-based HIV/STD and pregnancy prevention program for adolescents. *Journal of School Health*, **66**, 89–94.

Coyle, K., Basen-Engquist, K., Kirby, D., *et al.* (1999). Short-term impact of Safer Choices: a multicomponent, school-based HIV, other STD, and pregnancy prevention program. *Journal of School Health*, **69**, 181–188.

Coyle, K., Basen-Engquist, K., Kirby, D., *et al.* (2001). Safer choices: reducing teen pregnancy, HIV, and STDs. *Public Health Report*, **116** (Suppl. 1), 82–93.

Crosby, R. A., DiClemente, R. J., Wingood, G. M., *et al.* (2002). Participation by African-American adolescent females in social organizations: associations with HIV-protective behaviors. *Ethnicity and Disease*, **12**, 186–192.

D'Angelo, L. & DiClemente, R. (1996). Sexually transmitted diseases including human immunodeficiency virus infection. In R. J. DiClemente, W. B. Hansen, & L. E. Ponton (eds.), *Handbook of Adolescent Health Risk Behavior*, (pp. 333–367). New York: Plenum Press.

Deas-Nesmith, D., Brady, K. T., White, R., & Campbell, S. (1999). HIV-risk behaviors in adolescent substance abusers. *Journal of Substance Abuse Treatment*, **16**, 169–172.

Dévieux, J. G., Malow, R., Stein, J., *et al.* (2002). Impulsivity and HIV risk among adjudicated alcohol and other drug (AOD) abusing adolescent offenders. *AIDS Education and Prevention*, **14** (Suppl. B), 24–35.

DiClemente, R. J., Lanier, M. M., Horan, P. F., & Lodico, M. (1991). Comparison of AIDS knowledge, attitudes, and behaviors among incarcerated adolescents. A public school sample in San Francisco. *American Journal of Public Health*, **81**, 628–630.

DiClemente, R. J., Crosby, R. A., & Wingood, G. M. (2002). Enhancing STD/HIV prevention among adolescents: the importance of parental monitoring. *Minerva Pediatrica*, **54**, 171–177.

Dilorio, C., Denzmore, P., Wang, D. T., *et al.* (2000). Keepin' it REAL! In W. Pequegant & J. Szapocznik (eds.), *Working with Families in the Era of HIV/AIDS*, (pp. 113–132). London: Sage.

Ethier, K. & St. Lawrence, J. (2002). The role of early, multilevel youth development programs in preventing health risk behavior in adolescents and young adults. *Archives of Pediatrics and Adolescent Medicine*, **156**, 429–430.

Fisher, J. & Fisher, W. (1992). Changing AIDS-risk behavior. *Psychological Bulletin* **111**, 455–474.

Fisher, J. D., Fisher, W. A., Bryan, A. D., & Misovich, S. J. (2002). Information–motivation–behavioral skills model-based HIV risk behavior change intervention for inner-city high school youth. *Health Psychology*, **21**, 177–186.

Fortenberry, J. D. (1995). Adolescent substance use and sexually transmitted diseases risk: a review. *Journal of Adolescent Health*, **16**, 304–308.

Fraiberg, S. (1987). Enlightenment and confusion. In L. Fraiberg (ed.), *Selected Writings of Selma Fraiberg* (pp. 205–216). Columbus, OH: Ohio State University Press.

Gardner, W. & Herman J. (1990). Adolescents' AIDS risk taking: a rational choice perspective. *New Directions in Child Development*, **Winter**, 17–34.

Gillmore, M. R., Morrison, D. M., Lowery, C., & Baker, S. A. (1994). Beliefs about condoms and their association with intentions to use condoms among youths in detention. *Journal of Adolescent Health*, **15**, 228–237.

Giordano, P. C. (2003). Relationships in adolescence. *Annual Review of Sociology*, **29**, 257–281.

Grosskurth, H., Mosha, F., Todd, J., *et al.* (1995). Impact of improved treatment of sexually transmitted diseases on HIV infection in rural Tanzania: a randomised controlled trial. *Lancet*, **346**, 530–536.

Hingson, R. W., Strunin, L., Berlin, B. M., & Heeren, T. (1990). Beliefs about AIDS, use of alcohol and drugs, and unprotected sex among Massachusetts adolescents. *American Journal of Public Health*, **80**, 295–299.

Hobfoll, S. E., Jackson, A. P., Lavin, J., Johnson, R. J., & Schroder, K. E. (2002). Effects and generalizability of communally oriented HIV-AIDS prevention versus general health promotion groups for single, inner-city women in urban clinics. *Journal of Consulting and Clinical Psychology*, **70**, 950–960.

Hoff, C. C., Kegeles, S. M., Acree, M., *et al.* (1997). Looking for men in all the wrong places . . . : HIV prevention small-group programs do not reach high risk gay men. *AIDS*, **11**, 829–830.

Jemmott, J. & Jemmott, L. (2000). HIV behavioral interventions for adolescents in community settings. In J. L. Peterson & R. J. DiClemente (eds.), *Handbook of HIV Prevention*, (pp. 103–127). New York: Kluwer Academic/Plenum Press.

Jemmott, L. S., Outlaw, F., Jemmott, J. B., III, *et al.* (2000). Strengthening the bond: the mother–son health promotion project. In W. Pequegnat & J. Szapocznik (eds.), *Working with Families in the Era of HIV/AIDS* (pp. 133–151). London: Sage.

Joffe, A. & Radius, S. M. (1993). Self-efficacy and intent to use condoms among entering college freshmen. *Journal of Adolescent Health*, **14**, 262–268.

Kalichman, S. C., Rompa, D., & Coley, B. (1997). Lack of positive outcomes from a cognitive–behavioral HIV and AIDS prevention intervention for inner-city men: lessons from a controlled pilot study. *AIDS Education and Prevention*, **9**, 299–313.

Kalichman, S., Stein, J., Malow, R. M., *et al.* (2002). Predicting protected sexual behavior using the information–motivation–behavior skills (IMB) model among adolescent substance abusers in court-ordered treatment. *Psychology Health and Medicine*, **7**, 327–338.

Kamb, M. L., Fishbein, M., Douglas, J. M., *et al.* For the Project RESPECT Study Group (1998). Efficacy of risk-reduction counseling to prevent human immunodeficiency virus and sexually transmitted diseases. *Journal of the American Medical Association*, **280**, 1161–1167.

Kelly, J. A., Murphy, D. A., Sikkema, K. J., *et al.* (1997). Randomised, controlled, community-level HIV-prevention intervention for sexual-risk behaviour among homosexual men in US cities. *Lancet*, **350**, 1500–1505.

Kim, N., Stanton, B., Li, X., Dickersin, K., & Galbraith, J. (1997). Effectiveness of the 40 adolescent AIDS-risk reduction interventions: a quantitative review. *Journal of Adolescent Health*, **20**, 204–215.

Kirby, D. (2000). School-based interventions to prevent unprotected sex and HIV among adolescents. In J. L. Peterson & R. J. DiClemente (eds.), *Handbook of HIV Prevention*, (pp. 83–101). New York: Kluwer Academic/Plenum Press.

(2001a). Understanding what works and what doesn't in reducing adolescent sexual risk-taking. *Family Planning Perspectives*, **33**, 276–281.

(2001b). *Emerging Answers: Research Findings on Programs to Reduce Teen Pregnancy.* Washington, DC: National Campaign to Prevent Teen Pregnancy.

Krauss, B. J., Godfrey, C., Yee, D., *et al.* (2000). Saving our children from a silent epidemic: the PATH program for parents and preadolescents. In W. Pequegnat & J. Szapocznik (eds.), *Working with Families in the Era of HIV/AIDS* (pp. 89–112). London: Sage.

Leigh, B. C. (1990). The relationship of substance use during sex to high-risk sexual behavior. *Journal of Sex Research*, **27**, 199–213.

(2002). Alcohol and condom use: a meta-analysis of event-level studies. *Sexually Transmitted Disease*, **29**, 476–482.

Lonczak, H. S., Abbott, R. D., Hawkins, J. D., Kosterman, R., & Catalano, R. F. (2002). Effects of the Seattle social development project on sexual behavior, pregnancy, birth, and sexually transmitted disease outcomes by age 21 years. *Archives of Pediatric Adolescent Medicine*, **156**, 438–447.

Lucenko, B. A., Malow, R. M., Dévieux, J. G., Sanchez-Martinez, M., & Jennings, T. (2003), Negative affect and HIV risk in alcohol and other drug (AOD) abusing adolescent offenders. *Journal of Child and Adolescent Substance Abuse*, **13**, 1–17.

Lyon, M. E., Trexler, C., Akpan-Townsend, C., *et al.* (2003). A family group approach to increasing adherence to therapy in HIV-infected youths: results of a pilot project. *AIDS Patient Care and STDs*, **17**, 299–308.

Malow, R. M., McMahon, R., Cremer, D. J., Lewis, J. E., & Alferi, S. M. (1997). Psychosocial predictors of HIV risk among adolescent offenders who abuse drugs. *Psychiatric Services*, **48**, 185–187.

Malow, R. M., Devieux, J. G., Jennings, T., Lucenko, B. A., & Kalichman, S. C. (2001). Substance-abusing adolescents at varying levels of HIV risk: psychosocial characteristics, drug use, and sexual behavior. *Journal of Substance Abuse*, **13**, 103–117.

Malow, R. M., Dévieux, J. G., Rosenberg, R., Capp, L., & Schneiderman, N. (2002). A cognitive–behavioral intervention for HIV-positive recovering drug abusers: the 2000–05 NIDA-funded AIDS Prevention Center Study. *Psychology and AIDS Exchange*, **30**, 23–26.

Masterman, P. W. & Kelly, A. B. (2003). Reaching adolescents who drink harmfully: fitting intervention to developmental reality. *Journal of Substance Abuse Treatment, 24*, 347–345.

McKay, M., Baptiste, D., Coleman, D., *et al.* (2000). Preventing HIV risk exposure in urban communities. The CHAMP Family Program. In W. Pequegnat & J. Szapocznik (eds.), *Working with Families in the Era of HIV/AIDS* (pp. 133–151). London: Sage.

Moatti, J. P. & Souteyrand, Y. (2000). HIV/AIDS social and behavioural research: past advances and thoughts about the future. *Social Science and Medicine, 50*, 1519–1532.

Moos, R. H. (2003). Social contexts: transcending their power and their fragility. *American Journal of Community Psychology, 31*, 1–13.

Murphy, R., Tobias, C., Rajabiun, S., & Abuchar, V. (2003a). HIV case management: a review of the literature. *AIDS Education and Prevention, 15*, 93–108. Retrieved August 8, 2003 from http://www.bu.edu/hdwg/reports/DPH-lit-rev.pdf.

Murphy, D. A., Sarr, M., Durako, S. J., *et al.* (2003b). Barriers to HAART adherence among human immunodeficiency virus infected adolescents. *Archives of Pediatric Adolescent Medicine, 157*, 249–255.

Neighbors, C. J. & O'Leary, A. (2003). Responses of male inmates to primary requests of condom use: effects of message content and domestic violence history. *AIDS Education and Prevention, 15*, 93–108.

Newman, P. A. & Zimmerman, M. A. (2000). Gender differences in HIV-related sexual risk behavior among urban African American youth: a multivariate approach. *AIDS Education and Prevention, 12*, 308–325.

NIDA (National Institute for Drug Abuse) (1996). *Advances in Research on Women's Health and Gender Differences.* Rockville, MD: National Institute on Drug Abuse. Retrieved August 8, 2003 from www.drugabuse.gov/WHGD/WHGDAdvance.html, p. 2.

O'Hara, P., Messick, B. J., Fichtner, R. R., & Parris, D. (1996). A peer-led AIDS prevention program for students in an alternative school. *Journal of School Health, 66*, 176–182.

O'Leary, A. (2002). *Beyond Condoms: Alternative Approaches to HIV Prevention.* New York: Kluwer Academic/Plenum Press.

Palmquist, E. (1992). The fastest growing AIDS population: adolescents. In G. W. Lawson & A. W. Lawson (eds.), *Adolescent Substance Abuse: Etiology, Treatment, and Prevention.* Gaithersburg, MD: Aspen Publishers.

Paul, J. P., Catania, J., Pollack, L., & Stall R. (2001). Understanding childhood sexual abuse as a predictor of sexual risk-taking among men who have sex with men: the Urban Men's Health Study. *Child Abuse and Neglect, 25*, 557–584.

Pequegnat, W. & Szapocznik, J. (2000). The role of families in preventing and adapting to HIV/AIDS: issues and answers. In W. Pequegnat & J. Szapocznik (eds.), *Working with Families in the Era of HIV/AIDS*, (pp. 3–26). London: Sage.

Plichta, S. B, Weisman, C. S., Nathanson, C. A., Ensminger, M. E., & Robinson, J. C. (1992). Partner-specific condom use among adolescent women clients of a family planning clinic. *Journal of Adolescent Health, 13*, 506–611.

Purcell, D. W., DeGroff, A. S., & Wolitski, R. J. (1998). HIV prevention case management: current practices and future directions. *Health and Social Work, 23*, 282–289.

Purcell, D., Malow, R., Dolezal C., & Carballo-Dieguez, A. (2005). Sexual abuse of boys: associations with adult HIV risk behavior and implications for HIV prevention. In L. Koenig, L. Doll, W. Pequegnat, & A. O'Leary (eds.), *Childhood Sexual Abuse and HIV*. Washington, DC: American Psychological Press.

Rapkin, B. D. & Dumont, K. A. (2000). Methods for identifying and assessing groups in health behavioral research. *Addiction*, **95** (Suppl. 3), 395–417.

Rogers, E. M. (2002). Diffusion of preventive innovations. *Addictive Behaviors*, **27**, 989–993.

Rolf, J., Nanda, J., Baldwin, J., Chandra, A., & Thompson L. (1990). Substance misuse and HIV/AIDS risks among delinquents: a prevention challenge. *International Journal of the Addictions*, **25**, 533–559.

Rotheram-Borus, M. J. (2000). Expanding the range of interventions to reduce HIV among adolescents. *AIDS*, **14** (Suppl. 1), S33–50.

Rotheram-Borus, M. J., O'Keefe, Z., Kracker, R., & Foo, H. H. (2000). Prevention of HIV among adolescents. *Prevention Science*, **1**, 15–30.

Sanderson, C. A. & Jemmott, J. B. (1996). Moderation and mediation of HIV prevention interventions: relationship status intentions and condom use among college students. *Applied Social Psychology*, **26**, 2076–2099.

Schaalma, H., Kok, G., & Paulussen, T. (1996). HIV behavioural interventions in young people in the Netherlands. *International Journal of STD and AIDS*, **7** (Suppl. 2), 43–46.

Shoveller, J. & Pietersma, W. (2002). Preventing HIV/AIDS risk behavior among youth. *AIDS and Behavior*, **6**, 123–129.

Sikkema, K. J., Winett, R. A., & Lombard, D. N. (1995). Development and evaluation of an HIV-risk reduction program for female college students. *AIDS Education and Prevention*, **7**, 145–159.

Sikkema, K. J., Kelly, J. A., Winett, R. A., *et al.* (2000). Outcomes of a randomized community-level HIV prevention intervention for women living in 18 low-income housing developments. *American Journal of Public Health*, **90**, 57–63.

Simoni, J. (2000). Safer sex among HIV+ women: the role of relationships. *Sex Roles*, **42**, 691–708.

Smith, M. D. (2001). HIV risk in adolescents with severe mental illness: literature review. *Journal of Adolescent Health*, **29**, 320–329.

St. Lawrence, J. S., Brasfield, T. L., Jefferson, K. W., *et al.* (1995). Cognitive–behavioral intervention to reduce African-American adolescents' risk for HIV infection. *Journal of Consulting and Clinical Psychology*, **63**, 221–237.

St. Lawrence, J. S., Crosby, R., & O'Bannon, R. E. (1999). Adolescents at high risk of HIV infection: a comparison of four samples. *Journal of HIV/AIDS Prevention and Education*, **3**, 63–86.

Stadler, J. & Hlongwa, L. (2002). Monitoring and evaluation of LoveLife's AIDS prevention and advocacy activities in South Africa, 1999–2001. *Evaluation and Program Planning*, **25**, 365–376.

Strunin, L. & Hingson, R. (1992). Alcohol, drugs, and adolescent sexual behavior. *International Journal of the Addictions*, **27**, 129–146.

Tapert, S. F., Aarons, G. A., Sedlar, G. R., & Brown, S. A. (2001). Adolescent substance use and sexual risk-taking behavior. *Journal of Adolescent Health*, **28**, 181–189.

Trad, P. V. (1994). A developmental model for risk avoidance in adolescents confronting AIDS. *AIDS Education and Prevention*, **6**, 322–338.

UNICEF (2002). Young people and HIV/AIDS: opportunity in crisis. Pu Geneva: UNICEF. Retrieved September 13, 2003 from http://www.unicef.org/publications/index_4447.html.

Valleroy, L. A., MacKellar, D. A., Karon, J. M., *et al.* (2000). HIV prevalence and associated risks in young men who have sex with men. Young Men's Survey Study Group. *Journal of the American Medical Association*, **284**, 198–204.

Walter, H. & Vaughan, R. (1993). AIDS risk reduction among a multiethnic sample of urban high school students. *Journal of the American Medical Association* **270**, 725–730.

Walter, H., Vaughan, R., & Cohall, A. (1991). Psychosocial influences on acquired immunodeficiency syndrome-risk behaviors among high school students. *Pediatrics*, **88**, 846–852.

Wasserheit, J. N. (1992). Epidemiological synergy. Interrelationships between human immunodeficiency virus infection and other sexually transmitted diseases. *Sexually Transmitted Diseases*, **19**, 61–77.

Wawer, M. J., Sewankambo, N. K., Serwadda, D., *et al.* (1999). Control of sexually transmitted diseases for AIDS prevention in Uganda: a randomised community trial (Rakai Project Study Group). *Lancet*, **353**, 525–535.

Weinhardt, L. S. & Carey, M. P. (2000). Does alcohol lead to sexual risk behavior? Findings from event-level research. *Annual Review of Sex Research*, **11**, 125–157.

Wingood, G. & DiClemente, R. J. (2000). Application of the theory of gender and power to examine HIV-related exposures, risk factors, and effective interventions for women. *Health Education and Behavior*, **27**, 539–565.

Part IV

Empirically based interventions for adolescent substance abuse: research and practical implications

15

Adolescent therapeutic communities: future directions for practice and research

Nancy Jainchill

National Development and Research Institutes, New York, USA

The therapeutic community (TC) began as a mutual-help approach for the treatment of substance abuse outside of mainstream psychiatry, psychology, and medicine. Today, the TC is a recognized treatment approach for individuals with substance use and abuse problems. The primary agent for change remains mutual help; however, the TC has evolved to incorporate the participation of professionals into the therapeutic and organizational structure to address the increasingly complex needs of clients admitted for treatment. The current chapter presents a case for the role of the TC as a critical treatment option for adolescents with substance use/abuse and concomitant problems. The model is described and a review of the empirical basis for the approach is presented. The question of "What's next?" will be addressed, both in terms of directions for research and for clinical innovations.

Background and history

The TC views substance abuse as a disorder of the whole person, involving the possibility of impeded personality development with associated deficits in social, educational, and economic/survival skills (De Leon, 1986, 2000). This global perspective of the problem supports a multidimensional rehabilitative approach that occurs in a 24-hour setting. The *community* itself, consisting of member–residents and staff, and all of the community activities, are designed to produce therapeutic and educational change in the participants, who are also the mediators of these changes (De Leon, 1997).

The basic components of the TC (see De Leon, 1997, 2000) include community separateness (a location apart from other institutions and the external environment); an environment that focuses on community rather than personal use of space; community activities (rather than individualized); peers who are community members as well as role models; staff who are rational authorities, role models,

Adolescent Substance Abuse: Research and Clinical Advances, ed. Howard A. Liddle and Cynthia L. Rowe.
Published by Cambridge University Press. © Cambridge University Press 2006.

facilitators, and guides; a structured day (i.e., a deliberately scheduled routine); a phased therapeutic process that emphasizes incremental learning; job functions that contribute to the maintenance of the community and that are both educational and therapeutic; and a variety of peer groups.

The TC has evolved in the range of services provided, the diversity of the population served, and in the composition of the staff. Although once dedicated to the treatment of substance abusers, primarily male and primarily those involved with opiates, the clients today are almost one-third female and reflect a diversity in terms of race/ethnicity, age, presenting drug problems, psychological problems, psychosocial status (e.g., homeless), and criminal justice involvement. The complex needs of the clients have necessitated modifications to the traditional treatment approach in terms of the range of services provided, the location of programs, and the clinical "tools" themselves.

A recent review of adolescent drug treatment (Drug Strategies, 2003) provided an overview of 144 different programs across the USA, of which 60% offered residential treatment, incorporating a variety of approaches. Approximately 25% of the residential programs identify themselves as TCs, while others were self-described as long-term residential, short-term residential, 12-step, cognitive – behavioral or reality models. Many of the programs reported utilizing more than one approach, and the overlap among approaches (e.g., TC and 12-step) was probably greater than indicated. There were differences in the planned treatment tenures for non-TC residential programs and TC residential settings: 34% of the non-TC residential programs had a planned treatment duration of over 90 days, compared with approximately 73% of TCs, and 50% of the TCs are 6 months or longer compared with 16% of the other residential programs. Non-TC residential settings are generally smaller than residential TCs: the majority of the former have a capacity for under 20 beds or 20–30 beds; among the TCs there are as many programs with 30 or less beds as with more than 30 beds. The majority of programs in both types of residential setting serve mixed gender populations. Although studies have implicated the relationship between treatment tenure and outcomes (i.e., longer time in the program is associated with more positive post-treatment behaviors), the author knows of no studies that have compared non-TC residential settings with TC residential settings for adolescents.

Approximately 20–25% of admissions to TCs are adolescents. Until the late 1980s, with rare exception, the treatment of adolescents was not differentiated from the treatment of adults as regards location, therapeutic process, and staffing. The need to accommodate developmental differences, to facilitate maturation, and to address differences in lifestyle, cultural, and psychosocial circumstances has become increasingly evident as the number of adolescents entering treatment has increased (Jainchill, 1997; Jainchill, Bhattacharya & Yagelka, 1995).

In response, TCs have established segregated facilities for adolescents, recognizing that the treatment structure must be adapted to deal with issues unique to young substance abusers. Modifications to treatment include shorter recommended lengths of stay, more participation by families in the therapeutic process, and limited use of peer pressure focusing on positive influences since pretreatment peer influences have generally been negative. There is also less reliance on the use of life experiences to foster understanding about one's self and one's behaviors, because, developmentally, the level of self-understanding and reflection is more rudimentary. The authority structure is also modified for adolescents. Although this structure is still considered a therapeutic tool that can teach responsibility and discipline, among other things, adolescents' participation in the vertical authority structure is limited; all activities are staff supervised and the staff have ultimate control over all decisions. The dynamic of community as family has particular relevance since many of the youth come from disruptive family environments. The relationship between staff and clients frequently appears parental, providing the opportunity for these youth to learn how to be in positive authority–parent and peer–sibling relationships (Jainchill, 1997, 2000).

Approximately 10% of adolescents who receive treatment for substance use/abuse problems enter long-term residential programs, the majority of these being TCs (Dennis *et al.*, 2003). These youth have severe substance abuse problems, which typically are correlated with other problems, and they manifest serious dysfunctionality in many areas of their lives. They are frequently at the extreme end of the continuum in terms of antisocial or conduct disorder problems, as well as emotional and psychiatric distress (Jainchill, 1997).

The empirical basis for the therapeutic community approach

Social learning and cognitive–behavioral theories provide the theoretical and philosophical basis for the TC. Knowledge is presumed to lie within the individual and through the process of social learning the individual will own this knowledge. Social learning draws on the skills of the whole group, and both requires and facilitates creativity, change, and flexibility (Ottenberg, 1984). Social learning is experiential and necessitates a movement from an external to an internal ownership of the attitudes, values, and beliefs that ultimately drive behaviors. For example, behaviors that are initially motivated by conformity are later driven by personal commitment.

The social learning that occurs in the TC reflects the concept of interpersonal learning (Yalom, 1975, p. 19), a key mechanism that mediates therapeutic change in the community context: three elements associated with interpersonal learning are interpersonal relationships, the corrective emotional experience, and the group as a social microcosm. The multiple group experiences offered by the TC on the larger scale of community interactions, as well as on the smaller level of encounter groups and other types of group, provide the opportunity to reprocess interactions and concomitant affective responses.

The cognitive–behavioral perspective emphasizes personal awareness of learned emotional responses, enhanced communication skills through self-disclosure and positive relationship building, and cognitive restructuring to change thinking patterns and reinforce positive values and self-esteem. Behaviorally, there is a shift from an external focus of control to an internalized focus of control, a trial-and-error learning approach with an emphasis on rewarding successful and successive approximations of expected behaviors. Although seemingly paradoxical because of the TC's focus on "act as if" (i.e., behave the behaviors even if you do not feel like it), this process provides the learning experience necessary for bringing about changes in beliefs. Thus, the underlying premise is consistent: that beliefs drive actions and without a change in beliefs, behaviors will not change.

Outcome studies

There have been relatively few studies that have reported on the effectiveness of residential TCs, and none to date that have included control or comparison groups with random assignment of youth to different treatment conditions. With this as a caveat, the findings nonetheless support the effectiveness of residential TCs. There is a significant relationship between a client's length of stay in treatment and post-treatment outcomes; longer treatment tenures are significantly related to reductions in drug use and criminal activity post-treatment (e.g., De Leon, Wexler & Jainchill, 1982; Hubbard *et al.*, 1985; Jainchill *et al.*, 2000; Sells & Simpson, 1979). These studies involved large samples and across multiple settings, lending confidence to the validity of the findings.

The earliest studies of adolescents in TC treatment programs involved samples of youth who were in adult TCs. The Drug Abuse Reporting Program (DARP) was the first comprehensive multimodality study of the drug abuse treatment industry, evaluating programs in the 1960s and 1970s. One-third of the TC sample in the DARP study was adolescents; their treatment was incorporated with that of adults in the various programs (Sells & Simpson, 1979). The planned duration of treatment for most of these programs averaged between 18 months and 2 years; almost 25% of the youth left treatment within the first month, and about 15% completed treatment. Post-treatment outcomes were mixed: while opioid use decreased, marijuana use increased, and there was no change in alcohol consumption. There were changes in other behaviors indicating a more prosocial lifestyle, specifically increased employment and decreased criminal activity. Improved behaviors at follow-up were related to longer time in treatment (Sells & Simpson, 1979).

A second large, multisite national initiative was the Treatment Outcome Prospective Study (TOPS), which included admissions to 14 TCs from 1979 to 1981, of which adolescents constituted 14% of the treatment population (Hubbard *et al.*, 1985). The length of treatment recommended by programs was still at least 18 months; about one-third of the adolescents dropped out within the first month and approximately 10% completed treatment (Pompi, 1994). By this time, the drug abuse profile was changing, with fewer opioid abusers among admissions to TCs, and increasing numbers of cocaine and marijuana abusers. Treatment outcomes after 1 year showed positive behavior changes associated with longer time in treatment, including reductions in drug use and criminal activity, and increased employment.

More recently, the Drug Abuse Treatment Outcome Studies of Adolescents (DATOS-A) was conducted in the mid to late 1990s and reported findings on a sample of adolescents admitted to long-term residential treatment (TC and non-TC) who also completed a 1-year post-treatment follow-up interview. A caveat with regard to these findings is that the definition of long term was fairly inclusive, referring to all residential programs that were 90 days or longer. Most adolescents in the sample were marijuana abusers, and there were significant declines in drug use and criminal activity related to longer time in program (e.g., Grella *et al.*, 2000; Hser *et al.*, 2001).

Research conducted by Jainchill and colleagues (e.g., Hawke, Jainchill, & De Leon, 2000; Jainchill *et al.*, 1999, 2000) has constituted the largest study to date focused on this area of inquiry. The study, funded by NIDA (grant P50-DA-0770), involved all clients admitted to six programs (nine different sites) during the period from April 1992 through April 1994. Over 900 adolescents were interviewed at admission to treatment, and a subsample completed a 1-year post-treatment follow-up data. The method and findings are described by Jainchill and colleagues (2000).

Findings revealed that adolescents improved as a result of TC treatment. However, compared with adults, adolescents who entered TCs had poorer outcomes (i.e., higher drop-out rates) and more drug use and criminal activity post-treatment (e.g., Jainchill *et al.*, 2000). These findings appear to be related to various factors that have been associated with post-treatment outcomes in other studies. Specifically, previous studies of adults in TCs involved programs with an average duration of treatment of 18 months. These studies showed there was a consistent significant relationship between the length of time an individual remained in treatment and post-treatment outcomes: longer time in program was associated with reductions in drug use and criminal activity during the follow-up period (e.g., De Leon, Wexler & Jainchill, 1982). The programs in the current study had planned durations of stay that averaged between 6 and 9 months, primarily because of funding vicissitudes rather than clinical recommendations. Another factor that may be pertinent is that adolescents present with lower intrinsic motivation for treatment than adults (e.g., Melnick *et al.*, 1997); consequently, engaging them in the treatment process is more difficult. These factors, among others, contribute to reduced treatment engagement and lower motivation to change problem behavior, resulting in poorer retention and less than optimal post-treatment outcomes.

A 5-year follow-up study of a representative subsample (approximately 440) of these youth was the first to provide information for such an extended post-treatment time period. A typology was developed that described subtypes of adolescent during the 5 years following their separation from TC treatment. This typology differentiated lifestyle categories based on behavioral profiles during this period, including months of drug use (cocaine, opiates, marijuana), criminal activity (drug possession or sales, violent crimes, property crimes, and "miscellaneous" illegal activities), episodes of incarceration, prosocial behaviors (employment, school, long-term relationships, time with family), and multiple sexual partners. The findings revealed that the majority of the sample were "occasional drug users" (41%), a group that also was described by very little criminal activity and more prosocial behaviors, followed by "chronic marijuana users" (21%), who were similar to the occasional users except for their higher level of marijuana use. The remainder were classified as "drug-dependent criminals" (10%), whose greater involvement with cocaine and opiates distinguished them from those classified as "serious criminals" (29%) (Jainchill, Hawke, & Holland, 2001). Comparisons with other studies are limited in terms of the length of the outcome period. Winters (1999) has summarized outcome studies involving adolescents, including those studies in which youth met formal criteria for substance abuse or dependence, received treatment on either an outpatient (approximately 20 sessions) or short-term residential (4 weeks) basis involving a multidisciplinary staff, with 6 months or 1 year (or both) outcomes reported. There was considerable variability in abstinence/lapse rates at 6 months (16–54%), and at 1 year (25–62%). In a study of outcome at 4 years after intake, the progression from conduct disorder to antisocial personality disorder was examined; a poorer prognosis was obtained when conduct disorder is diagnosed independent of drug use (Myers, Stewart & Brown, 1998).

The prototypical adolescent therapeutic community

A recurrent finding across modalities and age ranges is that a longer treatment episode is significantly related to more-positive post-treatment outcomes; however, the TC, like other treatment modalities, determines treatment tenure as much by funding sources as by clinical criteria. The recommended length of treatment varies among programs and even within programs. The majority of adolescent TCs provide for a planned duration of treatment of 6–9 months, although a minority still provides a 12-month residential therapeutic curriculum.

Treatment is sequenced into phases or stages, no matter what the absolute length of the program is, and the length of time in a respective phase is dependent upon an adolescent's therapeutic process. An individual must meet specific criteria reflective of progress along behavioral, emotional, and developmental dimensions prior to advancement to the next phase (Jainchill, 2000).

Treatment protocol

A critical emphasis in adolescent TCs is to provide a psychologically and physically safe environment, which is often counter to the youth's social ecology of origin. The TC milieu is highly structured in terms of scheduled activities and behavioral expectations, providing a context for learning more adaptive personal and social behaviors. The structure provides the opportunity for these youth, who typically are from environments that lack structure or any kind of routine, to learn to follow a regime and to self-regulate their behavior. They learn that, as part of a community, their actions have social as well as personal consequences. This reality is not unique to the social microcosm of the TC, but has relevance to the external society. Therefore, the daily schedule and range of activities provide a forum for the adolescent to practice new behaviors and emotional responses, and to be evaluated and supported in these efforts, in preparation for participation in a prosocial lifestyle after residential treatment (Jainchill, 1997).

The typical day is structured around a variety of communal activities that reflects the essential component of *community as healer*. The day begins and ends with a community-wide meeting, involving the participation of all residents and reflecting the philosophy of personal and social responsibility. Seminars occur several times a week, conducted by a senior resident or counselor, providing a collective forum for informal learning and for the development of language and communication skills, a critical need among many of the adolescents.

The essential therapeutic tool is not the traditional dyadic relationship but is a group process, again reflecting the emphasis on community. The therapeutic role of the group evolved out of a history of unsuccessful experiences with more traditional therapeutic approaches with these clients. The TC peer groups are characterized by distinctive elements that are designed to strengthen the therapeutic alliance between the individual and the group (De Leon, 2000). In contrast to the negative influences that have often characterized these adolescents' peer relationships, the TC group process demonstrates a positive restructuring of peer interactions and relationships.

Most TCs incorporate a variety of groups into the therapeutic protocol, including, for example, the caseload group (individuals with the same primary counselor), the encounter group, gender groups, and tutorial groups (usually organized around a theme). The encounter group, which is the primary therapeutic group, has moderated over the years and provides an opportunity for the adolescent to deal with the here-and-now, learning how to address conflicts and express feelings appropriately and safely. Key features of the TC encounter group, in contrast with other peer groups that have demonstrated negative iatrogenic effects (e.g., Dishion, McCord, & Poulin, 1999; Poulin, Dishion, & Burraston, 2001), are that participants have varying lengths of treatment experience and a staff person serves as a facilitator to moderate interactions as needed.

Most of the day is spent in school, usually on-site; the classroom experience is both educational and therapeutic and is considered to be an integral part of the community and therapeutic process. Increasingly, adolescent TCs are requiring that teachers become a part of the community, demonstrating familiarity with TC concepts, integrating with and maintaining relationships with other staff, and even participating in case conferences (Jainchill, 1997; Riddle, 1994). It is important that adolescents have a positive academic experience, in contrast to their pretreatment school history, and that they attain a level of education that will facilitate further training and preparation for successful functioning as an adult in society. It is also critical that they be enabled to integrate with their home school upon returning there.

The role of family

Historically, TCs excluded families (or other guardian figures) from the treatment of the target client, particularly during the first several months of treatment, on the premise that the individual had to have minimal "external" distractions to focus on personal recovery. Inclusion of the family in the therapeutic process was incremental, and the level of involvement depended upon the individual's progress in treatment. More recently, the importance of involving the family in the treatment process has been recognized as critical to a successful recovery (e.g., CASA, 2002; Drug Strategies, 2003; Liddle & Dakof, 1995; PLNDP, 2002). However, the family's role in the treatment process varies considerably among TCs, because of such factors as the distance of the program from the home, the level of resources, and the family itself (e.g., their level of functionality and willingness to participate in activities).

Family activities range from drug education workshops and parent support groups to multifamily groups involving the adolescent and individual family sessions. The last are sometimes planned early in treatment to help to identify relational issues that need to be addressed; subsequent individual sessions are scheduled as needed (e.g., crisis intervention). Contact between parents and children is regulated, with minimal contact permitted during the first weeks of treatment (i.e., phone calls), family visits to the program initiated within the first month, and home visits beginning after several months. Initial visits are day passes and the adolescent is escorted home by a senior resident; the length of the visit extends to overnight as the youth and family demonstrate their ability to manage these experiences. Most programs require a minimum of two successful overnight stays prior to considering the adolescent ready to complete the residential phase of treatment.

Continuity of care/after-care

Adolescent TCs recognize the complexity and difficulty involved in the transition back into the youth's home community. The theme of relapse prevention receives increased attention during the reentry level of residential treatment with both residents and their families, and it is reinforced during the post-residential continuing care phase. However, there are generally very limited resources available to provide for additional support with the intensity and structure that is needed as they make the final transition to their family, school, and community environment.

In summary, the unique impact of the TC on the adolescent drug treatment field is manifest in several ways. Typically, youths who enter residential TCs for treatment need to be removed from their home environments for reasons ranging from the severity of their drug use and other behavioral problems to family issues. The clients served by TCs are distinguished by the severity of their problems, reflected in the fact that the large majority would be incarcerated if they did not enter residential TCs. The treatment model is distinguished by its communal approach to healing: with the emphasis on mutual help and the use of community and all of its members (staff and clients) as agents of therapeutic change. In the social learning context of the TC, adolescents are *habilitated* as much as rehabilitated, in a process that teaches "right living," guiding how they relate to themselves as individuals, to peers, to significant others, and to the larger society (De Leon, 2000). The tools of the TC emphasize the emotional, educational, and psychological strengths of community to facilitate personal maturation and recovery, in a physically and psychologically safe therapeutic context. Although the model typically has been identified as a stand-alone residential approach for this high-risk population, its potential for dissemination is being demonstrated through its adaptation and transportation to a variety of settings, including, for example, schools and juvenile justice facilities.

Adolescent therapeutic communities in the twenty-first century

Adolescents who enter drug-free residential TCs include young people with the most severe substance abuse problems, for whom drug use has already precipitated serious dysfunctionality in their lives. As reflected in the American Society of Addiction Medicine's (1996) patient placement criteria, those assigned to residential treatment must present with serious resistance to accepting treatment or a recovery environment and have high relapse potential. As a number of investigators have reported, adolescents in residential treatment manifest a greater severity of problems across a range of dimensions, such as psychological, substance use, environmental, legal, and developmental (e.g., Dennis *et al.*, 2003; Jainchill *et al.*, 2000). Consequently, there are challenges that are unique to the treatment of adolescents in TCs. First, most of the adolescents who enter treatment do so reluctantly, often under legal pressure, and they lack intrinsic motivation for personal change (e.g., Jainchill *et al.*, 1995; Szapocznik *et al.*, 1988). Second, they typically present with more problems both in terms of their drug use history and their level of antisocial behavior and psychopathology (e.g., Hawke *et al.*, 2000; Jainchill, 1997; Jainchill *et al.*, 1995). Third, these youth are particularly unprepared for the developmental demands they face; they are at a developmental stage when ideally they should be initiating steps toward autonomy and independence from parents (e.g., O'Malley, 1990); however, functionally they remain dependent and most often must return to their families of origin after treatment. Treatment programs assume the role of facilitating/guiding the range of developmental transitions including (a) physical/cognitive, (b) affiliative (i.e., changes in relationships with peers, parents, partners), (c) achievement (i.e., school, work), and (d) identity transitions (i.e., self-definition, self-regulation) (Schulenberg *et al.*, 2001).

The TCs for adolescents range in terms of their size (20–200), their location (rural, urban, suburban), their planned duration of treatment (6 months to over 1 year), and the demographic profile of the clients served (gender, race, ethnicity, and age at admission). There is also variability in the primary drug problem reported by admissions to treatment. Males make up approximately 70–75% of admissions to residential TCs and about 50% is Euro-American; however, the race and ethnic distribution among programs varies. The age range of the youth is 13–18 years, with a minority of programs having a ceiling age of entry to treatment of 20 years of age. The majority report marijuana as their primary substance of abuse upon entry into treatment; however, there are geographic differences in the distribution of drugs used. For example, use of amphetamines and other "uppers" is more commonly found among admissions to programs located on the west coast.

Many high-risk youth come from communities and homes that are not supportive of a prosocial lifestyle, and to address their substance use and concomitant problems it is necessary to remove them from their home environments and communities of origin. Although there has been growing opposition among service providers from other orientations to the idea that it is ever necessary to remove a young person from the family environment, residential TCs are a necessary and credible option for treatment for a significant proportion of youth. Clinical input, research, funding, and policy will influence the evolution of the adolescent TC in the twenty-first century. It is incumbent upon those involved with this treatment modality to address the unanswered questions that remain pertaining to the efficacy and effectiveness of the TC approach in order to assure continued support for these programs.

Following is a presentation of several of the critical methodological and clinical issues that should be the focus of future studies related to the client and the treatment, derived from the literature and from data obtained from a study of adolescent admissions to TC treatment conducted by the author and colleagues (e.g., Dennis *et al.*, 2003; Jainchill *et al.*, 1995, 1999, 2000; Onken, Blaine & Battjes, 1997).

Methodological issues

The major methodological issue that persists is that, to date, there have been no studies that have utilized random assignment of adolescents to residential TC treatment versus other treatment conditions, residential or otherwise. A number of important questions need to be addressed that require random assignment, including the comparative effectiveness of residential TCs versus other residential treatments for youth, the optimal planned length of stay in residential TCs for adolescents (treatment conditions can vary by planned duration), the comparative effectiveness of different TC programs, and the comparative effectiveness of residential TCs versus non-residential TCs.

The Adolescent Treatment Models project was launched by SAMHSA to support evaluations of 10 different treatment programs. The goals, as elaborated by Dennis and colleagues (2003), are relevant to the TC: to identify currently existing potentially exemplary models; to develop manuals that can be disseminated and utilized by other programs; to collaborate on cross-site comparisons; and to evaluate the effectiveness, cost and cost-effectiveness of these programs. This effort involves program evaluation rather than controlled studies and includes several residential TC programs. As a "demonstration" project, it can serve as a template for similar studies involving a range of TCs, to identify the exemplary TCs in the field, to develop manuals, and to conduct controlled studies of these programs.

Clinical issues

Process studies are needed to address the questions of what works, and for whom does it work. Studies utilizing random assignment within a residential TC to assess the efficacy or effectiveness of specific clinical interventions are needed. For example, the provision of individual counseling is relatively new to TCs, and staffing constraints still limit its use. An unanswered question is whether adolescents who participate in regularly scheduled individual counseling sessions do better than those who do not, taking into consideration therapeutic alliance, counseling protocols, etc. A corollary question is what are the components of effective encounter groups and are some youth more susceptible to the possibly negative iatrogenic effects of the peer group process than others?

Below are other issues that need to be addressed, which relate more to specific client and treatment process issues.

Client issues

Several key issues highlight the multivariate and complex needs of youth who enter residential TCs for treatment of substance use. First, aside from their substance use, the majority of youth also presents with serious juvenile justice involvement. About 70% are mandated to treatment by the judicial system. Their average age of first involvement with any kind of illegal activity is 11.8 years; the literature suggests that the earlier onset of criminal activity is associated with a poorer prognosis for an adulthood lifestyle described by prosocial attitudes and behaviors (e.g., Elliot, 1994). Corollary antisocial behaviors are indicated by the high percentage (87%) of youth who have been suspended or expelled from school, with an average of nine occurrences.

Second, the peer network of these adolescents is a classically deviant one; for example, 75% reported that they have friends who have gone to jail, and almost 47% stated that their friends "always/almost always" use street drugs. In this sample 95% were sexually active, reporting multiple partners (usually with a known person), and at least half of the activity was unprotected (Jainchill *et al.*, 1999).

Finally, these youth enter treatment with a variety of psychological and psychiatric problems in addition to their drug use. Although they typically do not present with severe DSM (American Psychiatric Association (1987)) axis I disorders (e.g., schizophrenia, bipolar disorder), most (85–90%) enter treatment with at least one psychiatric diagnosis not related to substance use (Jainchill, De Leon, & Yagelka, 1997). The most frequently occurring diagnoses are conduct disorder (~57%), oppositional defiant disorder (49%), separation anxiety (32%), attention-deficit hyperactivity (~25%), overanxious disorder (23%), current major depression (~21%), and dysthymia (~21% each). There are significant gender and race/ethnicity differences in diagnostic profiles. A significantly greater proportion of females yield diagnoses across all dimensions of disturbance (developmental/behavioral, affective, and anxiety disorders), and Euro-Americans who enter treatment present with a level of psychiatric disturbance that is significantly greater than Hispanics/Latinos and African-Americans.

Studies need to examine whether different clinical protocols need to target different "types" of client who enter treatment. For example, adolescents whose drug involvement is accompanied by more severe psychiatric and emotional disturbance can be distinguished from those who manifest more antisocial behaviors (e.g., poor school performance, negative peer networks, more criminal activity). Within the context of a TC approach, modifications to the therapeutic protocol to address these differences need to be implemented and evaluated.

Treatment issues

The evolution of the TC in general, and the adolescent TC specifically, has been in response to a number of factors, for example a changing client profile, funding exigencies, and policy recommendations. Many high-risk youths have entered residential TCs for treatment as a result of the need to remove them from their home environments. Up to now, TCs have been seen as a stand-alone and well-established treatment modality that targets a range of risk factors that are critical to the recovery process. However, a growing body of literature, including studies that have focused on long-term residential programs, have shown that a large percentage of youth leave residential treatment before completion, and others who complete TC treatment do not necessarily maintain their recovery (e.g., Jainchill *et al.*, 1995, 2000). Although there are significant reductions in drug use and criminal activity after treatment compared with pretreatment among those who complete treatment, as well as improvements (though smaller) among youth who leave prior to completion, often the gains experienced during residential treatment are not sustained (e.g., Jainchill *et al.*, 2000).

There are several possible explanations. First, these youth may not have attained the therapeutic goals necessary to maintain abstinence upon their return to the natural environment because they were in treatment for an insufficient period of time. Second, the therapeutic program may not address all of the issues relevant to enhancing the possibility for a stable recovery. Third, the post-residential environment may be embedded with a number of risk factors that require further intervention. For example, a disturbed family milieu (e.g., parental or sibling drug use, conflict), neighborhoods with social norms that are favorable to drug use, or school settings that are insufficiently resourced to work effectively with these youth will challenge the maintenance of prosocial behaviors and attitudes. These findings suggest that the optimal treatment tenure is not yet established and that TCs alone may not be sufficient for successful treatment of a large number of high-risk, drug-involved youth.

The planned duration of treatment has been steadily reducing since the early 1990s. The amount of time required to address the spectrum of issues with which an adolescent presents, and to attain the identified therapeutic goals, is unknown and likely variable. Although one of the most consistent findings across more than 20 years of research on adult TCs is the positive relationship between treatment tenure and post-treatment outcomes (e.g., De Leon, 1991; De Leon et al., 1982; Pompi, 1994), the relationship between treatment process variables, client factors, and treatment tenure needs further understanding. This is especially true for adolescents, for whom there have been few if any controlled studies involving TCs, and for whom similar though less-consistent findings have been obtained (e.g., DATOS; Jainchill et al., 2000). Among treatment programs that have been established for adolescents, the question of treatment tenure is critical for several reasons. First, there is the concern that adolescents are removed from their family of origin for the minimal length of time needed to affect positive and stable change. Second, the larger context of adolescent development presents unique challenges and developmental tasks, such as learning essential social skills, acquiring the emotional maturity necessary for successful relationships, and achieving necessary educational and vocational goals to move forward into productive adulthood (Drug Strategies, 2003). On the one hand, the demands of adolescent habilitation as elaborated suggest that a longer treatment tenure may be required; on the other hand, an extended out-of-home placement may not be recommended.

Policy issues

The future of TCs for adolescents requires that the parameters of treatment, both in terms of the structure and the kinds of service, be reconsidered. In particular, TCs need to be conceptualized not as a "stand alone" intervention but as a part of a more holistic and integrated treatment recovery process. The therapeutic model needs to provide a continuity-of-care approach that extends and enhances the therapeutic process beyond the residential context, and that redefines the role of the residential experience. Although a reintegration component is typically part of the residential treatment plan, it is also typical that only a few adolescents attend such programs and even fewer complete them (e.g., Alford, Koehler & Leonard, 1991, Godley, Godley and Dennis, 2001). This may be related to several factors, such as inherently low motivation on the part of the adolescent; the geographic distance from the adolescent's home community to the after-care setting; and the array of problems in addition to substance abuse, including family problems, that present challenges to continuing in treatment (e.g., Godley et al., 2001).

Furthermore, historically transitional programs have been considered secondary to the residential phase of treatment, resulting in a serious lack of funding and minimal services. Efforts to engage youth and their significant others in a post-residential intervention have lacked commitment and resources. An effective multidimensional after-care strategy must be an integral part of the therapeutic process, addressing the diversity of factors related to the individual and to the social environment. Reintegration must focus on issues of engagement and motivation, psychiatric problems, family relations, social skills and peer relationships, and linkages with community agencies to support recovery (e.g., schools, mental health settings, medical services).

The residential TC provides the foundation necessary toward establishing and maintaining a prosocial lifestyle; however, the transition back to the family and community of origin, with the subsequent involvement of the family, the original social environment, and associated institutions, is essential for appropriate personal and social development. The length of time in residential treatment required to ready the adolescent for successful reintegration into the outside community depends on the severity of an individual's problems as well as the available support system (e.g., family, after-care services).

The role of the *family* in the treatment process has been identified as critical (e.g., Drug Strategies, 2003; PLNDP, 2002; Williams & Chang, 2000), and TCs must identify the type of family involvement that will be most effective during the residential phase of treatment compared with family participation during the continuity-of-care phase. Strategies for working with families with varying levels of dysfunction or problems, including parental or sibling substance use, physical or sexual abuse, and other antisocial behaviors, are essential and further the evolutionary development of the TC clinically and philosophically. Many programs encounter challenges in working with adolescents' families: the home may be distant from the program, making it difficult for parents or others to attend activities; parents may be non-compliant for a variety of reasons such as their own substance use or other personal issues, work schedules, or the demands of other children who are at home; and sometimes they have been worn down and do not want contact with their child. Consequently, the challenge of the TC is to educate, engage, and motivate family members to understand and become a part of the treatment process.

Family therapy approaches that have theoretical and clinical origins external to the TC, for example Functional Family Therapy (Sexton & Alexander, 2002), Multidimensional Family Therapy (Rowe & Liddle, 2003), and brief strategic family therapy (Szapocznik *et al.*, 1988), offer evidence-based treatment strategies that can be integrated with TC treatment, particularly as continuity-of-care protocols. Current studies initiated by the author are investigating the efficacy and effectiveness of this kind of integrative strategy. For example, family interventions are being introduced subsequent to the primary residential treatment phase to facilitate the youth's transition to the home community and support a sustained recovery. The TC is not regarded as a stand-alone intervention but is part of a therapeutic continuum. The involvement of the family is incremental and becomes the focus of the therapeutic process when the youth returns home to his/her community of origin. An issue that is raised is how to incorporate approaches that have conflicting perspectives without violating their respective philosophies. As an example, on the one hand, the TC will not work with a parent or significant other who attends any therapy session or meeting under the influence of drugs or alcohol; on the other hand, most family therapy approaches will involve the individual in the session and incorporate the drug use into the therapeutic activity. The resolution of these differences (i.e., whether modifications to extant treatment protocols are implemented) needs to be delineated and assessed.

Family therapy approaches offer an ideal "after-care" component to be integrated with residential TC treatment, addressing the serious *continuity of care* needs of youth and their families. As the average planned duration of stay has decreased, adolescents are returning to their families, and less frequently to independent living situations, with an increasing need for continuing treatment services. In the past, these services have received neither the funding nor the attention now recognized as critical to a sustained recovery.

An ideal after-care program may be phased in the intensity of services provided, beginning with almost daily attendance by the adolescent, involving two or three groups each week as well as an individual counseling session and recreational activities. Adolescents reduce their involvement in after-care services (e.g., once weekly group and individual sessions) after demonstrating continued abstinence from drugs and a pattern of prosocial behaviors. A critical component of an after-care program is to facilitate access to other services that might be needed by the adolescent (e.g., mental health, vocational training) and to maintain communication with the youth's school and other relevant institutions.

Conclusions

The clinical and policy issues that have been reviewed and reflected in the proposed set of research directions identify the gaps that remain in the knowledge base, and what specific studies need to be done for the TC approach to have continued impact on the field. These priorities, in summary, include the need to (a) establish the effectiveness of the approach using randomized controlled trial designs; (b) conduct economic evaluations to address funding/policy questions; (c) examine moderators/mediators of immediate and long-term outcomes (e.g., typologies that differentiate youth along dimensions of psychiatric disturbance and antisocial behavior); (d) explore treatment process questions; and (e) design studies of integrative continuum-of-care models.

The TCs for adolescents vary along a number of dimensions including, for example, the size of the static population, treatment tenure, location (rural, urban, suburban), and resources (staff:client ratio, school facilities, etc.). There is also considerable variability among the youth who are admitted to residential TCs in terms of race/ethnic distribution, socioeconomic status, and primary drug abused; these differences generally reflecting regional differences of the programs. More importantly, perhaps, is that there is heterogeneity among the adolescents who enter treatment, irrespective of the program, that needs to be identified and responded to in terms of clinical interventions within the TC.

There is a critical need to codify the adolescent TC and to formalize the model through the development of a treatment manual that can both guide practice and serve as a research tool for assessment of adherence and fidelity to its implementation. Studies need to be conducted that utilize random assignment procedures to address key questions concerning effectiveness and cost-effectiveness, and that compare the residential TC with other treatment options. Studies must also investigate the key process components of the treatment to answer questions regarding optimal length of treatment, the impact of group and individual interventions, the role of the therapeutic alliance, the role of family therapy and aftercare interventions, and how modifications to the "standard" model can be applied to subgroups of youth entering TC treatment with particular needs. The future of the TC will depend upon and be guided by the implementation and outcomes of such studies.

REFERENCES

Alford, G. S., Koehler, R. A., & Leonard, J. (1991). Alcoholics Anonymous/Narcotics Anonymous inpatient treatment of chemically dependent adolescents: a 2-year outcome study. *Journal of Studies on Alcohol*, **52**, 118–126.

American Psychiatric Association (1987). *Diagnostic and statistical manual of mental disorders: DSM-III-R* (3rd ed.). Washington, DC: American Psychiatric Press.

American Society of Addiction Medicine (1996). *Patient Placement Criteria (ASAM-PPC-2) Assessment Dimensions*. Chevy Chase, MD: American Society of Addiction Medicine.

CASA (National Center on Addiction and Substance Abuse) (2002). *National Survey of American Attitudes on Substance Abuse VII: Teens, Parents and Siblings*. New York: Columbia University Press.

De Leon, G. (1986). The therapeutic community for substance abuse: perspective and approach. In G. De Leon & J. T. Zeigenfuss (eds.), *Therapeutic Communities for Addictions: Readings in Theory, Research and Practice* (pp. 8–18). Springfield, IL: Charles C. Thomas.

  (1991). Retention in drug free therapeutic communities. In R. W. Pickens, C. G. Leukefeld, & C. R. Schuster (eds.), *Research Monograph* No. 106: *Improving Drug Abuse Treatment* (pp. 218–244). Rockville, MD: National Institute on Drug Abuse.

  (1997). Therapeutic communities: is there an essential model? In G. De Leon (ed.) *Community as Method: Therapeutic Communities for Special Populations and Special Settings* (pp. 3–18). Westport, CT: Praeger.

(2000). *The Therapeutic Community: Theory, Model, and Method.* New York: Springer.

De Leon, G., Wexler, H. K., & Jainchill, N. (1982). Success and improvement rates 5 years after treatment in a therapeutic community. *International Jounal of Addictions,* **17,** 703–742.

Dennis, M. L., Dawus-Noursi, S., Muck, R. D., & McDermeit, M. (2003). The need for developing and evaluating adolescent treatment models. In S. J. Stevens & A. R. Morral (eds.), *Adolescent Substance Abuse Treatment in the United States: Exemplary Models from a National Evaluation Study.* Binghamton, NY: Haworth Press.

Dishion, T. J., McCord, J., & Poulin, F. (1999). When interventions harm: peer groups and problem behavior. *American Psychologist,* **554,** 755–764.

Drug Strategies (2003). *Treating Teens: A Guide to Adolescent Drug Programs.* Washington, DC: Drug Strategies.

Elliot, D. S. (1994). Serious violent offenders: onset, developmental course, and termination. *Criminology,* **32,** 1–22.

Godley, S. H., Godley, M. D., & Dennis, M. L. (2001). The Assertive Aftercare Protocol for adolescent substance abusers. In E. Wagner & H. Waldron (eds.), *Innovations in Adolescent Substance Abuse Interventions* (pp. 313–331). New York: Elsevier Science.

Grella, C. E., Hser, Y. I., Joshi, V., & Rounds-Bryant, J. (2000). Drug treatment outcomes for adolescents with comorbid mental and substance use disorders. *Journal of Nervous and Mental Disease,* **189,** 384–392.

Hawke, J., Jainchill, N., & De Leon, G. (2000). The prevalence of sexual abuse and its impact on the onset of drug use among adolescents in therapeutic community drug treatment. *Journal of Child and Adolescent Substance Abuse,* **9,** 35–49.

Hser, Y. I., Grella, C. E., Hubbard, R. L., *et al.* (2001). An evaluation of drug treatments for adolescents in four USA cities. *Archives of General Psychiatry,* **58,** 689–695.

Hubbard, R. L., Cavanaugh, E. A., Craddock. S. F., & Rachal, J. V. (1985). Characteristics, behaviors and outcomes for youth in the TOPS. In A. S. Friedman & G. M. Beschner (eds.), *Treatment Services for Adolescent Substance Abusers* (pp. 49–65). Rockville, MD: National Institute on Drug Abuse.

Jainchill, N. (1997). Therapeutic communities for adolescents: the same and not the same. In G. De Leon (ed.), *Healing Communities* (pp. 161–177). Westford, CT: Greenwood Press.

(2000). Substance dependency treatment for adolescents: practice and research. *Substance Use and Misuse,* **35,** 2031–2060.

Jainchill, N., Bhattacharya, G., & Yagelka, J. (1995). Therapeutic communities for adolescents. In E. Rahdert & D. Czechowicz (eds.), *Research Monograph* No. 156: *Adolescent Drug Abuse: Clinical Assessment and Therapeutic Interventions* (pp. 190–217). Rockville, MD: National Institute on Drug Abuse.

Jainchill, N., De Leon, G., & Yagelka, J. (1997). Ethnic differences in psychiatric disorders among adolescent substance abusers in treatment. *Journal of Psychopathology and Behavioral Assessment,* **19,** 133–148.

Jainchill, N., Yagelka, J., Hawke, J., & De Leon, G. (1999). Adolescent admissions to residential drug treatment: HIV risk behaviors pre- and post-treatment. *Psychology of Addictive Behaviors,* **13,** 163–173.

Jainchill, N., Hawke, J., De Leon, G., & Yagelka, J. (2000). Adolescents in TCs: one year post-treatment outcomes. *Journal of Psychoactive Drugs*, **32**, 81–94.

Jainchill. N., Hawke, J., & Holland, S. (2001). Adolescent drug abuse: long-term post-treatment outcomes. In *Proceedings of the 2001 Annual Meeting of the College on Problems of Drug Dependence*, Tucson.

Liddle, H. A. & Dakof, G. A. (1995). Efficacy of family therapy for drug abuse: promising but not definitive. *Journal of Marital and Family Therapy*, **21**, 511–543.

Melnick, G., De Leon, G., Hawke, J., Jainchill, N., & Kressel, D. (1997). Motivation and readiness for therapeutic community treatment among adolescent and adult substance abusers. *American Journal of Drug and Alcohol Abuse*, **23**, 485–506.

Myers, M. G., Stewart, D. G., & Brown, S. A. (1998). Progression from conduct disorder to antisocial personality disorder following treatment for adolescent substance abuse. *Journal of Psychiatry*, **155**, 479–485.

O'Malley, F. (1990). Developing a therapeutic alliance in the hospital treatment of disturbed adolescents. *Bulletin of the Menninger Clinic*, **54**, 13–24.

Onken, L. S., Blaine, J. D., & Battjes, R. J. (1997). Behavioral therapy research: a conceptualization of a process. In S. W. Henggeler & A. B. Santos (eds.), *Innovative Approaches for the Difficult-to-treat Populations* (pp. 477–485). Washington, DC: American Psychiatric Press.

Ottenberg, D. (ed.) (1984). The therapeutic community today: A moment of reflection on its evolution. In *Proceedings of the First World Institute of Therapeutic Communities*, Castel Gandolfo, Italy. Montréal: Portage Press.

PLNDP (Physician Leadership on National Drug Policy (2002)). *Adolescent Substance Abuse: A Public Health Priority*. Providence, RI: Brown University.

Pompi, R. F. (1994). Adolescents in therapeutic communities: retention and post-treatment outcome. In F. M. Tims, G. De Leon, & N. Jainchill (eds.), *Research Monograph* No. 144: *Therapeutic Community: Advances in Research and Application* (pp. 128–162). Rockville, MD: National Institute on Drug Abuse.

Poulin, F., Dishion, T. J., & Burraston, B. (2001). Three-year iatrogenic effects associated with aggregating high-risk adolescents in cognitive-behavioral preventive interventions. *Applied Developmental Science*, **5**, 214–224.

Riddle, K. (1994). Adaptations of the therapeutic community model for adolescents. In *Proceedings of the Therapeutic Communities of America 1992 Planning Conference: Paradigms: Past, Present and Future*. Providence, RI: Manisses Communications.

Rowe, C. L. & Liddle, H. A. (2003). Substance abuse. *Journal of Marital and Family Therapy*, **29**, 97–120.

Schulenberg, J., Maggs, J. L., Steinman, K., & Zucker, R. A. (2001). Development matters: taking the long view on substance abuse etiology and intervention during adolescence. In P. M. Monti, S. M. Colby, & O'Leary, T. A. (eds.), *Adolescents and Substance Abuse* (pp. 19–57). New York: Guilford Press.

Sells, S. B. & Simpson, D. D. (1979). Evaluation of treatment outcomes for youths in the Drug Abuse Reporting Program (DARP): a followup study. In G. M. Beschner & A. S. Friedman (eds.), *Youth Drug Abuse* (pp. 571–628). Lexington, MA: Lexington Books.

Sexton, T. L. & Alexander, J. F. (2002). Functional family therapy for at-risk adolescents and their families. In T. Patterson & F. Kaslow (series eds.), *Comprehensive Handbook of Psychotherapy*, Vol II: *Cognitive–Behavioral Approaches* (pp. 117–140). New York: John Wiley.

Szapocznik, J., Perez-Vidal, A., Brickman, A., *et al.* (1988). Engaging adolescent drug abusers and their families into treatment: a strategic structural systems approach. *Journal of Consulting and Clinical Psychology*, **56**, 552–557.

Williams, R. J. & Chang, S. Y. (2000). A comprehensive and comparative review of adolescent substance abuse treatment outcomes. *Clinical Psychology: Science and Practice*, **7**, 138–166.

Winters, K. C. (1999). Treating adolescents with substance use disorders: an overview of practice issues and treatment outcomes. *Substance Abuse*, **20**, 203–225.

Yalom, I. D. (1975). *The Theory and Practice of Group Psychotherapy*. New York: Basic Books.

16

School-based group treatment for adolescent substance abuse

Eric F. Wagner and Mark J. Macgowan

Florida International University, Miami, FL, USA

The extant empirical literature indicates that treatment for adolescent alcohol and other drug (AOD) abuse (a) can succeed for adolescents with AOD use problems, (b) produces treatment outcomes comparable to those found among adults with AOD use problems, (c) yields varied improvement across different domains of functioning (e.g., school performance, emotional distress, family relations), and (d) does not differ substantially among treatments in the probability of success, with the possible exception of outpatient family therapy, which might lead to better outcomes in outpatient populations (Brown *et al.*, 1996; Catalano *et al.*, 1990–1991; Wagner, Myers, & Mclninch, 1999a; Williams *et al.*, 2000). The literature also indicates that half of teenagers treated for substance use problems will relapse within 3 months of the completion of treatment, and two-thirds will relapse within 6 months (Brown, Mott, & Myers, 1990; Brown, Vik, & Creamer, 1989). Therefore, treatment can be effective for teenagers with AOD use problems, but relapse rates remain high, with most treated adolescents returning to substance use between 3 and 6 months after the completion of treatment.

While there is empirical support for the effectiveness of several adolescent AOD abuse treatments, many studies document the high level of unmet needs among substance abusers. Recent estimates suggest that only one out of every ten adolescents with a substance use problem receives treatment (Clark *et al.*, 2002; Dennis *et al.*, 2003). Part of the reason why so few adolescents in need of treatment actually receive it is a reliance on "the traditional service-delivery model" (Wagner, Swensen, & Henggeler, 2000). The traditional service-delivery model involves trained professionals treating teenagers with AOD problems and their families in clinics located in hospitals, universities, or other institutional settings. In the traditional service-delivery model, clients first must present to the clinic to receive services. Since substance-abusing adolescents rarely recognize the need for treatment, parents and other influential adults bear the responsibility for pursuing treatment. For some adults and for many reasons (e.g., time conflicts, lack of

Adolescent Substance Abuse: Research and Clinical Advances, ed. Howard A. Liddle and Cynthia L. Rowe.
Published by Cambridge University Press. © Cambridge University Press 2006.

knowledge, estrangement from the adolescent, personal substance use problems, reluctance to accept the label "substance abuser" for their child), the steps for accessing traditional treatment can be daunting and a barrier to receiving services. Ultimately, a reliance on the traditional service-delivery model substantially contributes to the high level of unmet treatment needs among adolescents with AOD abuse. This is especially true for ethnic minority and economically disadvantaged teenagers and their families, which are groups even less likely than their non-Hispanic White counterparts to utilize available services (Aguirre-Molina & Caetano, 1994; Giachello, 1994; Neighbors, 1985). One reason ethnic minority teenagers and their families may avoid the traditional services available to them is because they perceive them to be culturally insensitive.

Why use schools for delivery of substance abuse treatment

Given the inherent limitations of the traditional clinic-based service delivery model, alternative community-based approaches to providing adolescent AOD treatment are receiving increasing attention (Brown, 2001; Wagner, Kortlander, & Leon Morris, 2001a). A community-based treatment approach growing rapidly in popularity is the school-based service-delivery model. School-based treatments can take place at one or multiple levels, including individuals, classrooms, existing social groups (e.g., the football team, the marching band), purposely assembled social groups (e.g., students with substance use problems, children of alcoholics), and/or the entire school. Emory Cowen (1977), a pioneer in school-based mental health service delivery, has described the school-based treatment approach as the practice of community mental health with the school being the "community."

An important strength of the school-based treatment model is that it goes where most adolescents spend most of their weekday mornings and early afternoons most of the time. This approach circumvents many of the potential barriers to accessing more traditional services and should result in more adolescents in need of treatment actually receiving it. In addition, the school-based treatment model is ecologically stronger than traditional service-delivery model. School-based treatments provide an unique opportunity to assess and influence directly the proximal determinants and consequences of substance abuse in one of the more important natural environments in which such problems occur (for more detail on this perspective, see Wagner *et al.* [2000]). Finally, the school-based treatment model, relative to the traditional service-delivery model, has developmental advantages in that services are provided in a very high-impact social environment for influencing the psychosocial growth and adaptation of youth (Cowen, 1977).

A number of other potential advantages of school-based treatments relative to traditional clinic-based treatments are also noteworthy. First, by meeting teenagers and their families in a familiar environment (i.e., the school that the adolescent attends on a daily basis), therapeutic engagement may be enhanced. While not all adolescents like being at school, they do know where the school is and where specific rooms are within the school, and they can contact the main office for information about available services. Second, clinical assessment in school contexts may have greater validity for identifying the causes and consequences of substance use specific to the school environment, which, in turn, can lead to more valid and individualized treatment plans than those that do not take the immediate peer environment into account. Third, clinical outcome data may better reflect actual day-to-day functioning, as clinicians and researchers can directly evaluate behavioral changes in the school settings in which some of the target problem behaviors occurred. Finally, school-based treatments may be more responsive to the clients' individual needs, as both the treatment and the individual reside in, contribute to, and are influenced by the same school community.

The major disadvantage of school-based treatments is that adolescents need to be attending school to receive treatment. School-based treatments necessarily do not reach school drop-outs or school truants, who constitute groups at particularly high risk for alcohol and other drug involvement (McCluskey *et al.*, 2002). However, school-based surveys indicate that a small but significant proportion of students at middle and high school uses substances frequently enough and in large enough quantities to lead to negative consequences (Harrison, Fulkerson, & Beebe, 1998; Lewinsohn *et al.*, 1993). For example, Harrison *et al.* (1998) found that 13.8% of school-attending ninth graders and 22.7% of school-attending twelfth graders in Minnesota met DSM-IV criteria (American Psychiatric Association, 1994) for substance use problems at some point during the previous year. This translates to more than one of out of every eight ninth-grade students and more than one out of every five twelfth-grade students demonstrating diagnosable substance use disorders each year. Most of these students do not receive any formal substance abuse assessment or treatment, either in school or elsewhere. A second possible disadvantage of school-based treatments is the potential for stigmatization of substance-abusing youth within the school environment, though this can be substantially reduced by taking care in when and where treatment takes place during the school day.

Based on the putative strengths and advantages of school-based treatment described above, our research group has begun to explore the effectiveness of school-based treatments for addressing substance use problems among teenagers. The current chapter describes this recent work, with particular attention to current knowledge about successful school-based treatments for a range of problem behaviors, student assistance programs (SAPs; the most popular school-based treatment for adolescent substance use problems), the development and testing of a standardized SAP, the putative mechanisms of change in SAPs, and the future directions for research in this area.

What is known about effective school-based treatments?

There is a large and varied literature regarding the effectiveness of school-based treatments for psychosocial problems experienced by teenagers (for greater detail, see Wagner, Tubman, & Gil [2004]). The literature includes both single-focus programs (i.e., interventions designed to address a single problem, for example depression) and cross-cutting programs (i.e., interventions designed to address several interrelated problems simultaneously, for example substance abuse, truancy, and delinquency), as well as programs targeting individuals, classrooms, or entire schools (Durlak, 1997). While school-based treatment programs vary widely on a number of parameters (e.g., scope, targets for change, core change-producing procedures), a recent review of effective school-based treatments identified 10 key factors shared by effective school-based treatment programs (Wagner et al., 2004). Five of these factors involve conceptual and methodological issues associated with launching treatment programs in school environments, and five additional factors concern issues related to "buy-in" from stakeholders, consumer satisfaction, and the generalization of skills and competencies to "real life" domains.

First, effective school-based treatments possess a strong theoretical foundation and a clear conceptual basis for describing, predicting, and interpreting normative and non-normative patterns of development (i.e., they have the capacity to account for change in patterns of adaptive and maladaptive behavior) (Cicchetti & Toth, 1992). Second, effective school-based treatment programs incorporate rigorous evaluation plans in order to document the impact of treatment on participants and to identify areas in need of further development (Lipsey & Cordray, 2000). Third, effective school-based treatments combine educational components regarding the development, maintenance, and consequences of problem behavior with therapeutic components targeting the development of skills and competencies intended to replace targeted behaviors or to protect adolescents when confronted with high-risk situations (Bruvold, 1993; Cuijpers, 2002; Hansen, 1992; Tobler & Stratton, 1997; Tobler et al., 1999, 2000). Fourth, effective school-based treatments are carefully conceived in terms of the timing, duration, frequency, and intensity of exposure to treatment, each of which is a critical parameter in determining the ultimate effectiveness of treatment (Kirby, 1997). Fifth, effective school-based treatment programs incorporate standard procedures such as treatment manuals, therapist supervision, and systematic session review for ensuring fidelity in the implementation of core program components.

The sixth factor, and the first of the second set of factors identified, is that successful school-based treatment programs encourage full participation from, and provide training opportunities for, professional staff, teachers, and other school personnel in program development, implementation, and evaluation (Cowen *et al.*, 1983; Glynn, 1989; Perhats *et al.*, 1996; Rohrbach *et al.*, 1996; St. Pierre, 2001). Seventh, effective school-based programs are designed to engage consumers (e.g., adolescents with substance use problems) through the use of developmentally congruent and culturally relevant materials (Wagner, 2003). Eighth, staff of effective school-based treatment programs constantly seek program-related feedback from school and other program stakeholders and make appropriate adjustments to their programs in response to negative feedback or lack of interest (Gingiss, Gottlieb, & Brink, 1994). Ninth, effective treatment programs, and in particular those seeking to reduce current levels of harmful behavior (e.g., substance use and abuse), are most effective when backed by school-wide structures such as written policies or other organizational changes that are enforced at all levels of the school (e.g., CDC, 1994, 1999). Finally, effective school-based treatment programs promote the practice, assimilation, and generalization of socially competent and appropriate behaviors in key domains in which children are developing (e.g., family, neighborhood, and peer networks).

The student assistance program

The most commonly employed school-based treatment approach for adolescent AOD problems is the SAP. It has been estimated that well over 1500 USA school systems employ SAPs (Wagner *et al.*, 1999b). Schools with SAPs number in the thousands, and tens of thousands of students come in contact with SAPs each year. SAPs are modeled after employee assistance programs (Foote & Erfurt, 1991; Walsh *et al.*, 1991) and include (a) mechanisms for early identification of students with AOD problems and (b) methods for secondary and tertiary prevention of adverse consequences associated with those problems. SAPs were developed to address substance use and related problems among middle and senior high school students, and they involve procedures for identifying substance-abusing students, motivating these students to enter the program, intake and assessment, direct assistance (i.e., intervention) or referral for treatment, and follow-up. SAPs focus primarily on behavior and performance problems and intoxication at school as indicators of substance-related problems, and they tend to be somewhat eclectic in their assessment framework, conceptualization of dysfunction, theory of change, and intervention targets in terms of risk and protection. This eclecticism is reflected in basic conceptualizations of addiction (e.g., disease versus acquired habit), processes of change (e.g., working the 12-step program versus functional analysis of the "pros" and "cons" of using), and successful outcomes (e.g., abstinence versus harm reduction). However, SAPs are consistent in targeting substance use, academic performance, and school conduct for change, and in working with adolescents relatively early in their development of problems with alcohol and other drugs.

Given how widespread the use of SAPs is, it is probably not surprising that SAPs vary substantially in how they are run. Generally speaking, most SAPs fall into one of two categories. "Core team model" SAPs rely on trained school personnel to assess and identify students with AOD problems, and to refer students to outside treatment providers for treatment. These school personnel function as addiction treatment paraprofessionals, who for any of a number of reasons (e.g., personal interest, increased salary, assignment by superiors) become members of the SAP core team. In contrast, the "Westchester County, New York, model SAPs" rely on SAP specialty counselors, who assess and treat AOD-involved students at school. These counselors collaborate with school staff but are not themselves school employees, and they are professionals with specialized degrees in substance abuse and/or mental health treatment. Typically, in-school group counseling is the form of treatment provided by Westchester model SAPs (Morehouse, 1984). In addition to whether they follow one or other of these models, SAPs differ from one another in their descriptions, philosophies, staffing arrangements, student-processing procedures, and other structural and procedural features (e.g., the "Pennsylvania model" [Newman *et al.*, 1988–1989; DiRenzio, 1990]; the "Center of Alcohol Studies, Rutgers University SAP" [Milgram, 1989], "Project SCOPE" [Forman & Linney, 1988], the "Alcohol and Drug Defense Program" [Palmer & Paisley, 1991], the "Iowa Connection" [Simmering, 1991], and the "Westchester County, New York, model" [Morehouse, 1984]).

Because of the substantial variation across SAPs, it is difficult to ascertain their overall effectiveness for addressing AOD use problems. Moreover, the SAP literature generally has been devoted to reports concerning the specifics of conducting SAPs rather than to studies concerning the effectiveness of SAPs. Nonetheless, there are a few investigations that have evaluated SAP effectiveness, and provided preliminary evidence that certain SAPs can reduce AOD use and improve academic performance among substance-abusing adolescents (Carlson, Hughes, & Deebach, 1996; Carlson *et al.*, 1994; Morehouse, 1984; Wagner *et al.*, 1999b).

With funding from NIAAA, Morehouse (1984) developed and evaluated the Westchester County, New York, model SAP. Morehouse found that 63% of students who reported using alcohol and 94% of students who reported using marijuana at initial SAP referral reported abstinence from these drugs after SAP participation. Moreover, 50% of students who reported being drunk while in school prior to SAP participation treatment reported stopping this activity after

SAP participation. Finally, among those students who reported alcohol use at initial SAP referral, Morehouse found a statistically significant increase in school attendance from the 50-day marking period before SAP participation (less than 90% attendance) to the 50-day marking period after SAP participation (96% attendance).

Carlson and colleagues (1994, 1996) evaluated a Washington State SAP that utilized school-based treatment groups. SAP participant outcomes were assessed by counselors' ratings of improvement via a structured interview and by student self-reports. Based on counselors' reports, the majority of SAP participants ended their AOD involvement by the time they completed the program. Specifically, 57% of high school students, 51% of middle school students, and 24% of alternative school students were judged to be abstinent from AOD by the end of the school year in which they participated in the SAP. Middle school and alternative school students with the most serious AOD problems seemed to show the greatest response to SAP participations. By the end of the school year, 58% of the heaviest users (i.e., those judged to be substance dependent by the SAP counselors) in middle school were judged to be abstinent, and 73% of those in alternative schools were judged to be abstinent. However, the counselors concluded the program did not improve school attendance, academic performance, or school behavior. On a confidential survey concerning their AOD use conducted at the end of the school year, 65% of SAP participants reported no recent (i.e., within the last 30 days) alcohol use and 79% reported no recent use of drugs.

Finally, Wagner *et al.* (1999a) conducted a preliminary test of the Westchester model SAP treatment described later in this chapter. These investigators found that 86% of high school students who participated in the SAP reported stopping or significantly decreasing their substance use, and 73% rated their experience in the SAP as positive (Wagner *et al.*, 1999b). In addition, frequency of pretreatment alcohol use did not predict either the impact of the program or the participants' ratings of the SAP.

At least 37% of alcohol-abusing adolescents in Westchester County (Morehouse, 1984) and 56% of substance-abusing adolescents in Washington State (Carlson *et al.*, 1994, 1996) did not decrease their alcohol use in response to SAP participation. Unfortunately, neither group of investigators considered why SAPs were effective for some adolescents but not for others. Also, although these studies are promising in their attempts to evaluate the effectiveness of specific SAPs, all three investigations are marred by methodological weaknesses. None of these studies included a comparison or control group; utilized an experimental design; engaged in systematic, repeated, long-term follow-up of students who took part in the SAP; or evaluated students on standardized measures for alcohol and/or other drug use. Moreover, none of these studies included objective (i.e., biochemical) or collateral (e.g., parent) verification of self-reports or coun-selors' ratings of substance use. Furthermore, none of these studies attempted to isolate the mechanisms of change associated with their treatment or to investigate why certain students responded positively to SAP participation while others did not. In sum, published evaluations of SAPs suggest that these school-based treat-ments can be effective in reducing AOD use among some students; however, rigorous studies of the effectiveness of SAPs are sorely needed.

The Teen Intervention Project

Development of a standardized Westchester model student assistance program

Ellen Morehouse's (1984) original explication of the Westchester model laid the foundation for the development of similar SAPs across the country. While existing Westchester model SAPs have much in common with one another, they often vary in how counseling groups are assembled; the actual content, number, and sequen-cing of group sessions; and the supporting materials used by therapists and student participants. Such variation has represented a considerable challenge to conducting a rigorous clinical trial of SAP intervention, given that no manual or standardized materials have been available for systemically studying the approach. Consequently, standardization and manual development was the first necessary step in this research.

The theoretical basis of the standardized Westchester model group counseling intervention includes social learning theory (Bandura, 1977) and problem behavior theory (Jessor & Jessor, 1977). We hypothesized that multiple factors contribute to the development of substance use problems among teenagers, though we focused our intervention efforts on potentially modifiable environmental influences, beliefs and expectancies, and learned behaviors associated with AOD abuse among teen-agers. As a result, our standardized intervention includes student exercises exploring environmental influences, beliefs and expectancies, and learned behaviors associated with AOD abuse. In regard to the etiology and treatment of adolescent substance abuse, the intervention takes into consideration developmental factors with regard to AOD involvement. Therefore, it is acknowledged that some experimentation with drugs and/or alcohol may be normative (Johnston, O'Malley, & Bachman, 2002; Shedler & Block, 1990). However, teens deficient in coping skills to handle negative moods, to engage in comfortable social interactions, to generate positive feelings in the absence of alcohol and drug use, or to manage social pressures for substance involvement effectively are at a greater risk for developing problems (e.g., Bentler, 1992; Pandina & Schuele, 1983; Wagner et al., 1999a). These types of deficit characterize AOD-involved adolescents who are referred to SAPs and, therefore, are a focus of our treatment approach.

Like many current SAPs, our standardized intervention also incorporates material from motivational treatments that recognize the importance of client motivation to change in determining treatment engagement and treatment outcome (Miller & Rollnick, 1991). One way to enhance substance abusers' commitment to treatment is to allow them choices in approaches to, and goals for, treatment (Sobell & Sobell, 1993). Given most teenagers' preoccupation with the degree to which they, rather than others, are making choices about their lives, permitting adolescents to make choices in certain aspects of treatment may be especially important for increasing motivation to change. Therefore, our SAP materials incorporate motivational components designed to encourage student participants (a) to assess where they believe they are in regard to their current readiness to change and (b) to set both short- and long-term goals in regard to changing substance use and managing other areas of their lives (e.g., relationships, academics, career goals).

The intervention involves 10 weekly sessions, which sequentially present didactic material, discussion topics, and workbook exercises with the following objectives: (a) to educate participants about substance use and abuse, (b) to raise participants' awareness of the reasons underlying their use, (c) to understand the antecedents, consequences, and patterns associated with their personal use habits from a functional analysis perspective, (d) to set and meet goals for reduction or cessation of AOD use, and (e) to develop coping skills to manage stress and other factors related to use. The specific components of the intervention are presented in Table 16.1, and a session-by-session outline is presented in Table 16.2.

Like most Westchester model SAPs, we employ clinicians with at least a Masters degree who work collaboratively with school staff but who are not school employees. As often as possible, we hire therapists with experience in working with adolescents, conducting group therapy, and treating AOD use problems. We provide extensive training in implementing the treatment model and conduct weekly group supervision to address specific clinical concerns and help to ensure that our treatment is being implemented with fidelity. In the first week of training, therapists receive didactic instruction in how to conduct the treatment. In the second week of training, therapists conduct mock group sessions to practice intervention skills and receive feedback from the clinical supervisor as to areas of strength and areas in need of improvement. In the third week, therapists typically are assigned their first group. It should be noted we audiotape every therapy session and these audiotapes are rated on a session-by-session basis for adherence to the treatment manual. Drift from the manual is addressed according to need with our therapists in individual meetings with our clinical supervisor, as well in the weekly group supervision meetings.

Table 16.1 Specific components of the standardized Westchester model group counseling

Component	Content
Substance abuse education	Students are educated about substance use and the development of substance use problems
Recognition and acknowledgement of personal substance use problems	Students learn to connect current difficulties with substance use
Self-monitoring	Students monitor their own use of alcohol and other drugs
Commitment generation	Students commit to reducing or eliminating their alcohol and other drug use
Identification of high-risk situations	Students identify high-risk situations for substance use
Alternatives to substance use	Students develop alternative behaviors to substance use, with emphasis on high-risk for alcohol and other drugs use situations
Coping with stress	Students learn to recognize stress and develop strategies for coping with stress that do not involve substance use
Family conflict resolution	Students learn and rehearse ways to manage conflicts within their families
Relationship building	Students are given guidelines for initiating and developing reciprocal relationships with others
Abstinence-violation effect	Students learn to anticipate and cope with the negative emotional reaction that is likely to follow a slip and to prevent the slip from becoming a relapse
Practicing resistance/refusal	Students learn and rehearse ways to manage peer-related substance use situations
Social support	Students identify groups and individuals who will support their efforts to change their substance use behavior

Students may be referred to the SAP from any of a number of sources including teachers, administrators, school counselors, parents and/or the students themselves. Once a student has been referred, a clinical assessment specialist contacts parents and explains the intervention research program. Students whose parents consent to have their child involved in the program meet during school hours with the clinical assessor, who explains the program and seeks student assent. Those students who agree to participate are then assessed for AOD problems using standardized measures including the Drug-use Screening Inventory (Tarter & Hegedus, 1991) and the Time Line Follow-Back (Sobell & Sobell, 1992). To be

Table 16.2 Session-by-session outline of standardized Westchester model group counseling

Session No.	Session topic(s)
1	Group introduction and guidelines
2	Substance abuse education
3	Recognition and acknowledgment of personal substance use problems; self-monitoring of substance use
4	Identifying high-risk situations; assessing motivation to change
5	Commitment generation;[a] identifying alternatives to substance use
6	Specific plan for change; long- and short-term goals for change
7	Coping with stress
8	Improving relationships and communication skills
9	Abstinence-violation effect; practicing resistance/refusal
10	Final commitment to change: social support; closing exercises

[a] Repeated through the remaining sessions.

included in the program, a student must report five or more substance use occasions during the past 3 months. Qualifying students are assigned to mixed gender groups that include no less than four and no more than ten students from the same middle school or high school. Sessions are sequential and hierarchical, and thus enrollment is closed once a group begins. This approach is consistent with that employed in "abusers groups" in the Westchester model.

Study design and preliminary results

With funding from NIAAA (R01 AA10246), we conducted a randomized controlled trial of our standardized Westchester model group counseling. The study involved 289 students referred for school-based substance abuse counseling. Group counseling subjects (180) participated in the intervention and were assessed immediately before and after intervention and at follow-up at 1, 3, and 12 months. The comparison condition (i.e., 109 students for assessment/referral-only) subjects participated in substance abuse assessment and were offered referrals to self-help groups and local treatment providers, which is treatment-as-usual for substance-abusing students in the school system in which the study took place. Assessment/ referral-only subjects were assessed on the same schedule as the groupcounseling subjects. In terms of sample demographics, 53% of participants were in middle school, 47% were in high school, 39% were female, 62% were white, 20% were hispanic, 14% were black, and 4% were "other." The mean age of participants was 15.3 years. There were no significant differences between participants in the groups on any demographic variable.

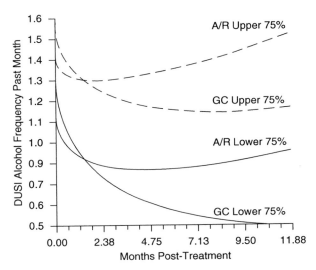

Fig. 16.1   Post-treatment growth curve models of past month alcohol use frequency by treatment condition and level of baseline alcohol involvement. A/R, assessment/referral only; GC, group counseling; DUSI, Drug Use Screening Inventory.

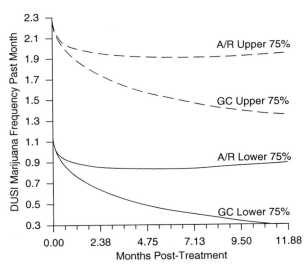

Fig. 16.2   Post-treatment growth curve models of past month marijuana use frequency by treatment condition and level of baseline marijuana involvement. Abbreviations as in Fig. 16.1.

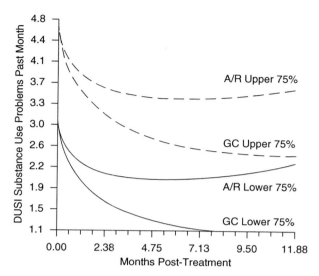

Fig. 16.3   Post-treatment growth curve models of number of past month substance use problems by treatment condition and level of baseline substance use problems. Abbreviations as in Fig. 16.1.

While the study had a number of different hypotheses, its primary hypotheses was that group counseling would be more effective in achieving and maintaining reductions in AOD use than the assessment/referral approach. The hierarchical linear model (Bryk & Raudenbush, 1987) was used (a) to model how participants change over time in their substance use and their substance use problems from immediately after treatment to 12 months after treatment and (b) to determine if group counseling affected the trajectory of change across time. Three separate trajectory or growth curve models were examined, with the respective dependent measures of past month alcohol use frequency, past month marijuana use frequency, and past month number of substance use problems as measured by the Drug Use Screening Inventory (Tarter & Hegedus, 1991). Participants within both groups were further subdivided at the 25th percentile of intensity of use, giving preliminary evidence of differential effects of SAPs based on degree of substance use involvement (see Carlson *et al.*, 1994, 1996) and the bimodal distribution use patterns in this sample.

Results from preliminary analyses generally confirmed our primary hypothesis (E. F. Wagner & C. N. Marti unpublished data 2003). Results of the hierarchical linear model analyses of post-treatment trajectories are presented in Figs. 16.1–16.3. Both approaches led to initial improvement in substance use status, but response to group counseling was significantly greater and longer lasting than response in the assessment/ referral only group, which demonstrated decreasing impact over time. Moreover, response in both groups was not significantly influenced by the level of baseline substance use or substance use problems (i.e., the lower 25% did not differ in response to treatment from the upper 75%). In short, these results support the contention that school-based group counseling, when conducted according to our model, leads to significant and sustained reductions in alcohol and marijuana use and substance use problems among AOD-involved middle and senior high school students.

Mechanisms of change in group counseling

Group counseling, like that offered in our Westchester model SAP, is commonplace in the treatment of AOD problems (Khantzian, 2001; Matano & Yalom, 1991; O'Leary *et al.*, 2002; Stinchfield, Owen, & Winters, 1994). Practitioners and treatment agencies often considered it the treatment of choice for adolescent AOD abusers because of its cost-effectiveness, the importance of peer factors in influencing behavior among adolescents, and the appeal of groups to adolescents (O'Leary *et al.*, 2002). Several meta-analyses have supported the efficacy of group methods for treating adolescents exhibiting a variety of problems (Hoag & Burlingame, 1997; Prout & DeMartino, 1986; Tillitski, 1990). However, there have been relatively few studies of group methods for treating adolescents with substance use problems, especially in comparison with other empirically established approaches. In general, the literature supports the preliminary conclusion that group treatment can be effective in reducing adolescent AOD problems (Dennis & White, 2002; Duehn, 1978; Kaminer & Burleson, 1999; Kaminer *et al.*, 1998a; Liddle *et al.*, 2001; Waldron *et al.*, 2001b), though it should be noted that the empirical literature on the effectiveness of group interventions with substance-abusing teenagers is quite limited.

The evidence from group-based research indicates that there are identifiable therapeutic factors that affect outcomes (Budman *et al.*, 1994; Greene, 2000; Kivlighan & Tarrant, 2001; Lewin, Lippitt, & White, 1939; Lieberman, Yalom, & Miles, 1973; Stinchfield *et al.*, 1994; Yalom, 1995). Although popularized by Yalom (Lieberman *et al.*, 1973; Yalom, 1985), others, such as Bloch and Crouch (1985), have further researched group therapeutic factors, which are defined as "an element of group therapy that contributes to improvement in a patient's condition and is a function of the actions of the group therapist, the other group members, and the patient himself" (Bloch & Crouch, 1985, p. 4). Group therapeutic factors have been examined mostly with adults (Cierpialkowska, 1994). In their extensive review of the literature, Bloch and Crouch (1985) found that insight, acceptance, and self-disclosure were the most important therapeutic factors in group psychotherapy with adults. There has been only one empirical study of therapeutic factors in adolescent groups. Shechtman, Bar-El, and Hadar, (1997) found that catharsis, interpersonal learning, and social skills learning were the most important therapeutic factors in group psychotherapy with teenagers. Their findings suggest that a different set of therapeutic factors may be at work in adolescent groups compared with adult groups. Additional research is needed to assess the relevance and impact of therapeutic factors in group work for substance-abusing youth.

While many adolescents with AOD problems seem to respond well to group treatment, there have been reports of iatrogenic effects among youths with conduct problems. Several studies have suggested that treating aggressive, delinquent youth in groups can have negative outcomes (e.g., Catterall, 1987; Dishion, McCord, & Poulin, 1999; Feldman, Caplinger, & Wodarski, 1983; Poulin, Dishion, & Burraston, 2001; Romig, 1978). The aggregation of delinquent youth in treatment groups may both exacerbate normative social pressures for conformity during adolescence and reduce access to the protective effects of less-deviant peers. Dishion *et al.* (1999) have argued that adolescent peer networks formed on the basis of deviance, such as treatment groups, provide a context where problem behaviors may be reinforced. However, it is important to note that (a) only a few studies of group intervention with delinquent youth have reported iatrogenic effects (noted above), (b) numerous empirical studies have not reported iatrogenic effects but instead have reported substantial reductions in delinquent behavior (e.g., Handwerk, Field, & Friman, 2000; Hoag & Burlingame, 1997; Shechtman & Ben-David, 1999; Wood *et al.*, 2001), and (c) none of the studies reporting iatrogenic effects included samples of AOD-abusing youth without other conduct problems. Overall, the findings from the studies on iatrogenic effects do not support the elimination of group services for youth with AOD and conduct problems. Rather, they point to the need to be thoughtful about group composition (i.e., not to have a majority of antisocial youth in groups) and to have experienced leaders who do not inadvertently promote deviance and who intervene quickly in the presence of such behavior (Dishion, Poulin, & Burraston, 2001; Feldman *et al.*, 1983). These and other recommendations for minimizing the possible iatrogenic effects of groups are further described below. Whether iatrogenic effects influence outcomes among youths with AOD problems remains an unresolved issue in need of further empirical study.

Conclusions and future directions

Given the importance of SAPs for treating adolescent substance abuse, empirical tests of their effectiveness are clearly needed. Preliminary results from the Teen Intervention Project are encouraging and speak to the need for additional research exploring both the overall impact of different SAPs as well as investigating the specific "active ingredients" of treatment. We are currently in the process of investigating such factors but would like to advocate for additional research on the topic by other research groups.

Adolescents with AOD use problems are a heterogeneous group, with individual differences for factors such as the anticipated effects and consequences of substance use; the context and motivations in which use occurs; and the risk factors that contribute to, or accompany, substance use (Wagner & Kassel, 1995). These differences may help to explain why certain substance-abusing adolescents may be more or less amenable to treatment. Amenability to treatment concerns the identification of individuals in a target population who are likely to respond to a treatment (Kazdin, 1995). To date, very few studies have examined the differential amenability of adolescents to various treatments. The variables we currently are examining as possible factors affecting amenability to treatment include psychiatric comorbidity, alcohol expectancies, social support, delinquency, motivation to change, history of abuse or maltreatment, family conflict, and parental substance use. Preliminary analyses have indicated that co-occurring psychopathology plays a moderating role in response to our school-based group counseling program (J. Gonzalez & E. F. Wagner, unpublished data). Specifically, adolescents with two or more disorders were significantly less likely to improve on measurements of average drinks per drinking day and total number of drinks ($p < 0.05$), and marginally less likely to improve in maximum number of drinks in 1 day ($p = 0.06$) and number of days alcohol used ($p = 0.07$). As knowledge develops about amenability to treatment factors in relation to SAPs, algorithms may be developed for matching substance AOD-abusing adolescents to the specific SAP program or program component(s) with the greatest chance of success.

Another important direction for future research is to examine the effectiveness of SAPs with other student populations and for other domains of adolescent problem behavior. For example, students who have been placed in alternative schools are more likely to be involved with substance use and have substance use problems than students enrolled in regular high schools. This population clearly is in need of substance abuse treatment and may benefit from SAP services. Regarding other domains of problem behavior, AOD-abusing adolescents often demonstrate additional problem behaviors such high-risk sexual practices and recklessness; SAPs, with some modifications, may be effective in also reducing these problems.

Future research should examine group processes as an active component of treatment (Rose, Tolman, & Tallant, 1985; Stinchfield *et al.*, 1994). Along this line, both helpful and harmful group processes could be measured and documented, which would not only provide useful descriptive information but also provide information about mediating, moderating, or side effect variables (Eddy, Dishion, &

Stoolmiller, 1998). For example, researchers could examine group engagement (e.g., using the Group Engagement Measure; Macgowan, 1997, 2000; Macgowan & Levenson, 2003) as a mediator of outcomes. Researchers also might explore how directive leadership (e.g., using the Therapist Intentions Scale, adapted for groups [Kivlighan & Tarrant, 2001; Stiles *et al.*, 1996]) moderates the effects of deviant peer training in groups. Some of the processes that AOD researchers have examined include adherence (Getter *et al.*, 1992; Kaminer *et al.*, 1998b), group alliance and cohesion (Gillaspy *et al.*, 2002), communication (Sandahl, Lindgren, & Herlitz, 2000), and interaction (Campbell & Page, 1993; Page *et al.*, 1989). Examining these types of group process is an important step towards looking into the "black box" of group-based AOD research with adolescents (Stinchfield *et al.*, 1994).

Finally, since at least some studies have suggested that treating aggressive, delinquent youth in groups can have negative outcomes (e.g., Catterall, 1987; Dishion *et al.*, 1999; Feldman *et al.*, 1983; Poulin *et al.*, 2001; Romig, 1978), we want to offer suggestions about how to mitigate the potential negative effects of aggregating youth with AOD and related problems. Group leaders should have education/ training and experience in leading groups with youth with conduct problems. Researchers have noted that effective groups have leaders who are well-trained and experienced in group methods (Feldman & Caplinger, 1977; Feldman *et al.*, 1983; Fors & Jarvis, 1995). In addition, group leaders need ongoing supervision that includes the use of observers or questionnaires to monitor disruptive group process, including deviance training (Galinsky & Schopler, 1977). Finally, although the evidence suggests that experienced group leaders can affect positive outcomes with both antisocial and prosocial youth (Feldman *et al.*, 1983), the leader's work is substantially helped by the group's composition (Feldman & Caplinger, 1977). Consequently, interventionists should thoughtfully compose treatment groups.

In summary, interest in school-based approaches to delivering substance abuse intervention is growing. For practical, conceptual, ecological, and developmental reasons, the school-based service-delivery model has many advantages over a more traditional clinic-based service-delivery model. There exists a reasonably large literature concerning school-based interventions for a variety of child and adolescent problems, and a review of the most effective of these interventions reveals several cores features related to their success. Among current approaches to school-based AOD intervention, SAPs are the most popular. Research on the effectiveness of SAPs has been supportive, though the few studies published to date share many methodological weaknesses. A more rigorous NIAAA-funded, randomized clinical trail of a SAP has provided initial evidence that SAPs are efficacious, and we are currently in the process of conducting additional analyses of these data, which we plan to disseminate as soon as possible. Moreover, an emerging focus of our research is group process factors that may influence adolescents' responses to substance abuse treatment. It is our hope that this chapter will encourage researchers into adolescent substance abuse intervention to become more interested in and have more success with working in school settings.

ACKNOWLEDGEMENTS

Supported by NIAAA grants R01 AA10246 and R01 AA12180. Special thanks to Ms. Jessica Gonzalez for her editorial help with this chapter.

REFERENCES

Aguirre-Molina, M. & Caetano, R. (1994). Alcohol use and alcohol-related issues. In C. W. Molina & M. Aguirre-Molina (eds.), *Latino Health in the US: A Growing Challenge* (pp. 393–424). Washington, DC: American Public Health Association.

American Psychiatric Association (1994). *The Diagnostic and Statistical Manual*, 4th edn (*DSM-IV*). Washington, DC: American Psychiatric Association.

Bandura, A. (1977). *Social learning theory*. Englewood Cliffs, NJ: Prentice-Hall.

Bloch, S. & Crouch, E. (1985). *Therapeutic Factors in Group Psychotherapy*. New York: Oxford University Press.

Budman, S. H., Simeone, P. G., Reilly, R., & Demby, A. (1994). Progress in short-term and time-limited group psychotherapy: evidence and implications. In A. Fuhriman & G. M. Burlingame (eds.), *Handbook of Group Psychotherapy: An Empirical and Clinical Synthesis* (pp. 319–339). New York: John Wiley.

Bentler, P. M. (1992). Etiologies and consequences of adolescent drug use: implications for prevention. *Journal of Addictive Diseases*, **11**, 47–61.

Brown, S. A. (2001). Facilitating change for adolescent alcohol problems: a multiple options approach. In E. F Wagner & H. B. Waldron (eds.), *Innovations in Adolescent Substance Abuse Intervention* (pp. 169–188). Oxford: Elsevier Science (pp. 169–188).

Brown, S. A., Cleghorn, A., Schuckit, M. A., Myers, M. G., & Mott, M. A. (1996). Conduct disorder among adolescent alcohol and drug misusers. *Journal of Studies on Alcohol*, **57**, 314–324.

Brown, S. B., Vik, P. W., & Creamer, V. A. (1989). Characteristics of relapse following adolescent substance treatment. *Addictive Behaviors*, **14**, 291–300.

Brown, S. B., Mott, M. A., & Myers, M. G. (1990). Adolescent alcohol and drug treatment outcome. In R. R. Watson (ed.), *Drug and Alcohol Abuse Prevention* (pp. 373–403). Totowa, NJ: Humana.

Bruvold, W. H. (1993). A meta-analysis of adolescent smoking prevention programs. *American Journal of Public Health*, **83**, 872–880.

Bryk, A. S. & Raudenbush, S. W. (1987). Application of hierarchical linear models to assessing change. *Psychological Bulletin*, **101**, 147–158.

Campbell, L. & Page, R. (1993). The therapeutic effects of group process on the behavioral patterns of a drug-addicted group. *Journal of Addictions and Offender Counseling*, **13**, 34–45.

Carlson, K. A., Hughes, J. D., Lachapelle, J. K., Holayter, M. C., & Deebach, F. M. (1994). Student assistance programs: do they make a difference? *Journal of Child and Adolescent Substance Abuse*, **4**, 1–16.

Carlson, K. A., Hughes, J. D., & Deebach, F. M. (1996). Proof positive: a student assistance program evaluation. *Student Assistance Journal*, **8**, 14–18.

Catalano, R. F., Hawkins, J. D., Wells, E. A., Miller, J., & Brewer, D. (1990–1991). Evaluation of the effectiveness of adolescent drug abuse treatment, assessment of risks for relapse, and promising approaches for relapse prevention. *International Journal of the Addictions*, **25**, 1085–1140.

Catterall, J. S. (1987). An intensive group counseling drop-out prevention intervention: some cautions on isolating at-risk adolescents within high schools. *American Education Research Journal*, **24**, 521–540.

CDC (Centers for Disease Control and Prevention) (1994). Guidelines for school health programs to prevent tobacco use and addiction. *Morbidity and Mortality Weekly Report*, **43**, 1–18.

   (1999). *Compendium of HIV Prevention Interventions with Evidence of Effectiveness*. Atlanta, GA: CDC HIV/AIDS Prevention Research.

Cicchetti, D. & Toth, S. L. (1992). The role of developmental theory in prevention and intervention. *Development and Psychopathology*, **4**, 489–493.

Cierpialkowska, L. (1994). Therapeutic factors in AA and Al-Anon groups. *Polish Psychological Bulletin*, **25**, 59–73.

Clark, H. W., Horton, A. M., Dennis, M., & Babor, T. F. (2002). Moving from research to practice just in time: the treatment of cannabis use disorders comes of age. *Addiction*, **97** (Suppl. 1), 1–3.

Cowen, E. L. (1977). Baby-steps toward primary prevention. *American Journal of Community Psychology*, **5**, 1–22.

Cowen, E. L., Spinell, A., Wright, S., & Weissberg, R. P. (1983). Continuing dissemination of a school-based mental health program. *Professional Psychology: Research and Practice*, **14**, 118–127.

Cuijpers, P. (2002). Effective ingredients of school-based drug prevention programs. *Addictive Behaviors*, **27**, 1009–1023.

Dennis, M. L. & White, M. K. (2002). The effectiveness of adolescent substance abuse treatment: a brief summary of studies through 2001. Bloomington, IL: Chestnut Health Systems. Available at http://www.drugstrategies.org.

Dennis, M. L., Dawud-Noursi, S., Muck, R., & McDermeit, M. (2003). The need for developing and evaluating adolescent treatment models. In S. J. Stevens & A. R. Morral (eds.), *Adolescent Substance Abuse Treatment in the United States: Exemplary Models from a National Evaluation Study* (pp. 3–34). Binghamton, NY: Haworth Press.

DiRenzio, P. M. (1990). A success story: SAP development in Pennsylvania. *Student Assistance Journal*, 2, 25–29.

Dishion, T. J., McCord, J., & Poulin, F. (1999). When interventions harm: peer groups and problem behavior. *American Psychologist*, 54, 755–764.

Dishion, T. J., Poulin, F., & Burraston, B. (2001). Peer group dynamics associated with iatrogenic effects in group interventions with high-risk young adolescents. *New directions for Child and Adolescent Development*, 91, 79–92.

Duehn, W. D. (1978). Covert sensitization in group treatment of adolescent drug abusers. *International Journal of the Addictions*, 13, 485–491.

Durlak, J. A. (1997). *Successful Prevention Programs for Children and Adolescents*. New York: Plenum Press.

Eddy, J. M., Dishion, T. J., & Stoolmiller, M. (1998). The analysis of intervention change in children and families: methodological and conceptual issues embedded in intervention studies. *Journal of Abnormal Child Psychology*, 26, 53–69.

Feldman R. A. & Caplinger, T. E. (1977). Social work experience and client behavioral change: multivariate analysis of process and outcome. *Journal of Social Service Research*, 1, 5–33.

Feldman, R. A., Caplinger, T. E., & Wodarski, J. S. (1983). *The St. Louis Conundrum: The Effective Treatment of Antisocial Youths*. Englewood Cliffs, NJ: Prentice-Hall.

Foote, A. E. & Erfurt, J. C. (1991). Effects of EAP follow up on prevention of relapse among substance abuse clients. *Journal of Studies on Alcohol*, 52, 241–782.

Forman, S. G. & Linney, J. A. (1988). School-based prevention of adolescent substance abuse: programs, implementation, and future directions. *School Psychology Review*, 17, 550–558.

Fors, S. W. & Jarvis, S. (1995). Evaluation of a peer-led drug abuse risk reduction project for runaway/homeless youths. *Journal of Drug Education*, 25, 321–333.

Galinsky, M. J. & Schopler, J. H. (1977). Warning: groups may be dangerous. *Social Work*, 22, 89–94.

Getter, H., Litt, M. D., Kadden, R. M., & Cooney, N. L. (1992). Measuring treatment process in coping skills and interactional group therapies for alcoholism. *International Journal of Group Psychotherapy*, 42, 419–430.

Giachello, A. L. M. (1994). Issues of access and use. In C. W. Molina & M. Aguirre-Molina (eds.), *Latino Health in the US: A Growing Challenge* (pp. 83–111). Washington, DC: American Public Health Association.

Gillaspy, J. A., Wright, A. R., Campbell, C., Stokes, S., & Adinoff, B. (2002). Group alliance and cohesion as predictors of drug and alcohol abuse treatment outcomes. *Psychotherapy Research*, 12, 213–229.

Gingiss, P., Gottlieb, N. H., & Brink, S. G. (1994). Increasing teacher receptivity toward use of tobacco prevention education programs. *Journal of Drug Education*, 24, 163–176.

Glynn, T. J. (1989). Essential elements of school-based smoking prevention programs. *Journal of School Health*, 59, 181–188.

Greene, L. R. (2000). Process analysis of group interaction in therapeutic groups. In A. P. Beck & C. M. Lewis (eds.), *The Process of Group Psychotherapy: Systems for Analyzing Change*. (pp. 23–47). Washington, DC: American Psychological Press.

Handwerk, M. L., Field, C. E., & Friman, P. C. (2000). The iatrogenic effects of group intervention for antisocial youth: premature extrapolations? *Journal of Behavioral Education*, **10**, 223–238.

Hansen, W. B. (1992). School-based substance abuse prevention: a review of the state of the art in curriculum, 1980–1990. *Health Education Research*, **7**, 403–430.

Harrison, P. A., Fulkerson, J. A., & Beebe, T. J. (1998). DSM-IV substance use disorder criteria for adolescents: a critical examination based on a statewide school survey. *American Journal of Psychiatry*, **155**, 486–492.

Hoag, M. J. & Burlingame, G. M. (1997). Evaluating the effectiveness of child and adolescent group treatment: a meta-analytic review. *Journal of Clinical Child Psychology*, **26**, 234–246.

Jessor, R. J. & Jessor, S. L. (1977). A final perspective. In R. J. Jessor, (ed.), *Problem Behavior and Psychosocial Development: A Longitudinal Study of Youth* (pp. 231–253). New York: Academic Press.

Johnston, L. D., O'Malley, P. M., & Bachman, J. G. (2002). Ecstasy use among American teens drops for the first time in recent years, and overall drug and alcohol use also decline in the year after 9/11. Ann Arbor, MI: University of Michigan News and Information Services National Press Release.

Kaminer, Y. & Burleson, J. A. (1999). Psychotherapies for adolescent substance abusers: 15-month follow-up of a pilot study. *American Journal on Addictions*, **8**, 114–119.

Kaminer, Y., Burleson, J. A., Blitz, C., Sussman, J., & Rounsaville, B. J. (1998a). Psychotherapies for adolescent substance abusers: a pilot study. *Journal of Nervous and Mental Disease*, **186**, 684–690.

Kaminer, Y., Blitz, C., Burleson, J. A., Kadden, R. M., & Rounsaville, B. J. (1998b). Measuring treatment process in cognitive–behavioral and interactional group therapies for adolescent substance abusers. *Journal of Nervous and Mental Disease*, **186**, 407–413.

Kazdin, A. E. (1995). Scope of child and adolescent psychotherapy research: limited sampling of dysfunctions, treatments, and client characteristics. *Journal of Clinical Child Psychology*, **24**, 125–140.

Khantzian, E. J. (2001). Reflections on group treatments as corrective experiences for addictive vulnerability. *International Journal of Group Psychotherapy*, **51**, 11–20.

Kirby, D. (1997). *No Easy Answers: Research Findings on Programs to Reduce Teen Pregnancy*. Washington, DC: National Campaign to Prevent Teen Pregnancy.

Kivilighan, D. M. & Tarrant, J. M. (2001). Does group climate mediate the group leadership–group member outcome relationship: a test of Yalom's hypotheses about leadership priorities. *Group Dynamics*, **5**, 220–234.

Lewin, K., Lippitt, R., & White, R. K. (1939). Patterns of aggressive behavior in experimentally created "social climates." *Journal of Social Psychology*, **10**, 271–299.

Lewinsohn, P. M., Hops, H., Roberts, R. E., Seeley, J. R., & Andrews, J. A. (1993). Adolescent psychopathology: I. Prevalence and incidence of depression and other DSM-III-R disorders in high school students. *Journal of Abnormal Psychology*, **102**, 133–144.

Liddle, H. A., Dakof, G. A., Parker, K., *et al.* (2001). Multidimensional family therapy for adolescent drug abuse: results of a randomized clinical trial. *American Journal of Drug and Alcohol Abuse*, **27**, 651–688.

Lieberman, M. A., Yalom, I. D., & Miles, M. B. (1973). *Encounter Groups: First Facts*. New York: Basic Books.

Lipsey, M. W. & Cordray, D. S. (2000). Evaluation methods for social intervention. *Annual Review of Psychology*, **51**, 345–375.

Macgowan, M. J. (1997). A measure of engagement for social group work: the groupwork engagement measure (GEM). *Journal of Social Service Research*, **23**, 17–37.

 (2000). Evaluation of a measure of engagement for group work. *Research on Social Work Practice*, **10**, 348–361.

Macgowan, M. J. & Levenson, J. S. (2003). Psychometrics of the group engagement measure with male sex offenders. *Small Group Research*, **34**, 155–169.

Matano, R. A. & Yalom, I. D. (1991). Approaches to chemical dependency: chemical dependency and interactive group therapy – a synthesis. *International Journal of Group Psychotherapy*, **41**, 269–293.

McCluskey, C. P., Krohn, M. D., Lizotte, A. J., & Rodriguez, M. L. (2002). Early substance use and school achievement: an examination of Latino, White, and African-American youth. *Journal of Drug Issues*, **32**, 921–943.

Milgram, G. G. (1989). Impact of a student assistance program. *Journal of Drug Education*, **19**(4), 327–335.

Miller, W. R. & Rollnick, S. (eds.), (1991). *Motivational interviewing: Preparing people to change addictive behavior*. New York: Guilford Press.

Morehouse, E. R. (1984). *A study of Westchester County's Student Assistance Program participants' alcohol and drug abuse prior to and after counseling during the school year 1982–1983* (Tech. Rep. No. MHa s65 15–1). White Plains, NY: Westchester County Department of Community Mental Health.

Neighbors, H. W. (1985). Seeking professional help for personal problems: Black americans' use of health and mental health services. *Community Mental Health Journal*, **21**(3), 156–166.

Newman, L., Henry, P. B., DiRenzio, P., & Stecher, T. (1988–1989). Intervention and student assistance: the Pennsylvania model. *Journal of Chemical Dependency Treatment*, **2**, 145–162.

O'Leary, T. A., Brown, S. A., Colby, S. M., *et al*. (2002). Treating adolescents together or individually? Issues in adolescent substance abuse interventions. *Alcoholism, Clinical and Experimental Research*, **26**, 890–899.

Page, R. C., Davis, K. C., Berkow, D. N., & O'Leary, E. (1989). Analysis of group process in marathon group therapy with users of illicit drugs. *Small Group Behavior*, **20**, 220–227.

Palmer, J. H. P. & Paisley, P. O. (1991). Student assistance programs: a response to substance abuse. *School Counselor*, **38**, 287–293.

Pandina, R. J. & Schuele, J. A. (1983). Psychosocial correlates of alcohol and drug use of adolescent students and adolescents in treatment. *Journal of Studies on Alcohol*, **44**, 950–973.

Perhats, C., Oh, K., Levy, S. R., Flay, B. R., & McFall, S. (1996). Role differences in gatekeeper perceptions of school-based drug and sexuality education programs: a cross-sectional survey. *Health Education Research*, **11**, 11–27.

Poulin, F., Dishion, T. J., & Burraston, B. (2001). Three-year iatrogenic effects associated with aggregating high-risk adolescents in cognitive–behavioral preventive interventions. *Applied Developmental Science*, **5**, 214–224.

Prout, H. T. & DeMartino, R. A. (1986). A meta-analysis of school-based studies of psychotherapy. *Journal of School Psychology*, **24**, 285–292.

Rohrbach, L. A., D'Onofrio, C. N., Backer, T. E., & Montgomery, S. B. (1996). Diffusion of school-based substance abuse prevention programs. *American Behavioral Scientist*, **39**, 919–934.

Romig, D. A. (1978). *Justice for our Children: An Examination of Juvenile Delinquent Rehabilitation Programs*. Lexington, MA: Lexington Books.

Rose, S., Tolman, R., & Tallant, S. (1985). Group process in cognitive behavioral therapy. *Behavior Therapist*, **8**, 71–75.

St. Pierre, T. L. (2001). Strategies for community/school collaborations to prevent youth substance abuse. *Journal of Primary Prevention*, **21**, 381–398.

Sandahl, C., Lindgren, A., & Herlitz, K. (2000). Does the group conductor make a difference? Communication patterns in group-analytically and cognitive–behaviourally oriented therapy groups. *Group Analysis*, **33**, 333–351.

Shechtman, Z. & Ben-David, M. (1999). Individual and group psychotherapy of childhood aggression: a comparison of outcomes and processes. *Group Dynamics*, **3**, 263–274.

Shechtman, Z., Bar-El, O., & Hadar, E. (1997). Therapeutic factors in counseling and psychoeducational groups for adolescents: a comparison. *Journal for Specialists in Group Work*, **22**, 203–214.

Shedler, J. B. & Block, J. (1990). Adolescent drug use and psychological health. *American Psychologist*, **45**, 612–630.

Simmering, K. F. (1991). A team approach to drug-free schools: the Iowa connection. *Student Assistance Journal*, **3**, 26–31.

Sobell, L. C. & Sobell, M. B. (1992). Timeline follow-back: a technique for assessing self-reported alcohol consumption. In R. Z. Litten & J. P Allen (eds.), *Measuring Alcohol Consumption: Psychosocial and Biochemical Methods* (pp. 41–72). Clifton, NJ: Humana Press.

Sobell, M. B. & Sobell, L. C. (1993). *Problem Drinkers: Guided Self-change Treatment*. New York: Guilford Press.

Stiles, W. B., Startup, M., Hardy, G. E., *et al.* (1996). Therapist session intentions in cognitive–behavioral and psychodynamic-interpersonal psychotherapy. *Journal of Counseling Psychology*, **43**, 402–414.

Stinchfield, R., Owen, P. L., & Winters, K. C. (1994). Group therapy for substance abuse: a review of the empirical literature. In A. Fuhriman & G. M. Burlingame (eds.), *Handbook of Group Psychotherapy: An Empirical and Clinical Synthesis* (pp. 458–488). New York: John Wiley.

Tarter, R. & Hegedus, A. M. (1991). The Drug Use Screening Inventory: its application in the evaluation and treatment of alcohol and drug abuse. *Alcohol Health Research World*, **15**, 65–75.

Tillitski, C. J. (1990). A meta-analysis of estimated effect sizes for group versus individual versus control treatments. *International Journal of Group Psychotherapy*, **40**, 215–224.

Tobler, N. & Stratton, H. (1997). Effectiveness of school-based drug prevention programs: a meta-analysis of the research. *Journal of Primary Prevention*, **18**, 71–128.

Tobler, N. S., Lessard, T., Marshall, D., Ochshorn, P., & Roona, M. (1999). Effectiveness of school-based drug prevention programs for marijuana use. *School Psychology International*, **20**, 105–137.

Tobler, N. S., Roona, M. R., Ochshorn, P., *et al.* (2000). School-based adolescent drug prevention programs: 1998 meta-analysis. *Journal of Primary Preventions*, **20**, 275–337.

Wagner, E. F. (2003). Conceptualizing alcohol treatment research for Hispanic/Latino adolescents. *Alcoholism: Clinical and Experimental Research*, **27**, 1349–1352.

Wagner, E. F. & Kassel, J. D. (1995). Substance use and abuse. In R. T. Ammerman & M. Hersen (eds.), *Handbook of Child Behavior Therapy in the Psychiatric Setting* (pp. 367–388). New York: John Wiley.

Wagner, E. F., Myers, M. G., & McIninch, J. L. (1999a). Stress-coping and temptation coping as predictors of adolescent substance use. *Addictive Behaviors*, **24**, 769–779.

Wagner, E. F., Brown, S. A., Monti, P. M., Myers, H. G., & Waldron, H. B. (1999b). Innovations in adolescent substance abuse intervention. *Alcoholism: Clinical And Experimental Research*, **23**, 236–249.

Wagner, E. F., Swensen, C. C., & Henggeler, S. W. (2000). Practical and methodological challenges in community-based interventions. *Children's Services: Social Policy, Research, and Practice*, **3**, 211–231.

Wagner, E. F., Kortlander, S. E., & Leon Morris, S. (2001a). The Teen Intervention Project. In E. F. Wagner & H. B. Waldron (eds.), *Innovations in Adolescent Substance Abuse Intervention*, pp. 189–203. Oxford: Elsevier Science.

Waldron, H. B., Slesnick, N., Brody, J. L., Turner, C. W., & Peterson, T. R. (2001b). Treatment outcomes for adolescent substance abuse at 4- and 7-month assessments. *Journal of Consulting and Clinical Psychology*, **69**, 802–813.

Wagner, E. F., Tubman, J. G., &. Gil, A. G. (2004). Implementing school-based substance abuse interventions: methodological dilemmas and recommended solutions. *Addiction*, **99** (Suppl. 2), 106–119.

Walsh, D. A., Hingson, R. W., Merrigan, D. M., *et al.* (1991). A randomized trial of treatment options for alcohol-abusing workers. *New England Journal of Medicine*, **325**, 775–782.

Williams, R., J., Chang, S, Y. for the Addiction Centre Adolescent Research Group. (2000). A comprehensive and comparative review of adolescent substance abuse treatment outcome. *Clinical Psychology: Science and Practice*, **7**, 138–166.

Wood, A., Trainor, G., Rothwell, J., Moore, A., & Harrington, R. (2001). Randomized trial of group therapy for repeated deliberate self-harm in adolescents. *Journal of the American Academy of Child and Adolescent Psychiatry*, **40**, 1246–125.

Yalom, I. D. (1985). *The Theory and Practice of Group Psychotherapy*, 3rd edn. New York: Basic Books.

(1995). *The Theory and Practice of Group Psychotherapy*, 4th edn. New York: Basic Books.

17

Profiles of change in behavioral and family interventions for adolescent substance abuse and dependence

Holly Barrett Waldron, Charles W. Turner, and Timothy J. Ozechowski
Oregon Research Institute, Eugene, OR, USA

Clinical research has yielded considerable empirical support for the efficacy of treatments for adolescent substance abuse and dependence (Dennis *et al.*, 2003a; Liddle *et al.*, 2001; Kaminer & Burleson, 1999; Kaminer *et al.*, 1998; Wagner *et al.*, 1999; Wagner & Waldron, 2001; Waldron *et al.*, 2001). Findings from controlled clinical trials have revealed consistent patterns, signaling initial, albeit preliminary, steps toward consensus regarding promising treatment models (Deas & Thomas, 2001; Liddle & Dakof, 1995; Muck *et al.*, 2001; Ozechowski & Liddle, 2000; Stanton & Shadish, 1997; Waldron, 1997; Waldron & Kaminer, 2004; Williams & Chang, 2000). Nevertheless, this body of findings has also revealed marked individual variability in treatment response. Even within the most efficacious models, in which the majority of adolescents achieve significant reductions in substance use, reductions vary widely, and fewer than half of treated youth remains drug or alcohol free during the year following treatment (Brown, Vik, & Creamer, 1989; Dennis *et al.*, 2003a; Spear, Ciesla, & Skala, 1999; Waldron *et al.*, 2001; Winters, 1999). Such differential treatment outcomes point to the importance of developing and testing treatments tailored to the unique developmental needs and substance use patterns of adolescents (Deas *et al.*, 2000; Winters, 1999). Yet, little is currently known about how substance abuse treatments work, for whom various treatments are effective, and how the durability of treatment effects over time might be enhanced. Without a better understanding of how individuals may differ in their response to treatment, we cannot effectively adapt and refine our interventions to serve adolescents better.

Encouragingly, a variety of novel analytic approaches have been developed that have the capacity to elucidate patterns of change across treated adolescents. Although the empirical support for adolescent substance abuse treatments has, thus far, been documented almost exclusively at the group level, these new strategies have considerable potential for treatment outcome research. Indeed,

Adolescent Substance Abuse: Research and Clinical Advances, ed. Howard A. Liddle and Cynthia L. Rowe.
Published by Cambridge University Press. © Cambridge University Press 2006.

without the implementation of more advanced analytic strategies to examine differential treatment responses, important effects between individuals that might serve as a guide for tailoring treatments to individual adolescents are likely to go undetected. Such effects could help to address critical questions associated with treatment mechanisms, moderators, and long-term outcomes, including patterns of relapse. One promising avenue of research focuses on identifying individual differences in profiles of change that are likely to occur over the course of treatment. The identification of individual change profiles shared by subgroups of individuals and the predictors of such profiles would enhance our ability to modify and fit existing treatments to specific groups of adolescents.

Studies of risk and protective factors may also offer important clues concerning variability in treatment outcome. Theoretical perspectives commonly view adolescent substance abuse as resulting from the impact of a variety of heightened risk factors and diminished protective factors associated with the social systems to which a youth is exposed. Substance abuse interventions typically are designed to enhance protective factors in the youth's social system and to reduce the impact of risk factors. Each adolescent can have a unique set of risk and protective factors, so that any one adolescent coming into treatment may be quite different from others receiving the same treatment. An important cause of variable treatment outcomes, then, may be that the therapeutic intervention failed to address appropriately all of the important risk factors impinging upon a particular adolescent. These unaddressed risk factors may serve to inhibit change in drug use and/or they may influence a return of drug use following treatment. One approach for identifying potential areas of improvement in therapy is to examine the relationships between various risk and protective factors across different profiles of change over the course of treatment. If we discover which risk and/or protective factors predict unsatisfactory change profiles, we may be able to identify new strategies specifically designed to target those factors.

A number of risk and protective factors have already been identified as predictors of treatment outcome, including pretreatment substance use, deviant behavior, peer and family influence, family relationships, and type and intensity of treatment (Broome, Joe, & Simpson, 2001; Brown *et al.*, 1989; Coatsworth *et al.*, 2001; Crowley *et al.*, 1998; Dobkin *et al.*, 1998; Latimer *et al.*, 2000a,b; Orwin *et al.*, 2000). Researchers focusing on mechanisms of change in adolescent treatment have also provided some initial support for the link between improvements in family functioning resulting from family therapy and subsequent reductions in adolescent problem behavior (Eddy & Chamberlain, 2000; Huey *et al.*, 2000). Similar links for family interventions and substance abuse treatment have also been found (H. B. Waldron *et al.*, unpublished data). The focus of this chapter is on identification of different patterns of responding to treatment and on predictors of these change patterns, in order to provide a basis on which interventions might be tailored to improve our response to the needs of various subgroups of adolescents.

Classifying patterns of change

Examinations of relapse patterns have figured prominently in research on adolescent response to substance abuse treatment. Relapse rates reported in the literature have ranged as high as 93%, with evidence that only 7–8% of treated adolescents maintain abstinence over extended follow-up periods (Brown *et al.*, 1989, 1994, 2001; Catalano *et al.*, 1990–1991; Friedman, Glickman, & Morrissey, 1990; Godley, Godley, & Dennis, 2001; Spear *et al.*, 1999; Winters, 1999). Such high rates of relapse profiles for adolescent substance abuse treatment are particularly disappointing in light of significant and meaningful reductions in substance use seen immediately after the end of treatment (Spear *et al.*, 1999; Williams *et al.*, 2000). Family-based treatments, which have garnered some of the strongest empirical support across numerous clinical trials, have not been spared the relapse problem (Ozechowski & Liddle, 2000; Stanton & Shadish, 1997; Waldron, 1997; Waldron *et al.*, 2001).

Recently, studies focusing on patterns of change across the course of treatment and beyond have begun to appear in the literature. In one such study, Spear and her colleagues (1999) documented post-treatment drug use for 113 adolescents who had participated in a 28-day residential drug abuse treatment program. At 12 months following treatment, 19% were either abstinent or had only isolated incidents of use, 20% were using one to three times per month, and 61% had returned to using at baseline levels of one or more times per week. They found that males were more likely to return to higher levels of use, and that somewhat different patterns emerged for specific drugs and drug use combinations. In addition, the findings indicated that 6 to 12 weeks following treatment appears to be a time of particular risk. The gender differences, drug-specific patterns, and timing of relapse all point to several important factors that could be addressed in the design of tailor-made interventions.

The a-priori definitions of relapse categories used by Spear *et al.* (1999), however, lacked specificity across levels of relapse, obscuring the extent to which some youth may have experienced clinically meaningful gains. Taking a different approach, Maisto *et al.* (2001) examined diagnostic status and post-treatment functioning of 131 youth treated for alcohol abuse and dependence, where the adolescents were classified into four categories: abstainers, drinkers without diagnosis, drinkers diagnosed as alcohol abusers, and drinkers diagnosed as alcohol dependent. Using this diagnostic taxonomy, the investigators were able to differentiate between non-problem and problem use. They showed that more that half of the youth in their sample no longer met criteria for an alcohol diagnosis

12 months after treatment. Within this group, only one-third were abstainers, revealing a high rate of non-problem drinking outcomes in adolescents. Baseline differences in levels of coping skills and resources among the groups suggest that the acquisition of these skills should be a focus of intervention programs.

In a third study, Brown and her colleagues (2001) followed 162 adolescents treated for alcohol abuse and dependence over a 4-year period. They were able to classify the longitudinal post-treatment patterns of substance use of almost all of the youth (98%) into five mutually exclusive categories. These operationally defined categories included 10% abstainers, 8% users (one to seven occasions per month), 10% slow improvers (those who failed to abstain initially but significantly reduced their use or became abstinent), 27% youth who became worse with time, and 48% continuous heavy users (18–25 use episodes per month). The findings highlight the variability in substance use over time and further underscore the disadvantages inherent in a "one size fits all" approach to intervention.

Taken together, the three studies revealed generally consistent patterns of improvement and maintenance of treatment gains and relapse. One important issue raised in these studies, however, is whether the different categorizations of post-treatment responding are valid or if the differentiation of response patterns are distinct. Youth in each of the three studies were classified conceptually on an a-priori basis, rather than the classification being empirically driven. Possibly, the differences between subgroups could have been produced by a limited number of individuals in each subgroup. Consequently, while these three studies represent a valuable first step in examining profiles of change, an empirical validation of the classification of change profiles is needed. In addition, a better understanding of the predictors of different patterns of treatment responding, of how treatment could be tailored to particular change profiles, and of the types of treatment support for adolescents with alcohol and drug problems are also needed (Latimer et al., 2000a; Wagner et al., 1999). In particular, the identification of different patterns of responding across treatment modalities could identify treatments that are differentially efficacious for youth at risk for relapse. Offering specific treatment regimens or selected intervention strategies for subgroups of youth who appear to be on different trajectories of recovery could serve to enhance protective factors associated with better outcomes and to anticipate risks that emerge over time. This could, in turn, significantly enhance post-treatment outcomes and guide a more efficient allocation of scarce treatment resources.

An examination of differences in individual outcomes

In this chapter, we examine trajectories of change using cluster analysis as an illustration of one analytic procedure investigators can apply to replicate and extend conceptually derived classifications of post-treatment responding. Cluster analysis is an approach used to identify, empirically, a relatively small number of distinct, homogeneous groups comprising individuals who display common internally consistent patterns of change over the course of outpatient treatment. Using data from one of our own clinical trials, we describe the steps involved in conducting a cluster analysis, the types of decisions researchers must make along the way, and some criteria for arriving at conceptually and clinically valid cluster solutions. We also attempt to identify pretreatment measures to predict which individuals are likely to manifest these various profiles of change. Therefore, our analytic strategy is designed (a) to identify different profiles of change throughout the therapeutic intervention, and (b) to examine hypotheses concerning the relationships among clinical processes that may account for these diverse trajectories. The purpose of this illustration is to demonstrate the application of innovative analytic procedures that can address a more diverse set of research questions regarding adolescent substance abuse treatment and that can provide a context for the development of new intervention strategies tailored to the unique treatment needs of youth.

The current examination is based on data collected for a randomized clinical trial of drug abuse treatment efficacy for 129 adolescents (Waldron *et al.*, 2001). Families of adolescents referred for outpatient treatment of marijuana abuse and dependence were randomly assigned to family therapy, individual cognitive–behavioral therapy (CBT), or a skills-based psychoeducation group therapy intervention. The study also included a combined intervention in which participants received both the individual CBT and the family treatment, with two sessions per week across the 12-week intervention period. Families participated in assessments from baseline through a 19-month follow-up period.

While the family and CBT intervention models we investigated have been shown to be efficacious in reducing problem behaviors in adolescents, the approaches are not successful with all individuals (Dennis *et al.*, 2003a; Kaminer & Burleson, 1999; Liddle *et al.*, 2001; Wagner & Waldron, 2001; Waldron *et al.*, 2001). In our previous research, for example, substance use and family relationship outcomes were initially examined at 4 and 7 months after the initiation of treatment using traditional repeated measures analysis of variance (ANOVA). These analyses demonstrated that family therapy produced rapid reductions in substance use from pre- to post-treatment for most youths, but those reductions were not consistently maintained at the 7-month assessment point (Waldron *et al.*, 2001). The group intervention revealed significant reductions in substance use only at the 7-month assessment, and the CBT intervention did not produce significant reductions in drug use at either time point. Recently, collected 19-month follow-up assessments have demonstrated similar findings when analyzed using repeated measures ANOVA procedures.

Our analyses provide tentative evidence that the three treatment interventions produced different average profiles of change. The findings also indicated that substantial variability existed in change profiles both within and between profiles. Adolescents treated with family and CBT interventions manifested a variety of profiles of change; consequently, an examination of these models provides an opportunity to demonstrate the utility of our proposed analytic approach for examining change profiles. We will now focus upon an analysis of the individual variability in these change profiles.

Cluster analysis procedures

Cluster analysis permits the classification of individuals who are assessed on a common set of dependent measures into groups that appear similar (Aldenderfer & Blashfield, 1984; Everitt, 2001). Generally speaking, cluster analysis is a family of procedures for identifying homogeneous subgroups of individuals based on response patterns across a set of variables. This procedure has been widely used across many research disciplines to create classification systems or taxonomies. In adolescent research, cluster analysis has been used to identify longitudinal patterns in the development of high-risk behavior (Gorman-Smith *et al.*, 1998; Wills *et al.*, 1996) as well as in response to clinical intervention (Hanish & Tolan, 2001). An important goal of the procedures is to create these groups such that the members within a group have very similar response profiles on the dependent measures, while the identified groups are distinct from each other in response profiles.

Cluster analysis often involves two procedures: *hierarchical* and *k*-means clustering. The hierarchical clustering procedure is useful as a preliminary step in determining the number of clusters that may be required to establish homogeneous groups. The first step in a hierarchical cluster procedure is to create a "proximity" matrix that represents the similarity of each individual to all other individuals.[1] The next step in hierarchical clustering is to insert these between-pair distances into a "proximity" matrix where both the rows and columns represent all of the individuals, and the cell entries represent the distance between the individual represented by the row and the individual represented by the column. This matrix is similar to a mileage chart, which represents all possible distances between pairs of cities. We can

---

[1] Propensity scores were used to control statistically for differential attrition biases, as well as other systematic missing data mechanisms (Little & Rubin, 1989; Rosenbaum & Rubin, 1985). Propensity scores were used to estimate the likelihood of completing or dropping out of a study based on sets of variables that may predict the participant's attrition status, including treatment group membership. Specifically, the predictor variables were incorporated in a logistic regression analysis with attrition status as the dependent variable. The logistic regression yielded a probability estimate of an individual dropping out of the study as a linear function of the predictor variables in the equation. These probability estimates, or propensity scores, were then used as covariates in subsequent statistical tests to control for differential attrition biases.

use computer algorithms to rearrange the rows and columns so that the adjacent columns have individuals with the smallest distance separating them.

Cluster analysis programs use a variety of statistics (sometimes called linkages) to provide an estimate of the number of distinct groups that exist within the proximity matrix. The linkage measures combine scores across individuals in the proximity matrix and provide an estimate of the average distance between groups of individuals rather than pairs of individuals. By examining plots (called dendrites) of these linkage scores, we can identify the number of distinct groups that appear to exist in the dataset.

Typically, the second analysis phase builds on the first phase, and it is called the k-means cluster procedure. In this procedure, the investigator starts with an assumption about the number (k) of clusters that are appropriate for the classification task. Sometimes, investigators can use the results of the hierarchical clustering criteria, but they also may have theoretical or practical reasons for selecting a specific number of groups to estimate. The k-means procedures can be viewed as a variant of the ANOVA procedures in which the program tries to sort individuals into "k" groups so as to minimize the within-cluster variance across all dependent variables, and to maximize the between-group variance across all measures. The program keeps rearranging each person's group membership so that the within-group variance is minimized by the specific allocation of individuals to groups. A descriptive index that reflects the effectiveness of the sorting procedure is an "F" test computed from the ratio of the within-cell to the between-cell variances. When the procedure is successful, all of the members of each group will have similar response profiles across the dependent variables, and these response profiles will be different from those obtained for other groups.

Morral *et al.* (1997) provided a valuable set of guidelines for evaluating cluster solutions involving treatment response data. According to Morral *et al.* (1997), the first criterion for evaluating cluster solutions is cluster size. If the investigator's choice of k is too small, then each group will be composed of heterogeneous profiles that inflate the within-cell variability. If the investigator has chosen too large a value for k, the number of individuals within a cluster may be very small, yielding unreliable clusters. The investigator can evaluate these possibilities by repeating the clustering procedure using $k+1$ groups, or by estimating a solution with $k-1$ groups and reevaluating the appropriateness of the solutions. A second evaluation criterion utilized by Morral *et al.* (1997, p. 675) is face validity: that is, differences between cluster profiles should be readily interpretable on theoretical and clinical grounds without any "tortuous reasoning." A third evaluation criterion is discriminability, which means that cases assigned to separate clusters should have significantly different responses on variables theoretically related to cluster membership.

Once an appropriate cluster solution has been achieved, a convenient technique for describing each cluster is to calculate the means and standard deviations of each cluster on each dependent variable. However, the discriminability of cluster solutions can be assessed using a variety of standard techniques for studying differences between groups (e.g., t-tests, MANOVA), and predicting the probability of group membership (e.g., discriminant function analysis, logistic regression).

Individual profiles of change

For our cluster analysis to identify individual differences in patterns or profiles of change in marijuana use, we initially performed a hierarchical clustering procedure with the four marijuana use assessment points (i.e., baseline and 4, 7, and 19 months) as dependent variables (H. B. Waldron *et al.*, unpublished data). The hierarchical solution suggested that solutions of three, four, or five groups might provide good classification profiles for the marijuana use. Based on theory and prior studies (e.g., Brown *et al.*, 2001; Latimer *et al.*, 2000b; Maisto *et al.*, 2001), we initially chose a four groups solution in our k-means procedure: continuous low use, gradual improvement, continuous heavy use, and gradual deterioration. Although prior research did not use cluster analysis procedures, the investigations provided a theoretical rationale for expecting four profiles of change, rather than the three- or five-cluster solutions.

Using the reasoning of Morral *et al.* (1997) to evaluate our proposed solution, we determined that each of our clusters was of a sufficient size (at least 15 individuals) to provide a reliable estimate of the cluster. Moreover, the cluster groups made theoretical sense and were consistent with prior classification solutions. Our initial four group cluster analysis (Fig. 17.1) provided evidence of change profiles in marijuana use that are somewhat similar to profiles previously described: continuous heavy use (24.8%), rapid improvement and continuous low use (36.8%), rapid improvement followed by deterioration (24.8%), and gradual improvement (13.7%). Finally, the results of this analysis indicated that a four-group cluster solution provided a very strong discrimination among the individuals. Each of the time points contributed substantially to the discrimination among the cluster types. An inspection of the effect size estimates for each time point revealed that the four-group solution had substantially larger effect sizes for the follow-ups than for the baseline assessment. Therefore, the four-group solution appears to be particularly sensitive to the individual variability in responding during the post-treatment periods (H. B. Waldron *et al.*, unpublished data).

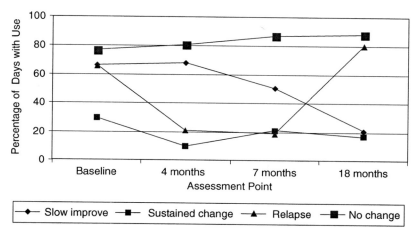

Fig. 17.1   Depiction of four marijuana drug use profiles across assessment points for the complete sample of 120 adolescents.

Predictors of profiles

In order to extend our understanding of the marijuana response profiles, we assessed differences among the clusters on measures of risk and protective factors at the baseline assessment point to determine whether the pretreatment assessments would discriminate among the different response profiles. For each family, the primary caregiver (usually the mother) and the adolescent were assessed on a variety of measures that should be related to the classifications, such as anxiety, depression, other adolescent problem behaviors, family conflict, relationships satisfaction, and negative drug use consequences. A comparison among profiles on parents' report of conflict was statistically significant, with *post hoc* comparisons indicating that the "no change" profile group had statistically significantly higher levels of parent reports of family conflict than the other profiles, which did not differ. The parents' report of adolescent anxiety and depression were marginally different across the profiles, with *post hoc* comparisons indicating that the "sustained change" profile group had higher levels of anxiety and depression than the other three profiles, which were not different from each other.

The adolescents' reported conflict and levels of anxiety and depression were not different across the four profiles, although the adolescents did report higher levels of conflict, anxiety, and depression, averaged across all four profiles, than the parents reported for their children. Statistically significant differences among profiles did occur on the adolescents' report of parent–adolescent relationship satisfaction. *Post hoc* comparisons on this measure indicated that adolescents with a profile reflecting sustained changes reported the lowest levels of satisfaction at baseline, and the other conditions were not significantly different.

Profiles of change associated with family therapy

The present findings provide preliminary evidence that the profiles of change are predicted by pretreatment differences. For example, the "no change" group had elevated levels of parent-reported conflict, while the parents reported more anxiety and depression for youth in the "sustained change" profile. While these findings provide a provisional examination of individual differences in profiles, we also recognized that the differences in profile patterns could be a reflection of the different treatments the adolescents had received. To evaluate these possibilities, we examined the occurrence of the different profiles with our three types of treatment intervention (i.e, family, individual CBT, or group). The results indicated that the "no change" trajectory occurred in 32% of the youths for the CBT condition, 27% in the group condition, and 17% of the family condition. The "relapse" trajectory occurred in 16% of the CBT group, 17% of the group condition, and 27% of the family condition. Approximately 35% of the youths in each condition displayed the "quick response" profile, and 20% displayed the "gradual improvement" profile. Therefore, while our findings provided empirical validation for prior classification research, they also suggested that different treatment modalities may be associated with distinct profiles of change. Given confounding of the trajectories of change with treatment condition, it is important to examine factors of treatment response profiles and predictors of those profiles within treatment conditions.

We were unable to examine trajectories of change for the CBT and group conditions because the sample sizes in these treatment conditions were too small for such explorations (30 in each group). We were able, however, to examine specific profiles in the family intervention condition (with 59 participants). This was fortuitous, because the family represents one of the most important social systems contributing to the development and maintenance of alcohol and drug abuse (Catalano *et al.*, 1990–1991; Stanton & Todd, 1982; Szapocznik & Coatsworth, 2000). The family can also serve as a protective system to reduce drug use and can influence other domains of potential risk and protection, including the schools, communities, and peer group social systems that increase the likelihood of drug use. In our earlier study (Waldron *et al.*, 2001), we found that average profiles of change for adolescents in the family-based treatments reflected reductions in marijuana use from pretreatment to the follow-up assessments at 4, 7, and 19 months. However, further analyses suggested that nearly half of the youths in the study did not achieve long-term reductions in drug use.

In order to identify and understand more clearly treatment response patterns in family therapy, we conducted a second *k*-means cluster analysis of marijuana use across the four assessment periods including only the 59 individuals receiving family therapy (H. B. Waldron *et al.*, unpublished data). We found that the most stable solution was represented by two primary patterns of treatment response: "improvement" (64.4%) and "relapse" (35.6%). In contrast to the initial cluster analysis performed across all treatment conditions, we found no evidence of a treatment non-response cluster characterized by continuous heavy marijuana use.

As before, we then compared the two clusters on measures of risk and protective factors assessed at the baseline assessment point in an effort to identify pretreatment differences between responders and relapsers with family therapy. Differences between responders and relapsers were found for family measures, peer and school measures, adolescent depression, and youth drug use patterns. Adolescents who relapsed from family therapy entered treatment using marijuana on a substantially greater percentage of days compared with those who maintain treatment gains (77.5% versus 44.2%). The relapse group also had other indicators of more serious drug-related problems at baseline, as they reported a higher number of drugs used and more frequent negative consequences associated with drug use.

The group comparisons on other measures indicated that the relapsing youth exhibited significantly higher levels of delinquent behavior and depression, endorsed more negative attitudes toward school, and were more likely to have friends who used alcohol at pretreatment. The two profile groups did not differ in the number of peers who used marijuana, perhaps because all of these youths were associated with peer groups that frequently used marijuana. We did not find a difference between the two profile groups in terms of ethnic identification (Hispanic versus non-Hispanic) or gender.

These findings provide a tentative picture of the pretreatment pattern of risk and protective factors associated with treatment effects in family therapy. Both profiles indicate a pattern of reduced drug use following family therapy, but approximately one-third of these youths eventually relapsed to the level of use that occurred prior to treatment. The family-related variables did not differentially predict the drug use profiles, likely because youth in both profiles received family therapy, an intervention that had a strong focus on family relationship issues. Waldron *et al.* (2001) reported that the family-based interventions were associated with major improvement in indicators of family functioning, and that risk factors outside of the family may be responsible for relapse. For example, youths in the relapse profile were more likely to have a history of delinquent behavior; they used marijuana more frequently than the non-relapsing groups; they used more types of drugs; they had more negative consequences of their drug use; they were more disaffected with school; and they associated with a peer group that used both alcohol and marijuana. These, findings are consistent with prior research.

Implications for treatment

Differences in the profiles, as well as factors related to cluster membership, can provide insight into questions about tailoring treatment to enhance its effectiveness and matching it appropriately with different types of adolescent. One improvement might involve intensified levels of relapse prevention training during treatment when the youth has a strong prior history of drug use, delinquency, or other psychopathology (Dobkin *et al.*, 1998; Crowley *et al.*, 1998; Latimer *et al.*, 2000a,b). The therapeutic interventions also could provide more support to increase attachment to schools and could encourage reduced contact with delinquent peers through improved and persisting levels of parent monitoring. Integrating more treatment components from interventions shown to be effective for addictive behaviors, adolescent depression, attention-deficit hyperactivity disorder, conduct disorder, and other problem behaviors into existing adolescent substance abuse treatment models, and using "menu" approaches for tailoring treatments to individual adolescents, could enhance outcomes. Such modified interventions could then be evaluated through formal matching studies.

Prior research has also suggested that treatment intensity and participation in continuing care are important predictors of recovery (Brown *et al.*, 2001; Latimer *et al.*, 2000a,b; McKay *et al.*, 2001; Miller *et al.*, 1997; Orwin *et al.*, 2000). Therefore, more intensive after-care programs, or at least regular follow-up booster sessions, may be required for these higher-risk youths to support their engagement in school and other prosocial peer activities. Again, a better understanding of matching youth to treatments is particularly needed to guide the implementation of continuing care programs. Our findings suggested that risk factors such as family conflict, negative attitudes toward school, and having peers who were using alcohol and marijuana were associated with trajectories with poorer outcomes (i.e., failure to improve, relapse following family therapy). Similarly, Latimer and his colleagues (2000a) found that pretreatment psychosocial risk level predicted treatment outcome better than severity of substance use, and that post-treatment risk factors did not predict longer-term outcomes. Rather, youth who failed to develop protective factors by the end of treatment appeared to be most prone to relapse and hence, perhaps, most in need of continued after-care. Protective factors may take time to develop, and continuing treatment may foster growth of new psychosocial factors or buffer risks that develop over time (Brown *et al.*, 2001; Latimer *et al.*, 2000a). Consequently, targeting subgroups of youth with poorer profiles to give them more intensive treatment or extended after-care intervention is an important implication of this research.

Conclusions

By numerous accounts, the field of adolescent substance abuse treatment is entering a new stage in its development as a science-based clinical discipline (cf. Dennis *et al.*, 2003b). With nearly two decades of experimental research yielding compelling evidence for the overall efficacy of a variety of treatments, the field is now poised to pursue a more diverse and complex array of questions concerning the components, processes, and mechanisms of effective treatment; for whom treatment is effective; and how those effects unfold over time. Answers to such intricate and relatively subtle research questions are sure to reside at the level of individual differences (as opposed to group differences) in response to treatment. Research designs and analytic methods capable of elucidating differences between individuals are bound to be pivotal components in an expanded research agenda for the field.

As a step toward an individual-focused research agenda, this chapter demonstrates the utility of cluster analysis as an analytic strategy to address a more diverse set of research questions regarding adolescent substance abuse treatment, such as identifying profiles of treatment responding. In addition, we have illustrated how differences in the profiles themselves, as well as factors related to cluster membership, can provide insight into questions about tailoring treatment to enhance its effectiveness and matching it appropriately with different types of adolescent. Along with the advantages and potential applications of cluster analysis, however, researchers must also be mindful of several key limitations and caveats associated with this technique. Statistical guidelines and criteria for evaluating the accuracy and validity of cluster solutions are not well developed, and the potential for subjectivity on the part of the researcher is high. Researchers should not rely on any single cluster solution but rather should develop a range of plausible cluster solutions and conduct supplemental univariate and multivariate tests to assess the internal and external (i.e., predictive) validity of each solution using variables not included in the cluster analysis. Above all, the validity of any cluster solution should be measured against the yardstick of clinical theory and experience.

Although the cluster analysis strategy presented above provides a preliminary basis for the identification of areas of improvement in therapy, cluster analysis is a person-centered (rather than variable-centered) technique, not a true multilevel analysis. Ultimately, the study of individual change over time requires a multilevel modeling approach in which individual- and group-level effects can be statistically modeled simultaneously. Modeling of individual growth curves is gaining popularity in longitudinal substance use research (e.g., Chassin *et al.*, 2000; Duncan, Duncan, & Hops, 1998; Schulenberg & Maggs, 2002). A strong case can also be made for the importance of a hypothesized therapy change mechanism using latent growth curve model procedures (McArdle & Hamagami, 1996; Muthén & Curran, 1997; Muthén & Muthén, 2000; Raudenbush & Bryk, 2002; Willett & Sayer, 1994; see also Ch. 3).

Longitudinal or growth mixture modeling, the multilevel analog of cluster analysis, is concerned with discovering latent classes (i.e., clusters) of individual growth trajectories that may vary in terms of initial status, rate, or shape of change over time and may be associated with different sets of covariate or predictor (Muthén, 2001). The growth curve approach provides an analytic method for hypothesis testing and confirmatory analyses concerning different profiles of change. In addition, these latent growth curve modeling procedures enable the researcher to determine whether change profiles for one clinically targeted behavior, such as family relationships, provide a predictive association with other targeted change profiles, such as drug use behaviors. The cluster analysis procedures presented tentative evidence for a number of pretreatment predictors of profiles, such as failure to change or improvement followed by relapse. The latent growth curve modeling approach would allow for the refinement of our hypotheses to assess whether pre- to post-treatment changes, in particular risk or protective factors, are associated with different change profiles in drug use. As change patterns emerge over the course of treatment for individual adolescents, intervention strategies targeting specific risk and change patterns and implemented at earlier points in time could enhance treatment outcomes for youth poorly served by current treatment systems.

REFERENCES

Aldenderfer, M. S. & Blashfield, R. K. (1984). *Cluster Analysis*. Thousand Oaks, CA: Sage.

Broome, K. M., Joe, G. W., & Simpson, D. D. (2001). Engagement models for adolescents in DATOS-A. *Journal of Adolescent Research*, **16**, 608–623.

Brown, S. A., Vik, P. W., & Creamer, V. A. (1989). Characteristics of relapse following adolescent substance abuse treatment. *Addictive Behaviors*, **14**, 291–300.

Brown, S. A., Myers, M. G., Mott, M. A., & Vik, P. W. (1994). Correlates of success following treatment for adolescent substance abuse. *Applied Preventative Psychology*, **3**, 61–73.

Brown, S. A., D'Amico, E. J., McCarthy, D. M., & Tapert, S. F. (2001). Four-year outcomes from adolescent alcohol and drug treatment. *Journal of Studies on Alcohol*, **62**, 381–388.

Catalano, R. F., Hawkins, J. D., Wells, E. A., Miller, J., & Brewer, D. D. (1990–1991). Evaluation of the effectiveness of adolescent drug abuse treatment, assessment of risks for relapse, and promising approaches for relapse prevention. *International Journal of the Addictions*, **25**, 1085–1140.

Chassin, L., Presson, C. C., Pitts, S. J., & Sherman, S. J. (2000). The natural history of cigarette smoking from adolescence to adulthood in a midwestern community sample: multiple trajectories and their psychosocial correlates. *Health Psychology*, **19**, 223–231.

Coatsworth, J. D., Santisteban, D. A., McBride, C. K., & Saapocznik, J. (2001). Brief strategic family therapy versus community control: engagement, retention, and an exploration of the moderating role of adolescent symptom severity. *Family Process*, **40**, 313–332.

Crowley, T. J., Mikulich, S. K., MacDonald, M., Young, S. E., & Zerbe, G. O. (1998). Substance-dependent, conduct-disordered adolescent males: severity of diagnosis predicts 2-year outcome. *Drug and Alcohol Dependence*, **49**, 225–237.

Deas, D. & Thomas, S. E. (2001). An overview of controlled studies of adolescent substance abuse treatment. *American Journal on Addictions*, **10**, 178–189.

Deas, D., Riggs, P., Langenbucher, J., Goldman, M., & Brown, S. (2000). Adolescents are not adults: developmental considerations in alcohol users. *Alcoholism: Clinical and Experimental Research*, **24**, 232–237.

Dennis, M. L., Godley, S. H., Diamond, G., *et al.* (2003a). The Cannabis Youth Treatment (CYT) study: main findings from two radomized trials. *Journal of Substance Abuse Treatment*, **27**, 197–213.

Dennis, M. L., Dawud-Noursi, S., Muck, R. D., & McDermeit, M. (2003b). The need for developing and evaluating adolescent treatment models. In S. J.Stevens & A. R. Morrall (eds.), *Adolescent Substance Abuse Treatment in the United States: Exemplary Models from a National Evaluation Study* (pp. 3–34). Binghamton, NY: Haworth Press.

Dobkin, P. L., Chabot, L., Miliantovitch, K., & Craig, W. (1998). Predictors of outcome in drug treatment of adolescent inpatients. *Psychological Reports*, **83**, 175–186.

Duncan, T. E., Duncan, S. C., & Hops, H. (1998). Latent variable modeling of longitudinal and multilevel alcohol use data. *Journal of Studies on Alcohol*, **59**, 399–408.

Eddy, J. M. & Chamberlain, P. (2000). Family management and deviant peer association as mediators of the impact of treatment condition on youth antisocial behavior. *Journal of Consulting and Clinical Psychology*, **68**, 857–863.

Everitt, B. (2001). *Cluster analysis*, 4th edn. New York: Oxford University Press.

Friedman, A. S., Glickman, N. W., & Morrissey, M. R. (1990). What mothers know about their adolescents' alcohol/drug use and problems, and how mothers react to finding out about it. In A. S. Friedman & S. Granick (eds.), *Family Therapy for Adolescent Drug Abuse* (pp. 169–181). New York: Lexington Books.

Godley, S. H., Godley, M. D., & Dennis, M. L. (2001) The assertive aftercare protocol for adolescent substance abusers. In E. F. Wagner & H. B. Waldron (eds.), *Innovations in Adolescent Substance Abuse Interventions* (pp. 313–331). New York: Pergamon.

Gorman-Smith, D., Tolan, P. H., Loeber, R., & Henry, D. B. (1998). Relation of family problems to patterns of delinquent involvement among urban youth. *Journal of Abnormal Child Psychology*, **26**, 319–333.

Hanish, L. D. & Tolan, P. H. (2001). Patterns of change in family-based aggression prevention. *Journal of Marital and Family Therapy*, **27**, 213–226.

Huey, S. J., Henggeler, S. W., Brondino, M. J., & Pickrel, S. G. (2000). Mechanisms of change in multisystemic therapy: reducing delinquent behavior through therapist adherence and improved family and peer functioning. *Journal of Consulting and Clinical Psychology*, **68**, 451–467.

Kaminer, Y. & Burleson, J. A. (1999). Psychotherapies for adolescent substance abusers: 15-month follow-up of a pilot study. *American Journal on Addictions*, **8**, 114–119.

Kaminer, M. D., Burleson, J. A., Blitz, C., Sussman, J., & Rounsaville, B. J. (1998). Psychotherapy for adolescent substance abusers: a pilot study. *Journal of Nervous and Mental Disease*, **186**, 684–690.

Latimer, W. W., Newcomb, M., Winters, K. C., & Stinchfield, R. D. (2000a). Adolescent substance abuse treatment outcome: the role of substance abuse problem severity, psychosocial, and treatment factors. *Journal of Consulting and Clinical Psychology*, **68**, 684–696.

Latimer, W. M., Winters, K. C., Stinchfield, R., & Traver, R. E. (2000b). Demographic, individual, and interpersonal predictors of adolescent alcohol and marijuana use following treatment. *Psychology of Addictive Behaviors*, **14**, 162–173.

Liddle, H. A. & Dakof, G. A. (1995). Family-based treatment for adolescent drug use: state of the science. In Rockville, MD: National Institute for Drug Abuse. *Research Monograph*, **156**: 218–254.

Liddle, H. A., Dakof, G. A., Parker, K., *et al.* (2001). Multidimensional family therapy for adolescent drug abuse: results of a randomized clinical trial. *American Journal of Drug and Alcohol Abuse*, **27**, 651–688.

Little, R. & Rubin, D. B. (1989). The analysis of social science data with missing values. *Sociological Methods and Research*, **18**, 292–326.

Maisto, S. A., Pollock, N. K., Lynch, K. G., Martin, C. S., & Ammerman, R. (2001). Course of functioning in adolescents 1 year after alcohol and other drug treatment. *Psychology of Addictive Behaviors*, **15**, 68–76.

McArdle, J. J. & Hamagami, F. (1996). Multilevel models from a multiple group structural equation perspective. In G.Marcoulides & R. Schumacker (eds.), *Advanced Structural Equation Modeling Techniques* (pp. 89–124). Hillsdale, NJ: Lawrence Erlbaum.

McKay, J. R., Merikle, E., Mulvaney, F. D., Weiss, R. V., & Koppenhaver, J. M. (2001). Factors accounting for cocaine use two years following initiation of continuing care. *Addiction*, **96**, 213–225.

Miller, N. S., Ninonuevo, F. G., Klamen, D. L., Hoffmann, N. G., & Smith, D. E. (1997). Integration of treatment and posttreatment variables in predicting results of abstinence-based outpatient treatment after one year. *Journal of Psychoactive Drugs*, **29**, 239–248.

Morral, A. R., Iguchi, M. Y., Belding, M. A., & Lamb, R. J. (1997). Natural classes of treatment response. *Journal of Consulting and Clinical Psychology*, **65**, 673–685.

Muck, R., Zempolich, K. A., Titus, J. C., *et al.* (2001). An overview of the effectiveness of adolescent substance abuse treatment models. *Youth and Society*, **33**, 143–168.

Muthén, B. (2001). Second generation structural equation modeling with a combination of categorical and continuous latent variables: new opportunities for latent class/latent growth modeling. In A. Sayer and L. Collins (eds.), *New Methods for the Analysis of Change* (pp. 291–322). Washington, DC: American Psychological Press.

Muthén, B. & Curran, P. (1997). General longitudinal modeling of individual differences in experimental designs: a latent variable framework for analysis and power estimation. *Psychological Methods*, **2**, 371–402.

Muthén, B., & Muthén, L. (2000). The development of heavy drinking and alcohol-related problems from ages 18 to 37 in a US national sample. *Journal of Studies on Alcohol*, **61**, 290–300.

Orwin, R. G., Ellis, B., Williams, V., & Maranda, M. (2000). Relationships between treatment components, client-level factors, and positive treatment outcomes. *Journal of Psychopathology and Behavioral Assessment*, **22**, 383–397.

Ozechowski, T. J. & Liddle, H. A. (2000). Family-based therapy for adolescent drug abuse: knowns and unknowns. *Clinical Child and Family Psychology Review*, **3**, 269–298.

Raudenbush, S. W. & Bryk, A. S. (2002). *Hierarchical Linear Models: Applications and Data Analysis Methods*, 2nd edn. Newbury Park, CA: Sage.

Rosenbaum, P. R. & Rubin, D. B. (1985). Discussion of "On state education statistics": a difficulty with regression analyses of regional test score averages. *Journal of Education Statistics*, **10**, 326–333.

Schulenberg, J. E. & Maggs, J. L. (2002). A developmental perspective on alcohol use and heavy drinking during adolescence and the transition to young adulthood. *Journal of Studies on Alcohol*, **14**, 54–70.

Spear, S. F., Ciesla, J. R., & Skala. (1999). Relapse patterns among adolescents treated for chemical dependency. *Substance Use and Misuse*, **34**, 1795–1815.

Stanton, M. D. & Shadish, W. R. (1997). Outcome, attrition, and family/couples treatment for drug abuse: a review of the controlled, comparative studies. *Psychological Bulletin*, **122**, 170–191.

Stanton M. D. & Todd T. C. (1982). *The Family Therapy of Drug Abuse and Addiction*. New York: Guilford Press.

Szapocznik, J. & Coatsworth, J. D. (2000). An ecodevelopmental framework for organizing the influences on drug abuse: a developmental model of risk and protection. In M. D.Glantz & C. R. Hartel (eds.), *Drug Abuse: Origins and Intervention*. Washington, DC: American Psychological Press.

Wagner, E. F. & Waldron, H. B. (eds.) (2001). *Innovations in the Treatment of Adolescent Substance Abuse*. Philadelphia, PA: Elsevier Science.

Wagner, E. F., Brown, S., Myers, M., Monti, P. M., & Waldron, H. B. (1999). Innovations in adolescent substance abuse intervention. *Alcoholism*, **23**, 236–249.

Waldron, H. B. (1997). Adolescent substance abuse and family therapy outcome: a review of randomized trials. In T. H. Ollendick & R. J. Prinz (eds.), *Advances in Clinical Child Psychology*, Vol. 19 (pp. 199–234). New York: Plenum Press.

Waldron, H. B. & Kaminer, Y. (2004). On the learning curve: cognitive–behavioral therapies for adolescent substance abuse. *Addiction*, **99**, 93–105.

Waldron, H. B., Slesnick, N., Brody, J. L., Turner, C. W., & Peterson, T. R. (2001). Treatment outcomes for adolescent substance abuse at 4- and 7-month assessments. *Journal of Consulting and Clinical Psychology*, **69**, 802–813.

Willett, J. B. & Sayer, A. G. (1994). Using covariance structure analysis to detect correlates and predictors of individual change over time. *Psychological Bulletin*, **116**, 363–381.

Williams, R. J., Chang, S. Y., for the Addiction Centre Adolescent Research Group (2000). A comprehensive and comparative review of adolescent substance abuse treatment outcome. *Clinical Psychology: Science and Practice*, **7**, 138–166.

Wills, A. W., McNamara, G., Vaccaro, D., & Hirkey, A. E. (1996). Escalated substance use: a longitudinal grouping analysis from early to middle adolescence. *Journal of Abnormal Psychology*, **105**, 166–180.

Winters, K. C. (1999). Treating adolescents with substance use disorders: an overview of practice issues and treatment outcome. *Substance Abuse*, **20**, 203–225.

18

Behavioral management approaches for adolescent substance abuse

John M. Roll and Donnie Watson

Washington Institute for Mental Illness and Research Training , Pullman, WA, USA
UCLA Integrated Substance Programs and Friends Research Institute, Torrance, CA, USA

As described elsewhere in this volume, adolescent substance use and abuse is a pernicious problem. To a large extent, the problems of continued substance abuse by adolescents cuts across cultures and socioeconomic status, and the costs of untreated adolescent substance abuse are high on both societal and personal levels. This chapter is a modest attempt to describe a behaviorally based treatment (i.e., contingency management) of adolescent substance abuse based on the application of principles delineated by workers in the field of experimental analysis of behavior (e.g., Catania, 1980; Turner, Callhoun, & Adams, 1981; Ullman & Krasner, 1965). This chapter is not intended to provide a comprehensive review of contingency management nor to describe how to implement contingency management, as several excellent sources already exist to fill those needs (e.g., Higgins & Silverman, 1999; Petry, 2000; Stitzer & Higgins, 1995). The chapter will, instead, focus on the reasons we believe behaviorally oriented treatment approaches are likely to prove useful in the treatment of adolescent substance use disorders. We will describe two commonly used contingency management procedures, review the application of these two procedures to treat adolescent substance abuse, and discuss the issues surrounding their implementation.

Behavior analysis

Behavior analysis has a long and rich history. The basic premise that has guided clinicians and researchers is that behavior is controlled by its consequences. That is, behavior that results in the presentation of an appetitive consequence (e.g., food, water, etc.) or that removes a noxious stimulus (e.g., escaping from a loud noise) leads to increases in those behaviors in the future. Conversely, behavior that results in the withholding of an appetitive consequence or that results in the presentation of a noxious stimulus leads to decreases in

Adolescent Substance Abuse: Research and Clinical Advances, ed. Howard A. Liddle and Cynthia L. Rowe.
Published by Cambridge University Press. © Cambridge University Press 2006.

those behaviors in the future. This very simple observation has led to the development of successful treatment modalities, especially contingency management, for a number of adult and childhood/adolescent disorders. These treatments seem especially well suited for the treatment of chronic, relapsing disorders in which treatment success can be measured in concrete behavioral milestones. For example, behaviorally oriented procedures have been used to treat and/or manage a number of conditions, including drug abuse (Higgins & Silverman, 1999), elective mutism (Wulbert et al., 1973), hyperactivity (Wulbert & Dries, 1977), orofacial and neuromuscular disorders (Parker et al., 1984), stuttering (Ingham & Packman, 1977), obesity (Jeffrey & Christensen, 1975), childhood asthma (Dahl, Gustafsson, & Melin, 1990), hemodialysis (Mosley et al., 1993), phobic disorders (Nock, 2002), dysphagia, (Chadwick, Jolliffe & Goldbart, 2002), rumination (Olden, 2001), pressure ulcers (Mathewson et al., 1999), aggression in brain-injured individuals (Teichner, Golden, & Giannaris, 1999), obsessive–compulsive disorder (Piacentini, 1999), conduct disorder (Wells & Forehand, 1981), retentive encorporesis (Stark et al., 1997), psychogenic vomiting (Sloan & Mizes, 1996), and urinary incontinence (Maney, 1976). Contingency management has also been used extensively in the provision of care to severely disabled individuals (Reid, Phillips, & Green, 1991).

Additionally, these therapeutic approaches have been used to increase oral hygiene, (Lattal, 1969; Iwata & Becksfort, 1981), reduce disruptive verbal behavior (Petry et al., 1998), increase rates of learning in school settings (McMichael & Corey, 1969), promote prenatal care (Melnikow, Paliescheskey, & Stewart, 1997), increase rates of follow-up following abnormal pap smears (Marcus et al., 1998), increase breast cancer screening (Stoner et al., 1998), increase rates of prostate cancer screening (Weinrich et al., 2003), increase rates of immunization (Achat, McItyre, & Burgess, 1999), increase hearing screenings for newborns (Isaacson, 2000), increase compliance with exercise regimens (Stalonas, Johnson, & Christ, 1978), increase social competence (Pfiffner, Calzada, & McBurnett, 2000), assist with pain management (Johansson et al., 1998), and increase medication compliance for a number of disorders including hypertension (Swain & Steckel, 1981), tuberculosis (Elk et al., 1995), asthma (Burkhart et al., 2002), opioid dependence (Carroll et al., 2002), and HIV treatment (Rigsby et al., 2000).

Focusing specifically on the treatment of problems of childhood/adolescence, it would be difficult to find a technique that has enjoyed such widespread success and application as behaviorally oriented therapies. Perhaps one of the greatest success stories is the use of behavior analytic techniques to treat autism. Despite occasional popular press claims to the contrary, data clearly indicate that autism is amenable to treatment by the judicious application of behavior analytic techniques (Lovas et al., 1973; Schriebman & Koegel, 1981). Additionally, these techniques have shown efficacy in the treatment of a variety of adolescent disorders, as indicated above. Of course, responsible clinicians would never suggest using a behavior analytic technique as a sole treatment for a disorder where safe and effective pharmacological treatment alternatives exist (e.g., asthma); however, the behaviorally based techniques may still prove to be a useful adjunctive therapy in such situations.

Techniques derived from behavior analysis are also commonly used to help in the day-to-day supervision of adolescents and adults. For example, the techniques are commonly used to manage classroom behavior, ranging from reaching learning goals, to promoting cohesive group cooperation, to the management of individual adolescents who are disruptive (Jones & Kazdin, 1981). The techniques are also successful in helping adolescents to adhere to pharmacotherapy or exercise regimens (Costa *et al.*, 1997; De Luca & Holborn, 1992). They have also proven successful in managing the seemingly more esoteric classes of behavior such as increasing seat belt use, increasing recycling behavior, and promoting community service (e.g., Lehman & Greller, 1990; Ludwig, Gray, & Rowell, 1998). Again, this incomplete list of situations in which techniques derived from behavior analysis have been utilized to manage the behavior of adolescents demonstrates that the techniques work in an adolescent population and that they are acceptable to a number of practitioners across a wide range of occupations.

Further support for the use of behavior analytic techniques to treat disorders common to adolescence can be found if the environment in which adolescents exist is carefully examined. Adolescents do not have the same freedom of behavior as adults. Said differently, adolescents are not able to alter their environment to avoid punishment and seek reinforcement as much as can adults. For example, adolescents generally have to stay in school for a portion of the day, are given rules by their caregivers to which they must adhere, and have fewer legally guaranteed rights than do adults. This relatively controlled environment may make the treatment of adolescent disorders easier than comparable adult disorders because the adolescents are more severely constrained by their environment, which may facilitate the engineering of this environment via the use of reinforcement and punishment. This, in turn, may make the use of behaviorally oriented techniques more feasible.

Given the acceptability and effectiveness of these behaviorally oriented treatment strategies, the stage is set to explore the use of such techniques in the treatment of adolescent substance abuse disorders. Data suggest that a technique based on the principles of the field of behavior analysis – contingency management – is an effective treatment for substance use disorders in adults (e.g., Higgins & Silverman, 1999). This treatment strategy is based on a conceptualization of drugs of abuse as reinforcers. In other words, the consumption of drugs with abuse potential increases the frequency of behaviors leading up to their acquisition and consumption. This is based on a wide body of research utilizing both human and animal laboratory models, which has demonstrated that drugs with abuse potential will be readily self-administered (e.g., Fischman & Foltin, 1991), often to the exclusion of other biologically relevant sources of reinforcement such as food. An active area of research is underway to attempt to understand the mechanism by which drugs of abuse assert their reinforcing effects in the central nervous system. Current thinking is that drugs with abuse potential "hijack" the motivational system (Leshner, 2001). That is, the brains of mammals are arranged such that certain biologically relevant stimuli, such as food, water, and access to mates, activate neural circuitry that produces a hedonically positive effect (Caine, 1998). This has often been termed the reward pathway. Such a pathway seems to exist and it ensures that mammals will continue to eat, drink, and reproduce because these activities produce pleasurable sensations. Most drugs with abuse potential seem also to activate this neural pathway by virtue of their affinity for certain receptors in this system. It is likely that when this pathway is activated by drugs with abuse potential, it is much more strongly activated or activated for a longer period of time than when activated by food or water. This results in these drugs becoming extremely potent reinforcers that, under certain circumstances, individuals will go to extremes to acquire and use.

Further subversion of the natural pathway occurs when drugs with abuse potential are used in combination with other natural sources of reinforcement. For instance, many drugs of abuse are used concurrently with sexual activity (e.g., alcohol, cocaine, and methamphetamine). Thus, the individual gets not only the enhanced response in their neural circuit from the drug but also the added activity of the natural behavior (i.e., sexual activity). As an aside, this association has been studied and it has been suggested that such a combination may be responsible for the initiation of adolescent substance abuse (Alessi *et al.*, 2002). For example, consider an adolescent who has recently moved into a new neighborhood. If all of the other adolescents in the neighborhood smoke marijuana on a regular basis, they will not likely be comfortable with a newcomer's presence unless the adolescent smokes marijuana. Thus, access to a potential peer group and the social reinforcement it has to offer is contingent on smoking marijuana. A situation like this would likely confer some reinforcing efficacy on marijuana use above and beyond that which can be accounted for by the pharmacology of the drug. This, in turn, may lead to more frequent use.

The pharmacology of abused drugs and their common association with naturally occurring reinforcers results in drugs functioning as extremely potent reinforcers, which can cause individuals, in certain circumstances, to engage in extreme behavior to acquire the drug and to use it compulsively. In this way, the behavior of the drug-abusing individual neatly fits into the behavior analytic conception outlined above in that the drug-taking behavior results in the production of a pleasurable state and, consequently, the behavior increases in frequency. Adding to the problem is the observation that after periods of continued use individuals often develop an actual dependency on the drug so that they need it to avoid withdrawal symptoms. This too fits into the above conceptualization in that consumption of the drug results in the removal of a noxious state of affairs (withdrawal symptoms) and drug use increases. Viewing substance abuse in this behavioral context suggests that changing the environment of the drug-abusing individual so that they receive reinforcement for abstaining from drugs of abuse and receive minimal or no reinforcement from using the drugs of abuse would assist the drug abuser in initiating and maintaining abstinence. This is, in fact, the heart of the various contingency management approaches to treating substance abuse. Data suggest that several contingency management protocols commonly used in the treatment of adult's substance use disorders are effective with adolescents. Therefore, we will first review these protocols as they have been much more thoroughly studied in the adult population than in the adolescent population.

Principles of contingency management for the treatment of substance abuse

A common type of contingency management intervention was popularized by Higgins and colleagues (e.g., Higgins et al., 1994). In this procedure, patients receive "vouchers" for the provision of biological samples (urine or breath) that indicated no recent drug use. Hence, the procedure is often called voucher-based reinforcement therapy (VBRT). These vouchers are withheld when the biological sample indicates recent drug use. As originally conceived, these vouchers were to be for goods or services that would help the patient to initiate or reestablish behavior that resulted in non-drug-based reinforcement. For example, if, prior to becoming dependent on cocaine, a person had spent considerable time fishing with his or her father, he or she might use any vouchers earned in treatment to purchase a fishing license and equipment, or even to take his or her father on a fishing trip. Thus, the vouchers could be conceptualized as tools for acquainting or reacquainting individuals in treatment to non-drug sources of reinforcement in the community, which might then serve to compete with drug use.

The VBRT approach has proven successful compared with standard treatment regimens (Higgins & Silverman, 1999) and has been shown to produce clinically significant periods of abstinence (Higgins, Badger, & Budney, 2000). Many individuals achieve some period of sobriety with this approach. Importantly, when the technique is used in conjunction with other psychosocial interventions, this period of abstinence allows clinicians to conduct psychotherapy with a sober patient.

The other contingency management technique that is becoming quite popular was developed by Petry (e.g., Petry *et al.*, 2000) and has been termed the "fishbowl" procedure; however, it is more properly called the variable magnitude of reinforcement procedure. This technique has many similarities to VBRT. Participants receive "draws," often from a number of slips of paper kept in a fishbowl, for providing a biological specimen that indicates no recent drug use. Provision of a sample indicating recent drug use results in the withholding of draws. Each draw has a chance of winning a "prize," the size of which varies. Typically, about half of the draws result simply in receiving a slip of paper that says "good job." Approximately half of the draws, though, result in the earning of a prize. The majority of the prizes are "small" and are valued at about $1.00; some prizes are "large" and are worth about $20.00, and typically there is one "jumbo" prize, which is worth about $100.00. Each time a participant draws a prize, they have a small chance of winning a jumbo prize, a moderate chance of winning a large prize and a 50/50 chance of winning a small prize.

The main impetus for developing the variable magnitude of reinforcement procedure was a desire to minimize the cost of the contingency management interventions, which can be prohibitive for a community-based treatment provider (Petry *et al.*, 2000). Early results suggest that VBRT and variable magnitude of reinforcement procedures are approximately equivalent in their ability to initiate and maintain abstinence if reinforcement schedules are kept comparable (Petry *et al.*, 2004). However, long-term outcome data for the variable magnitude of performance procedure have not yet been analyzed.

Several other variations on these procedures have been utilized, in which take-home doses of methadone have been arranged contingently on the provision of a drug-free urine test (Stitzer & Bigelow, 1978) or access to affordable housing and work opportunities have been made contingent on the provision of a drug-free test (e.g., Schuhmacher *et al.*, 1999; Silverman *et al.*, 2001). However, these latter procedures appear to have limited utility in the treatment of adolescent drug abusers since they are rarely maintained on methadone or in need of their own housing or employment. However, similar strategies could be adopted for potential sources of reinforcement that occur in the adolescent's natural environment, such as access to sporting events or participation in social activities. Similarly, behaviors other than the provision of drug-free tests could be targeted for reinforcement in treating adolescents. Several investigators have demonstrated some efficacy for reinforcing the completion of behaviors that are thought to compete with drug use, such as seeking employment or engaging in family-oriented activities (Iguchi *et al.*, 1997; Petry, Tedford, & Martin, 2001). This may be worth investigating with adolescents as well.

Contingency management for the treatment of adolescent substance abuse

Given the efficacy of other behavioral interventions in the treatment of adolescent disorders and the efficacy of contingency management in the treatment of adult substance abuse disorders, it seems appropriate to investigate the utility of the procedure in the treatment of adolescent substance abuse. This strategy has been clearly elucidated by Kaminer (2000), who outlined a strategy, based largely on the work of Petry (2000), for bringing contingency management into the treatment armamentarium of those providing adolescent substance abuse treatment.

The first study of which we are aware that systematically investigated the use of contingency management in the treatment of a substance use disorder in adolescents was conducted by Brigham and colleagues (1981). They used contingency management to treat alcohol abuse in three adolescents. They provided access to activities such as movie passes and camping trips contingent on not consuming alcohol. They also provided small monetary reinforcers for abstinence. This group reported positive outcomes, with one of the adolescents refraining entirely and two decreasing alcohol consumption while the intervention was in effect. However, they also reported a rebound to preintervention levels of drinking once the intervention was discontinued, raising important questions about the durability of the treatment effects.

Subsequently, we conducted a trial investigating the feasibility of using contingency management in the treatment of adolescent substance abuse disorders. We studied eight adolescent cigarette smokers using a within-participant design (Corby *et al.*, 2000). This is a powerful experimental design because it uses each participant as his or her own control, thereby greatly reducing the between-participant variability and permitting the use of smaller sample sizes (Johnston & Pennypacker, 1993; Sidman, 1960). In this study, we attempted to answer a fundamental question: is adolescent substance use sensitive to contingent environmental consequences? The study was designed to analyze, in an experimentally rigorous fashion, whether monetary reinforcement could be used to promote short-term abstinence from cigarette smoking in adolescents. The study was conducted strictly as a feasibility test. The primary question was whether abstinence from cigarette smoking in this population could be increased via the application of positive reinforcement.

A word about the tactic of using cigarette smokers is in order. Using cigarette smoking as a model for experimentally examining issues related to contingency management interventions is well established (e.g., Roll *et al.*, 1998; Stitzer & Bigelow, 1984; Stitzer, *et al.*, 1986). We believe that studies of this type represent a pragmatic use of resources, provide valuable information on which subsequent clinical trials can be based, and that results from such studies are generally applicable to other drugs of abuse (e.g., Higgins *et al.*, 1999; Roll, Higgins, & Badger, 1996; Roll & Higgins, 2000). However, it does still remain an empirical question as to how generalizeable these initial results obtained with cigarette smokers will be to other adolescent substance use disorders.

We recruited eight adolescent cigarette smokers (three female and five male) to participate in this study. These participants were volunteers recruited from the greater Detroit area via flyers. The population had no specific disease state and were not dependent on other drugs with abuse potential. Participants came to our laboratory twice daily, in the morning and evening, on weekdays for 3 weeks. At each of these visits, participants provided a breath sample that was analyzed for carbon monoxide (CO) levels. This is easily accomplished by having the participant blow through a small hand-held device that measures CO. Measures of CO represent a well-established (e.g., Roll & Higgins 2000) means of measuring recent smoking behavior. Levels above 6–8 parts per million (ppm) represent recent cigarette smoking while lower levels are indicative of a recent period of abstinence. During the first and third week, we asked the participants to use their will power to try and quit smoking. During both of these weeks, participants were paid for providing breath samples for CO analysis regardless of CO level. Payment for weeks 1 and 3 totaled $40.00 for each week. During the second week, the intervention week, we provided payment to participants only if their breath sample indicated recent abstinence. Thus, we modeled a VBRT intervention. Payment during the intervention week also totaled $40.00 if the participant was abstinent on all 10 occasions. Results from this feasibility study indicated that rates of total and continuous abstinence increased by approximately 90% from the first week to the intervention week, and that abstinence was largely maintained during the third week. Because this study was conducted strictly as a feasibility study, rigorous follow-up procedures were not used. Therefore, we are unable to make any statements about the durability of the treatment effect.

The results of this study indicated that it would perhaps be fruitful to proceed with further investigations of the efficacy of contingency management in treating adolescent substance abuse. Several investigations evaluating the efficacy of contingency management in the treatment of adolescent substance abuse support this position. One of these trials utilizes VBRT (Roll, 2005) and one utilizes a variable magnitude of reinforcement procedure (Roll *et al.*, 2003).

In the first of these trials, adolescent cigarette smokers who wanted to quit smoking were randomly assigned to one of two groups: the abstinence group or the attendance group. During the first 2 weeks of participation, all participants, regardless of group assignment, visited the clinic once weekly. Participants did not receive any incentives for either of these two visits. They were told to smoke in their normal fashion and to begin preparing to quit smoking at the beginning of the third week of their participation.

During weeks 3–6, all participants visited our office once daily on Mondays to Fridays after school (3–6 p.m.). As in our previous research on contingency management for smoking cessation, no visits occurred on the weekends (e.g., Roll & Higgins, 2000). At each of these visits, participants provided a breath sample for CO analysis. Participants received immediate feedback concerning their CO reading (whether or not they were abstinent). All participants received brochures during the 4 week intervention. These brochures were designed to explore a number of the negative consequences associated with cigarette smoking. This is comparable to treatments offered to adolescents in other smoking cessation trials (Hurt *et al.*, 2000). The frequent monitoring of smoking (daily CO monitoring) is an important treatment component as many studies have shown that simply providing feedback to an individual about a behavior they are engaging in can assist them in modifying that behavior (Green, 1978). More rigorous psychosocial programs are certainly available; however, the proposed psychosocial component we were using is pragmatic in that it is easily delivered and not time consuming to the participants. Furthermore, it is more intensive than the normally available cessation programs (most do not involve daily CO monitoring).

During weeks 3–6, the two treatment groups differed in that participants in the abstinence group receive monetary incentives if their CO levels were less than 6 ppm, a level indicative of recent abstention from smoking. Since we were only measuring CO levels once a day, we elected to use this very stringent abstinence criteria, as have other investigators when conducting similar investigations using infrequent CO sampling (Shoptaw *et al.*, 1996). Payment was arranged according to a derivative of a schedule that has proven effective in reducing the cigarette smoking for a variety of individuals (Corby *et al.*, 2000; Roll & Higgins, 2000; Roll *et al.*, 1996, 1998). The schedule was as follows. For each CO reading that was ≤ 6 ppm, the participant earnt $5.00. In addition, every time a participant produced five consecutive breath samples that had CO values of ≤ 6 ppm they received a bonus. The first bonus was $10.00, the second $20.00, the third $30.00 and the fourth $40.00. Finally, whenever a participant produced a breath sample with a CO of ≥ 6 ppm, or they fail to provide a CO sample, they received nothing. The monetary incentives used in this study were paid immediately in the form of gift certificates for a local department store that could be exchanged for merchandise such as CDs, radios, bicycle gear, etc. The maximum total value of the incentives a participant could earn was $200.00 for a total of 20 visits at the rate of five visits per week for 4 weeks.

Participants in the attendance group also received monetary incentives during weeks 3–6; however, they received them contingent on attendance rather than abstinence. The schedule of payment was the same as for the abstinence group. For example, a participant in the attendance group would receive a $5.00 incentive for attending the clinic after school and providing a CO sample. In addition, the participant would receive a $10.00 bonus for attending five consecutive sessions. The bonuses would escalate in value as outlined above. Finally, failure to attend would result in non-payment.

The duration of 4 weeks for the intervention was selected for several reasons. First, it is somewhat unrealistic to ask adolescents to attend a smoking cessation program for 10–15 minutes a day, after school, for much longer than a month. It was hoped that the 4 weeks would be long enough to gather meaningful data and exert an influence over the cigarette smoking of the participants, while not being so long as to discourage them from participating. Second, in another study using contingency management to treat cigarette smoking, Shoptaw and colleagues (1996) had also employed a 4-week intervention period during which they observed reductions in cigarette smoking.

The design of this trial allowed for an initial assessment of the utility of contingency management in the treatment of adolescent cigarette smoking. Participants in the attendance group had equal access to the educational and motivational cessation aids and had the opportunity to earn the same amount of monetary incentives as participants in the abstinence group. Therefore, by comparing these two groups, it is possible to determine directly whether or not contingent reinforcement of abstinence promotes abstinence above and beyond the provision of educational and motivational smoking cessation aids. Additionally, as described earlier, we believe results obtained with cigarette smokers are directly relevant to treating other types of substance use problem.

Results from this study demonstrated that contingency management reduced smoking relative to the comparison group. Specifically, participants receiving contingency management were approximately three times as likely to remain abstinent for the duration of the intervention as participants in the comparison group (Roll, 2005).

In the other ongoing investigation, which utilized the variable magnitude of reinforcement procedure, substance-abusing adolescents were enrolled in an intensive outpatient program that involved cognitive–behavioral therapy and family systems therapy. In addition, the adolescents received "draws" for prizes when they provided once-weekly biological samples that were negative for alcohol, marijuana, amphetamine, phencyclidine, cocaine, opioids, benzodiazepines, and barbiturates. If their test for any of these substances was positive, they received no "draws". Participants made their draws at the time they received their weekly drug test results. A bowl was used, containing tokens with labels corresponding with varying magnitudes of reinforcement. Half of the tokens were labeled "good job" and were not exchanged for any prizes; 41.8% of the tokens were labeled "small" and could be exchanged for a small item such as a candy bar, snack or drink item; 8% of the tokens were labeled "large" and could be exchanged for a $10.00 gift certificate to a variety of department stores; 0.2% of the tokens were labeled "jumbo" and could be exchanged for a $60.00 gift certificate. Participants received two "draws" the first time they tested negative for the listed drugs of abuse and each subsequent negative test increased the number of draws by two. The incentive procedure was in effect for 6 weeks. If an adolescent tested negative for all 6 weeks, he or she would receive 12 draws during the final week of participation. If a participant tested positive for any drug of abuse, he or she received no draws and was reset back to the initial two-draw level for their next negative test results.

Results from this pilot study are encouraging. When comparing the first 10 individuals to go through this program with a randomly selected group of 10 individuals who recently went through the identical program without the contingency management component (i.e., historical control group), we find that those participants in the contingency management group were three times as likely to be abstinent for the entire 6 weeks of the trial. Additionally, 30% of the historical control group dropped out of treatment prior to completing 6 weeks of the program, while none of the participants in the contingency management group have dropped out prior to completing 6 weeks of treatment.

Implementation issues

Given the promising results from these investigations, we do not believe it is premature to begin implementing contingency management into existing clinical practices for the treatment of adolescent substance abusers. However, several issues need to be considered when initiating these procedures. Foremost, careful attention must be paid to the clinical culture. The behavior of those who provide substance abuse treatment in community settings is controlled by the unique environment in which they operate. Practitioners receive reinforcement for providing quick and pragmatic treatment to substance abusers. Frequently, their treatment must be provided in financially rarefied settings that dictate that cost, in terms of both time and actual money spent, must be carefully managed. The monitoring of patients' behavior and their response to clinical interventions is done on an individual and not collective basis. The patients are often more heterogeneous than those included in research studies, and the interventions applied are similarly more likely to be idiosyncratically designed and applied. Therefore, it is absolutely essential to consider carefully the impact of instituting a new treatment paradigm into the day-to-day functioning of a substance abuse treatment clinic, paying special attention to the points mentioned above (J. M. Roll, R. A. Rawson, & N. M. Petry, unpublished data).

One issue that deserves special attention is the value of the vouchers or prizes used in contingency management interventions. There is no set monetary amount that a reinforcer has to attain to be effective. In many of the voucher studies that have been conducted to develop and refine contingency management procedures for treating adult substance use disorders, high-magnitude vouchers have been employed as a means to delineate the most efficacious procedures. However, there is nothing inherent to any reinforcer magnitude. Several researchers have published lists of potential reinforcers that can be used in contingency management interventions, some of which are quite inexpensive (e.g., Chutuape, Silverman, & Stitzer, 1998). For example, Amass and colleagues (1996) found that a number of items (restaurant gift certificates, movie passes or rentals) and activities (barbecues, hiking trips, etc.) would likely serve as effective reinforcers. Using these or similar reinforcers could reduce the cost of contingency management procedures. This may be especially true for adolescents, given the early work of Brigham and colleagues (1981), who showed that access to social activities was effective in reducing alcohol consumption among adolescents. Other potential sources of reinforcement could be related to extracurricular school activities such as participating in sports, band or other activities. Similarly, caregivers exert tremendous control over the adolescent's home life and could make a number of activities (e.g., telephone use, television viewing, and internet access) contingent on abstinence.

Another way in which the cost of contingency management interventions can be reduced is to reinforce behavior with the variable magnitude of reinforcement procedure in which participants earn "draws" for prizes (Petry *et al.*, 2000). In this way, clients occasionally draw high-magnitude "prizes" but generally earn either nothing or very low-magnitude "prizes." Thus, the programmed cost is generally reduced relative to many other procedures (e.g., VBRT) in which each instance of behavior is reinforced. Related to this, different reinforcement schedules for disbursing vouchers or prizes are being investigated (Roll & Higgins, 2000; Roll *et al.*, 1996). While simpler scheduling arrangements may eventually be developed that are as effective, or more effective, than the commonly used escalating reinforcement schedules in which consecutive instances of abstinence result in the delivery of higher magnitude reinforcers and failure to abstain results in a reset in reinforcer magnitude, none has yet been identified. Escalations in reinforcer magnitude for consecutive abstinences and resets in reinforcer magnitude for failures to abstain appear to optimize the efficacy of contingency management procedures (Roll & Higgins, 2000; Roll *et al.*, 1996).

While some lower-cost reinforcers or reinforcement systems can be arranged, it is important to keep in mind that a large body of literature also demonstrates that the more valuable a reinforcer is to an individual (e.g., the larger the magnitude), the more effective it will be at competing with drug use (Roll, Reilly, & Johanson, 2000; Stitzer & Bigelow, 1984). Therefore, academicians and clinicians have the common challenge of determining high-salience, yet low-cost, reinforcers. Each individual has a unique set of potential reinforcers in his or her life. A skillful clinician can arrange the environment so that access to one or more of these reinforcers is made contingent on engaging in a specific behavior (e.g., not using drugs). This is contingency management.

Concerns

There are several concerns that should be raised about contingency management interventions for adolescents. The first deals with the effect of reinforcement-based therapies on an individual's motivation. A commonly held position is that reinforcing the occurrence of high-probability behaviors reduces an individual's intrinsic motivation to engage in those behaviors in the future (Deci, Koestner, & Ryan, 1999). However, more recent evidence has called this generalization into question (Cameron, Banko, & Pierce, 2001). To date, no empirical evidence has been presented which indicates that the provision of reinforcement for abstinence decreases an individual's motivation to initiate or maintain abstinence. However, clinicians should pay careful attention to changes in motivation that they may observe clinically, as any such changes could have profound consequences on the subsequent achievements of adolescents.

Second, the issue of the durability of treatment effects merits brief discussion. To date, one of the best predictors of long-term abstinence in adults is short-term abstinence (Higgins *et al.*, 2000). That is, those individuals who are able to initiate and maintain abstinence for longer periods during treatment are more likely to be abstinent at subsequent follow-up assessments. Given this finding, support for contingency management is increased as a means of achieving long-term abstinence because it is an effective behavioral intervention for achieving short-term abstinence. Nonetheless, the generality of these findings to adolescents is an open question. We are unaware of any studies that have incorporated appropriate follow-up periods to address this issue.

Another potential limitation relates to generality of in-treatment contingency management effects. To what extent can changes inculcated via contingency management-based interventions be expected to persist after the intervention has ended and the participant is out of treatment? To the extent that being in treatment and out of treatment are easily discriminated by the individual, why would we expect changes acquired in treatment to persist? While it is clearly beyond the scope of this chapter to attempt to explore this question thoroughly, we would simply point out that this is a possible criticism of all psychosocial treatments for behavioral disorders. We suspect that individual participant motivation to change accompanied by the psychosocial interventions may help individuals to bridge the conceptual gap between being in and out of treatment. Additionally, because adolescents do exist in a relatively controlled environment, it may be possible for parents, educators, coaches, and similar figures to engineer the post-treatment environment so that access to naturalistic reinforcers becomes contingent on continued abstinence. Clearly, this is a very important area for future research.

Conclusions

The field of adolescent substance abuse treatment generally is relatively young and the use of contingency management in the treatment of adolescent substance abuse is in its infancy. Such a state of affairs poses more questions than answers. While we are encouraged by the initial results of the studies of contingency management for the treatment of adolescent substance use disorders, we clearly recognize that further replications and evidence are needed before the external validity of the procedures can be firmly established. Several important questions about the use of contingency management are readily apparent. First, to what extent is the efficacy of contingency management either enhanced or degraded by combining it with other interventions? In adults, contingency management is often combined with pharmacotherapies and is a useful adjunct (Bickel *et al.*, 1997). The extent to which this holds for adolescents remains an empirical question.

Contingency management has often been used in conjunction with psychosocial treatments including cognitive–behavioral therapy, relapse prevention, and the community reinforcement approach (Higgins & Silverman, 1999). For the most part, it remains an empirical question as to whether the combination of these therapies provides a benefit relative to contingency management alone (Rawson, *et al.*, 2002). However, we suspect that for adolescents, who exist in a relatively controlled environment, these other types of therapy may be crucial in helping them to maintain their abstinence. The community reinforcement approach may be especially important in this regard as may other types of family therapy (e.g., Rowe & Liddle, 2003) that seek to help the adolescent to derive reinforcement from readily available, non-drug sources that exist in their environment (e.g., home, school, etc.).

Finally, it seems that the success of the contingency management interventions in treating substance abuse disorders suggests an obvious prevention strategy. If we can arrange an individual's environment such that he or she receives reinforcement for not abusing drugs as a treatment strategy, it seems equally plausible that we should be able to engineer the environment so that the individual is in contact with these other sources of reinforcement prior to their developing a substance abuse disorder. Potentially this would block the development of a substance abuse disorder. Empirical support from such a strategy comes from both human and non-human research. Carroll and colleagues (1989) have shown that a rat will readily acquire a cocaine self-administration behavior but will either not acquire it or acquire it at a greatly retarded rate if you simply place a bottle of sweetened water in the rat's chamber. The provision of an alternative source of reinforcement can block the acquisition of drug-taking behavior. Similarly, it has been demonstrated that individuals can be prevented from taking drugs in the laboratory by providing them with a choice between taking a drug or receiving cash (Higgins, Roll, & Bickel, 1996; Roll *et al.*, 2000). Therefore, providing individuals with access to alternative, non-drug sources of reinforcement (i.e., cash) can prevent their self-administering the drug. Using such a strategy to prevent drug abuse would entail helping adolescents to access readily available sources of reinforcement (e.g., reading, after-school programs, religious activities, extracurricular activities, etc.) in the hopes that these sources of reinforcement would compete effectively with drug-taking behavior.

The behavioral approach to treating adolescent substance abuse outlined in this chapter represents the considered application of well-researched techniques for promoting and maintaining behavior change. Our belief is that further research will strengthen the techniques and make them more pragmatic in terms of cost and application. We believe that thoughtful application of these techniques is warranted in clinical settings and that their use will help adolescents to quit abusing drugs and to maintain sobriety, thereby aiding them in developing into productive members of society.

Clearly, future research is needed on all aspects of this approach. Currently, research suggests that the approach has efficacy in initiating and maintaining short-term (e.g., up to a month) abstinence. Important questions remain to be address concerning the maintenance of abstinence, the generality of the findings across drug classes, the nature of the sources of alternative reinforcement to be employed, how the alternatives are presented, and the effects of individual differences. Finally, it will be important to determine the most efficacious way to deliver contingency management. It will be necessary to determine if it should be delivered alone or in conjunction with psychosocial interventions or pharmacotherapy.

ACKNOWLEDGEMENTS

Preparation of this chapter was supported by NIDA grants 13941, 14392, 017084, 017407, and 14871. The authors would like to thank Drs MaryAnn Chapman, Joy

Chudzynski, Jimmy Anderson and Debbie Green for their assistance. Dr. Roll is now at Washington State University.

REFERENCES

Alessi, S. M., Roll, J. M., Reilly, M. P., & Johanson, C. E. (2002). Establishment of a diazepam preference in human volunteers following a differential-conditioning history of placebo versus diazepam choice. *Experimental and Clinical Psychopharmacology*, **10**, 77–83.

Achat, H., Mcintyre, P., & Burgess, M. (1999). Health care incentives in immunization. *Australian and New Zealand Journal of Public Health*, **23**, 285–288.

Amass, L., Bicket, W. K., Crean, J. P., & Higgins, S. I. (1996). Preferences for clinic privileges, retail items, and social activities in an outpatient buprenorphine treatment program. *Journal of Substance Abuse Treatment*, **13**, 43–49.

Bickel, W. K., Amass, L., Higgins, S. T., Badger, G. J., & Esch, R. A. (1997). Effects of adding behavioral treatment to opioid detoxification with buprenorphine. *Journal of Consulting and Clinical Psychology*, **65**, 803–810.

Brigham, S. L., Rekers, G. A., Rosen, A. C., *et al.* (1981). Contingency management in the treatment of adolescent drinking problems. *Journal of Psychology*, **109**, 73–85.

Burkhart, P. V., Dunbar-Jacob, J. M., Fireman, P. & Rohay, J. (2002). Children's adherence to recommended asthma self-management. *Pediatric Nursing*, **28**, 409–414.

Caine, S. B. (1998). Neuroanatomical bases of the reinforcing stimulus effects of cocaine. In S. T. Higgins & J. L. Katz (eds.), *Cocaine Abuse: Behavior, Pharmacology, and Clinical Applications* (pp. 21–50). New York: Academic Press.

Cameron, J., Banko, K. M., & Pierce, W. E. (2001). Pervasive negative effects of rewards on intrinsic motivation: the myth continues. *Behavior Analyst*, **24**, 1–44.

Carroll, K. M., Sinha, R., Nich, C., Babuscio, T., & Rounsaville, B. J. (2002). Contingency management to enhance naltrexone treatment of opioid dependence: a randomized clinical trial of reinforcement magnitude. *Experimental and Clinical Psychopharmacology*, **10**, 54–63.

Carroll, M. E., Lac, S. T., & Nygaard, S. L. (1989). A concurrently available nondrug reinforcer prevents the acquisition or decreases the maintenance of cocaine-reinforced behavior. *Psychopharmacology*, **97**, 23–29.

Catania, A. C. (1980). Operant theory: Skinner. In G. M. Gazada & R. J. Corsini (eds.), *Theories of Learning: A Comparative Approach*. Itasca, Il: Peacock.

Chadwick, D. D., Jolliffe, J., & Goldbart, J. (2002). Career knowledge of dysphasia management strategies. *International Journal of Language Communication Disorders*, **37**, 345–357.

Chatuape, M. A., Silverman, K., & Stitzer, M. L. (1998). Survey assessment of methadone treatment services as reinforcers. *American Journal of Drug and Alcohol Abuse*, **24**, 1–16.

Corby, E. A., Roll, J. M., Ledgerwood, D. M., & Schuster, C. R. (2000). Contingency management interventions for treating the substance abuse of adolescents: a feasibility study. *Experimental and Clinical Psychopharmacology*, **8**, 371–376.

Costa, I. G. D., Rapoff, M. A., Lemanek, K., & Goldstein, G. L. (1997). Improving adherence to medication regimens for children with asthma and its effects on clinical outcome. *Journal of Applied Behavior Analysis*, 30, 687–691.

Dahl, J., Gustafsson, D., & Melin, L. (1990). Effects of behavioral treatment program on children with asthma. *Journal of Asthma*, 27, 41–46.

Deci, E. L., Koestner, R., & Ryan, R. M. (1999). A meta-analytic review of experiments examining the effects of extrinsic rewards on intrinsic motivation. *Psychological Bulletin*, 125, 627–668.

De Luca, R. V. & Holborn, S. W. (1992). Effect of a variable-ratio reinforcement schedule with changing criteria on exercise in obese and nonobese boys. *Journal of Applied Behavior Analysis*, 25, 671–679.

Elk, R., Schmitz, J., Spiga, R., Rhoades, H., Andres, R., & Grabowski, J. (1995). Behavioral treatment of cocaine-dependent pregnant women and TB-exposed patients. *Addictive Behaviors*, 20, 533–542.

Fischman, M. W. & Foltin, R. W. (1991). Utility of subjective-effects measurements in assessing abuse liability of drugs in humans. *British Journal of Addiction*, 86, 1563–1570.

Green, L. (1978). Temporal and stimulus factors in self-monitoring by obese persons. *Behavior Therapy*, 9, 328–341.

Higgins, S. T. & Silverman, K. (eds.) (1999). *Motivating Behavior Change among Illicit-drug Abusers: Research on Contingency Management Interventions*. Washington, DC: American Psychological Press.

Higgins, S. T., Budney, A. J., Bickel, W. K., *et al.* (1994). Incentives improve outcome in outpatient behavioral treatment of cocaine dependence. *Archives of General Psychiatry*, 51, 568–576.

Higgins, S. T., Roll, J. M., & Bickel, W. K. (1996). Alcohol increases human cocaine self-administration. *Psychopharmacology*, 123, 1–8.

Higgins, S. T., Roll, J. M., Wong, C. J., Tidey, J. W., & Dantona, R. (1999). Clinic and laboratory studies on the use of incentives to decrease cocaine and other substance use. In S. T. Higgins & K. Silverman (eds.), *Motivating Behavior Change Among Illicit-drug Abusers: Contemporary Research on Contingency-management Interventions* (pp. 33–56). Washington, DC: American Psychological Press.

Higgins, S. T., Badger, G. J., & Budney, A. J. (2000). Initial abstinence and success in achieving longer term cocaine abstinence. *Experimental and Clinical Psychopharmacology*, 8, 377–386.

Hurt, R. D., Croghan, G. A., Beede, S. D., *et al.* (2000). Nicotine patch therapy in 101 adolescent smokers: Efficacy, withdrawal symptom relief, and carbon monoxide and plasma cotinine levels. *Archives of Pediatric and Adolescent Medicine*, 154, 337.

Iguchi, M. Y., Belding, M. A., Morral, A. R., Lamb, R. J., & Husband, S. D. (1997). Reinforcing operants other than abstinence in drug abuse treatment an effective alternative for reducing drug use. *Journal of Consultative Clinical Psychology*, 65, 421–428.

Ingham, R. J. & Packman, A. (1977). Treatment and generalization effects in an experimental treatment for a stutterer using contingency management and speech rate control. *Journal of Speech and Hearing Disorders*, 42, 394–407.

Isaacson, G. (2000). Universal newborn hearing screening in an inner-city, managed care environment. *Laryngoscope*, **110**, 881–894.

Iwata, B. A. & Becksfort, C. M. (1981). Behavioral research in preventative dentistry: educational and contingency management approaches to the problem of patient compliance. *Journal of Behavior Analysis*, **14**, 111–120.

Jeffrey, D. B. & Christensen, E. R. (1975). Behavior therapy versus "will power" in the management of obesity. *Journal of Psychology*, **90**, 303–311.

Johansson, C., Dahl, J., Jannert, M., Melin, L., & Anderson, G. (1998). Effects of a cognitive–behavioral pain-management program. *Behavior Research and Therapy*, **36**, 915–930.

Johnston, J. M. & Pennypacker, H. S. (1993). *Strategies and Tactics of Behavioral Research*, 2nd edn. Hillsdale, NJ: Lawrence Earlbaum.

Jones, R. T., & Kazdin, A. E. (1981). Childhood behavior problems in the school. In S. M. Turner, K. S. Calhoun, & H. E. Adams (eds.), *Handbook of Clinical Behavior Therapy* (pp. 568–606), New York: John Wiley.

Kaminer, Y. (2000). Contingency management reinforcement procedures for adolescent substance abuse. *Journal of the American Academy of Child and Adolescent Psychiatry*, **39**, 1324–1326.

Lattal, K. A. (1969). Contingency management of tooth brushing behavior in a summer camp for children. *Journal of Applied Behavior Analysis*, **2**, 195–198.

Lehman, G. R. & Greller, E. S. (1990). Participative education for children: an effective approach to increase safety belt use. *Journal of Applied Behavior Analysis*, **23**, 219–225.

Leshner, A. I. (2001). Understanding and treating drug abuse and addiction. *Business Health*, **19**, 27–30.

Lovas, O. I., Koegel, R. L., Simmons, J. Q., & Long, J. S. (1973). Some generalization and follow-up measures on autistic children in behavior therapy. *Journal of Applied Behavior Analysis*, **6**, 131–166.

Ludwig, T. D., Gray, T. W., & Rowell, A. (1998). Increasing recycling in academic buildings: a systematic replication. *Journal of Applied Behavior Analysis*, **31**, 683–686.

Maney, J. Y. (1976). A behavioral therapy approach to bladder retraining. *Nursing Clinics of North America*, **11**, 179–188.

Marcus, A. C., Kaplan, C. P., Crane, L. A., *et al.* (1998). Reducing loss-to-follow-up among women with abnormal Pap smears. Results from a randomized trial testing an intensive follow-up protocol and economic incentives. *Medical Care*, **36**, 397–410.

Matthewson, C., Ayllon, T., Adkins, V. K., Lenyoun, M., & Jones, M. L. (1999). Using contingency management to reduce the incidence of pressure ulcers in a patient with a history of related surgeries. *Rehabilitative Nursing*, **24**, 234–235.

McMichael, J. S. & Corey, J. R. (1969). Contingency management in an introductory psychology class produces better learning. *Journal of Applied Behavior Analysis*, **2**, 79–83.

Melnikow, J., Paliescheskey, M., & Stewart, G. K. (1997). Effect of a transportation incentive on compliance with the first prenatal appointment: a randomized trial. *Obstetrics and Gynecology*, **89**, 1023–1027.

Mosley, T. H., Jr., Eisen, A. R., Bruce, B. K., Brantley, P. J., & Cocke, T. B. (1993). Contingent social reinforcement for fluid compliance in a hemodialysis patient. *Journal of Behavior Therapy and Experimental Psychiatry*, **24**, 77–81.

Nock, M. K. (2002). A multiple-baseline evaluation of the treatment of food phobia in a young boy. *Journal of Behavior Therapy and Experimental Psychiatry*, **33**, 217–225.

Olden, K. W. (2001). Rumination. *Current Treatment Options for Gastroenterology*, **4**, 351–358.

Parker, L. H., Cataldo, M. F., Bourland, G., *et al.* (1984). Operant treatment of orofacial dysfunction in neuromuscular disorders. *Journal of Applied Behavior Analysis*, **17**, 413–427.

Petry, N. M. (2000). A comprehensive guide to the application of contingency management procedures in clinical settings. *Drug and Alcohol Dependence*, **58**, 9–25.

Petry, N. M., Bickel, W. K., Tzanis, E., *et al.* (1998). A behavioral intervention for improving verbal behaviors of heroin addicts in a treatment clinic. *Journal of Applied Behavior Analysis*, **31**, 291–297.

Petry, N. M., Martin, B., Cooney, J. L., & Kranzler, H. R. (2000). Give them prizes, and they will come: contingency management for treatment of alcohol dependence. *Journal of Consulting and Clinical Psychology*, **68**, 250–257.

Petry, N. M., Tedford, J. & Martin, B. (2001). Reinforcing compliance with non-drug-related activities. *Journal of Substance Abuse Treatment*, **20**, 33–44.

Petry, N. M., Tedford, J., Austin, M., *et al.* (2004). Prize reinforcement contingency management for treating cocaine users: How low can we go, and with whom? Addiction, **99**, 349–360.

Pfiffner, L. J., Calzada, E., & McBurnett, K. (2000). Interventions to enhance social competence. *Child and Adolescent Psychiatric Clinics of North America*, **9**, 689–709.

Piacentini, J. (1999). Cognitive behavioral therapy of childhood OCD. *Child and Adolescent Psychiatric Clinics of North America*, **8**, 599–616.

Rawson, R. A., Huber, A., McCann, M., *et al.* (2002). A comparison of contingency management and cognitive–behavioral approaches during methadone maintenance treatment for cocaine dependence. *Archives of General Psychiatry*, **59**, 817–824.

Reid, D. H., Phillips, J. F., & Green, C. W. (1991). Teaching persons with profound multiple handicaps: a review of the effects of behavioral research. *Journal of Applied Behavioral Analysis*, **24**, 319–336.

Rigsby, M. O., Rosen, M. I., Beauvais, J. E., *et al.* (2000). Cue-dose training with monetary reinforcement: pilot study of an antiretroviral intervention. *Journal of General Internal Medicine*, **15**, 841–847.

Roll, J. M. (2005). Using contingency management to modify the smoking behavior of adolescents. *Journal of Applied Behavior Analysis*, in press.

Roll, J. M. & Higgins, S. T. (2000). A within-subject comparison of three different schedules of reinforcement of drug abstinence using cigarette smoking as an exemplar. *Drug and Alcohol Dependence*, **58**, 103–109.

Roll, J. M., Higgins, S. T., & Badger, G. J. (1996). An experimental comparison of three different schedules of reinforcement of drug abstinence using cigarette smoking as an exemplar. *Journal of Applied Behavior Analysis*, **29**, 495–504.

Roll, J. M., Higgins, S. T., Steingard, S., & McGinley, M. (1998). Use of monetary reinforcement to reduce the cigarette smoking of persons with schizophrenia: a feasibility study. *Experimental and Clinical Psychopharmacology*, **6**, 157–161.

Roll, J. M., Reilly, M. P., & Johanson, C. E. (2000). The influence of exchange delays on cigarette versus money choice: a laboratory analog of voucher-based reinforcement therapy. *Experimental and Clinical Psychopharmacology*, **8**, 366–370.

Roll, J. M., Richardson, G., Prakash, S., Brethen, P., & Chudzynski, J. (2003). Contingency management for the treatment of adolescent substance abuse: pilot studies. In *Proceedings of the Annual Meeting of the College of Dmg Dependency*, Bal Harbor, FL.

Rowe, C. L. & Liddle, H. A. (2003). Substance abuse. *Journal of Marital and Family Therapy*, **29**, 97–120.

Sidman, M. (1960). *Tactics of Scientific Research*. Boston, MA: Authors Cooperative.

Schreibman, L. & Koegel, R. L. (1981). A guideline for planning behavior modification programs for autistic children. In S. M. Turner, K. S. Calhoun, & H. E. Adams (eds.), *Handbook of Clinical Behavior Therapy* (pp. 500–526). New York: John Wiley.

Schumacher, J. E., Milby, J. B., McNamara, C. L., *et al.* (1999). Effective treatment of homeless substance abusers: the role of contingency management. In S. T. Higgins & K. Silverman (eds.), *Motivating Behavior Change among Illicit-drug Abusers: Research on Contingency Management Interventions* (pp. 77–94). Washington, DC: American Psychological Press.

Shoptaw, S., Jarvik, M. E., Ling. W., & Rawson, R. A. (1996). Contingency management for tobacco smoking in methadone-maintained opiate addicts. *Addictive Behavior*, **21**, 409–412.

Silverman, K., Svikis, D., Robles, E., Stitzer, M. L., & Bigelow, G. E. (2001) . A reinforcement-based therapeutic workplace for the treatment of drug abuse: six-month abstinence outcomes. *Experimental and Clinical Psychopharmacology*, **9**, 14–23.

Sloan, D. M. & Mizes, J. S. (1996). The use of contingency management in the treatment of a geriatric nursing home patient with psychogenic vomiting. *Journal of Behavior Therapy and Experimental Psychiatry*, **27**, 57–65.

Stalonas, P. M., Jr., Johnson, W. G., & Christ, M. (1978). Behavior modification for obesity: the evaluation of exercise, contingency management, and program adherence. *Journal of Consulting and Clinical Psychology*, **46**, 463–469.

Stark, L. J., Opipari, L. C., Donaldson, D. L., *et al.* (1997). Evaluation of a standard protocol for retentive encopresis: a replication. *Journal of Pediatric Psychology*, **22**, 619–633.

Stitzer, M. & Bigelow, G. (1978). Contingency management in a methadone maintenance program: availability of reinforcers. *International Journal of Addiction*, **13**, 737–746.

  (1984). Contingent reinforcement for carbon monoxide reduction: within-subject effects of pay amount. *Journal of Applied Behavior Analysis*, **17**, 477–483.

Stitzer, M. L. & Higgins, S. T. (1995). Behavioral treatment of drug and alcohol abuse. In F. E. Bloom & D. J. Kupfer (eds.), *Psychopharmacology: The Fourth Generation of Progress* (pp. 1807–1819). New York: Raven Press.

Stitzer, M. L., Rand, C. S., Bigelow, G. E., & Mead, A. M. (1986). Contingent payment procedures for smoking reduction and cessation. *Journal of Applied Behavioral Analysis*, **19**, 197–202.

Stoner, T. J., Dowd, B., Carr, W. P., *et al.* (1998). Do vouchers improve breast cancer screening rates? Results from a randomized trial. *Health Services Research*, **33**, 11–28.

Swain, M. A. & Steckel, S. B. (1981). Influencing adherence among hypertensives. *Research in Nursing and Health*, **4**, 213–222.

Teichner, G., Golden, C. J., & Giannaris, W. J. (1999). A multimodal approach to treatment of aggression in a severely brain-injured adolescent. *Rehabilitation Nursing*, **24**, 207–211.

Turner, S. M., Calhoun, K. S., & Adams, H. E. (1981). *Handbook of Clinical Behavior Therapy.* New York: John Wiley.

Ullman, L. P. & Krasner, L. (1965). *Case Studies in Behavior Modifications.* New York: Holt, Rinehard & Winston.

Weinrich, S. P., Weinrich, M. C., Priest, J., & Fodi, C. (2003). Self-reported reasons men decide not to participate in free prostate cancer screening. *Oncology Nursing Forum*, **30**, E12–E16.

Wells, K. C. & Forehand, R. (1981). Childhood behavior problems in the home. In S. M. Turner, K. S. Calhoun, & H. E. Adams (eds.), *Handbook of Clinical Behavior Therapy* (pp. 527–567). New York: John Wiley.

Wulbert, M. & Dries, R. (1977). The relative efficacy of methylphenidate (Ritalin) and behavior-modification techniques in the treatment of a hyperactive child. *Journal of Applied Behavior Analysis*, **10**, 21–31.

Wulbert, M., Nyman, B. A., Snow, D., & Owen, Y. (1973). The efficacy of stimulus fading and contingency management in the treatment of elective mutism: a case study. *Journal of Applied Behavior Analysis*, **6**, 435–441.

19

Evidence-based cognitive–behavioral therapies for adolescent substance use disorders: applications and challenges

Yifrah Kaminer and Holly Barrett Waldron

University of Connecticut Health Center, Farmington, CT, USA
Oregon Research Institute, Eugene, OR, USA

The effectiveness of cognitive–behavioral therapy (CBT) has been tested extensively and its effectiveness has been demonstrated in randomized trials since the 1970s for adult alcohol and other substance use disorders (SUD). Morgenstern and Longabaugh, (2000), indicated that although these intervention packages have differed in modality (i.e., individual, group, couples, family), format, and content (e.g., exclusively CBT, CBT as a component of integrative psychosocial treatment, CBT in combination with psychopharmacology), a strong theoretical base and impressive efficacy data made CBT either the standard to which other treatments were compared or the primary technique or component in a variety of intervention conditions (e.g., family, 12-step therapies). By contrast, research conducted to evaluate CBT for adolescents has been limited and, while the evidence supporting CBT is promising, formal controlled clinical efficacy and effectiveness trials have only recently begun to emerge in the literature. Latest innovations in the management of treatment protocols for adolescent SUD and the recent completion of several randomized clinical trials examining manual-guided CBT, have established empirical support for CBT in youth (Dennis *et al.*, 2004; Kaminer, Burleson, & Goldberger, 2002; Waldron & Kaminer, 2004; Waldron *et al.*, 2001a). The purpose of this chapter is to review (a) the theoretical models underlying intervention approaches based on CBT; (b) the evidence-based literature on CBT for the most prevalent psychiatric disorders and behaviors accompanying SUD in youth; and (c) the empirical studies addressing CBT for youth with SUD. Mechanisms and therapeutic processes of CBT associated with change are examined in adults and youth, and future research directions and treatment implications conclude the chapter.

Theoretical models underlying cognitive–behavioral intervention approaches

Intervention approaches based on CBT have varied, with most approaches integrating strategies derived from classical conditioning, operant, and social learning

Adolescent Substance Abuse: Research and Clinical Advances, ed. Howard A. Liddle and Cynthia L. Rowe.
Published by Cambridge University Press. © Cambridge University Press 2006.

perspectives. Each of these perspectives view substance use and related problems as learned behaviors that are initiated and maintained in the context of environmental factors. Yet, experimental research within each theoretical perspective has focused on unique aspects of substance use behavior, resulting in the development of distinct interventions techniques that are often combined into a multicomponent CBT intervention. For example, animal and human research examining the classically conditioned acquisition of preferences and aversions for alcohol and drugs, tolerance, and urges and cravings has led to the development of stimulus-control interventions such as identifying stimulus cues for drug or alcohol use and learning to avoid high-risk situations as a means to facilitate sobriety (Dimeff & Marlatt, 1995; Monti *et al.*, 1995). Such interventions typically involve identifying contextual factors, such as the setting, time, or place, which may serve as potential "triggers." Strategies to manage urges and cravings, once stimulus cues have been identified, may involve techniques from different learning perspectives, such as self-control, reinforcers for competing behaviors, or other coping-skills training. Operant perspectives view alcohol and drug use behaviors in the context of the antecedents and consequences surrounding the behavior. In addition to the powerful reinforcement associated with the physiological effects of drugs that serve to maintain use, reinforcers can also include the reduction of tension, attenuation of negative affect, or enhancement of social interactions. Intervention strategies based on operant learning often include identifying alternative reinforcers that compete with drug use and other applications of contingency management (Gilchrist & Schinke, 1985; Higgins *et al.*, 1995; Stitzer, Bigelow, & Liebson, 1979; Stitzer & Kirby, 1991). The social learning model incorporates the influence of environmental events on the acquisition of behavior but also recognizes the role of cognitive processes (e.g., how environmental influences are perceived and appraised) in determining behavior (Bandura, 1977). Within this perspective, substance use can be influenced through a variety of cognitive and behavioral factors including modeling parents, siblings, or peers; social reinforcement; the expectation of the effects of drug use; self-efficacy beliefs about one's ability to refrain from use; and physical dependence (Abrams & Niaura, 1987). The stress-coping model, one example of a social learning-based approach, views substance use as a maladaptive response to stress, acquired through modeling drug use by others as a means of coping with stress and used in the absence of alternative appropriate coping models.

Multicomponent CBT approaches for substance abuse often include such components as self-monitoring, avoidance of stimulus cues, altering reinforcement contingencies, and coping-skills training to manage and resist urges to use. Drug and alcohol refusal skills, communication skills, problem-solving skills, assertiveness, relaxation training, anger management, modifying cognitive distortions, and relapse prevention are often incorporated to promote sobriety

(Marlatt & Gordon, 1985; Monti *et al.*, 1989, 1993). Therapy sessions characteristically include modeling, behavior rehearsal, feedback, and homework assignments. Behavioral targets of change usually include the adolescent's family relationships and school or work-related issues. Specific targets of change, however, such as negotiating privileges or identification of contingencies, must take into account the age and developmental level of the adolescent. Moreover, many adolescents may not have had sufficient opportunity to acquire certain social and coping skills normally developed during adolescence because of their heavy drug use, and components may need to be incorporated to address basic skill deficits.

Randomized clinical trials for adolescent substance abuse treatment

Early treatment-outcome research on CBT interventions for adolescent SUD, while providing an important impetus for later efficacy and effectiveness trials, was limited in a variety of ways. Methodological limitations included small samples, inadequate control or comparison conditions, non-randomized assignment to treatment, poor measures of variables of interest, absence of attrition data, limited descriptions of treatments, and the absence of treatment manuals and fidelity measures (Catalano *et al.*, 1990–1991; Kaminer, 2000; Waldron, 1997). Wide variations in selection criteria, measures of substance use outcome, and number and latency of follow-up assessments also characterized the research. The mixed findings in the literature likely derived from this methodological variability across studies. The emergence of formal randomized controlled trials and field experiments, however, has added significantly to the base of empirical support for CBT. These recent studies have employed more rigorous designs, with larger samples, random assignment, direct comparisons of two or more active treatments, improved measures of substance use and other variables, manual-guided interventions, and longer-term outcome assessments (Dennis *et al.*, 2004; Kaminer *et al.*, 1998a, 2002; Kaminer & Burleson, 1999; Waldron *et al.*, 2001a). These findings, taken together, establish the foundation for the effectiveness of CBT for adolescent SUDs.

Kaminer and his colleagues (1998a) have conducted several studies evaluating a group CBT intervention for outpatient adolescents with SUD. The intervention was originially developed in the context of a patient–treatment matching study for adults (Cooney *et al.*, 1991; Kadden *et al.*, 1989). In this adolescent patient–treatment matching study, 32 adolescents between the ages of 13 and 18 years were randomly assigned to 12 sessions of CBT or to a similar number of interactional group therapy sessions. Youth were all dually diagnosed. No patient–treatment matching effects between psychopathologies (i.e., externalizing, internalizing disorders) and treatment modalities (i.e., CBT, interactional therapy) were found (Kaminer *et al.*,

1998b). However, the short-term efficacy of CBT was significant. Adolescents assigned to CBT showed a greater short-term improvement than those assigned to interactional therapy. As in other adolescent treatment-outcome studies, however, relapse was a problem for many youth, and differences between the groups were no longer significant a year later (Kaminer & Burleson, 1999).

In a larger-scale controlled, randomized trial, Kaminer *et al.* (2002) compared the efficacy of CBT with psychoeducational therapies for adolescent substance abusers. It was hypothesized that participants in both conditions would improve from pretreatment to follow-up at 3 and 9 months, but that youth assigned to the CBT condition would have better retention rates in treatment and follow-up and superior short- and long-term outcomes, relative to those who had received psychoeducational therapy. The 88 predominantly dually diagnosed adolescents were randomly assigned to one of the two 8-week group interventions. Participants were between the ages of 13 and 18 years (mean, 15.4; standard deviation, 1.3), and included 62 males and 26 females. The majority (79) were White. For older youth and for males, the CBT group showed significantly lower rates of positive urinalysis than the psychoeducational therapy group at the 3-month follow-up. Moreover, self-report drug use measures revealed significant improvement from baseline to follow-up at both 3 and 9 months across conditions. There was also a trend toward improvement for adolescents who received CBT at the 3-month follow-up, with significant improvement for males and older subjects. Similar patterns were not found for psychoeducational therapy. Contrary to hypotheses, CBT did not produce any long-term differential relapse rate compared with psychoeducational therapy, as a result of the increase in relapse among CBT participants at the 9-month follow-up. However, most of the participants improved substantially in a variety of domains. The majority of the substance use-related problems assessed showed improvements at follow-up at 3 months and continued to improve at 9 months, relative to baseline, regardless of assigned treatment condition.

Waldron and her colleagues (2001a) have evaluated the efficacy of CBT and family-based treatments in two studies of substance abuse treatment for youth referred for outpatient services. In the first study, adolescents were randomly assigned to one of four interventions: individual CBT, group CBT, family therapy, and a combined intervention including both individual CBT and family therapy. The 129 adolescents ranged in age from 13 to 17 years (median, 15.54), with 77% of the sample male. Participants included 35% Hispanic, 41% Anglo, 6% Native-American, and 15% mixed ethnicity. Substance use was measured at four points in time: pretreatment and at 4, 7, and 19 months after the initiation of treatment. At pretreatment, adolescents reported using alcohol or drugs (excluding tobacco) on an average of 61.11% of the days in the 6 months prior to treatment. Substance use varied little with age or between single and two-parent families. The average percentage days of substance use reported for the past 6 months was 67.78% for girls and 57.78% for boys. Adolescents completed an average of 85% of their available treatment sessions, with no significant differences between groups.

Youth who were assigned to family therapy, individual CBT, or group CBT received 12 hours of therapy, while adolescents assigned to the combined condition received 24 hours of treatment (12 family therapy, 12 individual CBT). The individual CBT condition was patterned after coping-skills training programs developed by Monti and colleagues (1989) and Project MATCH (Kadden, Carroll, & Donovan, 1992). The underlying model was designed to teach the individual adolescent self-regulation and coping skills for avoiding substance use (Hester & Miller, 1989; Wilkinson & LeBreton, 1986). The CBT intervention included a two-session motivational-enhancement intervention (Miller & Rollnick, 1991) and 10 skills modules focusing on such topics as communication training, problem solving, peer refusal, negative-mood management, social support, work and school-related skills, and relapse prevention. The group CBT included some psychoeducational material, focusing on drug and alcohol effects and expectancies and consequences of substance use, but focused primarily on communication skills training, assertiveness, and substance-refusal skills. There was some content overlap between the individual and group CBT, although individual CBT involved a flexible treatment plan based on each adolescent's needs while the group was more structured and emphasized group interaction and feedback more than individual skill acquisition.

The 30 adolescents who received group CBT showed significant reductions in their percentage days of marijuana use from a pretreatment to 7 months and then further to the assessment at 19 months. The positive outcomes for the CBT group treatment were delayed, but substantial: the effect size for the group intervention at 19 months was 0.93, compared with 0.67 for the family-based intervention. A somewhat different pattern of findings emerged when examining clinically meaningful change, with the proportion of youth achieving abstinence or minimal levels of use (i.e., reported use on fewer than 10% of the days) as the outcome measure. Pretreatment to 4-, 7-, and 19-month change in clinically significant marijuana use was assessed using a Wilcoxon sign test procedure within each treatment condition. As with the measure of percentage days of use overall, a significantly greater number of youth in the CBT group treatment had achieved abstinence or minimal use at the 7-month and 19-month follow-up assessments, but not at the 4-month assessment. For individual CBT, however, a significant proportion of youth had become abstinent by 4 months. This pattern was only a trend by 7 months and did not persist at 19 months. However, the findings revealed that some youth did benefit from individual CBT, and understanding who will benefit has critical implications for client–treatment matching.

In another study, Waldron *et al.* (2003) evaluated the efficacy of individual CBT for 31 adolescents who were initially treatment refusers but later entered treatment as a result of a parent-focused engagement intervention. The CBT intervention was the same as in the previous trials (Waldron *et al.*, 2001a). Adolescents in this study completed an average of five therapy sessions, half the number of sessions completed by youth in the earlier studies, but they were using drugs or alcohol an average of 80.39% of the days in the past 3-month period. The CBT was associated with a significant decrease in percentage days of substance use from pre- to post-treatment (F, 9.42 [degrees of freedom 1, 27]; $P < 0.005$). Although reduction in use was statistically significant, adolescents' continued heavy use at post-treatment suggests that more intensive engagement and intervention strategies may be needed to increase the dosage of treatment received and enhance the impact of the intervention for this difficult treatment-resistant population.

Liddle and his colleagues (2001) also conducted a study comparing family therapy with CBT. A group of 182 adolescent substance abusers were randomly assigned to one of three treatment conditions: Multidimensional Family Therapy, an adolescent skills-based group therapy, and a family-education group intervention. The group intervention was based on a CBT model and focused on social-skills training (e.g., communication, self control, and problem solving). Group therapy was preceded by two family sessions to enhance cooperation and participation. All three conditions showed reductions in substance use and improvement in other areas of functioning, with clinically significant reductions in drug use at post-treatment in 45% of youth in family therapy, 32% in group, and 26% in the family-education group. Although the investigators reported the most consistent pattern of improvements in the family-therapy condition, the findings also provided support for the CBT group intervention. In a second study, 224 adolescents were randomly assigned to either multidimensional family therapy (Liddle, 2002) or individual CBT. The CBT and family interventions both included individual and conjoint family sessions. However, the CBT condition emphasized self-monitoring, communication and problem-solving skills training, contingency contracting, and substance-refusal skills. Both interventions produced significant decreases in substance use from pretreatment to follow-up assessments at 6 and 12 months, although there appeared to be continued improvement over time in the family-therapy condition compared with some leveling off in substance-use reductions in the CBT condition after the 6-month follow-up. Again, the authors concluded that support for family therapy was relatively stronger, although the efficacy of CBT for adolescent substance abuse was also supported.

The Cannabis Youth Treatment study was a randomized field experiment that compared a total of five interventions, in various combinations, across four implementation sites (Dennis *et al.*, 2004). The study was designed to address the differential efficacy of the treatment modalities implemented and the effect of treatment dose contribution to outcome. The interventions included two family-based treatments and three CBT treatments: a five session CBT group intervention (Sampl & Kadden, 2001; Webb *et al.*, 2002), a 12 session CBT group intervention, and a 12 session individual CBT intervention (adolescent community reinforcement approach; Godley, Meyers, & Smith, 2002). The five treatment models were evaluated in two arms. The replication of the five session CBT intervention across all four sites made it possible to study site differences and conduct quasi-experimental comparisons of the interventions across study arms. This study is described comprehensively in Ch. 5 and so will only be briefly reviewed here with emphasis on the CBT interventions.

According to Dennis *et al.* (2004), all five interventions produced significant reductions in both cannabis use and negative consequences of use from pretreatment to the 3-month follow-up. These reductions were sustained through to the 12-month follow-up. Some findings, however, were unanticipated. For example, the five session CBT appear to produce outcomes on par with the 12-session CBT and the 12-session CBT combined with a 12-session family support intervention, findings not consistent with a simple dose–response relationship. Also, the individual community reinforcement approach and the individual/group (motivational enhancement with five CBT sessions) behavioral interventions produced better outcomes than the family approach in terms of days of substance use at 3 months, although these initial differences were not sustained. Overall, support was found for each of the CBT interventions, with initial level of change emerging as the best predictor of long-term outcomes.

Cognitive–behavioral therapy for common comorbid psychiatric disorders

Diagnosis of comorbid disorders for adolescents with SUDs is the rule rather than the exception. Bukstein, Glancy, and Kaminer (1992) found that 62% of adolescents receiving inpatient treatment were dually diagnosed. DiMilo (1989) found that 42% of adolescents presenting for treatment of substance abuse also met criteria for conduct disorder, the most common disorder co-occurring with substance abuse, and 35% also had a major depressive disorder. In a most recent outpatient study utilizing DSM criteria, 90% of youth had comorbid diagnoses (Kaminer *et al.*, 2002): 54% had an externalizing disorder and 32% were diagnosed with an internalizing disorder. The comorbidity issue adds a level of complexity to understanding substance abuse. Whether substance abuse is primary or occurs secondary to another disorder, and how the interaction of coexisting disorders influence the onset, identification, course, and treatment of substance abuse problems, remains in question.

Research evaluating CBT for behavioral problems and disorders associated with adolescent substance abuse, such as depression (Birmaher *et al.*, 2000; Brent *et al.*, 1997; Clarke *et al.*, 1999; Wood, Harrington, & Moore, 1996), anxiety (Barrett *et al.*, 2001; Kendall, 1994; Kendall *et al.*, 1997; Spence, Donovan, & Brechman-Toussaint, 2000), and conduct problems (Kazdin, 1995; Kendall & Wilcox, 1980; Kendall *et al.*, 1990), is well established. Empirical support for CBT with adolescent disorders known to co-occur with adolescent substance use would seem to lend support to CBT for adolescents with comorbid disorders including SUD. Surprisingly, few systematic studies have been conducted evaluating CBT for such youth. Research evaluating CBT for other psychiatric disorders, then, provides a critical foundation for future clinical trials.

Depression

Several randomized controlled studies have found positive effects of CBT for youth depression (Birmaher *et al.*, 2000; Brent *et al.*, 1997; Clarke *et al.*, 1999; Wood *et al.*, 1996). Brent's group (1998, 1999) reported that CBT was more efficacious than alternative psychosocial interventions such as systematic behavioral family therapy and non-directive supportive therapy. The patients treated with CBT showed a more rapid and complete symptomatic relief of depression. Wood and colleagues (1996) found a clear advantage of brief CBT compared with a control treatment, relaxation training. None of these studies however, showed significant differences in long-term outcome (Birmaher *et al.*, 2000). A study by Kroll and colleagues (1996) suggested that monthly booster sessions of CBT may substantially reduce the rate of depressive relapse. Therefore, one reason for the high rate of recurrence and for the lack of sustained differential effect of CBT may have been the absence of a vigorous continuation treatment component (i.e., continued care or aftercare). The positive outcomes for CBT with youth diagnosed with depression lends support to the notion that CBT is likely to be particularly beneficial for depressed youth with a co-occurring SUD.

Offspring of depressed parents are considered to be more severely depressed than those with negative family history for depression. Beardslee, Wright, & Salt, (1997) conducted a randomized, controlled trial of a family-based, cognitive intervention for offspring of depressed parents. They found positive intervention effects on child and parent outcomes but did not report outcomes for depressive episodes. Clarke and colleagues (2002) conducted a randomized, controlled effectiveness trial of group CBT for depressed adolescent offspring of depressed parents in the Health Maintenance Organization. However, group CBT did not appear superior to the usual care offered, which included any non-study mental health care. Similar poor outcomes for this population have been reported in another CBT trial (Brent *et al.*, 1998). Considering that significant treatment effects are much more often detected in efficacy trials than in effectiveness trials (Weisz *et al.*, 1995), these results should not be viewed as evidence for the overall ineffectiveness of CBT. Rather they may suggest the need for more aggressive treatments, including combinations of antidepressant medications, for a more severely affected subpopulation of juvenile patients. Only one pilot study examining the feasibility and preliminary symptomatic efficacy of CBT for depressed, substance-abusing adolescents has been reported so far (Curry *et al.*, 2003).

Finally, CBT as a treatment modality or as a significant component of a treatment manual was successfully implemented with youth manifesting self-harm behaviors such as a suicide attempts (Rotheram-Borus *et al.*, 1994) and repeated deliberate self-harm (Wood *et al.*, 2001). These studies however, did not include a comparison group. Therefore, no definitive conclusions regarding efficacy of CBT for these problems can be drawn.

Anxiety disorders

There have been promising developments in the treatment of anxiety disorders with CBT for youth diagnosed with anxiety disorders showing considerable promise (Kazdin & Weisz, 1998; Ollendick & King, 1998; Pina *et al.*, 2003). Kendall's group have reported significant improvements based on parent-, child-, and teacher-reported measures post-treatment for an approach employing a manual-based CBT for children with anxiety disorders (Kendall, 1994; Kendall *et al.*, 1997). Manassis *et al.* (2002) reported that children with anxiety disorders improved with CBT whether administered in a group or individual format. Group setting of CBT for anxious adolescents has also shown promising results (Albano *et al.*, 1995; Hayward *et al.*, 2000). A study on CBT for social phobia in female adolescents showed significant short-term gains for subjects assigned to treatment compared with the no-treatment groups; however, these differences were not maintained at 1-year follow-up (Hayward *et al.*, (2000)). Other reports further support the efficacy of CBT for childhood anxiety disorders, including benefits from adding a family anxiety-management component to the child's treatment (Barrett, Dadds, & Rapee, 1996; Spence *et al.*, 2000). Follow-up at 1, 3, and 6 years showed maintenance of long-term gains (Barrett *et al.*, 2001; Kendall & Southam-Gerow, 1996). We are not aware of any reports of efficacy studies comparing different treatment modalities for anxiety disorders in youth.

Post-traumatic stress disorder

Despite the paucity of empirical treatment outcome studies in youth with post-traumatic stress disorder, clinical consensus among experts in the field suggests empirical support for the use of CBT among the essential components of treatment. This treatment modality include components such as direct discussion of the trauma, desensitization and relaxation techniques, cognitive reframing, and contingency-reinforcement programs for problematic behaviors (Deblinger & Heflin, 1996). Deblinger, Lipman, & Steer, (1996) used trauma-focused CBT to treat sexually abused children. Subjects were randomly assigned to one of four treatment conditions: child-only receiving CBT, parent-only receiving CBT, child and parent receiving CBT, or assignment to a community treatment control. Results indicated that, although all groups improved, the two conditions in which the child received direct treatment demonstrated significantly greater improvement in stress disorder symptoms than the other two conditions. Cohen and Mannarino, (1996) reported a significant decrease of symptoms of post-traumatic stress disorder in a CBT group compared with non-directive supportive therapy. In conclusion, cognitive interventions and skills training may be helpful in the treatment of post-traumatic stress disorder, but their long-term efficacy is still untested.

Conduct disorders/antisocial behavior

Deficits in problem-solving skills, perceptions, self-statements, and attributions have been shown to be associated with disruptive and antisocial behavior (Offord & Bennett, 1994). The set of techniques variously termed cognitive–behavioral interpersonal social skills training have proved to be quite successful with these problems (Lipsey & Wilson, 1998). For example, Kazdin, Siegel, & Bass, (1992) reported that random assignment of children with antisocial behavior to cognitive problem-solving skills and/or parent management training have shown reduced overall deviance and aggressive, antisocial, and delinquent behavior, and increased social competence. The combination of both interventions was superior to each component alone. The "reasoning and rehabilitation" program developed by Ross and Ross (1995) for juvenile delinquents resulted in reduced recidivism (i.e., reoffending). This program included social skills training, lateral thinking (to teach creative problem solving), critical thinking, values education, assertiveness training, negotiation skills training, interpersonal cognitive problem solving, and social perspective training. Role playing and modeling are important ingredients employed in this successful training program. Based on meta-analysis techniques, it appears that the evidence for effectiveness is mixed and that the link between cognitive change and behavioral change has not been fully demonstrated for adolescents with conduct disorders (Farrington, 1999).

A number of investigators have shown that youth diagnosed with conduct disorder and SUD are at increased risk of not completing treatment (Kaminer *et al.*, 1992, 2002; Myers, Stewart, & Brown, 1998). This is particularly true for those youth who do not also have concurrent depression or anxiety (Kaminer *et al.*, 1992). The link between treatment completion and better treatment outcomes suggests that more treatment development is required.

Client–treatment matching

There has been growing interest in the possibility that treatment efficacy may depend upon characteristics of the client being treated (Kadden *et al.*, 2001; Project MATCH Research Group, 1997; Snow, Tebes, & Arthur, 1992). In earlier work by Kadden and colleagues (1989), client sociopathy and global psychopathology were effective variables for treatment matching: adult clients with low severity of both sociopathy and psychopathology were likely to benefit from interactional group therapy, whereas those scoring high on either of these dimensions benefited more from a CBT coping skills intervention. Furthermore, these findings were sustained in a 2-year follow-up study (Cooney *et al.*, 1991). In a recent study by Kadden and colleagues (2001), adult clients were assigned to group treatments prospectively based on a matching theory derived from the previous findings. All participants met criteria for alcohol dependence or abuse. About half were prospectively assigned to either CBT coping skills training or interactional therapy: those with higher levels of psychiatric severity or sociopathy were given CBT and those who were less severely affected in both dimensions were given interactional therapy. The other half were randomly assigned to those treatments. It was concluded that the matching effects from their previous study were not replicated; nevertheless, prospective matching did reduce the negative consequences of drinking, consistent with their previous results. Kadden and colleagues (2001) concluded that it might be necessary to determine client variables related to treatment responsiveness and the treatment variables that best addressed the particular client needs. Project MATCH (1997), which included CBT, motivational interviewing, and a 12-step intervention, did not find any matching effects in adult alcoholics.

Because CBT does not appear to be equally efficacious for all youth, research focused on understanding who might benefit from CBT is needed. The finding of Kaminer *et al.* (2002) that older and male subjects had better outcomes is intriguing but difficult to explain. Perhaps boys respond more positively to the structured context of CBT interventions compared with girls. Older youth may be in a more advanced stage of cognitive development. Babor and colleagues (2002) analyzed the data from the Cannabis Youth Treatment study using a unidimensional subtyping approach. This included psychopathology, gender, age of onset, family history positive for substance abuse, and difficult temperament. The powerful discrimination provided by the externalizing disorders subtype suggested that CBT and family therapy models may be particularly suited to the most severely problematic adolescent marijuana users. The CBT approach may provide needed structure and coping skills, while family interventions may help to address the coercive cycle of parent–child interactions that can contribute to substance abuse as an "acting out" coping strategy. Evidence for treatment matching was found and indicated that adolescents with early-onset problems do better in family support networks, as do youth with internalizing disorders. Adolescents with difficult temperament do best in Multidimensional Family Therapy whereas those without difficult temperament do better in motivational enhancement therapy plus CBT.

Other youth-treatment matching variables for future investigation should include co-occurring psychological problems, parenting and family factors, capacity to form a therapeutic alliance, and motivation. Treatment outcome may also be influenced by timing and magnitude of readiness to change; motivation for engagement in treatment; differences in number, quality, and magnitude of coping-skills deficits; level of vulnerability and opportunity for exposure to different situations posing high-risk for relapse; self efficacy; negative moods; and treatment expectancies (Morgenstern & Longabaugh, 2000; Waldron, Miller, & Tonigan, 2001b; J. A. Burleson & Y. Kaminer, unpublished data).

Treatment modality: group or individual intervention

Questions have also been raised as to whether CBT is best implemented with groups of adolescents or individually. Taken together, studies conducted by the authors and their colleagues provide support for the benefits of behavioral group therapy, with modest additional support for the efficacy of individual CBT, in reducing youth substance abuse and related problems in outpatient settings. The empirical support for the efficacy of CBT with adolescents is also similar to evidence found for treatment studies for adult drinking and drug use (Graham, Annis, & Brett, 1996; Kadden *et al.*, 1989; Marques & Formigoni, 2001; Project MATCH Research Group, 1997; Woody, Luborsky, & McLellen, 1983).

The results of the recent clinical trials for adolescents are particularly important because of the enhanced design and methodological features of these trials, which represent significant improvements over previous studies. Although the absence of untreated control groups represents a limitation in the recent clinical trials, the differential efficacy of treatments across multiple studies provides compelling evidence that the reductions in substance use were a direct function of the treatments clients received, rather than an artifact of the passage of time or involvement in a clinical trial.

It is important to note, however, that despite the advances of recent clinical trials over previous studies, none of these interventions sufficiently addressed the adolescents' problems. Relapse was a consistent problem for youth across studies. In the Cannabis Youth Treatment study, for example, approximately a third of the adolescents were in a state of early recovery (i.e., in the community without any marijuana use or problems) during the follow-up period, but another third of received additional treatment during the rest of the year. The single best predictor of 12-month outcomes was not baseline client characteristics or components of the intervention but whether the adolescent initially responded to treatment at 3 months.

This consistent empirical support of group CBT for substance-abusing adolescents stands in contrast to the iatrogenic effects reported for group interventions (Dishion, McCord, & Poulin, 1999; Dishion, Poulin, & Barreston, 2001). However, their research focused on preventative interventions for youth who were at risk for substance use but had not yet developed a SUD. The negative consequences experienced by adolescents diagnosed with substance abuse or dependence would be expected to influence treatment motivation. A number of features associated with group approaches to treatment may also facilitate cognitive, affective, and behavioral changes. These factors include the realization that others share similar problems, the development of socializing techniques, modeling, rehearsal, and peer/therapist feedback. The opportunity to try out new behaviors in a social environment and the development and enhancement of interpersonal learning and trust may also be influential.

In studies of group versus individual CBT conducted with adults, both conditions were similarly successful in reducing drinking and drug use at 12-month follow-up (Graham, Annis, & Brett, 1996; Marques & Formigoni, 2001). Furthermore, Graham and colleagues (1996) reported that the group condition demonstrated its superiority in improving social skills deemed important for relapse prevention in many patients, including adolescents. Because teenagers typically use alcohol or drugs when in the company of other users, and they are easily influenced in group settings (Myers & Brown, 1996), group treatment has the benefit of mirroring their daily experience. Role playing, an effective component employed in CBT, takes advantage of the group setting by allowing the participants to practice scenes of high-risk experience.

Mechanisms of change in cognitive–behavioral therapy for substance abuse disorders

Establishing support for CBT for SUDs is complicated by the wide variations in treatment components in different CBT models. These variations also make the identification of mechanisms of change more difficult. That is, intervention approaches often include a diverse array of modules and can range from those involving a select few components to those with a full complement of distinct components. While there is virtually no research aimed at elucidating mechanisms of change for therapy process variables associated with adolescent outcomes, researchers have begun to wrestle with the mechanisms and therapeutic processes of CBT associated with change in adults with SUDs (Litt *et al.*, 2003;

Morgenstern & Longabaugh, 2000; Maisto, Connors, & Zywiak, 2000; Wilson, 1999). This research may point the way to similar research for adolescent substance abuse treatment.

Litt and colleagues (2003) conducted a matching study comparing the efficacy of CBT and interactional therapy for adult alcoholics. Contrary to expectations, neither treatment effected greater increases in coping than the other. Furthermore, although higher levels of coping appear to be related to better outcomes, it is not clear that coping skills per se were responsible for those outcomes, that CBT improved coping, and that increased coping was associated with abstinence or reduction of substance use. Increased use of coping skills was predicted by baseline readiness for change and abstinence self-efficacy. These results were interpreted as suggesting that those with high readiness and/or self-efficacy are able to take advantage of any treatment offered to increase their ability to cope and thereby improve their outcomes. Training in coping skills per se does not appear essential for increasing the use of coping skills. These results raise the question of how to identify existing causal effects of specific mediators of CBT to improve treatment outcome differentially.

These findings lend support to the "critical period" hypothesis: those with high self-efficacy and motivation to change at baseline sought treatment at a time when they could capitalize on the treatment provided. Litt and colleagues (2003) findings fit nicely with the literature on initiation of health behavior change in which self-efficacy and motivation are seen as necessary mediators.

Cognitive and behavioral coping has a central role in the hypothesis that deficits in the ability to cope with life stress in general and substance cues in particular serve to maintain substance use or lead to relapse. Therefore, all CBT packages use a standard set of techniques to teach coping skills, which includes identification of high-risk situations where these skills should be employed (Morgenstern & Longabaugh, 2000). No review has evaluated evidence supporting the hypothesized mechanisms of action through which CBT works. Evidence of efficacy does not demonstrate that a treatment works as purported, since other mechanisms of action are possible. Demonstrating that a treatment is effective without understanding how it works undermines the potential for replicability. If active ingredients can be identified, then the intervention might be modified to enhance these. Alternatively, effectiveness might be improved by patient–treatment matching or by combining treatments with different active ingredients. These last strategies are predicated on the assumption that different treatments work, at least in part, through distinct, non-overlapping mechanisms. Numerous process and matching studies have tested the hypothesis that CBT works through its specific effects on coping, but support has been absent (Litt *et al.*, 2003; Morgenstern & Longabaugh, 2000; Wilson, 1999).

It has been suggested that treatment acts at least partially through non-specific effects (Wampold *et al.*, 1999). Similarly, Wilson (1999) addressed the renewed attention to the "non-specifics" of therapy as mediators of rapid response to CBT. Rapid response to CBT by alcohol abusers resulted in 64% of the total improvement being evident during the first 4 weeks of treatment (Breslin *et al.*, 1997). This pattern appears to be a general phenomenon that might emerge before the presumed specific impact of CBT affects the client. Furthermore, rapid response is not limited to any specific disorder (e.g., depression, SUDs bulimia nervosa). The rapid treatment effect of CBT cannot be dismissed as a placebo or a non-specific response. CBT quickly becomes significantly more effective than equally credible, alternative psychological therapies, including interpersonal psychotherapy for adults (Jones *et al.*, 1993) and youth (Kaminer *et al.*, 1998a) and supportive psychotherapy (Wilson, 1999). Other therapies have a more gradual dose–response relationship and, according to the measure of treatment outcome used by Howard *et al.* (1986, p. 163), which is that at least 50% of patients improve: "subjects who have had less than 6–8 sessions should be considered, for purposes of research, as not having been effectively exposed to treatment and should be analyzed separately." Variables such as therapeutic alliance (Ilardi & Craighead, 1994) or patients' perception regarding what treatment is more suitable for their problems (Wilson, 1999) could not explain early response to CBT. Home assignments are unique to CBT and might enhance self-efficacy and have an early therapeutic effect in adults (Ilardi & Craighead, 1994). However, the rate of complete home assignment in youth has been very low and this cannot, therefore, provide a satisfactory explanation in this age group. It is plausible that enhancement of self-monitoring during early sessions of CBT, including prompting increased awareness of self-evaluative reactions (i.e., affect, behavior, cognition), improves self-regulation and problem solving (Bandura, 1986). However, this hypothesis must be empirically examined.

An opposite approach might be to focus on non-responders to CBT, who may provide therapists with the opportunity to explore more effective treatment modalities and/or dosage. This could be done by developing the analysis of time course of therapeutic change by illustrating different profiles of improvement in responders versus non-responders to CBT in general and to specific sessions in particular. Also, analyzing improvement as a function both of time (number of weeks) and therapy dose (treatment sessions) could be useful, as demonstrated in the Cannabis Youth Treatment outcome report (Dennis *et al.*, 2004). Treatment mediators identify possible mechanisms through which a treatment might achieve its effects. These mechanisms are causal link between treatment and outcome (Kraemer *et al.*, 2002). Therefore, studies designed to investigate mediators of the therapeutic change attributed to CBT must include early measures of proposed mediators that must operate prior to the achievement of the presumed outcome (Wilson, 1999). Morgenstern & Longabaugh (2000) indicated that there is a need to improve strategies for measuring CBT mediators. A comprehensive set of CBT mediators may include cognitive constructs such as negative expectancies. Measurement of the fidelity of administration of treatment components (e.g., role modeling) is necessary. The search for mediators responsible for symptom reduction in CBT for SUD has not been completed. Delineating causal mechanism is perplexing. The acquisition of problem-solving skills and the frequency of their application on a daily basis are constructs to be examined.

Determinants of relapse in patients who achieved complete abstinence from SUD following CBT would be useful to ascertain for several reasons, as noted by Halmi and colleagues (2002, p. 1105) in their CBT for bulimia nervosa: "The identification of variables associated with relapse may engender modifications leading to more effective treatment. If relapse predictors are known, it may be possible to design effective post-CBT intervention strategies for susceptible patients or modify CBT to prevent relapse."

Although little research addressing mechanisms of change associated with CBT has been conducted for the adolescent age group, Kaminer and colleagues (1998b) were able to identify several active ingredients characterizing CBT (i.e., problem solving, identification of high-risk situations, skills training, and role playing) and discriminate between them and ingredients characterizing interactional therapy. However, the efficacy of these components was not examined. In other research, Myers and Brown (1990a, 1990b) found that, following CBT, problem-solving coping strategies were more likely to be used by adolescent alcohol abstainers and minor relapsers than by major relapsers. Coping factors have also been identified as significant predictors of treatment outcome (Myers, Brown, & Mott, 1993). Research has been challenged, however, by the lack adequate measures for assessing pre- to post-treatment change in coping skills and, to date, no published studies of adolescent substance abuse treatment have examined critically the assumption that coping skills are actually acquired or enhanced in treatment. There is a need to determine to what extent outcome of adolescent treatment is a function of acquired or improved coping skills, and whether coping-skills acquisition is a function of specific treatment approaches. Factors such as readiness to change, expectancy, therapeutic alliance, and engagement in treatment may mediate change independently or interact to influence change.

Clinical implications and future research directions

Despite some prominent differences in design and methodology, the studies employing different treatment modalities in youth with SUDs, including CBT, have reported remarkably similar outcomes. Taken together, the findings represent significant developments in treatment outcome research (Waldron & Kaminer, 2004). Yet, many of the questions raised in this chapter are valid, including the contribution of the "placebo-assessment effect" and other "nonspecific" mediators that might be responsible for the similar results in outcome regardless of the specificity of the interventions. Future research should focus on improving short- and long-term outcomes, including maintenance of treatment gain in after-care programs (Kaminer, 2001) and examining the transportability of CBT into other treatment modalities such as telephone (Kaminer & Napolitano, 2004) or internet interventions, as well as into settings such as therapeutic communities, residential treatment, or the juvenile justice system facilities. The relationship of CBT with features such as enhancing motivation/readiness to change, improving engagement strategies, increasing self-efficacy, and identifying mechanisms and processes associated with positive change also requires investigation, particularly for youth with comorbid conditions.

The two most important clinical implications are to determine the point at which patients who have not improved will be unlikely to respond to more of the same treatment and should have their treatment changed and to decide what alternative treatment should be implemented. Innovative, sequential intervention treatment design is needed to address these issues.

ACKNOWLEDGEMENTS

This research was supported by grants to Dr. Kaminer from the National Institute on Alcohol Abuse and Alcoholism – (K24 AA13442), and (RO1 AA12187–01A2)- and to Dr Waldron from the National Institute on Alcohol Abuse and Alcoholism (R01AA12183) and the National Institute on Drug Abuse (RO1 DA11955).

REFERENCES

Abrams, D. B. & Niaura, R. S. (1987). Social learning theory. In H. T. Blane & K. E. Leonard (eds.), *Psychological Theories of Drinking and Alcoholism* (pp. 131–178). New York: Guilford Press.

Albano, A. M., Marten, P. M., Holt, C. S., Heimberg, R. G., & Barlow, D. H. (1995). Cognitive–behavioral group treatment for social phobia in adolescents: a preliminary study. *Journal of Nervous and Mental Disease*, **183**, 649–656.

Babor, T., Webb, C., Burleson, J., & Kaminer, Y. (2002). Subtypes for classifying adolescents with marijuana use disorders: construct validity and clinical implications. *Addiction*, **97** (suppl. 1), 58–69.

Bandura, A. (1977). *Social Learning Theory*. Englewood Cliffs, NJ: Prentice Hall.

(1986). *Self Foundations of Thought and Action: A Social Cognitive Theory*. Englewood Cliffs, NJ: Prentice Hall.

Barrett, P. M., Dadds, M. R., & Rapee, R. M. (1996). Family treatment of childhood anxiety: a controlled trial. *Journal of Consulting and Clinical Psychology*, **64**, 333–342.

Barrett, P. M., Duffy, A. L., Dadds, M. R., & Rapee, R. M. (2001). Cognitive behavioral treatment of anxiety disorders in children: long-term (6-year) follow-up. *Journal of Consulting and Clinical Psychology*, **69**, 1–7.

Beardslee, W. R., Wright, W. J., & Salt, P. (1997). Examination of children's responses to two preventive intervention strategies over time. *Journal of the American Academy of Child and Adolescent Psychiatry*, **36**, 196–204.

Birmaher, B., Brent, D. A., Kolko, D., *et al*. (2000). Clinical outcome after short-term psychotherapy for adolescents with major depressive disorder. *Archives of General Psychiatry*, **57**, 29–36.

Brent, D. A., Holder, D., Kolko, D., *et al*. (1997). A clinical psychotherapy trial for adolescent depression comparing cognitive, family, and supportive treatments. *Archives of General Psychiatry*, **54**, 877–885.

Brent, D. A., Kolko, D., Birmaher, B., *et al*. (1998). Predictors of treatment efficacy in a clinical trial of three psychosocial treatments for adolescent depression. *Journal of the American Academy of Child and Adolescent Psychiatry*, **37**, 906–915.

Brent, D. A., Kolko, D., Birmaher, B., Baugher, M., & Bridge, J. (1999). A clinical trial for adolescent depression: predictors of additional treatment in the acute and follow-up phase. *Journal of the American Academy of Child and Adolescent Psychiatry*, **38**, 263–270.

Breslin, F. C., Sobell, M. B., Sobell, L. C., Buchan, G., & Cunningham, J. A. (1997). Toward a stepped care approach to treating problem drinkers: the predictive utility of within treatment variables and therapist prognostic ratings. *Addiction*, **92**, 1479–1489.

Bukstein, O. G., Glancy, L. G., & Kaminer, Y. (1992). Patterns of affective comorbidity in a clinical population of dually diagnosed adolescent substance abusers. *Journal of the American Academy of Child and Adolescent Psychiatry*, **31**, 1041–1045.

Catalano, R. F., Hawkins, J. D., Wells, E. A., Miller, J., & Brewer, D. (1990–1991). Evaluation of the effectiveness of adolescent drug abuse treatment, assessment of risks for relapse, and promising approaches for relapse prevention. *International Journal of the Addictions*, **25**, 1085–1140.

Clarke, G. N., Rohde, P., Lewinsohn, P. M., Hops, H., & Seeley, J. R. (1999). Cognitive-behavioral treatment of adolescent depression: efficacy of acute group treatment and booster sessions. *Journal of the American Academy of Child and Adolescent Psychiatry*, **38**, 272–279.

Clarke, G. N., Hornbrook, M., Lynch, F., *et al*. (2002). Cognitive–behavioral treatment for depressed adolescent offspring of depressed parents in HMO. *Journal of the American Academy of Child and Adolescent Psychiatry*, **41**, 305–313.

Cohen, J. A. & Mannarino, A. P. (1996). Factors that mediate treatment outcome in sexually abused preschoolers. *Journal of the American Academy of Child and Adolescent Psychiatry*, **35**, 1402–1410.

Cooney, N. L., Kadden, R. M., Litt, M D., & Getter, H. (1991). Matching alcoholics to coping skills or interactional therapies: two-year follow-up results. *Journal of Consulting and Clinical Psychology*, **59**, 598–601.

Curry, J. F., Wells, K. C., Lochman, J. E., Craighead, W. E., & Nagy, P. D. (2003). Cognitive–behavioral intervention for depressed, substance-abusing adolescents: development and pilot testing. *Journal of the American Academy of Child and Adolescent Psychiatry*, **42**, 656–665.

Deblinger, E. & Heflin, A. H. (1996). *Cognitive Behavioral Interventions for Treating Sexually Abused Children*. Thousand Oaks, CA: Sage.

Deblinger, E., Lipman, J., & Steer, R. (1996). Sexually abused children suffering posttraumatic stress symptoms; initial treatment outcome finding. *Child Maltreatment*, **1**, 310–321.

Dennis, M. L., Godley, S. H., Diamond, G., *et al.* (2004). The Cannabis Youth Treatment (CYT) study: main findings from two randomized trials. *Journal of Substance Abuse Treatment*, **27**, 197–213.

Dimeff, L. A. & Marlatt, G. A. (1995). Relapse prevention. In R. K. Hester & W. R. Miller (eds.), *Handbook of Alcoholism Treatment Approaches: Effective Alternatives* (pp. 176–194). Boston: Allyn and Bacon.

DiMilo, L. (1989). Psychiatric syndromes in adolescent substance abusers. *American Journal of Psychiatry*, **146**, 1212–1214.

Dishion, T. J., McCord, J., & Poulin, F. (1999). When interventions harm: peer groups and problem behavior. *American Psychologist*, **54**, 755–764.

Dishion, T. J., Poulin, F., & Barraston, B. (2001). Peer group dynamics associated with iatrogenic effects in group interventions with high-risk young adolescents. *New Directions for Child and Adolescent Development*, **91**, 79–92.

Farrington, D. P. (1999). Conduct disorder and delinquency. In H. Sreinhausen & Verhulst, F. (eds.), *Risks and Outcomes in Developmental Psychopathology* (pp. 165–192). Oxford: Oxford University Press.

Gilchrist, L. D. & Schinke, S. P. (1985). Preventing substance abuse with children and adolescents. *Journal of Consulting and Clinical Psychology*, **53**, 121–135.

Godley, S. H., Meyers, R. S., & Smith, J. E. (2002). *Cannabis Youth Treatment (CYT) Manual Series* Vol. 4: *The Adolescent Community Reinforcement Approach for Adolescent Cannabis users*. Rockville, MD: Center for Substance Abuse, Substance Abuse and Mental Health Services Administration.

Graham, K., Annis, H. M., & Brett, P. J. (1996). A controlled field trial of group versus individual Cognitive–behavioral training for relapse prevention. *Addiction*, **91**, 1127–1139.

Halmi, K. A., Agras, S., Mitchell, J., *et al.* (2002). Relapse predictors of patients with bulimia nervosa who achieved abstinence through cognitive behavioral therapy. *Archives of General Psychiatry*, **59**, 1105–1109.

Hayward, C., Varady, S., Albano, A. M., *et al.* (2000). Cognitive–behavioral group therapy for social phobia in female adolescents: results of a pilot study. *Journal of the American Academy of Child and Adolescent Psychiatry*, **39**, 721–726.

Hester, R. K. & Miller, W. R. (1989). *Handbook of Alcoholism Treatment Approaches: Effective Alternatives*. Needham Heights, MA: Allyn & Bacon.

Higgins, S. T., Budney, A. J., Bickel, W. K., *et al.* (1995). Outpatient behavioral treatment for cocaine dependence: one-year outcome. *Experimental Clinical Psychopharmacology*, **3**, 205–212.

Howard, K. I., Kopta, S. M., Krause, M. S., & Orlinsky, D. E. (1986). The dose–effect relationship in psychotherapy. *American Psychologist*, **41**, 159–164.

Ilardi, S. S. & Craighead, W. E. (1994). The role of nonspecific factors in cognitive–behavior therapy for depression. *Clinical Psychology: Science and Practice*, **1**, 138–156.

Jones, R., Peveler, R. C., Hope, R. A., & Fairburn, C. G. (1993). Changes during treatment for bulimia nervosa: a comparison of three psychological treatments. *Behavior Research and Therapy*, **31**, 479–485.

Kadden, R. M., Cooney, N. L., Getter, H., & Litt, M. B. (1989). Matching alcoholics to coping skills or interactional therapies: posttreatment results. *Journal of Consulting and Clinical Psychology*, **57**, 698–704.

Kadden, R. M., Carroll, K., & Donovan, D. (eds.) (1992). *Cognitive–Behavioral Coping Skills Therapy Manual: A Clinical Research Guide for Therapists Treating Individuals with Alcohol Abuse and Dependence*. Rockville, MD: National Institute on Alcohol Abuse and Alcoholism.

Kadden, R. M., Litt, M. B., Cooney, N. L., Kabela, E., & Getter, H. (2001). Prospective matching of alcoholic clients to cognitive–behavioral or interactional group therapy, *Journal on Studies of Alcohol*, **62**, 359–369.

Kaminer, Y. (2000). Contingency management reinforcement procedures for adolescent substance abuse. *Journal of the American Academy of Child and Adolescent Psychiatry*, **39**, 1324–1326.

(2001). Adolescent substance abuse treatment: where do we go from here? *Psychiatric Services*, **52**, 147–149.

Kaminer, Y. & Burleson, J. (1999). Psychotherapies for adolescent substance abusers: 15-month follow-up. *American Journal of Addictions*, **8**, 114–119.

Kaminer, Y. & Napolitano, C. (2004). Dial for therapy: after-care for adolescent substance use disorders. *Journal of the American Academy of Child and Adolescent Psychiatry*, **43**, 171–174.

Kaminer, Y., Tarter, R. E., Bukstein, O., & Kabene, M. (1992). Comparison between treatment completers and noncompleters among dually diagnosed substance abusing adolescent. *Journal of the American Academy of Child and Adolescent Psychiatry*, **31**, 1046–1049.

Kaminer, Y., Blitz, C., Burleson, J., Sussman, J., & Rounsaville, B. J. (1998a). Psychotherapies for adolescent substance abusers: treatment outcome. *Journal of Nervous and Mental Disease*, **186**, 684–690.

Kaminer, Y., Blitz, C., Burleson, J. A., Kadden, R. M., & Rounsaville, B. J. (1998b). Measuring treatment process in cognitive–behavioral and interactional group therapies for adolescent substance abusers. *Journal of Nervous and Mental Disease*, **186**, 407–413.

Kaminer, Y., Burleson, J., & Goldberger, R. (2002). Psychotherapies for adolescent substance abusers: short- and long-term outcomes. *Journal of Nervous and Mental Disease*, **190**, 737–745.

Kazdin, A. E., (1995). *Conduct Disorder*. Newbury Park CA: Sage.

Kazdin, A. E. & Weisz, J. (1998). Identifying and developing empirically supported child and adolescent treatments. *Journal of Consulting and Clinical Psychology*, **51**, 504–510.

Kazdin, A. E., Siegel, T. D., & Bass, D. (1992). Cognitive problem solving skills training and parent management training in the treatment of antisocial behavior in children. *Journal of Consulting and Clinical Psychology*, **60**, 733–747.

Kendall, P. C. (1994). Treating anxiety disorders in children: results of a randomized clinical trial. *Journal of Consulting and Clinical Psychology*, **62**, 100–110.

Kendall, P. C., & Southam-Gerow, M. (1996). Long-term follow-up of treatment for anxiety disordered youth. *Journal of Consulting and Clinical Psychology*, **65**, 883–888.

Kendall, P. C. & Wilcox, L. E. (1980). A cognitive–behavioral treatment for impulsivity: concrete vs. conceptual training in non-self-controlled problem children. *Journal of Consulting and Clinical Psychology*, **47**, 1020–1029.

Kendall, P. C., Reber, M., McCleer, S. E. J., & Roman, K. R. (1990). Cognitive–behavioral treatment of conduct-disordered children. *Cognitive Therapy and Research*, **14**, 279–297.

Kendall, P. C., Panichelli-Mindel, S. M., Sugarman, A., & Callahan, S. A. (1997). Exposure to child anxiety: theory, research, and practice. *Clinical Psychology: Science and Practice*, **4**, 29–39.

Kraemer, H. C., Wilson, T., Fairburn, C. G., & Agras, A. S. (2002). Mediators and moderators of treatment effects in randomized clinical trials. *Archives of General Psychiatry*, **59**, 877–883.

Kroll, L., Harrington, R., Jayson, D., Fraser, J., & Gowers, S. (1996). Pilot study of continuation cognitive–behavioral therapy for major depression in adolescent psychiatric patients. *Journal of the American Academy of Child and Adolescent Psychiatry* **35**, 1156–1161.

Liddle, H. A. (2002). Advances in family-based therapy for adolescent substance abuse: findings from the multidimensional family therapy research program. In L. S. Harris (ed.), *Research Monograph No. 182: Problems of Drug Dependence 2001* (pp. 113–115). Bethesda, MD: National Institute on Drug Abuse.

Liddle, H. A., Dakof, G. A., Diamond, G. S., Parker, G. S., Barrett, K., & Tejeda, M. (2001). Multidimensional family therapy for adolescent substance abuse: results of a randomized clinical trial. *American Journal of Drug and Alcohol Abuse*, **27**, 651–687.

Lipsey, M. W., & Wilson, D. B. (1998). Effective intervention for serious juvenile offenders: a synthesis of research. In R. Loeber & D. P. Farrington (eds.), *Serious and Violent Juvenile Offenders: Risk Factors and Successful Interventions* (pp. 313–345). Thousand Oaks, CA: Sage.

Litt, M. B., Kadden, R. M., Cooney, N. L., & Kabela, E. (2003). Coping skills and treatment outcomes in cognitive–behavioral and interactional group therapy for alcoholism. *Journal of Consulting and Clinical Psychology*, **71**, 118–128.

Maisto, S. A., Connors, G. J., & Zywiak, W. H. (2000). Alcohol treatment, changes in coping skills, self-efficacy, and levels of alcohol use and related problems 1 year following treatment initiation. *Psychology of Addictive Disorders*, **14**, 257–266.

Manassis, K., Mendlowitz, S. L., Scapillato., D., & Avery, D. (2002). Group and individual cognitive–behavioral therapy for childhood anxiety disorders: A randomized trial. *Journal of the American Academy of Child and Adolescent Psychiatry*, **41**: 1423–1430.

Marlatt, G. A. & Gordon, J. R. (eds.) (1985). *Relapse Prevention: Maintenance Strategies in the Treatment of Addictive Behaviors.* New York: Gilford Press.

Marques, A. C. & Formigoni, M. L. (2001). Comparison of individual and group cognitive–behavioral therapy for alcohol and/or drug dependent patients. *Addiction,* **96,** 835–846.

Miller, W. R. & Rollnick, S. (1991). *Motivational Interviewing.* New York: Guilford Press.

Monti, P. M., Abrams, D. B., Kadden, R. M., & Cooney, N. L. (1989). *Treating Alcohol Dependence.* London: Gilford Press.

Monti, P. M., Rohsenow, D. J., Rubonis, A. N., *et al.* (1993). Cue exposure with coping skills treatment for male alcoholics: a preliminary investigation. *Journal of Consulting and Clinical Psychology,* **61,** 1011–1019.

Monti, P. M., Rohsenow, D. J., Colby, S. M., & Abrams, D. B. (1995). Coping and social skills training. In W. R. Miller & R. K. Hester (eds.), *Handbook of Alcoholism Treatment Approaches: Effective Alternatives,* 2nd edn (pp. 221–241). New York: Allyn & Bacon.

Morgenstern, J. & Longabaugh, R. (2000). Cognitive-behavioral treatment for alcohol dependence: a review of evidence for its hypothesized mechanisms of action. *Addiction,* **95,** 1475–1490.

Myers. M. G. & Brown, S. (1990a). Coping and appraisal in potential relapse situations among adolescent substance abusers following treatment. *Journal of Adolescent Chemical Dependency,* **1,** 95–115.

(1990b). Coping responses and relapse among adolescent substance abusers. *Journal of Substance Abuse,* **2,** 177–189.

(1996). The adolescent relapse coping questionnaire: psychometric validation. *Journal of Studies on Alcohol,* **57,** 40–46.

Myers, M. G., Brown, S., & Mott V. (1993). Coping as a predictor of adolescent substance abuse treatment outcome. *Journal of Substance Abuse,* **5,** 15–29.

Myers, M. G., Stewart, D. G., & Brown, S. A. (1998). Progression from conduct disorder to antisocial personality disorder following treatment for adolescent substance abuse. *American Journal of Psychiatry,* **155,** 479–485.

Offord, D. R. & Bennett, K. J. (1994). Conduct disorder: long-term outcomes and intervention effectiveness. *Journal of the American Academy of Child and Adolescent Psychiatry,* **33,** 1068–1078.

Ollendick, T. H. & King, N. J. (1998). Empirically supported treatments for children with phobic and anxiety disorders: current status. *Journal of Clinical Child Psychology,* **27,** 156–167.

Pina, A. A., Silverman, W. K., Fuentes, R. M., Kurtines, W. M., & Weems, C. F. (2003). Exposure-based cognitive–behavioral treatment for phobic and anxiety disorders: treatment effects and maintenance for Hispanic/Latino relative to European American youths. *Journal of the American Academy of Child and Adolescent Psychiatry,* **42,** 1179–1187.

Project MATCH Research Group (1997). Matching alcoholism treatments to client heterogeneity: Project MATCH post-treatment drinking outcomes. *Journal of Studies on Alcohol,* **58,** 7–29.

Ross, R. R. & Ross, R. D. (1995). *Thinking Straight; The Reasoning and Rehabilitation Programme for Delinquency Prevention and Offender Rehabilitation.* Ottawa: Air Training and Publication.

Rotheram-Borus, M. J., Piacentini, J., Miller, S., Graae, F., & Castro-Blanco, D. (1994). Brief cognitive–behavioral treatment for adolescent suicide attempters and their families. *Journal of the American Academy of Child and Adolescent Psychiatry*, **33**, 508–517.

Sampl, S. & Kadden, R. (2001). *Cannabis Youth Treatment Series, Vol. 1: Motivational Enhancement Therapy and Cognitive Behavioral Therapy for Adolescent Cannabis Users: 5 sessions.* Rockville, MD: Center for Substance Abuse Treatment, Substance Abuse and Mental Health Administration.

Snow, D. L., Tebes, J. K., & Arthur, M. W. (1992). Panel attrition and external validity in adolescent substance use research. *Journal of Consulting and Clinical Psychology*, **60**, 804–807.

Spence, S. H., Donovan, C., & Brechman-Toussaint, M. (2000). The treatment of childhood social phobia: the effectiveness of social skills training-base, cognitive–behavioral intervention, with and without parental involvement. *Journal of Child Psychology and Psychiatry*, **41**, 713–726.

Stitzer, M. L., & Kirby, K. C. (1991). Reducing illicit drug use among methadone patients. In C. G. L. R. W. Perkins & C. R. Schuster (eds.), *Improving Drug Abuse Treatment* (pp. 178–203). Rockville, MD: National Institute for Drug Abuse.

Stitzer, M. L., Bigelow, G. E., & Liebson, I. (1979). *Reinforcement of Drug Abstinence: A Behavioral Approach to Drug Abuse Treatment.* Rockville, MD: National Institute for Drug Abuse.

Waldron, H. B., (1997). Adolescent substance abuse and family therapy outcome: a review of randomized trials. In T. H. Ollendick & R. J. Prinz (eds.), *Advances in Clinical Child Psychology*, Vol. 19 (pp. 199–234). New York: Plenum Press.

Waldron, H. B. & Kaminer, Y. (2004). On the learning curve: cognitive–behavioral therapies for adolescent substance abuse. *Addiction*, **99**, 93–105.

Waldron, H. B., Slesnick, N., Brody, J. L., Turner, C. W., & Peterson, T. R. (2001a). Treatment outcomes for adolescent substance abuse at 4- and 7-month assessments. *Journal of Consulting and Clinical Psychology*, **69**, 802–813.

Waldron, H. B., Miller, W. R., & Tonigan, J. S. (2001b). Client anger as a predictor of differential response to treatment. In R. Longabaugh (ed.), *Research Monograph No. Client Treatment Matching.* Rockville, MD: National Institute on Alcohol Abuse and Alcoholism Administration, National Institutes of Health.

Waldron, H. B., Turner, C. W., Ozechowski, T., & Hops, H. (2003). Traditional outpatient versus "treatment-elusive" adolescent substance abusers: Baseline and treatment outcome differences. In *Proceedings of the 2003 Annual Meeting of the College on Problems of Drug Dependence*, Bal Harbour, Florida.

Wampold, B. E., Mondin, G. W., Moody, M., & Hyun-Nie, A. (1999). Meta-analysis of outcome studies comparing bona fide psychotherapies: empirically, "all must have prizes." *Psychological Bulletin*, **122**, 203–215.

Webb, C., Scudder, M., Kaminer, Y., & Kadden, R. (2002). *Cannabis Youth Treatment (CYT) Series, Vol. 1: Motivational Enhancement Therapy and Cognitive Behavioral Therapy for Adolescent Cannabis Users: 7 Sessions.* Rockville, MD: Center for Substance Abuse Treatment, Substance Abuse and Mental Health Administration.

Weisz, J. R., Donenberg, G. R., Hann, S. S., & Weiss, B. (1995). Bridging the gap between laboratory and clinic in child and adolescent psychotherapy. *Journal of Consulting and Clinical Psychology*, **63**, 688–701.

Wilkinson, D. A., & LeBreton, S. (1986). Early indications of treatment outcome in multiple drug users. In W. R. Miller & N. Heather (eds.), *Treating Addictive Behaviors: Processes of Change* (pp. 239–261). New York: Plenum Press.

Wilson, G. T. (1999). Rapid response to cognitive behavior therapy. *Clinical Psychology: Science and Practice*, **6**, 289–292.

Wood, A., Harrington, R., & Moore, A. (1996). Controlled trial of a brief cognitive–behavioral intervention in adolescent patients with depressive disorders. *Journal of Consulting and Clinical Psychology*, **37**, 737–746.

Wood, A., Trainor, G., Rothwell, J., Moore, A., & Harrington, R. (2001). Randomized trial of group therapy for repeated deliberate self-harm in adolescents. *Journal of the American Academy of Child and Adolescent Psychiatry*, **40**, 1246–1253.

Woody, G. E., Luborsky, L., & McLellan, A. T. (1983). Psychotherapy for opiate addicts: Does it help? *Archives of General Psychiatry*, **40**, 639–645.

Part V

Culturally based treatment development for adolescent substance abusers

20

Family-centered treatment for American Indian adolescent substance abuse: toward a culturally and historically informed strategy

Alison J. Boyd-Ball and Thomas J. Dishion

Child and Family Center of the University of Oregon, Eugene, OR, USA

Substance use in adolescence undermines normative development across all cultural communities. Onset before age 15–16 years predicts problematic substance use in young adulthood (Dishion & Owen, 2002; Robins & Przybeck, 1985). Early and sustained substance use contributes to a variety of young adult difficulties and negative consequences, including disengagement from education opportunities (Newcomb & Bentler, 1988a), delayed or troubled family commitments (Kandel et al., 1986; Newcomb & Bentler, 1988b), and continued substance use into the third decade of life (Chen & Kandel, 1995). The purpose of this chapter is to consider the application of our current thinking on the development and intervention of adolescent substance use to American Indian and Alaskan Native (AIAN) youth and families.

Research since the mid-1980s has produced abundant information regarding risk factors associated with adolescent substance use (Beauvais, 1992; Hawkins et al., 1992; Herring, 1994; Moncher, Holden, & Trimble, 1990; Walker et al., 1988). Only a handful of studies have measured risk factors in middle childhood, prior to the onset of substance use. By and large, these studies agree that a combination of family disruption and early problem behavior at home and school are antecedents to early-onset drug use (Baumrind, 1985; Block, Block, & Keyes, 1988; Dishion, Capaldi, & Yoerger, 1999; Kellam et al., 1983; McCord, 1988; Pulkkinen, 1983; Smith & Fogg, 1979).

The literature on substance use can be used to formulate a model that is a useful empirical guideline for the design of both substance use treatment and prevention protocols (Dishion, Reid, & Patterson, 1988). In Fig. 20.1, an ecological framework is used to organize the risk and protective factor data into a model for the development of problem behavior in general (e.g., Dishion & Patterson, 1999) and substance use in particular (e.g., Dishion & Medici Skaggs, 2000).

Adolescent Substance Abuse: Research and Clinical Advances, ed. Howard A. Liddle and Cynthia L. Rowe.
Published by Cambridge University Press. © Cambridge University Press 2006.

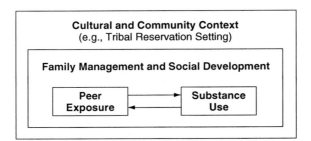

Fig. 20.1   An ecological framework for studying adolescent substance use.

The guiding principle of an ecological framework is that specific processes leading to substance use are *conditional* on community and cultural contexts. In this sense, the model development process is iterative, with an explicit effort to understand variation in developmental processes, as well as commonalities, across communities. In developing models that describe the onset and course of socialization and problem behavior in youth, and from an ecological perspective, it is critical to conceptualize and measure community and cultural factors that affect socialization, such as poverty (McLoyd, 1990), economic change (Conger *et al.*, 1992; Elder, Caspi, & van Nguyen, 1986), acculturation (Szapocznik, Kurtines, & Fernandez, 1980), community organization (Oetting *et al.*, 1998), and minority group oppression (Duran & Duran, 1995).

The model in Fig. 20.1 emphasizes that adolescent peers provide a proximal environment conducive to early adolescent substance use. For some time, the literature has strongly implicated involvement with substance-using peers as a major predictor of early-onset adolescent substance use (Oetting & Beauvais, 1987). In the massive and carefully conducted longitudinal research by Elliott, Huizinga, and Ageton (1985), peer deviancy was the major correlate of adolescent-onset substance use. Other investigators also documented the critical role of peers in the etiology of adolescent substance use (Dishion & Loeber, 1985; Jessor & Jessor, 1977; Newcomb, 1992).

Adult caregivers often structure environments in a manner that either prevents or reduces contact with substance-using peers. Analyses of the ecology of early adolescent drug use reveal that adult caregivers are crucial across multiple settings and communities, as well as across all phases of social development (see Dishion & McMahon, 1998; Kerr & Stattin, 2000). Their key role is in structuring the lives of their children and guiding their behaviors. For example, Dishion *et al.* (1991) found that lack of parental monitoring in middle childhood accounted for youngsters' increased involvement with antisocial peers by early adolescence, even when the analysis controlled for prior levels of contact, peer rejection, academic failure, and antisocial behavior. In addition, an ecological analysis of peer group pressure revealed that youth left unsupervised after school were most susceptible to peer group pressure (Steinberg, 1986). Consistent with these findings, Dishion and Loeber (1985) found that caregiver monitoring predicted adolescent exposure to deviant peers and uniquely accounted for much of the variance in marijuana use. Baumrind (1985) also found parent supervision practices to be predictive of adolescent substance use in girls.

A positive parent–child relationship suggests commitment to adult and family values, and a history of willingness to cooperate with adult leadership (Elliott *et al.*, 1985; Hawkins *et al.*, 1986; Hirschi, 1969; Oetting & Donnermeyer, 1998). We think that positive relationships with adults reduce the "flight to deviant peers," which is often observed among adolescents with troubled, disrupted, or conflicted family lives (Elder, 1980). The longitudinal data analyzed by Elliott and colleagues (1985) supported the hypothesis that the low quality of a parent–child relationship is directly related to adolescent association with substance-using peers, but not directly to substance use.

We hypothesize that a combination of positive family relationships, caregivers who attend to behavior management, and supervision is optimal for promoting health and well-being among adolescents. Dishion and McMahon (1998) made the case that a positive parent–child relationship and monitoring go hand in hand: parents have difficulty monitoring and supervising if their parent–child relationship is cold, distant, or conflictive. The key idea is that socialization is a bidirectional process that unfolds over time: as children become more involved in problem behavior, it becomes more difficult to monitor, to manage, and to maintain a positive relationship with the adolescent (Kerr & Stattin, 2000).

Communication is the first thing to break down when relationships become stressed and adolescent problem behavior increases. As might be expected, family communication skills with adolescents are highly related to substance use and other problem behaviors (Forgatch & Stoolmiller, 1994; Hops *et al.*, 1990; Oetting & Beauvais, 1987). Negative affect and conflict seem to be the hallmark of poor family communication practices, as well as avoidance, denial, or relinquishing the parental role (Dishion & Kavanagh, 2003).

Clearly, family socialization processes vary considerably across cultures and contexts (Deater–Deckard & Dodge, 1997; Dishion & Bullock, 2001; Kellam, 1990; Mason *et al.*, 1996; Masten & Coatsworth, 1998; McLoyd, 1997; Oetting *et al.*, 1998; Werner, 1995; Whiting & Whiting, 1975), although work in studying the variation in socialization systems and strategies across cultural communities has only just begun. We assume, however, that some form of adult involvement, caring, and structure is necessary for healthy social development in the adolescent transition period, including AIAN adolescents and their families.

American Indian communities

Today, AIANs are representative of over 500 different tribes and 200 different languages and have a unique social and political history. Unlike other ethnic groups, and despite colonization of genocidal proportions, many of their beliefs and values are traceable to indigenous, spiritual beliefs and practices that are embedded within the land, described in popular terms as "philosophy of deep ecology."

Within the tribes, there is considerable diversity in resources, culture, history, and child-rearing dynamics. To this extent, we make the argument that the peer and family processes associated with substance use are to be considered relative to the cultural and historical context of each tribe. Although indigenous practices across North American tribes provide some similarities with respect to the socialization "system," there is also considerable diversity in specific caregiving practices, embedded rituals, traditions, and stories that transmit the oral history and cultural system.

AIAN communities have long experienced poverty, inadequate education, high unemployment rates, discrimination, and cultural dislocation (Mitchell *et al.*, 1996). The Indian Health Service (IHS), a main health-care provider for many Indian people, has reported that chronic and behavioral-related diseases, including substance abuse, are posing new challenges (IHS, 2001a). The IHS has reported that AIAN adolescents aged 12–17 years have the highest rate of illicit drug use (31.2%) when compared with all other ethnic groups (IHS, 2001b).

Despite accumulating data citing high rates of substance use among AIAN adolescents, little research has been done on this vulnerable population. Survey research that includes people of color (Hispanic, AIAN, and African-American) does not generally find different causal processes than those summarized in the model described above (see Barrera, Castro, & Biglan, 1999; Oetting & Beauvais, 1990). Of note, the majority of this research does not include children and adolescents living within a "reservation" community.

This oversight in our program of research is noteworthy, as it is within the reservation community that a high rate of substance use and demoralization is found. Moreover, because of the lack of tribally specific epidemiological data, we cannot confirm the assumptions that tribes vary tremendously on the extent to which substances are problematic. Therefore, we need to extend research in order to understand the abstinence and abuse rates within the AIAN communities and to identify the profile of youth who are engaged in intervention services within those communities. This information will help in the design of long-term prevention and treatment strategies that build on existing community strengths and address risk processes.

Historical policies and events for AIANs have led to a dramatic disruption of the indigenous socialization processes for individuals, families, and communities (Institute for Government Research Studies in Administration, 1928; Nies, 1996). Policies in the USA for AIANs were first developed to annihilate this population and later to assimilate it into mainstream society (Hazzon-Hammond, 1997). The three major strategies were (a) to attenuate indigenous family influence and socialization by sending children to boarding schools when they were as young as 5 years of age; (b) to separate the Indians from their land base by creating reservations; and (c) to prohibit Indians' religious practices and replace them with European religious practices (Lomawaima, 1993).

These policies resulted in the disorganization of tribal structures and effectively replaced socialization with practices and beliefs inherent to the boarding school system. Compounded with race- and class-based barriers that are deepening between AIANs and the dominant society, families and communities appear to be struggling (Kavanagh *et al.*, 1999). Traditional family practices have been affected adversely, including basic skills of communication, monitoring, limit setting, and problem solving. Historically, the family structure represented an extension of the community-at-large and was the principal mechanism from which to garner support during difficult times. Today, the family structure itself is often fragmented and in need of support.

The macrolevel processes that influence substance use among families within AIAN communities are probably bidirectional. Substance abuse alone can disrupt a community in many ways. The health and well-being of the community are undermined, as evidenced by indicators of, among others, behavioral health, injury, violence, mental health, tobacco use, and social problems such as child abuse, family dysfunction, prison terms, and spousal abuse (Brave Heart & DeBruyn, 1998; Szasz, 1992). Because these effects are bound to sectors of the community, and with the magnitude of the problems being shrouded within marginalized communities (e.g., few mainstream research studies focus on the reservation community), it can be difficult for investigators to get specific information that guides the development of family interventions.

In order to improve our understanding of the causal relationships to substance abuse and associated problems of AIAN populations, it is necessary to investigate the historical and traumatic events that contribute to the force of addiction in these communities (Duran & Duran, 1995). For example, as stated above, adult involvement and monitoring are seen as protective factors for young adolescents, especially in high-risk environments. In the context of the probable influence of traditional boarding schools, attenuated intergenerational ties and socialization processes contributed to decreased adult influence on peer group formation and activities. The sequelae, according to current models of socialization, would be higher levels of problem behavior and decreased emotional maturation and well-being (First Nations House of Learning, 1991). Some hypothesize that, without countervailing forces, these past efforts of assimilation propagate across generations to the point where, in some families, the adults are not able to function as socialization agents within a traditional, indigenous context or within that of the "majority" cultural context. Several AIAN researchers emphasize the need to study the processes that differentiate resilient AIAN families from those who are more vulnerable (Fisher & Ball, 2002).

We hypothesize that identification and measurement of constructs that incorporate culturally relevant strengths of AIAN parents will lead to model development and testing that will help us to understand AIAN resilience and how best to support families with intervention services. Even so, the identification of unique historical and traumatic influences on the disruption of families and communities is more than an academic exercise in model building. This kind of research can inform us why services are underutilized and what kinds of intervention are likely to be accepted and effective in reducing existing substance use and in preventing future substance use (Brave Heart & DeBruyn, 1998).

Given this history of trauma and the oppression of cultural practices within AIAN communities, it is clear that a critical component of substance use treatment and prevention is cultural restoration and support (Fisher & Ball, 2002). Interventions that ignore historical and cultural issues may actually do harm because they undermine (explicitly and implicitly) the pain of the past and the peoples' pride. In fact, qualitative analyses of substance use in reservation communities suggest that these behaviors are a functional adaptation of the youth to the dynamics of the reservation community (O'Nell & Mitchell, 1996). To the extent that the reservation community represents the outcome of European intrusion, it is reasonable that peer drug use is not the sole mediating factor in the reservation community (Swaim *et al.*, 1993). The peer influence would become less salient when substance use occurs among family members, who experience poor social conditions, fewer opportunities, and a lack of resources.

Obviously, there is a moral imperative to acknowledge and redress the trauma to AIAN youth and families during the treatment and prevention of substance use (Duran & Duran, 1995). There is also a pragmatic rationale for supporting traditional cultural practices and cultural restoration of the individual and the family specifically. Outside of peyote use, drug and alcohol use are not found in any of the traditional cultural and spiritual practices indigenous to AIAN communities. Sweats, dancing, talking circles, and religious ceremonies are practices that promote abstinence.

We now turn to discuss three phases of research that address the development of a family-centered intervention strategy for AIAN adolescents who were referred for inpatient treatment of alcohol and drug problems, primarily from reservation communities across the western USA. In this research, we attempt to integrate the empirical literature, in its incomplete state, with the historical and political realities and cultural strengths of AIAN communities.

Toward a family-centered inpatient treatment

At present, the primary approach to addressing substance abuse among AIAN youth in reservation communities is inpatient treatment. In fact, youth are often sent away to other geographic locations, much like the externally imposed boarding school tradition, to participate in such treatment. There are 12 IHS Youth Regional Treatment Centers located throughout the USA. These centers often have large waiting lists; only under acute circumstances are youth referred to centers outside of IHS-funded treatment. The model we describe here involves a 7-year collaboration with an IHS-funded, tribally contracted treatment center we will refer to, for reasons of anonymity, as the Western American Indian Treatment (WAIT) Center for adolescents.

Youth who are treated at the WAIT Center identify as AIAN; they are eligible for treatment between the ages of 12 and 18 years. The youth and their families represent at least 44 different tribes, from both urban and rural settings. To access the WAIT Center, youth and families travel a range of under 1 mile up to 1466 miles, excluding distances from Alaska. The travel distance demonstrates the complexity of access owing to both geographic accessibility and the need to deliver culturally and historically sensitive treatment, given the diversity of tribal culture and history.

Before admittance to the WAIT Center, referrals are screened informally to assure a good fit between the needs of the adolescent and the treatment protocol. Youth with severe psychiatric disturbance or potential for violence are referred elsewhere. The intervention consists of a 7-week protocol (Table 20.1) that is gender specific, with successive cohorts of males and females throughout the year. In each year, there are six cycles passing through the treatments, with anywhere from 12 to 20 individuals admitted at one time.

The 7-week treatment protocol is a highly structured approach to promoting abstinence and emphasizing cultural pride, awareness, and educational engagement. The range of services to AIAN youth includes individual therapy, group therapy, 24-hour supervision, psychiatric and psychological services, assessment and referral, life-skills counseling, medical services, family program, and after-care planning. In addition to a 12-step program emphasis, the youth are offered American Indian culture and traditional services, such as outdoor outings,

Table 20.1 The 7-week protocol for intervention services

Week	Stage	Content
1	Orientation	Provide expectations of treatment, attitude, and behaviors
2	Detoxification process	Engage in treatment and response to detoxification process, mentally and physically
3	Attitudes and behaviors checklist	Deal with feelings of anger, denial, impulse control, and so forth
4	Immersion into program	Continue with behavior changes, motivation to change, coping mechanisms
5	Right-of-passage gathering	Participate in a wilderness outing that supports healthy life styles and provides a mechanism for spiritual reconnection through the environment
6	Maintenance and relapse prevention	Preparation in returning to communities and families
7	Family week	Family education and support

AIAN crafts, drumming and singing, cultural and traditional relaxation therapy, sweat lodges, and spiritual support. Other services include an educational program directed toward obtaining high school credit or a general education diploma and cultural and recreational activities.

A multidisciplinary team, comprising certified counselors in alcohol and substance abuse, a psychologist, a psychiatrist, a family therapist, and an educational specialist, provided direct services. To accompany the cultural and educational components, elders from local tribal communities and cultural specialists lead activities conducive to sobriety within an AIAN lifestyle and community. In general, a holistic approach to treatment is emphasized for adolescent substance abuse, incorporating traditional values, beliefs, ceremonies, and healing processes.

During the time of the pilot research described below, the treatment program increased the emphasis on family involvement. In the last week of the treatment protocol, adolescents' families were invited to come and stay at the WAIT Center and to attend all major treatment events. Diagnostic and treatment program issues were shared with caregivers, and individualized plans for the family to maintain sobriety were arranged collaboratively with the family and the community service providers. To maintain their connection to family and community, adolescents were allowed to return home for family traditional practices, ceremonial events, weddings, and funerals.

Effectiveness and enhancement research

Pilot research

The goal of the first phase of the pilot research was twofold (Boyd-Ball, 1997): to build a collaboration with the WAIT Center by analyzing existing data on the characteristics of the adolescents and families attending for treatment, predicting those factors that were related to initial levels of substance use; and to examine the substance use patterns of the AIAN youth who were served by the treatment center. To accomplish these goals, archival case file data were coded and analyzed. A chart review survey was developed to gather information on the substance use patterns, background factors, and the treatment outcomes. Boyd-Ball (1997) described, in detail, the procedures and findings from the archival analysis of the treatment data from the WAIT Center.

In Boyd-Ball's 1997 study, 50% of the participants were selected at random for analysis, chart review, and coding of intake data. The sample consisted of 73 adolescents (56% male) with an average age of 16 years and education at eighth grade; 30% of the youth had dropped out of school and 47% were on target for graduation from high school. The youth represented 44 different tribes, with 80% enrolled in a federally recognized tribe; 52% of the youth lived primarily in a reservation community.

Overall, adolescents who initiated treatment perceived themselves as having a positive support system of family, friends, peers, and other non-family adults. Substance use did not vary by gender, except for two findings. Males initiated use by a mean age of 8.4 years, in contrast to age 10.3 years in females. The age of first use for marijuana also showed a significant gender difference, with a mean age of 11.5 years for males and 12.9 years for females. No gender differences were found with first use of alcohol, nicotine, or speed. For the number of substances tried, no significant differences were found for gender (5.4 for male and 4.3 for female).

The analysis of background factors associated with substance use patterns of the adolescents revealed valuable results on which to build the foundation for the Shadow Project, which was the next phase of the pilot study. History of family substance use and the adolescent's trauma history were associated with age of onset and levels of substance use. In addition, gender (males more than females) and the interviewers' ratings on the number of DSM-III symptoms (American psychiatric Association, 1987) present at intake were positively correlated with substance use at intake.

A supportive finding for the WAIT Center was the relevance of traditional practices in the substance use patterns of the adolescent clients. Self-identification as a member of an American Indian religion was found to serve as a protective factor for substance use. Additionally, youth perception of positive adult support for abstinence served as a protective factor for substance use. If youth perceived they had positive adult support outside their family units, they used their drug of choice less frequently.

The entire treatment protocol of the WAIT Center was completed by 58% of the adolescents. In analyzing the relapse rates in this study, 34 out of 73 adolescents completed a self-report after leaving treatment. The voluntary responses regarding whether or not the youth had relapsed since discharge were collected at 3, 6, 9 and 12 months and revealed 68% self-reported substance use during the intervals. Given the small completion rate, the cursory nature of the outcome data, and the limited availability of staff to complete the follow-up reports, these findings are quite limited. Despite the preliminary nature of the data, we were encouraged to apply these ideas to improve our measurement of key theoretical constructs and to integrate cultural restoration further into the intervention program.

Enhancement research

Two years after initiating the pilot study, we met with the treatment staff to plan a collaboration to improve the evaluation of the effectiveness of the treatment program and to design a culturally responsive enhancement that would further increase the engagement of the family and utilize the strength of AIAN indigenous culture. The Shadow Project, a 3-year study funded by NIAAA, was conducted in three major phases: the design of the evaluation model; the design of the enhancement condition (FCI-E); and the comparison of family-centered intervention (FCI) relative to the FCI-E.

Evaluation model

To improve the potential for evaluating the impact of the WAIT treatment program, a multiagent, multimethod assessment battery was devised that included the latest strategies for assessing substance use, family interaction, and follow-up of substance use in distant communities.

To begin, in consultation with the treatment center and cultural experts, we formulated a quasi-experimental design for evaluating the intervention protocol. Because the adolescents are treated in groups, and many of the activities during family week were in groups, individual random assignment to the two intervention conditions was not pragmatically feasible or palatable to the treatment families and staff. For the first half of the study, we collected data on the FCI, and for the second half, we collaborated with the staff in implementing the FCI-E.

In general, the assessment battery described by Dishion and Kavanagh (2003) was used for this study. The family assessment included observation of family interactions, interviews, questionnaire packets, and a computerized questionnaire. Monthly follow-ups after completion of the treatment protocol were conducted for a period of 11 months, followed by a more intensive interview and question-naire assessment. The monthly follow-ups were conducted using structured telephone interviews (Chamberlain & Reid, 1987) with both the parent and the youth.

We adapted the direct observation of the family-interaction assessment to the strengths of AIAN families, in consultation with AIAN cultural and research experts. In the family observation tasks, five areas were assessed: relationship building, positive reinforcement, limit setting, monitoring, problem solving, and communication. We adapted two of these tasks for AIAN families.

Two legends were used to assess the caregivers' use of storytelling to promote norms, to set limits, to build relationships with youth, and to engage in problem solving and communication as a family unit. Lillian Tom-Orme (2000) explains storytelling among AIANs as a basic and valued means of communication that transmits information from one generation to the next. By incorporating Indian stories, families were afforded the opportunity to use indigenous practices for parenting. This also provided an opportunity for the research and intervention team to examine that the family's level of assimilation into the dominant culture had occurred (Hodge *et al.*, 2002).

The enhancement condition

An advisory board to design the FCI-E comprised AIAN cultural and intervention experts from within the geographical and cultural communities served by the WAIT Center: the authors (the first author is a tribal member of one of the tribes served by the treatment center), three AIAN treatment providers with doctorates and expertise in adolescent alcohol and drug treatment and research on historical trauma with AIAN communities and families, and one AIAN advisor with a Master's degree and one with a Bachelor's degree, who, both had experience working with AIAN adolescents in the social service and juvenile justice systems. The board also examined the assessment and design procedures for cultural sensitivity.

The FCI-E consisted of two components that were new to the WAIT Center. Motivational interviewing (Miller & Rollnick, 2002) was used in the form of the "family check-up," developed and described in detail by Dishion and Kavanagh (2003). During family week, family observation assessments were combined with the comprehensive multiagent, multimethod assessment to provide feedback to caregivers and motivation to support the youth in sobriety following completion of the WAIT Center treatment protocol.

Briefly, motivational interviewing is a systematic procedure for interacting with caregivers in order to build motivation to monitor and support sobriety in adolescents. The family check-up consists of an intake interview, a comprehensive assessment, and a feedback session with caregivers. The procedure was adapted during the WAIT Center family week, separate from the initial interview, and provided feedback without statistically comparing AIAN families with other AIAN families or non-native families. Direct social comparisons were deemed as inappropriate to the cultural backgrounds of many AIAN families by the Cultural Advisory Board.

The second level of adaptation to the family check-up and the WAIT Center treatment protocol was the design of the welcome home ceremony. This ceremony was designed to incorporate the cultural custom of public acknowledgement of a major accomplishment of a young person. In this situation, the welcome home ceremony was designed to coalesce tribal and family members to support publicly the youth's commitment to sobriety. Historically, many tribes mark important events, such as a boy's first hunting kill, a girl's first berry-picking experience, or puberty, with ceremonies. Today, many AIAN families retain this practice through both modern and traditional ceremonies, such as birthdays, baptisms, memorials, and puberty rites.

Both modern and traditional ceremonies have some things in common, like a respected person speaking on behalf of the honoree, a dinner, and giveaway to those who come to support and honor the individual. To accomplish the task of carrying out any ceremony requires the families to communicate with one another, agree, assign tasks, and problem solve. In this activity, the family communicates its desires, problem solves, and assigns tasks by deciding what will happen at this event. The family agrees on people to invite and determines how this activity will honor the youth.

Inviting family, spiritual advisors, and important community members further facilitates the mediation process to strengthen the individual's ability to regain control over the substance abuse behavior (Watts, 2001). Not only can kinship extend beyond non-biological relationships, but it remains a highly valued perception among AIANs. By utilizing these kinships as support, the family-centered model is adjusted to build on the strategies and strengths of indigenous practices (Tom-Orme, 2000).

Analysis of outcomes

The outcome research involved 57 youth and their families, distributed across eight treatment cohorts. Voluntary participation in the study was solicited during the intake at the WAIT Center. Youth were referred from the western region of the United States, including Alaska, Montana, Arizona, Nevada, Washington, Idaho, Oregon, and California.

In addition to soliciting the voluntary participation of each adolescent and family, we notified each tribe within which the youth and family were enrolled and requested passive consent. Of the 104 families initially recruited, 66 (63%)

Table 20.2 Demographics of the Shadow Project study

Characteristic	Treatment (%)
Gender	
Male	56.10
Female	43.90
Mean age (years [SD])	15.89 (1.44)
Live on/near reservation	70.00
Education	
High school drop-out	28.80
On-target for graduation	59.60
Referred for special education	18.90
Highest grade completed (mean [SD])	9.68 (1.49)

SD, standard deviation.

agreed to participate. The most frequent reason for declining participation was the lack of an identified caregiver to be available for participation in the research, or the caregivers' inability to attend the family week at the end of treatment. Of the 66 participants, one later declined participation, seven dropped out during treatment, and one youth became emancipated (86% retention through the 1-year follow-up).

The demographics of the sample, including the FCI and FCI-E are summarized in Table 20.2. Contrary to expectations, the sample was not evenly distributed by gender (56% male, 44% female). The youth represented 28 different tribes, with 83% enrolled in federally recognized tribes.

The level of substance use did not vary by condition (Table 20.3). As in the earlier pilot work, the sample participants tended to start using substances at a young age (11.5 years for males, 12.9 years for females). For an inpatient treatment sample at baseline, the percentage of days abstinent was higher than expected (74% alcohol, 56% marijuana, and 98% hard drugs).

Table 20.4 provides an overview of the level of post-treatment support for the youth in both the FCI and the FCI-E interventions. A trend is seen toward more adult support in the FCI-E situation. In general, however, considerable support for abstinence was observed in both conditions.

The level of alcohol and drug use for the two interventions from both the parent and youth perspective over the 11-month follow-up period is summarized in Table 20.5 and Fig. 20.2, respectively, which show the number of substances used as a summary index for both reports. In addition, we provided an index of parent awareness of teen alcohol and drug use at three different intervals after treatment (see Table 20.5). Parents were asked about their certainty of their child's

Table 20.3 Substance use patterns

Condition	Total		FCI		FCI-E	
	No. assessed	Mean(SD)	No. assessed	Mean(SD)	No. assessed	Mean(SD)
Number of drugs tried, lifetime	57	6.05 (1.99)	30	5.9 (1.86)	27	6.19 (2.17)
Age of first use, any substance (years)	57	12.28 (1.81)	30	12.55 (1.68)	27	11.97 (1.92)
Number of times used, last year						
Alcohol	55	70 (105)	29	81 (129)	26	59 (69)
Tobacco	53	313 (365)	28	244 (270)	25	391 (441)
Marijuana	56	218 (330)	29	173 (215)	27	267 (419)
Other hard drugs	42	32 (70)	22	37 (87)	20	26 (45)

FCI, family-centered intervention (treatment-as-usual); FCI-E, family-centered intervention enhanced; SD, standard deviation.

Table 20.4 Perceived support systems

	FCI	FCI-E
Support of positive adult (%)		
Family member	93	96
Non-family member	89	92
Support of positive peer (%)	64	68

FCI, family-centered intervention (treatment-as-usual); FCI-E, family-centered intervention enhanced.

substance use, with responses ranging from not knowing if their child was using at all, to uncertain about use, to certain that their youth used or did not use alcohol and other drugs.

Although there is a slight trend toward less substance use in the FCI-E over the FCI intervention, in general, we observed low rates of substance use in both conditions. These data suggest that the treatment was influential in reducing substance use among this high-risk AIAN adolescent sample. By follow-up at 1 year, as indicated for both conditions, we observed abstinence of 87% for alcohol, 77% for marijuana use, and 99% for hard drugs.

At the completion of treatment, adolescents who participated in FCI and FCI-E perceived themselves as having a positive family support system, support from

Table 20.5 Parent monitoring of adolescent alcohol and drug use

Condition	Follow-up month		
	1	6	11
Alcohol use (%)			
Do not know about child's alcohol use	5.4	3.6	9.6
Not certain about child's alcohol use	44.6	39.3	40.4
Certain about the amount of the child's alcohol use	50.0	57.1	50.0
Drug use (%)			
Do not know about child's alcohol use	8.9	10.7	11.5
Not certain about child's alcohol use	41.1	32.1	55.8
Certain about the amount of the child's alcohol use	50.0	57.1	32.7

other non-family adults, and positive peer support, with slight increases for the FCI-E group (Table 20.4). An interesting finding was the use of traditional versus the conventional support services youth accessed after treatment (Fig. 20.3). The traditional supports included Indian healers or spiritual advisors, elders, family and friends, and ancestral ceremonies. The conventional support services included support groups such as Alcoholics Anonymous, substance abuse treatment counselors, psychologists or psychiatrists, and mental health workers.

Conclusions

Our hope is that behavioral science could address the problems of substance abuse, mental health concerns, and problem behavior among some AIAN adolescents in various communities. Our preliminary work in this area suggests that some of the constructs that emerge from this literature, such as family management and peer clustering, are relevant for addressing substance abuse in AIAN adolescents and families. We believe this work will go forward, based on successfully incorporating our understanding of adolescent and family health and resilience within and across AIAN communities.

It is also clear that the behavior science community will need to step back and consider the historical and immediate effects of societal events on the AIAN communities. Relevant to this issue, perhaps, is the apparent low rates of substance use for the AIAN adolescents involved in inpatient treatment.

In an outpatient treatment sample (Waldron *et al.*, 2001), days of marijuana use at baseline were 57.5%, compared with our sample of 43.8%. Given that many of these youth are sent away from home, often hundreds and in some cases thousands of miles, these low rates of substance abuse among the treated youth

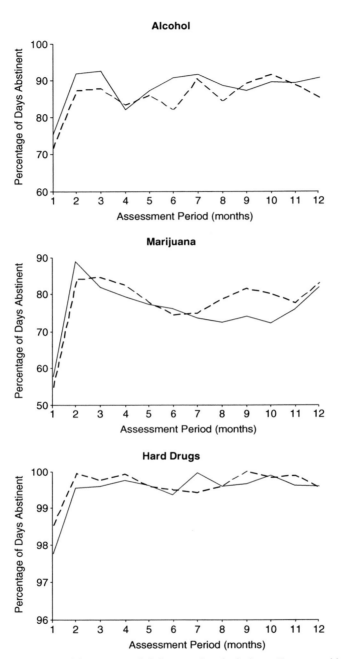

Fig. 20.2   Summary of the 11-month follow-up for alcohol, marijuana, and hard drugs for the usual family-centered intervention (- - -) and the enhanced intervention (—).

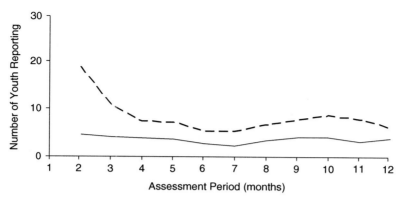

Fig. 20.3   Youth self-report of the use of traditional versus use of conventional support services at each month of follow-up across all participants for the usual family-centered intervention (---) and the enhanced intervention (—).

are somewhat paradoxical because it would be much less expensive to provide outpatient treatment in the community. Why are people sent so far away to manage a problem that, for a majority youth, would be handled on a community-based outpatient treatment program?

The AIAN communities may be relying on strategies that have been inculcated over the last 300 years by USA policy. AIAN communities are sending their troubled youth away to get "fixed," much as they have been sending youth to boarding schools to get "educated." This is a clear example of what Duran and Duran (1995) refer to as the AIAN population internalizing the message and strategies of oppression. The federal government no longer mandates the use of boarding schools, yet this remains a dominant strategy for education within the AIAN community. Inpatient treatment is a simple extension of this strategy. It is no accident that a boarding school is located less than 5 miles from the WAIT Center, and that many of the youth at the WAIT Center received referrals to and from the school.

It is reassuring that the WAIT Center promotes traditional and indigenous AIAN practices and culture. We found that the WAIT staff, who are predominantly AIANs themselves, were supportive of individual tribal culture and AIAN practices. Youth often emerge from treatment with a sense of pride and commitment to their AIAN heritage. Moreover, as evidenced by the high levels of adult support for sobriety at home, the AIAN communities and families effectively promote the health and well-being of these young people. The WAIT Center's cultural sensitivity, family orientation, and engagement appear to involve, mobilize, and empower the family communities effectively.

An implicit conclusion from this research is that high-risk youth and families living within AIAN communities can be engaged and retained in social science research when such research clearly is culturally sensitive and in their best interests. The youth and families involved in this treatment were highly stressed (81% experienced the death of a close friend or relative), but in general, they were cooperative in promoting follow-up assessments. Our efforts to recruit and retain this population are highly effective, given the isolated geographical origins of the participants, the high-risk nature of their referrals, and their occasional barriers to direct communication resources.

Families can be a major support in helping to reduce problem behaviors, which then leads to the increased good health of the adolescents. There also are impeding limitations, given the lack of understanding on how cultural norms, historical events, and family and community settings impact the problems (Bradley *et al.*, 2001). The key to conducting this research is to have the leadership team that guides the research come from within the AIAN community (Fisher & Ball, 2002).

It brings to question whether alcohol and drug abuse underlie the mental health problems for AIAN adolescents and their families or the reverse. There is a need to develop longitudinal models to determine the antecedents and sequelae of substance use within AIAN communities. Dishion and Patterson (1999) have discussed the process of developing models as an iterative process. Intervention research is a key step in testing models of etiology. Though it could be argued that models may vary by community, it is an empirical question.

There is a paradox, however. Clearly, research in AIAN communities is a delicate process, in light of the harm that has been done in the past. Research that simply observes youth and their families could be experienced as exploitative, especially if an outside team of researchers conducts the research.

It seems clear that applied research within the AIAN community is best received if it involves the development and evaluation of a service identified as a priority by the community. Fisher and Ball (2002) provided an overview of a culturally sensitive approach to working within AIAN communities to develop and test intervention services. The key point is that tribal ownership and involvement needs to be integrated into every step of the process, including publication of scientific reports.

Based on the work we describe in this chapter, future directions should include studies designed to prevent and reduce substance use among AIAN youth in the community, without sending them away to inpatient treatment. Family involvement is a strength within the AIAN community, given that a majority of the families of the inpatient youth traveled hundreds of miles to participate in the last week of treatment. Developing culturally sensitive family-centered interventions within the community would seem to be even more effective in preventing and treating high-risk youth.

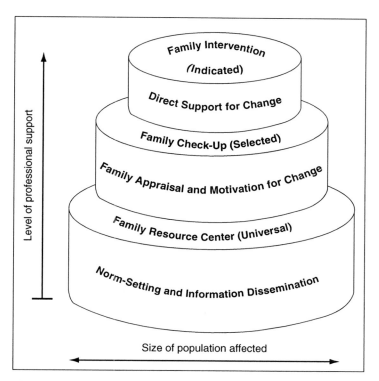

Fig. 20.4   The multilevel adolescent transitions program strategy.

We developed a multilevel, tiered strategy called the adolescent transitions program, which we have found to be effective in preventing and reducing problem behavior in high-risk, multiethnic communities. The program is implemented as a school-based program, with universal, selected, and indicated levels of intervention (Dishion *et al.*, 2002) (Fig. 20.4). The universal intervention involves establishing a family resource center within a public school environment run by a family-centered clinician who is effective in establishing collaborative relationships with school professionals and caregivers. We describe the interventions in detail elsewhere (Dishion *et al.*, 2002; Dishion & Kavanagh, 2003).

The adolescent transitions program would require serious adaptation to be useful to AIAN communities. One issue is the relation between the school and the AIAN community. In some areas, having a school-based intervention that targets AIAN youth would only reinforce experiences of stigmatization and misunderstanding in public schools. Another issue that should be considered is the historical context of each tribe. Although colonization was rampant and severe for all AIAN tribes, the specific experiences and extent of oppression varied by tribes (Duran & Duran, 1995). Tribal involvement in the intervention service and its evaluation is central for

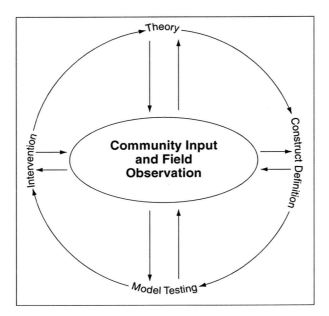

Fig. 20.5   The model-building process.

developing and maintaining a long-term collaboration that would truly benefit AIAN youth and families. We offer a revision of model building by Dishion and Patterson (1999) to illustrate that tribal leadership must guide such adaptations and evaluation of these intervention services, first and foremost (Fig. 20.5). This begins the process of taking into account the cultural dimensions that are often denied or ignored within the field (Koss–Chioino & Vargas, 1992).

The collective work in the field on the role of family management in the etiology of adolescent problem behavior and substance use, and the development of empirically sound family-centered interventions, is a practical catalyst for work within the AIAN communities. The next step is to develop funding sources that provide an infrastructure within AIAN communities that promotes true collaboration between AIANs and majority investigators. Such collaboration would build on the cultural strengths within AIAN communities that promote prosocial behavior and reduce substance use, mental health problems, and serious problem behavior among AIAN youth. Most important, these strategies should not inadvertently replicate or reinforce externally imposed strategies (e.g., geographically distant treatment centers) that, in the long run, further compromise tribal sovereignty and right of self-determination in the protection of AIAN youth and families.

When dealing with marginalized or excluded societies, we will need to explore and expand our research designs and methodologies to enhance engagement of these populations, thereby contributing to the reduction of health disparities. By validating, or invalidating, their theories, the process can be empowering to the researchers, the tribal leaders, and the participants of the study. This information can then be disseminated to the scientific community, as well as to the AIAN population, as reliable, valid research, and its usefulness can be incorporated into social, political, and mental processes.

ACKNOWLEDGEMENTS

The Shadow Project was supported by grant AA 12702 from NIAAA at NIH to T. J. Dishion. We would like to thank the families who participated in the Shadow Project and the Shadow Project American Indian Advisory Board: John Spence, Bob Ryan, Tom Ball, Debbie Oriero, and Donna Ralston–Lewis. We would also like to thank Renda Dionne, the Indian Family Wellness program, Charlotte Winter, and Bernadette Bullock for data analysis, and Ann Simas for editing and graphics preparation on the manuscript.

REFERENCES

American Psychiatric Association (1987). *Diagnostic and statistical manual of mental disorders: DSM-III-R* (3rd ed.). Washington, DC: American Psychiatric Press.

Barrera, M., Castro, F. G., & Biglan, A. (1999). Ethnicity, substance use and development: exemplars for exploring group differences and similarities. *Development and Psychopathology*, **11**, 805–822.

Baumrind, D. (1985). Familial antecedents of adolescent drug use: a developmental perspective. In C. L. Jones & R. J. Battjes (eds.), *Research Monograph* No. 56: *Etiology of Drug Abuse: Implication for Prevention* (pp. 13–44). Rockville, MD: National Institutes of Health.

Beauvais, F. (1992). The consequences of drug and alcohol use for Indian youth. *American Indian and Alaska Native Mental Health Research*, **5**, 32–37.

Block, J., Block, J. H., & Keyes, S. (1988). Longitudinally foretelling drug usage in adolescence: early childhood personality and environmental precursors. *Child Development*, **59**, 336–355.

Boyd-Ball, A. J. (1997). *How background factors impact substance use patterns among American Indian Youth in treatment*. Ph.D. thesis, University of Oregon (UMI Microform No. 9810009).

Bradley, R. H., Corwyn, R. F., McAdoo, H. P., & Garcia-Coll, C. (2001). The home environments of children in the United States. Part 1: Variations by age, ethnicity, and poverty status. *Child Development*, **72**, 1844–1867.

Brave Heart, M. Y. H., & DeBruyn, L. M. (1998). The American Indian holocaust: healing historical unresolved grief. *American Indian and Alaska Native Mental Health Research: The Journal of the National Center*, 8, 60–82.

Chamberlain, P. & Reid, J. B. (1987). Parent observation and report of child symptoms. *Behavioral Assessment*, 9, 97–109.

Chen, X. & Kandel, D. B. (1995). The natural history of drug use from adolescence to the mid-thirties in a general population sample. *American Journal of Public Health*, **85**, 41–47.

Conger, R. D., Conger, K. J., Elder, G. H., Jr., *et al.* (1992). A family process model of economic hardship and adjustment of early adolescent boys. *Child Development*, **63**, 526–541.

Deater-Deckard, K. & Dodge, K. A. (1997). Externalizing behavior problems and discipline revisited: nonlinear effects and variation by culture, context, and gender. *Psychological Inquiry*, **8**, 161–175.

Dishion, T. J. & Bullock, B. (2001). Parenting and adolescent problem behavior: an ecological analysis of the nurturance hypothesis. In J. G. Borkowski, S. Ramey, & M. Bristol-Power (eds.), *Parenting and the Child's World: Influences on Intellectual, Academic, and Social–Emotional Development* (pp. 231–249). Mahwah, NJ: Lawrence Erlbaum.

Dishion, T. J. & Kavanagh, K. (2003). *Intervening in Adolescent Problem Behavior: A Family-centered Approach*. New York: Guilford Press.

Dishion, T. J. & Loeber, R. (1985). Male adolescent marijuana and alcohol use: the role of parents and peers revisited. *American Journal of Drug and Alcohol Abuse*, **11**, 11–25.

Dishion, T. J. & McMahon, R. J. (1998). Parental monitoring and the prevention of child and adolescent problem behavior: a conceptual and empirical formulation. *Clinical Child and Family Psychology Review*, **1**, 61–75.

Dishion, T. J. & Medici Skaggs, N. (2000). An ecological analysis of monthly "bursts" in early adolescent substance use. *Applied Developmental Science*, **4**, 89–97.

Dishion, T. J. & Owen, L. D. (2002). A longitudinal analysis of friendships and substance use: bi-directional influence form adolescence to adulthood. *Developmental Psychology*, **38**, 480–491.

Dishion, T. J. & Patterson, G. R. (1999). Model-building in developmental psychopathology: a pragmatic approach to understanding and intervention. *Journal of Clinical Child Psychology*, **28**, 502–512.

Dishion, T. J., Reid, J. B., & Patterson, G. R. (1988). Empirical guidelines for a family intervention for adolescent drug use. *Journal of Chemical Dependency Treatment*, **1**, 189–194.

Dishion, T. J., Patterson, G. R., Stoolmiller, M., & Skinner, M. (1991). Family, school, and behavioral antecedents to early adolescent involvement with antisocial peers. *Developmental Psychology*, **27**, 172–180.

Dishion, T. J., Capaldi, D. M., & Yoerger, K. (1999). Middle childhood antecedents to progression in male adolescent substance use: an ecological analysis of risk and protection. *Journal of Adolescent Research*, **14**, 175–206.

Dishion, T. J., Kavanagh, K., Schneiger, A., Nelson, S., & Kaufman, N. (2002). Preventing early adolescent substance use: a family-centered strategy for the public middle-school ecology. *Prevention Science*, **3** (Special Issue), 191–201.

Duran, E. & Duran, B. (1995). *Native American Postcolonial Psychology*. Albany, NY: State University of New York Press.

Elder, G. (1980). *Family Structure and Socialization*. New York: Arno.

Elder, G. H., Caspi, A., & van Nguyen, T. (1986). Resourceful and vulnerable children: family influences in hard times. In R. K. Silbereisen, K. Eyferth, & G. Rudinger (eds.), *Development as Action in Context: Problem Behavior and Normal Youth Development* (pp. 167–186). New York: Springer-Verlag.

Elliott, D. S., Huizinga, D., & Ageton, S. S. (1985). *Explaining Delinquency and Drug Use*. Beverly Hills: Sage.

First Nations House of Learning (1991). Special issue. *Canadian Journal of Native Education*, **18**, issue 1/2.

Fisher, P. A. & Ball, T. J. (2002). The Indian Family Wellness Project: an application of the tribal participatory research model. *Prevention Science*, **3** (Special Issue), 235–240.

Forgatch, M. S. & Stoolmiller, M. (1994). Emotions as contexts for adolescent delinquency. *Journal of Research on Adolescence*, **4**, 601–614.

Hawkins, J. D., Lishner, D. M., Catalano, R. F., & Howard, M. O. (1986). Childhood predictors of adolescent substance abuse: toward an empirically grounded theory. *Journal of Children in a Contemporary Society*, **8**, 11–47.

Hawkins, J. D., Catalano, R. F., Morrison, D. M., *et al.* (1992). The Seattle Social Development Project: effects of the first four years on protective factors and problem behaviors. In J. McCord & R. Tremblay (eds.), *The Prevention of Antisocial Behavior in Children* (pp. 139–162). New York: Guilford Press.

Hazzon-Hammond, S. (1997). *Timelines of Native American history: Through the centuries with Mother Earth and Father Sky*. New York: Berkley.

Herring, R. D. (1994). Substance use among Native American Indian youth: a selected review of causality. *Journal of Counseling and Development*, **72**, 578–584.

Hirschi, T. (1969). *Causes of delinquency*. Berkeley CA: University of California Press.

Hodge, F. S., Pasqua, A., Marquez, C., & Geishirt–Cantrell, B. (2002). Utilizing traditional storytelling to promote wellness in American Indian communities. *Journal of Transcultural Nursing*, **13**, 6–11.

Hops, H., Tildesley, E., Lichenstein, E., Ary, D. & Sherman, L. (1990). Parent–adolescent problem solving interactions and drug use. *American Journal of Drug and Alcohol Abuse*, **16**, 239–258.

IHS (Indian Health Service) (2001a). *Health and Heritage Brochure: Indian Health Service: An Agency profile*. Retrieved October 23, 2001, from http://info.ihs.gov.

(2001b). *Health and Heritage Brochure: Alcoholism and Substance Abuse*. Retrieved October 23, 2001, from http://info.ihs.gov.Health/Health6.pdf.

Institute for Government Research Studies in Administration (1928). *The Problem of Indian Administration: Report of a Survey made at the request of Honorable Hubert Work, Secretary of the Interior*. [Submitted February 21 1928] Retrieved July 9, 2002, from http://www.alaskool.org.native_ed/research_reports/IndianAdmin/Indian_Admin_Problms.htm.

Jessor, R. & Jessor, S. L. (1977). *Problem Behavior and Psychosocial Development*. New York: Academic Press.

Kandel, D. B., Davies, M., Karus, D., & Yamaguchi, K. (1986). The consequences in young adulthood of adolescent drug involvement. *Archives of General Psychiatry*, **43**, 746–754.

Kavanagh, K., Absalom, K., Beil, W., Jr., & Schliessmann, L. (1999). Connecting and becoming culturally competent: a Lakota example. *Advances in Nursing Science*, **21**, 9–31.

Kellam, S. G. (1990). Developmental epidemiological framework for family research on depression and aggression. In G. R. Patterson (ed.), *Depression and Aggression in Family Interaction* (pp. 11–48). Hillsdale, NJ: Lawrence Erlbaum.

Kellam, S. G., Brown, C. H., Rubin, B. R., & Ensminger, M. E. (1983). Paths leading to teenage psychiatric symptoms and substance use: developmental epidemiological studies in Woodlawn. In S. R. Guze, F. J. Earns, & J. E. Barrett (eds.), *Childhood Psychopathology and Development* (pp. 17–51). New York: Raven.

Kerr, M. & Stattin, H. (2000). What parents know, how they know it, and several forms of adolescent adjustment: further support for a reinterpretation of monitoring. *Developmental Psychology*, **36**, 366–380.

Koss–Chioino, J. D. & Vargas, L. A., (1992). *Working with Culture: Psychotherapeutic Interventions with Ethnic Minority Children and Adolescents*. San Francisco, CA: Jossey-Bass.

Lomawaima, K. T. (1993). Domesticity in the federal Indian schools: the power of authority over mind and body. *American Ethnologist*, **20**, 227–240.

Mason, C. A., Cauce, A. M., Gonzales, N., & Hiraga, Y. (1996). Neither too sweet nor too sour: problem peers, maternal control, and problem behavior in African-American adolescents. *Child Development*, **67**, 2115–2130.

Masten, A. S. & Coatsworth, J. D. (1998). The development of competence in favorable and unfavorable environments: lessons from research on successful children. *American Psychologist*, **53**, 205–220.

McCord, J. (1988). Identifying developmental paradigms leading to alcoholism. *Journal of Studies on Alcohol*, **49**, 357–362.

McLoyd, V. C. (1990). The impact of economic hardship on Black families and children: psychological distress, parenting, and socioemotional development. *Child Development*, **61**, 311–346.

(1997). The impact of poverty and low socioeconomic status on the socioemotional functioning of African-American children and adolescents: mediating effects. In R. D. Taylor & M. C. Wang (eds.), *Social and Emotional Adjustment and Family Relations in Ethnic Minority Families* (pp. 7–34). Mahwah, NJ: Lawrence Erlbaum.

Miller, W. R. & Rollnick, S. (2002). *Motivational Interviewing: Preparing People to Change Addictive Behavior*, 2nd edn. New York: Guilford Press.

Mitchell, C. M., O'Nell, T. D., Beals, J., *et al.* (1996). Dimensionality of alcohol use among American Indian adolescents: latent structure, construct validity, and implications for development research. *Journal of Research on Adolescence*, **6**, 151–180.

Moncher, M. S., Holden, G. W., & Trimble, J. E. (1990). Substance abuse among Native American youth. *Journal of Consulting and Clinical Psychology*, **58**, 408–415.

Newcomb, M. D. (1992). Understanding the multidimensional nature of drug use and abuse: the role of consumption, risk factors, and protective factors. In M. Glantz & R. Pickens (eds.), *Vulnerability to Drug Abuse* (pp. 255–297). Washington, DC: American Psychological Press.

Newcomb, M. D. & Bentler, P. M. (1988a). Impact of adolescent drug use and social support on problems of young adults: a longitudinal study. *Journal of Abnormal Psychology*, **97**, 64–75. (1988b). *Consequences of Adolescent Drug Use*. Newbury Park, CA: Sage.

Nies, J. (1996). *Native American History: A Chronology of a Culture's Vast Achievements and their Links to World Events*. New York: Ballantine.

Oetting, E. R. & Beauvais, F. (1987). Peer cluster theory, socialization characteristics and adolescent drug use: a path analysis. *Counseling Psychology*, **34**, 205–213.

(1990). Adolescent drug use: findings of national and local surveys. *Journal of Consulting and Clinical Psychology*, **58**, 385–394.

Oetting, E. R. & Donnermeyer, J. F. (1998). Primary socialization theory: the etiology of drug use and deviance: I. *Substance Use and Misuse*, **33**, 995–1026.

Oetting, E. R, Donnermeyer, J. F, Trimble, J. E., & Beauvais, F. (1998). Primary socialization theory: culture, ethnicity, and cultural identification. The links between culture and substance use: IV. *Substance Use and Misuse*, **33**, 2075–2107.

O'Nell, T. D. & Mitchell, C. M. (1996). Alcohol use among American Indian adolescents: the role of culture in pathological drinking. *Social Science of Medicine*, **4**, 565–578.

Pulkkinen, L. (1983). Youthful smoking and drinking in a longitudinal perspective. *Journal of Youth and Adolescence*, **12**, 253–283.

Robins, L. N. & Przybeck, T. R. (1985). Age of onset of drug use as a factor in drug and other disorders. In C. L. Jones & R. J. Battjes (eds.), *Research Monograph* No. 56: *Etiology of Drug Abuse: Implications for Prevention* (pp. 178–193). Rockville, MD: National Institute on Drug Abuse.

Smith, G. M. & Fogg, C. P. (1979). Psychological antecedents of teenage drug use. *Research in Community Mental Health*, **1**, 87–102.

Steinberg, L. (1986). Latchkey children and susceptibility to peer pressure: an ecological analysis. *Developmental Psychology*, **22**, 433–439.

Swaim, R. C., Oetting, E. R., Thurman, P. J., & Beauvais, F. (1993). American Indian adolescent drug use and socialization characteristics: a cross-cultural comparison. *Journal of Cross-Cultural Psychology*, **1**, 53–70.

Szapocznik, J., Kurtines, W. M., & Fernandez, T. (1980). Bicultural involvement and adjustment in Hispanic American youths. *International Journal of Intercultural Relations*, **4**, 353–366.

Szasz, M. C. (1992). Current conditions in American Indian and Alaska Native communities. In P. Cahape & C. B. Howley (eds.), *Indian Nations at Risk: Listening to the People* (pp. 1–5). Charleston, WV: ERIC.

Tom-Orme, L. (2000). Native Americans explaining illness: storytelling as illness experience. In Whaley, B. B. (ed.), *Explaining Illness: Research, Theory, and Strategies* (pp. 237–257). Mahwah, NJ: Lawrence Erlbaum.

Waldron, H. B., Slesnick, N., Brody, J. L., Turner, C. W., & Peterson, T. R. (2001). Treatment outcomes for adolescent substance abuse at 4- and 7-month assessments. *Journal of Consulting and Clinical Psychology*, **69**, 802–813.

Walker, H. M., Severson, H., Stiller, B., Williams, G. J., Haring, N., Shinn, M. R., & Todis, B. (1988). Systematic screening of pupils in the elementary age range at risk for behavior disorders: development and trial testing of a multiple gating model. *Remedial and Special Education*, **9**, 8–20.

Watts, L. (2001). Applying a cultural models approach to American Indian substance dependency research. *American Indian and Alaska Native Mental Health Research: The Journal of the National Center*, **10**, 34–50.

Werner, E. E. (1995). Resilience in development. *Current Directions in Psychological Science*, **4**, 81–85.

Whiting, B. B. & Whiting, J. M. (1975). *Children of Six Cultures: A Psychocultural Analysis*. Cambridge, MA: Harvard University Press.

21

Using treatment development methods to enhance the family-based treatment of Hispanic adolescents

Daniel A. Santisteban, Maite P. Mena, and Lourdes Suarez-Morales

Center for Family Studies, University of Miami Miller School of Medicine, FL, USA

A growing emphasis on the utilization of empirically supported treatments for drug abuse and other psychiatric disorders (Barlow, 1996; SAMHSA, 2001) has also led to a need to specify treatments that have been developed and tested with Hispanics. Chambless and Hollon (1998, pp. 7–18) define empirically supported treatments as "clearly specified psychological treatments shown to be efficacious in controlled research with a delineated population." This and similar definitions have raised questions about the extent to which the "delineated populations" have consisted of large groups of minority clients (Bernal & Scharron-Del-Rio, 2001). In this chapter we will argue that (a) there is a severe shortage of empirically supported substance abuse treatment models that have been fully tested with Hispanics or that incorporate research on cultural processes; (b) that many of the commonly used ideas of cultural competence continue to be distal to the treatment processes therapists encounter and, therefore, often difficult to transfer to the front lines of practice; and (c) that the treatment-development mechanism (Rounsaville, Carroll, & Onken, 2001) can be a powerful tool for designing interventions for minority groups by systematically integrating findings on cultural processes with a treatment's theoretical change mechanisms. Based on this line of thought, we present an ongoing treatment development effort designed to produce an enhanced family-based treatment model with several innovative characteristics (e.g., a flexible treatment manual and thematic/psychoeducational modules) that facilitate the tailoring of the intervention package to the needs of each Hispanic adolescent/family.

Empirically supported treatments and Hispanics

The importance of establishing empirically supported treatments for Hispanics is timely given that minority ethnic groups now make up 27.2% of the USA population

Adolescent Substance Abuse: Research and Clinical Advances, ed. Howard A. Liddle and Cynthia L. Rowe. Published by Cambridge University Press. © Cambridge University Press 2006.

and Hispanics 13% (US Bureau of Census, 2000). Although Hispanics and other ethnic minorities are highly represented in the vast pool of drug-related research, there is little focus on their ethnic identity and the ethnicity-related factors that are the contexts for drug use (Tucker, 1985). The lack of focus on ethnicity-related issues among Hispanics may be partly because of the complexity and diversity within and between groups that fall under the "Hispanic" umbrella. Although the different Hispanic groups often share common linguistic, cultural, and family values, there are also substantial differences within Hispanics, including reasons for and route of migration, length of residence in the USA, level of acculturation, traditionalism, social class, education, and other life experiences (marginalization, immigration-related separations, etc.).

In assessing the availability of empirically supported treatments for Hispanics, it is important to question the assumption that an empirically supported treatment that has not been tested with a minority group is necessarily efficacious for that group. As Bernal and Scharron-Del-Rio (2001) argued, it would be a major contradiction if the field, on the one hand, called for the application of empirically supported treatments, and, on the other hand, supported the use of treatments for ethnic minorities with no strong empirical support. We should require that promising interventions be fully tested with major racial/ethnic groups. One might go a step further and argue that, even if a treatment has been shown to be efficacious with a minority population, it may have less than optimal efficacy if it has not incorporated the findings of basic research on cultural factors and culture-related processes (Santisteban et al., 2002). In the case of minority groups, the use of models that do not incorporate findings on culture-related variables ignores the individual differences and differences in life experiences that define ethnic minorities (Bernal & Scharron-Del-Rio, 2001). Just as one would expect that treatment models that work with adolescents incorporate the findings of developmental research (Liddle et al., 2000) and findings on family processes (Patterson, Reid, & Dishion, 1992), we believe that interventions with minority groups must be informed and enhanced by findings on key culture-related processes.

Shortcomings of current efforts to ensure "cultural competence"

Cultural competence, defined as a set of congruent behaviors, practices, and attitudes that enable professionals to function effectively in the context of cultural differences (Cross et al., 1989; Straussner, 2001), is a crucial aspect in the provision of substance abuse treatment with ethnic minorities. Cultural competence has been shown to influence client–clinician communication and trust, successful development of a therapeutic alliance, and the retention of culturally diverse clients in treatment (Bernal et al., 1998).

In an effort to establish a set of general guidelines for clinicians, the American Psychological Association (1993) and independent researchers (e.g., Sue, Arrendondo, & McDavis, 1992) have described cultural competencies in several areas. These guidelines recommend that clinicians develop competencies in the areas of personal, cultural, and professional knowledge, aptitude, and skills that they systematically integrate in their clinical work with ethnic minorities (Hansen, Pepitone-Arreola-Rockwell, & Greene, 2000). Personal knowledge involves an awareness of one's own cultural heritage, values, and biases related to identified minority groups, and the ability to self-assess accurately one's cultural competence to proceed ethically. Cultural knowledge is recommended for the areas of manifestations of prejudice, oppression, and discrimination in the USA; sociopolitical influences (e.g., poverty, marginalization, stereotyping) that impinge on the lives of identified minority groups; and normative values about illness, help-seeking behaviors, worldviews, and interactional styles of cultural groups. Professional knowledge is also required concerning culturally specific diagnostic categories; history of culturally bound psychological theory, research methods, and professional practice; culturally specific assessment tools and their empirical support; and family structures and gender roles. These will differ across identified groups in the USA. In addition, culturally relevant skills include the ability to evaluate culture-specific and universal hypotheses related to clients in order to develop accurate clinical conceptualizations, and to design and implement non-biased and effective treatment plans and interventions.

Although cultural competence guidelines provide clinicians with a comprehensive description of the competencies that should be developed for their clinical work with ethnic minorities, they are often general and cover very broad areas of clinical and cultural competency. Further, because current empirical treatments do not include culturally relevant applications of the intervention, clinicians are often left to adjust a treatment intervention creatively to a particular ethnic group by using available knowledge, many times stereotypical or anecdotal in nature. We believe that a developer or user of a model who is particularly knowledgeable about core change mechanisms is in the best position to articulate the *interaction* between these mechanisms and unique cultural characteristics.

The treatment-development process described later in this chapter attempts to counteract the limitations described above by integrating cultural competency into the content and process of a family-based treatment for substance-abusing Hispanic adolescents. Clinicians implementing this model are trained on specific culturally relevant areas (e.g., separations as a result of immigration; acculturation effects on parenting practices) that interact with drug abuse and family processes and learn to apply the intervention in a culturally congruent manner. We turn, next, to a brief description of the formal stages of treatment development to provide a background for our work in the development of a culturally informed treatment model for substance-abusing Hispanic adolescents and their families.

Utilizing basic research and treatment development mechanisms to enhance a family treatment

The stage model for the development and testing of behavioral treatments specifies a series of steps that help treatment to progress from the point where it is simply an idea to the point where it can be delivered in a clinical setting as an empirically supported treatment (Rounsaville *et al.*, 2001). During stage I, specific interventions are developed, formed into a manual, and pilot tested. As described by Rounsaville *et al.* (2001), stage I studies are designed to encourage innovation and specify the components of novel treatments in a manual form that can later undergo rigorous efficacy testing. The treatment-development work that is the focus of this chapter integrates research findings in the cultural domain with findings in the domains of family processes, developmental factors, and drug abuse treatment. Stage II will be the next important step: taking the treatment to the point where it can be successfully implemented in clinical settings. Stage II studies can serve two purposes. The primary purpose is to conduct rigorous randomized clinical trials on manual-guided and pilot-tested treatments that have demonstrated promise for becoming efficacious treatments (Rounsaville *et al.*, 2001). These studies can also help to identify key components that are necessary for the successful implementation of a treatment with a population (Rounsaville *et al.*, 2001). Once a treatment has been shown to have efficacy in at least two randomized clinical trials, a stage III study provides the avenue by which the treatment can be transported to clinical settings in the community. Research issues that are of primary focus during a stage III study include generalizability to different settings and different population, and implementation issues, such as training, cost-effectiveness, and how acceptable the new treatment is to clinicians, patients, community agencies, and insurance companies (Rounsaville *et al.*, 2001). One of the great benefits of articulating this stage model of treatment development and testing is that the importance of newer and less visible stage I research is highlighted.

Stage I research serves as a mechanism for incorporating basic research into clinical interventions. All too often, well-designed treatment-development endeavors do not fully link development/refinements to basic research (Onken & Bootzin, 1998). In the case of developing treatments for minorities, we believe that the stage I model of treatment development is particularly well suited for systematically incorporating basic research on culture-related factors into novel interventions, and testing the impact of enhancements. Basic research can be very effective at documenting the specific characteristics of subtypes of patients that research on "aptitude by treatment interaction" indicates must be addressed in a more focused manner if treatment impact is to be enhanced (Shoham & Rohrbaugh, 1995; Snow, 1991). The remainder of this chapter presents work based on the hypothesis that by linking this culture-specific information directly with hypothesized theories of problem development and problem change, we can improve outcomes and training for therapists to be culturally competent with Hispanic families.

Development of an integrative family therapy for Hispanic adolescents

The goal of the treatment-development effort reported in this chapter is to utilize established scientific methods, available research findings, and the findings of this project's basic research study to design a treatment that is highly efficacious with Hispanics. The model we are developing, culturally informed family therapy for adolescents (CIFTA), draws on structural family therapy (Minuchin & Fishman, 1981) and on an existing, empirically established version of structural family therapy, namely brief strategic family therapy, which was designed to modify the within-family interactions that have been linked to drug abuse in adolescents (Santisteban, et al., 2003; Szapocznik & Kurtines, 1989; Szapocznik et al., 1990). Like other models of structural family therapy, CIFTA also hypothesizes family interactions to be a major change mechanism that leads to a reduction in drug use and behavior problems in youth. Unlike many other systemic family models, however, CIFTA places strong emphasis on factors at the individual level relevant to drug abuse processes (e.g., triggers to use, relapse prevention, role of co-occurring disorders, adolescent's lack of knowledge of specific brain effects) and adolescent developmental processes (e.g., difficulties in skills development, decision making, relationships, and the creation of life goals). Further, in the treatment of Hispanics, CIFTA strongly emphasizes, and is informed by, findings on culture-related processes (e.g., acculturation processes, immigration and acculturation stress, immigration-related processes such as parent–child separations).

There are several "model enhancements" to the traditional systemic family therapy model that make CIFTA capable of addressing the important themes described above. Some of these major enhancements that extend from previous work in family therapy include (a) designing a flexible manual that assumes that one size *does not* fit all and that facilitates the tailoring of an intervention package to the needs of each Hispanic adolescent/family; (b) designing thematic/psycho-educational modules that provide families with educational content, a vocabulary, and a frame to link key culture-related, family process, and behavior problem themes; and (c) integrating individually oriented interventions that facilitate family change and help adolescents to handle successfully the many developmental challenges that they face (e.g., learning interpersonal skills, setting of life goals). These enhancements are described in detail in the next part of this chapter on manual development.

The activities of this treatment-development effort can be broken down into three major phases: (a) a manual development phase with refinement pilot cases, (b) a basic research phase, and (c) a small randomized trial phase. Within this design, there is an iterative process of treatment development in which the findings of each phase informs the activities of the subsequent phases. Each of the three phases is described below.

Developing a draft manual

The value of creating a manual to guide treatment has been well demonstrated in the clinical research literature (Luborsky & DeRubeis, 1984). Treatment manuals play a critical role by (a) highlighting the most salient features of treatments; (b) delineating replicable procedures that facilitate the training of therapists, the implementation of the therapy, and the further testing and refinement of an approach; (c) ensuring therapist fidelity/adherence and competence in implementing a given modality; and (d) facilitating the discovery of the active ingredients in psychotherapy (Lambert & Ogles, 1988; Moras, 1993).

The creation of the CIFTA manual began with a collaborative effort between researchers and clinical teams that focused on the development of the treatment. A goal was to incorporate as many aspects as possible from the findings on drug abuse treatment, the adolescent developmental literature, family process and treatment, and culture-related processes that can inform a framework for conceptualizing problem development and treatment. Below are some of the major research findings that informed CIFTA's design.

Adolescent developmental literature

The adolescent developmental stage is characterized by numerous changes, including biological, cognitive, and interpersonal changes. During the adolescent stage of development, children experience growth spurts, changes in body shape and facial features, and hormonal changes related to the emergence of sexuality (Weisz & Hawley, 2002). Perhaps more important than the actual changes that occur is how early or late they occur during the developmental stage (Weisz & Hawley, 2002). For example, both boys and girls who mature early may be at a greater risk for substance abuse and risky sexual behaviors (Flannery, Rowe, & Gulley, 1993; Williams & Dunlop, 1999). The way parents react to their child's physical maturation also plays a role in how the child reacts to the changes that are occurring (Liddle *et al.*, 2000).

During adolescence, the physical changes that the adolescent experiences are coupled with the sudden awareness of their sexuality. Research shows that what parents say to adolescents about sex and how they say it influences the adolescent's sexual behaviors (Dilorio, Kelley, & Hockenberry-Eaton, 1999). Parents, however, often shy away from the topic. This is particularly true for Hispanic parents, because sex is a topic that is considered taboo (Marin & Gomez, 1997). Baumeister, Flores and Marin (1995) have shown that Hispanic adolescents report less communication with their parents about sex than non-Hispanic adolescents.

Adolescents also experience changes at the cognitive level. Piaget (1972) used the concept of formal operations to define the adolescent stage as characterized by the development of abstract thinking and hypothetical reasoning. Holmbeck *et al.* (2000) identify three cognitive skills that develop during adolescence: abstraction, consequential thinking, and hypothetical reasoning. The development of the cognitive skills defined by Holmbeck *et al.* (2000) can be extremely useful to an adolescent, particularly during the course of any treatment (Weisz & Hawley, 2002). For example, consequential thinking allows them to consider different solutions to a problem and what consequences there may be for each solution. Skills training in the context of therapy is particularly important during the adolescent developmental stage. This is true because, at this stage, the development of new skills for adaptively handling personal and environmental challenges is expected and developmentally appropriate (Tilton-Weaver, Vitunski, & Galambos, 2001).

Changes in personal relationships are also characteristic of adolescence. More specifically, peers become increasingly important and have direct influences on adolescent choices. Most conflicts between parents and adolescents during this period are minor and revolve around differences in opinions about curfew, school grades, and peers (Keating, 1990). When adolescents learn to negotiate with parents around those issues and are able to compromise, they are developing their sense of self and autonomy, improving their self-competence and reasoning skills, and enabling healthy interpersonal relationships (Liddle *et al.*, 2000). When conflict between parents and adolescents becomes severe through failures in negotiation, the attachment between parent and child can be damaged. The literature on adolescent development shows that when adolescents do not have an emotional connection with their parents they are at greater risk for developing emotional symptoms (Papini & Roggman, 1992). Family therapists should consider the normative developmental processes occurring during adolescence and their impact on family relations while designing developmentally informed interventions.

Family process and treatment of adolescent drug abuse

Family functioning, often operationalized in terms of family conflict, support, communication, and parenting practices, has been shown to be critically important in the emergence and maintenance of adolescent behavior problems and drug use (Cauce et al., 1990; Loeber et al., 1998). In many cases, family conflict and communication problems maintain conduct problems and drug involvement by directing negativity toward the youth and/or inadvertently reinforcing undesirable behavior (Dishion, Capaldi, & Yoerger, 1999; Patterson, Bank, & Stoolmiller, 1990). Maladaptive parenting practices have also been linked with the emergence and/or maintenance of drug using and other delinquent behavior (Dishion & Andrews, 1995; Liddle & Dakof, 1995; Patterson, 1986). Parents of youth with behavior problems show overall poor family management, consisting of things such as absence of limit-setting and parental monitoring, and inconsistent parenting (Lindahl & Malik, 1999). The quality of parent–adolescent relationships or attachment has also been shown to play an important role in the emergence of adolescent substance abuse (Bailey & Hubbard, 1990; Newcomb & Felix-Ortiz, 1992). The important role of these specific family factors in emerging and continued drug use has led to the development of treatments that target and modify family functioning, and these approaches have shown considerable promise in ameliorating adolescent behavior problems and drug abuse (Alexander, Holtzworth-Munroe, & Jameson, 1994; Chamberlain & Rosicky, 1995; Henggeler, Pickrel, & Brondino, 1999; Santisteban et al., 2003; Schmidt, Liddle, & Dakof, 1996; Shadish et al., 1993; Szapocznik et al., 1990; Waldron, 1997). The family component in CIFTA utilizes this literature to refine the interventions and focus on parent–adolescent attachment issues, parenting practices (including parent–school and parent–peer functioning), family processes that reinforce problematic adolescent behaviors, family conflict/negativity, and conflict resolution.

Culture-related variables and processes

Acculturation and externalizing behavior

There appear to be unique aspects in the development and treatment of Hispanic adolescent drug abuse (Santisteban et al., 2002) that should be integrated in a treatment model for this population. For example, a number of studies with Hispanic adolescents have found a significant positive relationship between acculturation and drug use (Buriel, Calzada, & Vasquez, 1982; Junger & Polder, 1992; Oetting & Beauvais, 1991). Among Hispanic youth, years living in the USA and being acculturated have been linked to adolescents' engagement in delinquency and substance abuse (Fridrich & Flannery, 1995; Gil, Wagner, & Vega, 2000; Lovato et al., 1994; Sommers, Fagan, & Baskin, 1993; Vega et al., 1993). Conversely, those adolescents who maintain their Hispanic values and behaviors appear less likely to participate in delinquent activity (Buriel *et al.*, 1982). Vega *et al.* (1993) found that family factors, such as low levels of family pride, cohesion, and parental support, along with acculturation stress (i.e., psychological distress resulting from the clash between the family's culture of origin and American culture), can impact delinquent behavior among Hispanic adolescents.

Acculturation and parenting practices

Given the important role of parenting practices in the development and treatment of substance abuse, it is helpful to investigate possible links between culture-related factors and parenting practices. One study showed that acculturation was associated with less-effective types of parenting practices that directly impacted behavior problems in youth (Gil *et al.*, 2000). In our own basic research (D. A. Santisteban *et al.*, unpublished data), we found that families that remain high in Hispanicism[1] (independent of their level of Americanism) show parenting styles that appeared to protect their youth from becoming involved in delinquency and drug abuse. Hispanicism did not have a direct effect on externalizing behaviors but had its effect indirectly through parenting. Specifically, the mother's level of Hispanicism was positively related to higher parental involvement, higher disciplining behavior, and effective parenting; these, in turn, were associated with decreased likelihood of externalizing behaviors in youths. These findings suggest that the loss of Hispanic values by parents may lead to less-successful parenting practices than those common in their culture of origin, and this may shed light on a potential mechanism behind the acculturation–behavior problem relationship.

Immigration-related experiences and parent–adolescent attachment

In working with immigrant Hispanic families, one of the first and major considerations is the effect of immigration on the family (e.g., parent–child attachment). Immigration is a major life event (Silove *et al.*, 1997), and clinical experience tells us that immigration-related parent–child separations can also be a very powerful disruptive force to family relations and child development (Mitrani, Santisteban, & Muir, 2004). When parents emmigrate ahead of their children or must send their children ahead of them (Bemak & Greenberg, 1994; Foner, 1987), there is a breaking of ties with nuclear family members and resulting feelings of abandonment and loss. When children arrive in the USA years after the parents' immigration and problems emerge in the child's behavior, our clinical experience has demonstrated that there are a number of powerful family dynamics

---

[1] This work moves beyond the traditional view of acculturation as a unidimensional process (i.e., in which Hispanicism is replaced by Americanism) and instead investigated it as a bidimensional process (i.e., allowing for different and independent profiles on their adherence to Hispanicism and Americanism).

that seem to be operating. These include (a) child feelings of abandonment and resentment, as well as guilt for having these feelings; (b) dual loyalties toward the mother and the family member who was the primary caretaker during the separation; (c) a cultural pattern dictating that the emergence of strong negative emotions around these issues is disrespectful; (d) the mother's dual loyalty between newly established relationships and the separated children; (e) age-inappropriate parenting behavior, partly because the mother has not adjusted to the child's development that occurred during the separation; and (f) parental reluctance to set limits because of the guilt associated with the separation.

Preliminary findings from CIFTA's basic research study have suggested that a relatively high percentage (16%) of families reported at least one significant parent–child separation caused by migration. Of the adolescents separated from parents in this way, 13% were separated from both mother and father during the immigration. Another 57% were separated from their mother, who was the primary caretaker. This is particularly powerful given that many of these youngsters had never had their father as a significant caretaker. In these cases, losing the mother was a loss of their only parental figure. An additional 26% were separated at the time of immigration from their fathers and 4% from a sister. The average age of the child at the time of the separation was 7 years, and the average duration of the separation was slightly over 3 years. Later analyses will directly explore the empirical relationship between separations and key family processes (e.g., attachment).

Hispanic values and family processes

It is important for family therapists to consider the family's underlying value system when designing effective and culturally consistent interventions. Among the most commonly reported values among Hispanic families are "familismo" (familism) and "respeto" (respect), which impact the workings of the family (Marin, 1993; Sabogal et al., 1987). Familismo refers to the strong identification and attachment of individuals with their families (nuclear and extended), manifested by strong feelings of loyalty, reciprocity, and solidarity among members of the same family (Triandis et al., 1982). Research has identified three dimensions of familismo: familial obligations (e.g., the perceived obligations to provide material and emotional support to the members of the extended family), support from family (e.g., perceived support from relatives to solve problems), and family as referents (e.g., the perception of relatives as behavioral and attitudinal referents) (Marin, 1993; Sabogal et al., 1987).

It may at times be hard to understand or change the Hispanic family without understanding the important role of values and their manifestations within the family dynamics. For example, Hispanic children from a very early age are socialized to show highly respectful behavior to authority figures: parents, rela-tives, seniors, and professionals (Ramos-McKay, Comas-Diaz, & Rivera, 1988), which may decrease with age as a result of maturation and/or contact with American culture in the process of acculturation (Gil *et al.*, 2000). Hispanic's strong preference for markedly hierarchical family relations (Miranda, Estrada, & Firpo-Jimenez, 2000; Szapocznik *et al.*, 1978) may be related to the underlying value of *respeto*, and this can have powerful implications for family communica-tion and conflict resolution in treatment. Families expecting marked levels of authority (non-egalitarian) can perceive open disagreements between parents and adolescents as disrespectful and unacceptable. For example, an intervention that openly encourages the youngster to "speak his/her mind" and "tell parents what he/she really thinks" may be viewed by Hispanic families as incompetent or misguided, encouraging precisely that which is perceived to be the dysfunctional behavior (e.g., disrespectful challenging of authority). This view may clash with a mental health culture in which full conflict emergence with resolution is valued. Similarly, the cultural expectation that Hispanic adolescents defer completely to adults as a sign of respect may sometimes have disadvantages in an individualized environment where exercising critical thinking skills are needed in order to function (Padilla, 1997).

Research findings show that familismo decreases with increased levels of accul-turation (Cortes, 1995; Gil *et al.*, 2000; Marin, 1993; Sabogal *et al.*, 1987). Specifically, aspects of familism, such as family obligations and perceptions of relatives as referents, were found to decrease with acculturation, whereas, per-ceived family support remained constant at different levels of acculturation. Given that acculturation changes basic Hispanic values (Sabogal *et al.*, 1987), family therapists working with Hispanic families must understand the impact of accul-turation on family relations. Most importantly for family therapists, value changes caused by acculturation can be expected to occur differentially for different family members (e.g., youngsters acculturate faster and may change their values faster than their parents; Szapocznik *et al.*, 1978), creating an incongruence and stress within the family. Family therapists must understand the range family members can display, understand the strengths of a given family's stance on value dimen-sions, as well as the potential complications that may emerge with acculturation. Therapists must always be attentive to personal and cultural values and be careful not to undermine either the need for self-sufficiency *or* the reliance on other family members in those individuals for whom this is important and adaptive.

Designing interventions to integrate the relevant literature

Having identified many of the research findings that must be incorporated into the intervention, we embarked on the task of creating the types of link between these findings and the family processes we sought to modify. We refined the focus of our targets of change (e.g., improving parenting practices, parent–adolescent attachment, adolescent ability to meet developmental challenges, increasing family support and decreasing family conflict/negativity, increasing knowledge of drug effects and triggers to use) by considering them in their developmental and cultural context. For example, a goal was to discuss openly how difficult it is for many Hispanic families to talk about drugs (as it is difficult to have discussions of adolescent sexual behavior). Similarly, we highlighted how alcohol abuse among Hispanic youth and adults was often perceived as less problematic (more culturally syntonic) than drug abuse, although the reasons for use and the processes of addiction are similar. Another example was our focus on couching parent–adolescent relationship/attachment problems in the context of immigration-related parent–child separations and/or differential acculturation pressures, which regularly place the younger and older family members at odds with each other.

Creating thematic modules

The remaining challenge, however, was to create practical and focused manual-guided treatment components that would be most efficient at addressing the themes described above. Having selected the themes that would be at the core of the intervention, we were still left with decisions about the structure and process of the new treatment components. An early and important decision was that there was a benefit to providing clear and systematic information to parents and adolescents via the delivery of *thematic, psychoeducational-type modules.* Psychoeducational modules were deemed helpful because the free-flowing process of family therapy does not readily facilitate the family's learning of important facts that have accumulated in key areas relevant to adolescent drug abuse (e.g., drug education, parenting practices, risk of infection with the human immunodeficiency virus (HIV), interpersonal skills, crisis management). Further, the direct acquisition of knowledge and skills can facilitate the behavioral changes targeted by individual and family therapy sessions. Modules were developed that provided a structured and systematic presentation of important topics in a format and at a level that parents and the adolescent could understand. Furthermore, each module was informed by knowledge of culture-specific processes. Thematic modules were developed to provide important information (e.g., HIV risk, drug education), teach critical skills (e.g., parenting practices, HIV risk-reduction strategies, interpersonal skills, crisis management strategies), and highlight family interactions that can be targeted in family therapy (e.g., parent–adolescent negotiation, parent–adolescent attachment, movement to a bicultural position). Information delivered via thematic modules created "therapeutic frames" for the core problems, thereby increasing family readiness to seek more adaptive family relations.

For example, a hopeless and frustrated parent may be more willing to stay engaged in treatment if he perceives the relationship problem with his son as partly caused by the complex and normative acculturation processes, rather than a personal rejection of him and his beliefs.

Creation of a manual with a flexible design

The flexible features of a manual are particularly important for Hispanics because of the considerable heterogeneity both between and within groups under the Hispanic umbrella, and because of the different specific clinical profiles of adolescents/families seeking treatment. For these reasons, it is helpful to have flexible treatment (Beutler, 1999) with multiple treatment options. The goal is to have a menu of interventions from which to select in order to tailor the treatment to the specific needs of the families. Unique treatment needs may arise from the composition of the family (e.g., blended, single parent), different clinical pictures (e.g., co-occurring disorders requiring medication, severe skills deficiencies, court involvement), and different possible stressors/life experiences, which are more common in some subgroups of Hispanics than in others (parent–child separations, acculturation-related conflicts). Different profiles along these dimensions may all severely disrupt the adaptive family interactions needed to keep youth drug free but may be more central to some families than others; each would require different focused interventions.

A key development in designing a flexible manual was the creation of a systematic procedure for clinically assessing families and for facilitating the selection of modules and themes that should guide treatment for each adolescent and family. A comprehensive semi-structured interview was conducted with the adolescent and parents during the initial family sessions. Adolescent and parents are asked about mental health or substance abuse problems in the adolescent and other family members, and the history of these problems within the family. Family functioning and family patterns are assessed (e.g., what roles do members have, who is the primary disciplinarian, who is in charge of parenting). Families are also asked to share their immigration history with the therapist (e.g., where the family is from; when and why the family immigrated; were family members separated; if so for how long). After the initial sessions with the family, the therapist, based on the information gathered, can begin to formulate a treatment plan for the family. Part of the plan entails deciding which CIFTA enhancements are most relevant and will be most useful to the adolescent and the parents.

Integration of individual treatment

In addition to the two enhancements to the family-based model already mentioned (i.e., module development and flexible manual), a third modification involved the inclusion of individually oriented treatment sessions. Individual therapy sessions were designed to enhance the work of CIFTA by addressing challenges common during the adolescent developmental stage. First, these sessions focus on increasing the adolescent's engagement and motivation. This treatment goal involves getting to know the adolescent and her/his world in a way that does not focus on symptoms or dysfunction, and showing the adolescent how therapy can be relevant and helpful. An important part of this component includes the adolescent's establishment of personal goals and a vision of the future. These goals must be separate from the goals of parents, which at the time of therapy are often more behavior-control oriented. Setting of the adolescent's goals promotes engagement with the therapist and with the therapy processes, as the adolescent perceives that this process can help with personal and normative adolescent struggles. Individual sessions also are most effective at tracking/monitoring and addressing drug use and other risky behaviors that may be difficult to discuss in conjoint family sessions. Part of this work also includes preparing the adolescent to discuss these topics in mature and adaptive ways during family sessions. A final goal of individual sessions is to help adolescents to use the learned skills in their daily lives. It is the responsibility of the therapist to help the adolescent to identify daily situations in which the adolescent can implement more skillful and effective behavior.

Pilot cases to refine the interventions

The pilot phase of the intervention tests the newly developed treatment components with the intended population for the purpose of determining feasibility and acceptability, and for refinement of the interventions. The evaluation of these aspects of treatment components are achieved by assessing (a) the level of therapeutic alliance achieved in specific sessions, (b) the participant reports of satisfaction/usefulness of distinct therapy components, and (c) the attrition rates and missed sessions. For example, participant reports of satisfaction and ratings of alliance during a session focusing on a particular module was used to inform our treatment development team as to whether the module was useful and understandable to the family and adolescent. Evaluation of attrition rates and/or missed sessions were used as indicators of treatment acceptability or feasibility, and highlighted areas needing modification of treatment dosage and/or treatment intensity, as well as strengthening the engagement phase of treatment.

This phase was also used to refine the parameters and process of treatment, and for working through implementation challenges. An example was testing who in the family receives each thematic module, whether the family together, the adolescent alone, or the parents alone, and what process might enhance efficacy. In this example, we hypothesized that the drug education module must be given to the adolescent alone to facilitate the open disclosure of details regarding specific triggers and use patterns. However, a brief module was created for parents so that they could understand the process of addiction, the warning signs for certain drugs, and facilitate later parent–adolescent discussions around substance abuse in family therapy. Parents reported that this separate module, educating them on the warning signs of drug use and relapse, was a key to making them more competent in this area and better able to provide leadership to their adolescent. We subsequently strengthened that module and designed it to address parent-specific questions and concerns. Another challenge during the pilot phase was determining how educational material contained in thematic modules could be integrated in subsequent family and individual therapy sessions, such that the issues raised in the educational sessions could be addressed by several treatment components. Refinement of this process led to all treatment components maximizing the impact of the modules and vice versa. Lastly, issues of treatment implementation with Hispanic families were looked at closely during this phase. The appropriateness and acceptability of treatment materials provided in Spanish during delivery of thematic modules were examined. Based on feedback from therapists and clients, the materials were modified until all families understood them and felt they could put them into practice. Refinements to the treatment model accomplished during the pilot phase prepared the model for a stage I mini-randomized trial.

A basic research study to investigate empirically the links between culture-related factors and family process

In addition to integrating research findings that already existed in the literature, our treatment development effort included a small substudy that directly tested the relationship of key culture-related factors to important family processes and drug use. On the topic of immigration-related separations, our study showed that fully 16% of our Hispanic substance-abusing adolescent sample had experienced separations. Furthermore, these separations could be of long duration (up to 3 years) during a particularly vulnerable age (up to 7 years of age). Future analyses will allow us to test the relationships between these separations, the quality of attachment of parents and adolescent, and the degree of adolescent substance use and other externalizing behaviors. Our preliminary data have also pointed to the types of treatment characteristic that Hispanic parents wish to see in the treatment. Our survey of 106 parents of drug-abusing youth asked parents which of the following issues they would like to see addressed in their treatment sessions: parenting information, HIV/AIDS information, drug information, or acculturation/immigration information. The majority of parents (54%) of drug-abusing youth reported that they wanted more focus on parenting information and 38% reported wanting information on drug use. Interestingly, parents reported very little interest in HIV and immigration-related information. These findings are consistent with our observations that parents do not readily see the connection between HIV and acculturation stress and behavior problems of their youth. Implications for treatment are that we should be prepared to do more motivation enhancement around these particular issues if they appear to be central. In response to this finding, we have also removed the separate general acculturation module and instead included acculturation material as it relates specifically to the distinct module topics (e.g., acculturation relevance to parenting practices or immigration-related separations). Further, when parents were asked their feelings about a treatment specifically developed for Hispanics, 69% said they would be more likely to attend such a treatment, while the remaining parents said they would be less likely to attend (3%) or it wouldn't make a difference (28%).

Because parenting is a key area in which CIFTA places great emphasis, we want to understand more about how this looks for Hispanics; consequently, we are also testing such things as (a) whether there exists a relationship between levels of youth and parent acculturation, Hispanic parents' attitudes about speaking to adolescents about sex, and the adolescent engaging in risky sexual behaviors; and (b) whether level of acculturation of the parents is related to their parenting style (e.g., authoritarian, permissive) and involvement with school and peers.

A small randomized trial to test the efficacy of the intervention

The final step of the treatment development project included a mini-randomized trial of 24 participant families, who met the trial criteria and were randomized after intake to either CIFTA or traditional family therapy. Randomization was stratified by gender and drug use severity. Participant families in each condition were assessed at three time points throughout the course of therapy: intake and at 2 and 4 months. A final assessment at 8 months after intake was also conducted. Because of the small size of the sample, the data collected during the trial will be used to estimate (a) the preliminary indicators of the effect sizes of the CIFTA treatment model relative to traditional family therapy on engagement, retention, therapy alliance, and outcome (e.g., drug abuse and behavior problems); (b) the clinical significance of changes on indicators of outcome; and (c) the growth curves of the hypothesized family mechanisms and alliance in relation to successful outcome. Overall indicators of feasibility and acceptability are also central to this type of study.

In addition, the trial was an avenue for piloting and refining the treatment procedures developed during earlier stages of the treatment-development process. During the trial, particular attention was placed on how CIFTA is implemented and on treatment adherence of the therapists. Treatment adherence may present a particular challenge, particularly because the CIFTA model has several components (family, individual, and thematic modules) and several different modules (e.g., parenting, drug education, immigration separations, etc.). The stage I randomized trial described here is the avenue through which procedures will be refined in preparation for a larger stage II study.

Conclusions and implications for blending research and practice

In this chapter, we have argued that there is a serious shortage of empirically supported treatments for working with Hispanic drug abusers, that there is a body of research findings on culture-related variables that can inform the treatment of Hispanic drug-abusing adolescents, and that treatment-development studies are an excellent mechanism for fully integrating the diverse bodies of literature. We have also presented efforts at utilizing established scientific and treatment development methods to design and test a powerful intervention that is attractive and relevant to Hispanic drug-abusing adolescents and their families. This work is consistent with the belief that culture-related processes should be linked directly to core family and treatment processes if treatment models for minority populations are going to be enhanced (Santisteban *et al.*, 2002). The treatment-development process led to a CIFTA model that has a flexible manual and has expanded the focus of the treatment from a purely family-systems focus to one that emphasizes adolescent development, education on drug abuse and relapse processes, and culture-related content. In addition, CIFTA expanded the components of therapy from a family therapy modality to one that includes individual treatment and structured thematic modules presented in a psychoeducational format.

Currently, one of the very important areas in the field of drug abuse treatment involves the blending of research and practice. Among other efforts to bridge the gap between research and practice, NIDA has formed the Clinical Trials Network and SAMHSA has formed the Addiction Technology Transfer Centers. These efforts are attempting to bridge the gap that has existed over many years between what is known about effective treatment and what is deemed standard practice in community treatment agencies. In working with Hispanics, there is an even wider gap because of the lack of treatment models that have empirical support for their use with this minority population. It is critically important that models be tested with this population, and that models be made as user-friendly and relevant as possible for Hispanic-serving organizations, treatment providers, and Hispanic adolescents and their families. We believe that there are special aspects of CIFTA that will facilitate its utilization by front-line providers. First, there is the inclusion of thematic modules that clearly spell out culture-related processes and their specific impact on family dynamics, such as parenting and attachment, adolescent development, and drug use. This should make it easier for the drug abuse counselor to deliver family services to Hispanics in a culturally competent fashion. Second, we believe that the flexible manual allows the counselor to use good clinical decision making in the process of tailoring the treatment to the specific adolescent and family. This should lower the apprehension clinicians often express about the rigidity of treatment manuals. Third, by making drug abuse issues and processes prominent, the drug counselor can feel comfortable that the model is not assuming that family process changes alone will impact drug abuse without focusing specifically on the unique challenges they raise (e.g., triggers to use, relapse).

REFERENCES

Alexander, J. F., Holtzworth-Munroe, A., & Jameson, P. (1994). The process and outcome of marital and family therapy: research review and evaluation. In A. Bergin & S. L. Garfield (eds.), *Handbook of psychotherapy and behavior change*, 4th edn (pp. 595–630). New York: John Wiley.

American Psychological Association (1993). Guidelines for providers of psychological services to ethnic, linguistic, and culturally diverse populations. *American Psychologist*, **48**, 45–48.

Bailey, S. L. & Hubbard, R. L. (1990). Developmental variation in the context of marijuana initiation among adolescents. *Journal of Health and Social Behavior*, **31**, 58–70.

Barlow, D. H. (1996). Health care policy, psychotherapy research, and the future of psychotherapy. *American Psychologist*, **51**, 1050–1058.

Baumeister, L. M., Flores, E., & Marin, B. V. (1995). Sex information given to Latina adolescents by parents. *Health Education Research*, **10**, 233–239.

Bemak, F. & Greenberg, B. (1994). Southeast Asian refugee adolescents: implications for counseling. *Journal of Multicultural Counseling and Development*, **22**, 115–124.

Bernal, G. & Scharron-Del-Rio, M. R. (2001). Are empirically supported treatments valid for ethnic minorities? Toward an alternative approach for treatment research. *Cultural Diversity and Ethnic Minority Psychology*, **7**, 328–342.

Bernal, G., Bonilla, J., Padilla-Cotto, L., & Perez-Prado, E. (1998). Factors associated to outcome in psychotherapy: an effectiveness study in Puerto Rico. *Journal of Clinical Psychology*, **54**, 329–342.

Beutler, L. E. (1999). Manualizing flexibility: the training of eclectic therapists. *Journal of Clinical Psychology*, **55**, 399–404.

Buriel, R., Calzada, S., & Vasquez, R. (1982). The relationship of traditional Mexican American culture to adjustment and delinquency among three generations of Mexican American male adolescents. *Hispanic Journal of Behavioral Sciences*, **4**, 41–55.

Cauce, A. M., Reid, M., Landesman, S., & Gonzales, N. (1990). Social support in young children: measurement, structure, and behavioral impact. In B. R. Saranson, I. G. Saranson, & G. R. Pierce (eds.), *Social Support: An Interactional View* (pp. 64–94). New York: John Wiley.

Chamberlain, P. & Rosicky, J. G. (1995). The effectiveness of family therapy in the treatment of adolescents with conduct disorders and delinquency. *Journal of Marital and Family Therapy*, **21**, 441–459.

Chambless, D. L. & Hollon, S. D. (1998). Defining empirically supported therapies. *Journal of Consulting and Clinical Psychology*, **66**, 7–18.

Cortes, D. E. (1995). Variations in familism in two generations of Puerto Ricans. *Hispanic Journal of Behavioral Sciences*, **17**, 249–255.

Cross, T. L., Bazron, B. J., Dennis, K. W., & Isaacs, M. R. (1989). *Towards a Culturally Competent System of Care: A Monograph on Effective Services for Minority Children who are Severely Emotionally Disturbed.* Washington, DC: Georgetown University Child Development Center, CASSP Technical Assistance Center.

Dilorio, C., Kelley, M., & Hockenberry-Eaton, M. (1999). Communication about sexual issues: mothers, fathers, and friends. *Journal of Adolescent Health*, **24**, 181–189.

Dishion, T. J. & Andrews, D. W. (1995). Preventing escalation in problem behaviors with high-risk young adolescents: immediate and 1-year outcomes. *Journal of Consulting and Clinical Psychology*, **63**, 538–548.

Dishion, T. J., Capaldi, D. M., & Yoerger, K. (1999). Middle childhood antecedents to progressions in male adolescent substance use: an ecological analysis of risk and protection. *Journal of Adolescent Research*, **14**, 175–205.

Flannery, D. J., Rowe, D. C., & Gulley, B. L. (1993). Impact of pubertal status, timing, and age on adolescent sexual experience and delinquency. *Journal of Adolescent Research*, **8**, 21–40.

Foner, N., (1987). *New Immigrants in New York.* New York: Columbia University Press.

Fridrich, A. & Flannery, D. J. (1995). The effects of ethnicity and acculturation on early adolescent delinquency. *Journal of Child and Family Studies*, **4**, 69–87.

Gil, A. G., Wagner, E. F., & Vega, W. A. (2000). Acculturation, familism, and alcohol use among Latino adolescent males: Longitudinal relations. *Journal of Community Psychology*, **28**, 443–458.

Hansen, N. D., Pepitone-Arreola-Rockwell, F., & Greene, A. F. (2000). Multicultural competence: criteria and case examples. *Professional Psychology: Research and Practice*, **31**, 652–660.

Henggeler, S. W., Pickrel, S. G., & Brondino, M. J. (1999). Multisystemic treatment of substance abusing & dependent delinquents: outcomes, treatment fidelity and transportability. *Mental Health Services, Research*, **1**, 171–184.

Holmbeck, G. N., Colder, C., Shapera, W., et al. (2000). Working with adolescents: guides from developmental psychology. In P. C. Kendall (ed.), *Child and Adolescent Therapy: Cognitive–Behavioral Procedures*, 2nd edn (pp. 334–385). New York: Guilford Press.

Junger, M. & Polder, W. (1992). Some explanations of crime along four ethnic groups in the Netherlands. *Journal of Quantitative Criminology*, **8**, 51–78.

Keating, D. P. (1990). Adolescent thinking. In S. Feldman & G. Elliot (eds.), *At the Threshold: The Developing Adolescent* (pp. 54–89). Cambridge, MA: Harvard University Press.

Lambert, M. J. & Ogles, B. M. (1988). Treatment manuals: problems and promise. *Journal of Integrative and Eclectic Psychotherapy*, **7**, 187–204.

Liddle, H. A. & Dakof, G. A. (1995). Family-based treatments for adolescent drug abuse: state of the science. In E. Rahdert & D. Czechowicz (eds.), *Adolescent Drug Abuse: Clinical Assessment and Therapeutic Interventions* (pp. 218–254). Rockville, MD: National Institute on Drug Abuse.

Liddle, H. A., Rowe, C., Diamond, G. M., *et al.* (2000). Toward a developmental family therapy: the clinical utility of research on adolescence. *Journal of Marital and Family Therapy*, **26**, 485–500.

Lindahl, K. M. & Malik, N. M. (1999). Marital conflict, family processes, and boys' externalizing behavior in Hispanic American and European American families. *Journal of Clinical Child Psychology*, **28**, 12–24.

Loeber, R., Farrington, D. P., Stouthamer-Loeber, M., & van Kammen, W. B. (1998). Multiple risk factors for multiproblem boys: co-occurrence of delinquency, substance abuse, attention deficit, conduct problems, physical aggression, covert behavior, depressed mood, and shy/withdrawn behavior. In R. Jessor (ed.), *New Perspectives on Adolescent Risk Behavior* (pp. 90–149). New York: Cambridge University Press.

Lovato, C. Y., Litrownik, A. J., Elder, J., Nunez-Liriano, A., Suarez, D., & Talavera, G. A. (1994). Cigarette and alcohol use among migrant Hispanic adolescents. *Farm Community Health*, **16**, 18–31.

Luborsky, L. & DeRubeis, R. J. (1984). The use of psychotherapy treatment manuals: a small revolution in psychotherapy research styles. *Clinical Psychology Review*, **4**, 5–14.

Marin, G. (1993). Influence of acculturation on familism and self-identification among Hispanics. In M. E. Bernal & G. P. Knight (eds.), *Ethnic Identity: Formation among Hispanics and Other Minorities*. New York: State University of New York Press.

Marin, B. & Gomez, C. A. (1997). Latino culture and sex: implications for HIV prevention. In J. Garcia & M. C. Zea (eds.), *Psychological Interventions and Research with Latino Populations* (pp. 73–93). Boston, MA: Allyn & Bacon.

Minuchin, S. & Fishman, H. C. (1981). *Family therapy techniques*. Cambridge, MA: Harvard University Press.

Miranda, A. O., Estrada, D., & Firpo-Jimenez, M. (2000). Differences in family cohesion, adaptability, and environment among Latino families in dissimilar stages of acculturation. *Family Journal: Counseling and Therapy for Couples and Families*, **8**, 341–350.

Mitrani, V. B., Santisteban, D., & Muir, J. A. (2004). Addressing immigration-related separations in Hispanic families with a behavior-problem adolescent. *American Journal of Orthopsychiatry*, **74**, 219–229.

Moras, K. (1993). The use of treatment manuals to train psychotherapists: observations and recommendations. *Psychotherapy*, **30**, 581–586.

Newcomb, M. D. & Felix-Ortiz, M. (1992). Multiple protective and risk factors for drug abuse and abuse: cross-sectional and prospective finding. *Journal of Personality and Social Psychology*, **63**, 28–296.

Oetting, G. R. & Beauvais, F. (1991). Orthogonal cultural identification theory: the cultural identification of minority adolescents. *International Journal of the Addictions*, **25**, 655–685.

Onken, L. S. & Bootzin, R. R. (1998). Behavioral therapy development and psychological science: if a tree falls in the forest and no one hears it. *Behavior Therapy*, **29**, 539–543.

Padilla, F. (1997). *The Struggle of Latino/a University Students: In Search of a Liberating Education*. New York: Routledge.

Papini, D. R. & Roggman, L. A. (1992). Adolescent perceived attachment to parents in relation to competence, depression, and anxiety: a longitudinal study. *Journal of Early Adolescence*, **12**, 420–440.

Patterson, G. R. (1986). Performance models for antisocial boys. *American Psychologist*, **41**, 432–444.

Patterson, G. R., Bank, L., & Stoolmiller, M. (1990). The preadolescent's contributions to disrupted family process. In R. Montemayor, G. R. Adams, & T. P. Gullotta (eds.), *From Childhood to Adolescence: A Transitional Period*? (pp. 107–133). Newbury Park, CA: Sage.

Patterson, G. R., Reid, J. B., & Dishion, T. J. (1992). *Antisocial Boys*. Eugene, OR: Castalia.

Piaget, J. (1972). Intellectual evolution from adolescence to adulthood. *Human Development*, **15**, 1–12.

Ramos-McKay, J. M., Comas-Diaz, L., & Rivera, L. A. (1988). Puerto Ricans. In L. Comas-Diaz & E. E. H. Griffith (eds), *Clinical Guidelines in Cross-cultural Mental Health* (pp. 204–232). New York: John Wiley.

Rounsaville, B. J., Carroll, K. M., & Onken, L. S. (2001). A stage model for behavioral therapies research: getting started and moving on from stage I. *Clinical Psychology: Science and Practice*, **8**, 133–142.

Sabogal, F., Marin, G., Otero-Sabogal, R., Marin, B. V., & Perez-Stable, E. J. (1987). Hispanic familism and acculturation: what changes and what doesn't? *Hispanic Journal of Behavioral Sciences*, **9**, 397–412.

SAMHSA (Substance Abuse and Mental Health Services Administration) (2001). *Summary of Findings from the 2000 National Household Survey on Drug Abuse*. Rockville, MD: Department of Health and Social Services, Substance Abuse and Mental Health Services Administration Office of Applied Studies.

Santisteban, D., Muir-Malcolm, J. A., Mitrani, V. B., & Szapocznik, J. (2002). Integrating the study of ethnic culture and family Psychology Intervention Science. In H. Liddle, D. A. Santisteban, R. Levant, & J. Bray (eds), *Family Psychology Intervention Science*. Washington, DC: American Psychological Association Press.

Santisteban, D. A., Szapocznik, J., Coatsworth, D., *et al.* (2003). The efficacy of brief strategic/structural family therapy in modifying behavior problems and an exploration of the mediating role that family functioning plays in behavior change. *Journal of Family Psychology*, **17**, 121–133.

Schmidt, S. E., Liddle, H. A., & Dakof, G. A. (1996). Changes in parenting practices and adolescent drug abuse during multidimensional family therapy. *Journal of Family Psychology*, **10**, 12–27.

Shadish, W. R., Montgomery, L. M., Wilson, P., *et al.* (1993). Effects of family and marital psychotherapies: a meta-analysis. *Journal of Consulting and Clinical Psychology*, **61**, 992–1002.

Shoham, V. & Rohrbaugh, M. (1995). Aptitude X treatment interaction (ATI) research: sharpening the focus, widening the lens. In M. Aveline & D. A. Shapiro (eds.), *Research Foundations for Psychotherapy Practice* (pp. 73–95). New York: John Wiley.

Silove, D., Sinnerbrink, I., Field, A., Manicavasagar, V., & Steel, Z. (1997). Anxiety, depression and PTSD in asylum-seekers: associations with pre-migration trauma and post-migration stressors. *British Journal of Psychiatry*, **170**, 351–357.

Sommers, I., Fagan, J., & Baskin, D. (1993). Sociocultural influences on the explanation of delinquency for Puerto Rican youths. *Hispanic Journal of Behavioral Sciences*, **15**, 36–62.

Snow, R. E. (1991). Aptitude–treatment interaction as a framework for research on individual differences in psychotherapy. *Journal of Consulting and Clinical Psychology*, **59**, 205–216.

Straussner, S. L. A. (2001). *Ethnocultural Factors in Substance Abuse Treatment*. New York: Guilford Press.

Sue, D. W., Arrendondo, P., & McDavis, R. J. (1992). Multicultural counseling competencies and standards: a call to the profession. *Journal of Counseling and Development*, **70**, 477–486.

Szapocznik, J. & Kurtines, W. (1989). *Breakthroughs in Family Therapy with Drug Abusing Problem Youth*. New York: Springer.

Szapocznik, J., Scopetta, M. A., Aranalde, M. A., & Kurtines, W. M. (1978). Cuban value structure: clinical implications. *Journal of Consulting and Clinical Psychology*, **46**, 961–970.

Szapocznik, J., Kurtines, W., Santisteban, D. A., & Rio, A. (1990). The interplay of advances among theory, research and application in treatment interventions aimed at behavior problem children and adolescents. *Journal of Consulting and Clinical Psychology*, **58**, 696–703.

Tilton-Weaver, L. C., Vitunski, E. T., & Galambos, N. L. (2001). Five images of maturity in adolescence. What does "grown up" mean? *Journal of Adolescence*, **24**, 143–158.

Triandis, H. C., Marin, G., Betancourt, H., Lisansky, J., & Chang, B. (1982). *Dimensions of Familism among Hispanic and Mainstream Navy Recruits*. Chicago, IL: University of Illinois Press.

Tucker, M. B. (1985). USA Ethnic minorities and drug abuse: an assessment of the science and practice. *International Journal of the Addictions*, **20**, 1021–1047.

US Bureau of Census (2000). *Resident Population Estimates of the US by Sex, Race, and Hispanic origin: April 1, 1990 to July 1, 1999, with Short-term Projection to September 1, 2000*. http://www.census.gov.

Vega, W. A., Gil, A. G., Warheit, G. J., Zimmerman, R. S., & Apospori, E. (1993). Acculturation and delinquent behavior among Cuban American adolescents: toward an empirical model. *American Journal of Community Psychology*, **21**, 113–125.

Waldron, H. B. (1997). Adolescent substance abuse and family therapy outcome. In T. H. Ollendick & R. J. Prinz (eds.), *Advances in Clinical Child Psychology* (pp. 199–233). New York: Plenum Press.

Weisz, J. R. & Hawley, K. M. (2002). Developmental factors in the treatment of adolescents. *Journal of Consulting and Clinical Psychology*, **70**, 21–43.

William, J. M. & Dunlop, L. D. (1999). Pubertal timing and self-reported delinquency among male adolescents. *Journal of Adolescence*, **22**: 157–171.

Part VI

Building the future

22

The road ahead: achievements and challenges for research into the treatment of adolescent substance abuse

Howard A. Liddle and Arlene Frank

Center for Treatment Research on Adolescent Drug Abuse, University of Miami Miller School of Medicine, Miami, FL, USA

The preceding chapters have offered a grand tour of treatment science and related topics in the specialty of adolescent substance abuse. They provide evidence for the remarkable advances that have been made in understanding and treating adolescent substance abuse. These scientific and clinical developments reflect and have been propelled by changes in public perceptions about drug abuse generally, and that of youth in particular. More than ever before, in the USA and across Europe, adolescent substance abuse and related problems have come to be seen as enormous public health challenges that deserve increased attention and more informed policies from governments and jurisdictions (Burniston *et al.*, 2002; European Monitoring Centre for Drugs and Drug Addiction, 2003; Krausz, 2000; McArdle *et al.*, 2002; Plant & Miller, 2001; Rigter, 2004). This has resulted in no small part from the progressively more refined and comprehensive national and cross-national survey studies that have been carried out since the 1980s (McArdle *et al.*, 2002 and Chs. 6 and 7). These studies have documented the prevalence and varying patterns of substance use, abuse, and associated problems among adolescents of various ages and backgrounds. This is precisely the kind of benchmark information that is needed to establish national drug treatment policies for youth, set research and funding priorities, and improve service delivery, day-to-day clinical practice, and client outcomes.

The amount and quality of basic research in the adolescent substance abuse specialty has increased exponentially (Clark, 2004). Great strides have been made in elucidating the personal, familial, and environmental risk and protective factors that are related to the development of adolescent substance abuse and how these forces interact to affect the clinical course, outcomes, and post-treatment adjustment of adolescents (Ch. 2). This expanding knowledge base has established an important new reality: adolescent substance abuse is a heterogeneous, multifaceted and multidetermined disorder with antecedents in basic biology, early childhood development, intrapersonal developmental issues, family processes, and peer relations. Its clinical presentation takes many forms. For example, teens typically present for treatment with functional and developmental impairments in many realms and comorbidity is now known to be the rule rather than the exception (Ch. 13). Furthermore, on the basis of longitudinal research, substance abuse in the adolescent years is now understood to have broad and far-reaching consequences that can extend into adulthood and continue to impact numerous functional domains, including relationship, marital, and employment stability. This, in turn, has underscored the need for assessment, intervention, and prevention strategies that are similarly comprehensive, multivariate, and grounded in an understanding of developmental psychology and psychopathology (Newcomb & Bentler, 1989). Here too, impressive progress has been made.

A wide variety of valid and reliable methods and measures have now been developed for assessing the multiple problems, needs, risk factors, and protective factors evidenced by substance-abusing adolescents at specific developmental points, and tracking changes in them over time (Ch. 11). Many of these assessment tools are in the public domain and may become even more accessible to clinicians via the Internet, allowing for real-time collection and evaluation of treatment-relevant data and monitoring of client progress (e.g., Rahdert, 1990). Parallel advances have occurred in research methods and statistics so that it is now possible to examine simultaneously and longitudinally the multiple and interdependent factors that shape development and characterize the growth trajectories of individual adolescents (Ch. 3). These same data analysis models are now used to examine changes in response to treatment, as well as outcome predictors, moderators, and mediators (Huey *et al.*, 2004). The potential of these techniques has yet to be fully realized, but already investigators have begun to identify subgroups of adolescents with similar change and relapse profiles, revealing information that could lead to more targeted interventions and effective patient–treatment matching (Henderson *et al.*, 2004; Rowe *et al.*, 2004; Ch. 17).

A clear way to discern progress in adolescent treatment research is to examine the results achieved in rigorously controlled studies of specialized treatments for youth (see Brown, 2004). Although methodological flaws still recur, reviews of the literature concur that this specialty is surely moving in the right direction (Colby *et al.*, 2004) – witness the growing number of treatments for teen drug use and abuse with demonstrated efficacy (Rowe & Liddle, 2003; Waldron & Kaminer, 2004). It certainly is true that these treatments have not always been tested under conditions that give us confidence about their effectiveness in non-research settings. However, there is an accumulating body of research, some of which has attended to generalizability and transfer issues, that supports the claim for the existence of adolescent drug abuse interventions which are both effective and potentially trans-portable (e.g., Liddle *et al.*, 2002). These treatments have demonstrated effectiveness with a variety of clinical populations, including older and younger teens, males and females, teens from diverse ethnic groups, families and communities, those with a heterogeneous spectrum of drug use and abuse characteristics, and those with other impairments as well. They have also been shown to yield gains that are sustainable for follow-up periods of 1 to 4 years (Henggeler *et al.*, 2002). The effects are also broad based, including not only reductions in drug abuse and related problems, such as delinquency, aggression, and affiliation with drug using peers, but also improvements in important protective functional domains such as family and school functioning.

Process research, an important step in the evaluation and development of any treatment, has illuminated some of the mechanisms by which adolescent substance abuse interventions achieve their effects. This is a high priority area at present (NIDA, 2002a). Certain family-based treatments, for instance, have demonstrated a connection between the theory-based targets of change, such as family function-ing and parenting, and changes in target symptoms including drug use and delinquency (Huey *et al.*, 2000; Schmidt, Liddle, & Dakof, 1996). Other studies have linked core therapeutic activities, such as the development of the therapeutic alliance, with a variety of outcomes of interest (Robbins *et al.*, 2003; Robbins *et al.*, 2005; Shelef *et al.*, 2005).

Nowhere have advances in this specialty been more apparent than in the area of treatment development (Liddle, 2004; Stevens & Morral, 2002). Here, progress has been robust, diverse, and, in many cases, programmatic. A range of individual, group, school, community- and family-based interventions for adolescent sub-stance abusers have been and continue to be developed, codified into manuals, empirically evaluated, and refined in recent years (Chs. 16 and 18–21).

Several themes exemplify this work. The treatments being developed are generally well specified in terms of their connection to basic science, with interventions targeting known determinants of dysfunction, as well as known areas of health promotion and development facilitation. Increasingly, these treatments have an integrative spirit, with new models often combining theoretical premises and methods from more than a single theoretical framework (Liddle, 1999). They also are being developed with a view toward sensitivities of particular ethnic and cultural groups (Chs. 20 and 21). The newest wave of work in the treatment development area involves the attempt to adapt, transport, and test the effectiveness of research-developed interventions into regular community practice settings (NIDA, 2002b). Different versions of certain approaches, along with specialized adherence and fidelity measures (Hogue *et al.*, 1998) that compliment and work in tandem with the standardized training treatment protocols (Liddle, Diamond, & Becker, 1997), are being developed and gaining empirical support. These flexible treatment systems, in contrast to one-size-fits-all models, maximize the chances of adoption and dissemination in actual routine clinical settings. They directly address a common complaint, which is that research-based therapies lack flexibility and do not fit with the organizational structures or clinical procedures and regulations of non-research environments (Liddle, 2004).

Remaining gaps and future directions

One of the main challenges for the future is to narrow the gap further between research and practice. We have only begun to transfer lessons learned from controlled studies in research settings, with select and closely supervised clinicians and fairly homogeneous samples of adolescents, to the real-world settings where "average" community-based clinicians treat heterogeneous groups of teens under less than controlled conditions. Despite the availability of valid and reliable methods and instruments for assessing adolescent substance abuse and associated problems, treatment referral decisions and treatment plans are often not guided by, or even linked to, assessment data (Bukstein & Winters, 2004; Ch. 11). There also are a variety of barriers to the routine screening of adolescents for developing or emergent substance abuse problems, and the translation and use of developments in the area of primary care have been slow at best. It is also important to expand our perspective about the barriers to widely implementing, let alone sustaining, empirically supported treatments in community settings (Ch. 8). Essential first steps have been taken in identifying some of the clinical, organizational, and policy-level barriers to adoption. However, how best to overcome them still is not well understood, and there has been little research aimed specifically at addressing problems of workforce development, variations in treatment quality, fragmented systems of care, and lack of coordination among community agencies and providers serving adolescent substance abusers. Recent NIDA initiatives (e.g., NIDA, 2002b,c, 2003) should help in this regard. Surely more partnerships between clinicians (including pediatricians and primary-care practitioners), researchers, educators, policy makers, and funding agencies will need to be developed in order to realize fully the potential of available treatments for adolescent substance abusers.

As these initiatives proceed and as treatment dissemination efforts continue, the field will invariably have to confront a number of issues related to the contexts into which empirically supported treatments are transported. One critically important issue is the extent to which treatments for adolescent substance abusers are (or can be made) relevant to and demonstrate effects with the various racial/ethnic groups that make up the community; these groups may have unique cultural norms, values, and family characteristics and processes. While some progress has been made in this regard (Chs. 20 and 21), much remains to be learned about the effects of acculturation, traditionalism, immigration, and discrimination on the development of adolescent substance abuse and its treatment. Research is also needed to help therapists and researchers to develop cultural competencies and to tailor treatment models and manuals to take account of what we now know to be considerable diversity between and within minority groups. These challenges become all the more urgent given how marginalized and under-served some minority groups have been, and how explosive the growth of others has been as a percentage of the population (e.g., Hispanics). The NIH mandate to have "adequate representation" of minorities in all federally funded research has been helpful. However, without more minority-focused training and treatment initiatives (NIH, 2004a), work in this area will continue to lag. Even now, it is still the case that the numbers of ethnic minorities included in treatment trials are often too small to evaluate whether and in what ways the results apply to a specific minority group, let alone to distinct subgroups. Rectifying this problem may require some combination of large sample, multisite studies and multiple, small sample studies targeting specific high-need and high-risk minority groups. The availability of funding support for initiatives of these sorts is not clear, but it is certain that without increases in funding from federal and foundation sources, progress in adolescent substance abuse will be suboptimal.

Another issue relevant to the use of empirically supported treatments in community settings involves access. Getting providers to adopt such treatments is only half the battle. Adolescent substance abusers and their families must be able to access those and related services. In some instances, especially in rural communities, treatment cannot be accessed for logistical reasons. In other situations, adolescents and families in need of treatment do not access available services because of cultural taboos or the stigma of seeking help for substance abuse problems, the perception that their needs will not be met, or other barriers to treatment. While reflecting different historical periods and standards of care, the Drug Abuse Reporting Program (early 1970s), the Treatment Outcome Perspectives Study (early 1980s), and the Drug Abuse Treatment Outcome Studies for Adolescents (early 1990s) have all documented limits on access to care and shown that indeed the multiple service needs of substance-abusing teens too often go unmet (Ch. 7). We need to understand better the various sources of disparities in service delivery and in help-seeking behavior and be creative in developing solutions to the problem. For example, in rural settings, telemedicine techniques may prove especially useful, and indications are that Medicare and Medicaid are increasingly willing to pay for these services. In urban settings, more consideration could usefully be given to in-home and school-based rather than traditional office-based interventions, as has been used to good effect in some drug abuse treatment for adolescents (Henggeler, 2001) and in Student Assistance Programs (Ch. 16), respectively. For parents who themselves have substance abuse problems but who are reluctant to involve their children in any form of mental health or substance abuse treatment, behavioral couples therapy (Fals-Stewart, Birchler, & O'Farrell, 2005) may represent another viable option, and one that has considerable empirical support.

All of this suggests that we need to expand the context of care for substance-abusing teens, as well as points of access to treatment. One context in particular – the juvenile justice system – deserves and is getting more attention (see NIDA 2004a). Adolescent substance abuse and delinquency separately and together pose serious social and public health problems and enormous clinical and policy challenges (Teplin *et al.*, 2002). Recent national surveys (by the US Office of National Drug Control Policy, the National Institute of Justice and the Office of Justice Programs) have documented an alarming rise in juvenile drug offenders. If experience with adult substance abusers is any guide, juvenile and family drug courts may prove to be one useful intervention approach with these teens. However, research on such court programs has been slow in coming, and the value and essential features of these programs are in many cases unclear and in others only beginning to emerge (Belenko & Dembo, 2003). Other intervention development activities must also occur with these youths. Examinations of detention services, and the treatment that occurs in residential and long-term placement facilities, alone and in conjunction with reentry services, are areas where further studies are needed to improve the integration of empirically supported adolescent-specialized therapies into existing systems of care.

Nowhere are the issues of "context" and "access" to care more important than in confronting the challenges posed by the human immunodeficiency virus (HIV) and acquired immunodeficiency disease (AIDS); infection with HIV is increasing at an alarming rate among youth worldwide (Ch. 14). Adolescent substance abuse and HIV risk behavior (especially sexual risk behavior) are known to be related and multiply determined problems. With youth initiating sexual activity and substance use at earlier ages than ever before, it is all the more urgent that we develop, rigorously evaluate, and disseminate multilevel interventions that are effective in addressing the many facets and contextual factors that influence their risk behaviors and that the adolescents and their families can access (DiClemente, 1998).

Policy: learning how to use science to improve practice

Both juvenile delinquency and HIV/AIDS highlight another important challenge, and opportunity, facing those working in the field of adolescent substance abuse – namely, how to use the many scientific advances that have been made in this specialty to influence public policy. This chapter, and indeed this book as a whole, show how far we have come in understanding the basic science of adolescent substance abuse (e.g., drug properties, their mechanisms of action, and their impact on child development), its epidemiology (e.g., the prevalence of teen alcohol and drug abuse worldwide, comorbidity as the rule, the disproportionate number of teens in juvenile justice and mental health settings with drug problems), its multiple causes and correlates (e.g., biological, psychosocial, and familial), and its potentially serious long-term consequences (e.g., deepening substance abuse and psychopathology extending into adulthood, and involvement in criminal activity). Increasingly, and with the aid of the media, through public service announcements, private advertising campaigns, and government websites (http://www.mediacampaign.org/mg/television.html), as only a few examples, this science-based information is finding its way into the consciousness of the public at large and onto the agendas of those charged with making and implementing policies on drug treatment and prevention. More than ever before, policy makers, consumers, service providers, and researchers, both within and outside this field, are coming to view adolescent substance abuse as a major public health problem, yet one that can be understood and effectively addressed through research and through what is a growing array of empirically supported treatment and prevention approaches.

A call to action: policy development to address the research–practice gap

We believe that in order for the benefits of recent scientific advances in this specialty to be fully realized, and in order for further advances to be made, the scientific community will have to become more actively and proactively involved in the policy arena. This, in turn, will require something of a change in mindset. For too long, researchers and practitioners specializing in adolescent substance abuse have viewed the policy domain as being outside their purview. This is not surprising since the worlds of science, practice, and policy differ in many respects. As Shonkoff (2000) and Nutley (2003) have pointed out, these worlds have different values, priorities, and ways of thinking about the problems and needs of adolescents; they use different languages and are guided by different "rules of evidence;" they operate on different time scales; and they are subjected to different incentives/disincentives and pressures from different constituencies. Nonetheless, these worlds are by no means independent; in fact, they are highly interdependent.

Policy making and implementation exists in multiple contexts. Here we take policy to mean a framework, roadmap, or mandate for action with respect to program/service development, training, financing, and access that is intended to deal with a recognized public health problem (in this case adolescent substance abuse) and that is typically formalized through enactment of laws and/or regulations (per Jenkins, 2001; Shatkin & Belfer, 2004; Whiteford, 2001). Policy could be thought of as a statement of how "things ought to be." Better that policy be based on science than political expediency, ideology, or even popular cultural myths as to what can and should be done to improve the lives of young people (Shonkoff, 2000; Whiteford, 2001). Put simply, what we need is what many in the UK have termed "evidence-based" policy (Davies *et al.*, 2000; Wyatt, 2002: Young *et al.*, 2002) or what some have more modestly termed "evidence-informed/aware" policy (Nutley, 2003).

At the same time, it must be remembered that the road from research to policy is not a one-way street. The scientific community also must develop a greater appreciation for, and understanding of, the needs of policy makers, who operate under their own set of constraints and are influenced by the larger political, economic, historical, and social forces operating at any given point in time. Not the least of these constraints is the need of policy makers to answer to multiple and often competing constituencies and interest groups, who themselves are vying for a share of limited resources. They typically make decisions through a process of negotiation and compromise, and because of limits of time, money, and/or resources, they are often compelled to act even with incomplete information. Indeed, it might be said that, in addition to more evidence-informed policy, we need more policy-informed research on adolescent substance abuse, including studies (or at the least, systematic inquiries) of policy-making procedures, processes, and outcomes. The point we wish to emphasize here is that while policy influence/change and advances in the science of adolescent substance abuse are worthy ends in and of themselves, they also can be viewed as mediators of practice improvements. In fact, it is at the intersection or interface of the research, practice, and policy domains that we are apt to find the richest opportunities for lessening the research–practice divide and creating a true sense of a shared mission among scientists, service providers, and policy makers. In the remainder of this chapter, we offer some ideas about how, in practical terms, this goal can be achieved, and specifically what will be needed in order to make more progress in the area of adolescent substance abuse policy.

Doing our homework

The first task is to specify better the existing policy landscape. We know that advances in any given field are not always made in a linear or organized, "building blocks of science" manner. Advances often occur in fits and starts, by way of circuitous routes, and at variable rates. The field of adolescent substance abuse, with its many subspecialties, is no exception. For example, the progress that has been made in identifying risk and protective factors for teen substance abuse and in developing empirically supported therapies based on that framework has outpaced advances in the development and utilization of combined behavioral–pharmacological treatments, in clinician workforce training and quality control, and in widespread dissemination of science-based treatments to community settings. With a few exceptions (the California experience discussed below), advances in policy making and implementation in this area have lagged even further behind. Just as research has too frequently failed to influence the practice patterns of everyday clinicians, it also lags in its influence on policy in the youth treatment arena.

Creating a policy plan

We believe that the broad outlines of what evidence-informed policy in the adolescent substance abuse specialty would look like are becoming apparent. First and foremost, it would reflect the fact that teen substance abuse is a widespread and serious problem affecting all segments of society, including all social, economic, racial, and ethnic groups in a wide variety of Western countries (Johnston et al., 2003). In other words, using existing research that certifies the scope of the adolescent substance abuse public health problem, the policy would officially designate adolescent substance abuse as a priority area in and of itself, justifying a plan of action specifically devoted to teens. One might think that this is already a given and that it is the policy content and methods of implementation that are at issue. However, we need only look to the state of affairs with respect to child and adolescent mental health more generally to see that this is not the case. For example, in a review of international databases, Shatkin and Belfer (2004) found that only 35 of 191 member countries of the World Health Organization (WHO) (representing 18% of countries worldwide) had identifiable mental health policies that *might* impact – indirectly if not directly – children and adolescents. Only 14 of those (most in Europe, and the USA is not among them) had any sort of national policies/program plans that specifically recognized children and adolescents as a distinct group and the primary beneficiaries. Even then, the scope and adequacy of the policies varied. Some covered service delivery *and* plans for training professionals, conducting research, and educating the public, whereas others did not.

Yet in each of these areas, advances have been made that could shape or at least inform policy-making efforts. For example, in the service-delivery area, there is now ample evidence that (a) only a small minority of teens who need substance abuse services receive them; (b) many (if not most) who do, receive them as a result of entering the juvenile justice system, which itself is poorly equipped to meet their needs; and (c) the services that are available more generally are fragmented, uncoordinated, and underfunded, and they usually fail to offer the kind of comprehensive continuum of care that most consider essential for treating and preventing adolescent substance abuse problems. Effective policy would include provisions for addressing each of these.

Progress in any given area requires imagination: a plan of action. Successful models of how research, practice, and policy comingle productively to address pressing public health problems do exist; they can serve as a guide to those working in the field of adolescent substance abuse. Policy on HIV/AIDS is an excellent example (Institute of Medicine, 1989; Overseas Development Institute, 2004). Epidemiological studies documenting the scope and spread of the disease were instrumental in mobilizing public awareness and concern on a large scale: essentially putting the problem on the global map. With the assistance of front-line medical personnel, researchers from many fields came together and began to accumulate data on the routes of transmission and biology of the disease, its diverse manifestations, and fatal consequences. This helped to counter early public perceptions of HIV/AIDS as a circumscribed and largely social/moral problem. As the far-reaching socioeconomic implications of the HIV/AIDS epidemic became more apparent, researchers, practitioners, patients, and their families joined to form advocacy groups that proved highly effective in influencing policy makers and legislators to provide more funds for research on the basic science of HIV/AIDS and its prevention and treatment. Remarkable advances followed, notably including the development of potent antiviral medications that could forestall progression of the disease and its associated complications. Simultaneously, public education programs about HIV risk behaviors, including substance abuse, began to proliferate, offering real hope that further infections could be prevented.

No one would dispute the fact that there is much more to be done, especially in developing countries where access to effective HIV/AIDS treatments is still limited and where historical, political, and cultural factors combine to perpetuate the stigma of the disease and make difficult the dissemination and uptake of scientific information about how to prevent it. Nonetheless, this example shows how it is possible for scientists, service providers, policy makers, politicians, funding agencies, patients, their families, and the public at large to become mobilized and motivated to work together to confront public health problems.

At the same time, the parallels between the HIV/AIDS epidemic and adolescent substance abuse have their limits, even though both are global problems that will affect future generations. Obviously, in scope and consequences, HIV/AIDS represents a far greater public health challenge than substance abuse generally, and adolescent substance abuse in particular; in addition, the monies needed to address each are of such a different order of magnitude that they cannot really be compared. Both have had to deal with the problem of stigma, but at least today and in developed countries this problem may be worse with respect to substance abuse than HIV/AIDS.

Scientific advances in understanding how HIV/AIDS is transmitted combined with some well-publicized and poignant case examples of some of those afflicted with the virus (e.g., Ryan White, Arthur Ashe, Issac Asimov) did much to undercut the notion that HIV/AIDS results solely from voluntary moral lapses. The same has not yet occurred in the area of substance abuse. Drug use/abuse, especially among teens, is still widely seen as reflecting poor choices and as being more the fault of the adolescents than their circumstances, or as being something that "they got themselves into and should now suffer the consequences of their actions." With diseases that are more clearly recognized as such and that have the drama (in some cases promoted by Hollywood as in the case of the film *Philadelphia*) and the fatal consequences that HIV/AIDS has, it may be easier for people to overcome or set aside the stigma issues. With some notable exceptions (media campaigns by the Mothers against Drunk Driving [MADD] and the Students against Drinking and Driving [SADD] and periodic news reports of the tragic deaths of teens from overdoses or drunk-driving accidents), adolescent substance abuse is not routinely or consistently associated in the public's mind with death or disability. In fact, when licit substances (tobacco and alcohol) are involved, there is a tendency to downplay the serious consequences of their use/abuse, casting the latter as almost "normal" for teens or as "something they will grow out of."

The advocacy vacuum

These circumstances make it less likely that the kinds of influential advocacy group that have mobilized to support and raise money for treatment of and research on HIV/AIDS, and have shaped public policy in this area, would do the same for adolescent substance abuse. It is, therefore, all the more important that we in the scientific community take up that charge and act as advocates, drawing on the many scientific advances that have been made in this specialty to influence policy and generate funding for further work in both the research and the practice spheres. In fact, despite some major differences between these public health problems, they have enough in common (e.g., in their social, political, legal, cultural, economic, and scientific dimensions) that we ought to be able to use many of the lessons learned from experience with HIV/AIDS and apply them to adolescent substance abuse. Another aspect of facilitating policy change through advocacy efforts might include broadening our base of those who might serve as advocates for our issues. Although celebrities afflicted with a disease such as HIV (the case of Magic Johnson for instance) often accomplish impressive fund raising and public awareness feats (also see the history of the Scott Newman Foundation [http://www.scottnewman center.org/history/history.html] for a notable positive example in the youth drug abuse area), celebrities, given the nature of the problem we are discussing here, may not be a realistic advocacy cohort. Perhaps consideration of the potential of youths and families themselves as advocates for their own cause can yield fresh possibilities. The Youth Empowerment Movement (http://www.nllc.org/main.html), a grass roots citizen-led group, and the work in an area called Positive Youth Development (Catalano *et al.*, 2004) are examples of movements outside the classic prevention or treatment circles that might be included in our efforts to search for sources of potential influence in political and funding settings.

Another notable example of science affecting practice by way of influencing policy that has even more direct relevance to adolescent substance abuse can be found in what we term "the California experience." Over a period of 2 years, the Charles and Helen Schwab Foundation partnered with the Alcohol and Drug Policy Institute (ADPI) – a group comprising treatment providers, county administrators of substance abuse programs, researchers, and educators – combined to review the status of adolescent substance abuse treatment in California and to recommend steps that could be taken to establish a responsive system of care implementing best practices based on sound research and on collaboration among the agencies and entities, both private and public, that serve youth. The results of this remarkable effort are described in the Foundation's 2004 report, *The Need to Invest in Adolescent Treatment: Policy Recommendations for Adolescent Substance Abuse Treatment in California* (http://www.schwabfoundation.org/index.php/articles). Note the boldness and action orientation of the first part of the report's title. The report presents eight specific policy recommendations that provide a model of what can and should be done in other states and nationally to improve the lives of substance-involved young people. The following is a summary of those recommendations.

1. Establish a high level Governor's Council, comprising the heads of all state departments who work with youth, that will be responsible for the strategic planning, coordination, and allocation of resources for adolescent substance abuse treatment and will provide the technical and administrative supports needed to develop, implement, and evaluate evidence-based substance abuse services for adolescents.

2. Establish county coalitions of representatives from publicly funded youth service programs that will develop a comprehensive continuum of care for adolescent substance abusers and define the primary components needed to create a streamlined, integrated service system, will inventory existing county service capabilities and gaps, and will identify available funding resources that can be dedicated specifically to youth services.

3. Adopt and mandate adherence to state treatment guidelines for all programs that provide adolescent substance abuse services, using treatment models and interventions that research has found to be effective with youth.

4. Establish evidence-based, standardized screening and assessment protocols for adolescents who have been or are at risk for substance abuse problems, and

ensure that periodic screenings are done in the variety of settings where youth interact.

5. Establish new and sustainable funding streams specifically dedicated to adolescent substance abuse treatment.

6. Mandate that health insurance plans provide coverage for substance abuse and mental health problems that is "in parity" with that provided for other medical disorders and diseases.

7. Mandate statewide collection of a standardized set of adolescent-specific outcome measures on every teen entering substance abuse treatment to monitor their progress and ensure that the most effective treatment is being provided to them.

8. Sponsor a public information campaign to increase awareness of adolescent substance abuse as a serious public health problem that affects every community and to correct misconceptions about substance abuse that contribute to stigma and inhibit many from seeking treatment.

Particularly noteworthy is that some of these recommendations were incorporated into a recently proposed California State Senate bill, which unfortunately was not passed in 2004 because of the state's current budget crisis but may be reintroduced in the future (R. Richman, personal communication, 2004). Other private foundations (e.g., Robert Wood Johnson, Annie E. Casey Foundation, Drug Strategies [which generated a recent report on teen drug abuse and will develop a new report on juvenile justice and substance abuse]) are involved in similar efforts and in promoting their expansion through increased funding (both in-house and by the federal government) aimed at addressing substance abuse problems. The Drug Strategies report demonstrates how science has already influenced policy. In its recommendations to treatment providers, the public, and policy personnel, it highlights the importance of involving families in adolescent drug treatment as one of its nine key conclusions about needed treatment components. Reaching this conclusion would not have been possible even a few years ago. However, in a relatively short period of time, family-based treatments have come to be the most intensely and frequently researched intervention modality for adolescent drug abusers (Williams & Chang, 2000). The studies have consistently supported the conclusion that families, particularly parents or caregivers of drug-involved teens, should be involved in their treatment. The *Treatment Improvement Protocol Series* (TIPS) No. 32 on adolescent substance abuse treatment (CSAT, 1999) also shows the influence of science on policy and treatment recommendations. The 1999 edition includes major sections on family-based treatment, an area of focus virtually ignored in the previous edition of the same volume.

There are undoubtedly other examples of science influencing policy within and outside of the substance abuse field, although major reviews of what has (and has not) been done at the interface of these fields have been few and slow in coming. Yet the topic is receiving more attention in leading journals, such as *Addiction*, which in recent years has published an increasing number of articles on how science can influence substance abuse policy. One such article was the edited summary with invited commentaries (Anon., 1995) on a book entitled *Alcohol Policy and the Public Good* (Edwards *et al.*, 1994). That volume was the first product of an international review group convened under the auspices of WHO Europe specifically to assemble and examine the scientific evidence bearing on alcohol policies. As with the Schwab Foundation report, it identified a number of ways in which research can practically inform front-line policy choices.

A subsequent commentary series (Alcohol and Public Policy Group, 2003) on the successor book entitled *Alcohol: No Ordinary Commodity – Research and Public Policy* (Babor *et al.*, 2003) extended and updated that earlier discussion. Like its predecessor, this book represented a major international effort by 15 scientists specializing in alcohol abuse that reviewed the scientific evidence for and against various alcohol prevention and treatment strategies and policies. In it, the authors make the important point that evidence as to the effectiveness of a given intervention is not the only criterion for evaluating policy options. It also is necessary to consider the population reach and the political acceptability of the strategy; its applicability in various cultures and countries; and its relative costs in terms of time, resources, and money. They cite the example of policies designed to regulate the physical availability of alcohol (through sales restrictions, alcohol taxes, etc.) and to support drinking-and-driving countermeasures (such as sobriety checkpoints, lowered blood alcohol concentration limits, license suspension, and graduated licensing for new teen drivers). Not only is there strong evidence as to the effectiveness of such approaches, they also have broad reach, seem applicable in most countries, and are relatively inexpensive to implement and sustain. This makes their potential public health impact quite high and deserving of consideration as "best practice" policy options. By contrast, they see the likely impact of school-based alcohol education programs as being much lower. While shown effective in changing teens' attitudes toward alcohol, and while feasible to implement because schools provide a captive audience, such programs have produced only modest and generally short-lived effects on actual drinking behavior, rendering them not particularly cost-effective or beneficial. The impact at the population level of alcohol treatment and early intervention services is likewise seen as being somewhat limited. Despite accumulating scientific evidence that specialized alcohol treatment programs are at least moderately effective, they can only benefit the relatively small fraction of the population who seek treatment, and, therefore, are unlikely to alter problem drinking rates significantly in the population at large.

These examples from Babor *et al.* (2003) illustrate how the growing alcohol abuse research literature can be translated into a meaningful analysis of alcohol policy making, and how such an analysis can be informed by multiple scientific disciplines (in the above case by epidemiology, health-care economics, law enforcement, and education, as well as treatment and services research). The same type of review and analysis could usefully be done with respect to other substances frequently used (e.g., tobacco) and abused (e.g., cannabis) by adolescents. Particularly encouraging in this regard is the upcoming launch in the UK of a new peer-review journal, *Evidence and Policy: A Journal of Research, Debate, and Practice*. While not dealing specifically with substance abuse, this journal will be "dedicated to comprehensive and critical treatment of the relationship between research evidence and the concerns of policy makers and practitioners ... and will be international in scope and interdisciplinary in focus" (for further information see http://www.evidencenetwork.org/JournalOfResearch.html). Other organizational structures have been developed and are making progress in making the connections between research, practice, and policy come alive and yield tangible results (e.g., University of St. Andrew's Research Unit for Research Utilisation [http://www.st-andrews.ac.uk/~ruru], Reclaiming Futures [http://www.reclaimingfutures.org]. In addition a variety of governmental entities continue to support research and the enhancement of practice with science-based interventions (McKeganey *et al.*, 2003, NIDA, 2002b, 2003; Scottish Executive Effective Interventions Unit, 2003; UK Home Office Drug Strategy Directorate, 2002). All of this activity underscores the readiness of the field for further advances in evidence-informed substance abuse policy development.

Action items: recommendations to conceptualize and launch policy work

For those who would become involved in this endeavor – of bringing the science of adolescent substance abuse treatment to bear on policy – some cautionary comments are in order.

First, it is useful to keep in mind a point made earlier: the worlds of research, practice, and policy embody their own distinctive cultures. In the policy world, science represents only one point of view and frequently is not the most influential source of information (Shonkoff, 2000). Policy makers are often moved by "common sense," cultural norms, and social attitudes; they typically use scientific evidence selectively, to support an action agenda that may be based more on tradition (how things have always been done) than on data. A good example of this is the DARE program, whose efficacy was not substantiated empirically (Clayton *et al.*, 1991) but was kept in place because communities strongly supported it, because it "made sense," and because people liked the fact that police delivered the intervention, reinforcing the idea that scare tactics or at least an authoritarian, antidrug posture could prevent teen drug use. To enhance the likelihood that scientific evidence will be used in determining whether to adopt or continue (or not) a program such as the Drug Abuse Resistance Education (DARE) program, researchers cannot be purists in the sense of construing science only as the furthering of knowledge, and evidence only as established facts or theories. Informed hypotheses and reasonable inferences drawn from still incomplete information also can serve as "evidence" and science can legitimately be used to support advocacy – especially on behalf of children and adolescents, who generally have no direct political or economic influence and only limited rights. Advocacy is not something we should or need to shy away from. As Nutley (2003) and others have pointed out, the uptake of research findings by practitioners and policy makers is more likely to occur when those findings have strong advocates.

Second, even the most committed and advocacy-minded researchers in this field will have to face numerous challenges to taking action. In particular, they will have to compete with other constituencies and interest groups for legislators' attention, for the public's support, for governmental initiatives, and of course for funding. They will have to formulate a strategic plan and clearly communicate that plan in a way that is tailored and relevant to the needs of the policy community. They will have to go beyond existing dissemination efforts and partner with diverse groups to explore how scientific findings can be adapted to local practice contexts and different policy forums (see Gregrich, 2003, p. 235, "The importance of forum"). They will have to realize that not everything is possible all at once or at all times, that windows of opportunity for policy action will open and close, and that timing their initiatives accordingly will be critical. They will have to understand what the landscape of policy intervention work is like and also they will need to have their own "manual," something that may not be unlike how interventionists think of therapy manuals. Examples of manuals (Walter, Nutley, & Davies, 2003) and frameworks for action (Addiction Technology Transfer Centre Network, 2004; Nutley, Walter, & Davies, 2002) exist, and these excellent guides should be studied and adapted according to local needs and intentions. Finally, they will have to ask and answer some hard questions about the stage of development that the specialty of adolescent substance abuse has reached and the scientific "product(s)" that should be chosen for advocacy. Which research in this specialty is sufficiently developed and robust to present and use in policy forums? What are the bottom-line conclusions and recommendations we will offer and how have these been achieved? In a frank and practical presentation of "do's and don'ts" to researchers interested in impacting the world of policy, Gregrich (2003) focused not only on the quality of findings but also on the implementation barriers of findings for the average policy maker or policy influencer. He noted (p. 234) that "research is not often undertaken, or reported in a manner that directly takes into account the resource limitations faced by policy makers and practitioners." Gregrich also observed (p. 234) that improvements can be made in the very nature of research that seeks to impact policy. "Research is often not undertaken, or reported, in a manner that addresses the most pressing questions facing policy makers." Clearly these tasks are complex, and success in policy influence can only come from organized, intelligent, and broad-based effort. A concrete action step would be to follow what many fields and specialties have done in an effort to organize and summarize findings in a field at critical points in its development. Consensus conferences are a well-defined way of addressing a research area's contributions and gaps, and thus its policy implications and possibilities. Can the specialty of adolescent substance abuse, particularly in the light of its international attention, support a consensus conference in the same way that a NIH consensus event (2004b) was held on the topic of violence prevention? (Other models also exist, e.g., Edwards' [1997] discussion of the *European Conference on Health, Society and Alcohol.*)

Third, it must be recognized that our work does not end when policy is finally made and enacted into law or regulations. It is not enough to persuade policy makers through the use of research findings to mandate provision of particular services for adolescent substance abusers. We also must work to ensure that such policy mandates are effectively implemented, maintained over time, and further modified as teens' needs change and as new research findings emerge. As Shonkoff (2000, p. 185) pointed out, "Inconsistent implementation and variable quality control threaten any enterprise, regardless of its goals and demonstrated efficacy." To guard against this will require more attention by the adolescent substance abuse research community to what has been an underdeveloped area – namely, program evaluation. Especially in this era of limited resources, the public expects and public officials demand that allocated funds are well spent and that the institutions or programs receiving them are held accountable for how they are spent. Although there are exemplars in some jurisdictions, for example some states in the USA (Williams, 2005), it has been noted (see Little Hoover Commission, 2003) that the infrastructure needed to support program evaluation in this field is sorely lacking. We simply do not have uniform systems for tracking and monitoring the quality and effectiveness of programs serving adolescent substance abusers that are applicable across the various agencies and organizations involved in delivering these services. Most areas do not even have a common set of core outcome indicators by which to assess the performance of programs within that locality relative to their own objectives. The scientific community and policy-focused reports such as that issued by Drug Strategies (2003) can help to change this state of affairs. Again, however, this will require that researchers expand their horizons. Imagination and hard work are required. For example, the tasks that will need to be done in order to make progress may include activities such as the capacity to reach out to program administrators, not only to provide input to them but to seek input from them (as in the Clinical Trials Network [NIDA, 2004b]). It is likely that new publications and meeting contexts (as well as new kinds of meeting) will also be required, where the intersection of policy, research, and practice can be addressed.

Even with these cautionary comments in mind, there are immediate concrete steps that we can take to get more involved in the policy arena and to promote the development of evidence-informed policy with respect to adolescent substance abuse treatment and research.

Fact-finding

First and foremost, we need to do our homework and become aware. Significant literature sources exist (Neilson, 2001) and should be accumulated and studied. The adolescent substance abuse specialty is behind others in understanding the basics of policy making and implementation. We need to familiarize ourselves with policy procedures, processes, and expectable outcomes: the what, where, when, how, by whom, and to what end questions, drawing on successful models from various fields. Resources abound. We need only access them. For example, all of the major professional organizations involved in adolescent substance abuse treatment and research (e.g., the American Psychological Association, American Psychiatric Association, American Academy of Child and Adolescent Psychiatry) now have offices and websites specifically dedicated to helping scientists to learn about and partici-pate in the policy-making process (see http://www.apa.org/ppo/ppan/piguide.html, http://www.psych.org/advocacy_policy/leg_issues/research.cfm, http://www.aacap.org/legislation/ul.htm). They all offer written guidelines on how to communicate and work effectively with legislators to promote evidence-based policies and treatment options. They also issue periodic reports on particular substance abuse problems that need governmental attention (e.g., increasing treatment capacity for juvenile drug offenders, making screening for drug and alcohol problems a routine part of primary care and emergency room visits, etc.), as well as regular "action alerts" that serve to notify professionals in this field of current or pending policy and funding initiatives that urgently need the support of or input from the scientific community. In addition to these resources, and those available from NIDA, NIAAA, CSAT and the SAMHSAA Center for Substance Abuse Protection, there are a growing number of private, ad hoc organizations that have been formed to advance the adoption of evidence-based substance abuse policies. They too have a wealth of information at their disposal. Two notable examples are the Physicians and Lawyers for National Drug Policy, a non-partnership (funded by the Justice, Equality, Human Dignity and Tolerance Foundation, the Robert Wood Johnson Foundation, and the Charles and Helen Schwab Foundations [http://www.plndp.org]), and Join Together, a project of the

Boston University School of Public Health supporting community-based efforts to reduce and prevent substance abuse and crime (http://www. jointogether.org). Each of these organizations and offices have links to key consumer groups that are involved at the grassroots level in advocating for increased funding of services and research aimed at improving the lives of teens with drug and alcohol problems. Successful efforts such as the recent testimony given on adolescent drug abuse problems should be well publicized, written up, followed up, and evaluated in terms of their impact (American Psychological Association, 2004).

Political strategy 101: build coalitions

A second step that we can take to influence policy in this specialty is to build coalitions. The Physicians and Lawyers for National Drug Policy is an excellent example of this. Originally made up only of physicians, it now includes both physicians and lawyers, who, rather than squaring off as opponents in debates over national drug policies, have joined forces in a common cause to advance evidence-based substance abuse policies. That experience shows how it is possible to implement a suggestion made by MacIntyre (1997) – namely that professionals should form strategic partnerships and claim the "high ground" in policy discussions by avoiding professional turf issues. Another group of professionals who have similarly crossed disciplinary lines and banded together to work for improvements in the science and practice of adolescent substance abuse treatment is the Society for Adolescent Substance Abuse Treatment Evaluation (SASATE http://www.chestnut. org/LI/APSS/SASATE/). In addition to these coalitions of professionals, we can (and should) work to build coalitions with the adolescents and families who will be most directly affected by policy change. The fact that family-based therapies for adolescent substance abusers have gained widespread acceptance and empirical support presents obvious opportunities for coalition building with their parents similar to that which has been created by the National Alliance for the Mentally Ill, a potent consumer advocacy group for mental health issues. Mobilizing and partnering with the families of adolescent substance abusers is apt to be especially useful because, as MacIntyre (1997) also has pointed out, they are often seen by legislators as being more objective and less self-serving than scientists, and better representing the community of citizens/voters that legislators ultimately must answer to at election time. Ryder's (1996) estimation of the constituent ingredients of the policy-influencing process applies to this part of our discussion.

The adoption of policies in the public arena is essentially a political process. This is often not scientific, but neither does it exclude science. By understanding the politics of the policy process, and that this is a process with discernible stages, researchers can learn to work with it, thus raising the probability that policies on alcohol and other drugs will contribute to "the public good" (Ryder, 1996).

Plan strategically

Obviously, in order for such coalitions to be effective, it will be necessary to develop a common agenda and strategic plan specifying the short- and long-term goals we hope to achieve and how we might achieve them. The chapters in this book provide a good framework for action, but there is more that can be done to translate the scientific advances made to date into a viable strategic plan for the future. For example, in addition to pooling our knowledge and resources, it will be necessary to decide which "battles" need and should be waged first, and by whom. It is unrealistic to expect that most researchers and service providers, who already are busy (and getting paid) to do research and practice, will also make policy work a central part of their jobs. A more reasonable and we believe attainable goal is to identify and empower those individuals or groups in this specialty who would be willing to do some of the "heavy lifting." This might include activities such as working with legislators; being available to offer congressional testimony; speaking to the media; serving on local, state, or national boards or commissions that make policy; or simply preparing and distributing brief "fact sheets" on key issues related to adolescent substance abuse treatment and research. Treatment-development activities now proceed along reasonably systematic and, to some extent, stage-specific lines (e.g., Kazdin, 1994). Just as a process of treatment development can be articulated, a process of policy development can be and has been articulated (Hogwood & Gunn, 1984). Ryder (1996) offers an eight-stage process (agenda setting, issue filtration, issue definition, forecasting, options analysis, objective setting, monitoring, and maintenance/succession termination) by which research can influence government policies. We await application of policy-development procedures and indeed protocols to have the same influence in the adolescent drug treatment specialty.

Link to other initiatives

We make the above recommendation with full recognition that no one individual or group can do everything, or do it alone; which brings us to the fourth step that we in the scientific community can take to become more involved in and have an influence on policy making. We can link into and build upon other ongoing initiatives that already are having an impact on policy and are helping to bridge the gap between research and practice. Some excellent examples of this are the Reclaiming Futures and workforce development initiatives of the Robert Wood Johnson Foundation and Drug Strategies' new initiative on juvenile justice. Other examples include the NIDA (2004b) Clinical Trials Network, which through a nationwide partnership of scientists and practitioners is moving evidence-based substance abuse treatments into community settings. The more recently launched Criminal Justice–Drug Abuse Treatment Studies cooperative with NIDA is trying to do the same with adult and adolescent criminal justice populations (see www.cjdats.org). The CJ-DATS studies are aiming for (criminal and juvenile justice) systems-level change, as is the Reclaiming Futures initiative and the Charles and Helen Schwab Foundation project. Of course, the more that the results of those efforts and their policy implications are disseminated in public forums and in publications in journals with diverse readerships, the more likely it is that additional support for similar efforts will be forthcoming.

Train the next generation

Fifth, we can seek ways to incorporate policy issues and practices into our training programs. It currently is the case that outside of schools of public health and some social work programs, academic courses on policy analysis and the connection between policy and practice or research are rare. In non-academic settings, opportunities for learning about policy processes are equally if not more limited, and few trainees have the time or wherewithal to take advantage of those that do exist, especially given the many other skills and expanding knowledge base that they are expected to master. Even training directors may not be aware of opportunities that exist in this area, such as the American Psychological Association's public interest policy internship program, the purpose of which is "to provide graduate students with first-hand knowledge of the ways in which psychological research can inform public policy and the roles that psychologists can play in its formulation and implementation" (see http://www.apa.org/ppo/funding/pifell.html; also see the American Psychological Association Congressional Fellowship Program [http://www.apa.org/ppo/funding/congfell.html] as another model of facilitating skill in policy intervention efforts).

In our role as educators of the next generation of researchers in substance abuse, we can help to change this state of affairs by at least introducing policy study and analysis into our training curriculum. The teaching of activism in social policy for professionals is a bona fide specialty with a diverse and practically oriented literature (Pawar, 2004). Much has been done to good effect with health-care economics (http://www.healthpolicyscholars.org/). While once the province of select groups of health-services researchers, training in cost analysis has become more common throughout the substance abuse field. This, in turn, has spawned more interest in and research on the cost-effectiveness and cost–benefits of substance abuse treatment, providing policy makers with the kind of data that they desperately need. Training in other policy-related matters could be equally useful and have the added benefit of enticing more new investigators to enter this specialty by showing how their research can make a real difference in the lives of young people with drug and alcohol problems. As it is, the cohort of researchers going into this specialty is small and not keeping pace with what is needed to advance the science and practice of adolescent substance abuse treatment (http://www.iom.edu/project.asp?id=5084).

Seek more funding

Last, but by no means least, we can intensify our efforts to locate and obtain more funding for research into adolescent substance abuse treatment. Again there are a variety of resources to draw on. Examples include FundSource, an internet search tool created with support from the National Science Foundation and the American Psychological Association to help behavioral and social scientists to find research funding (http://www.decadeofbehavior.org/fundsource), and the American Association for the Advancement of Science's internet guide to organizations and advocacy groups (like Research!America) that are devoted to expanding and strengthening funding for health-care research and education (http://www.aaas.org/spp/cstc/wwc/resgroups.htm). Traditionally, efforts to secure more money for this specialty have revolved around lobbying for increases in the budgets of NIDA, NIAAA, and CSAT. While highly successful, we have to some extent overlooked other potential funding sources, such as private philanthropic organizations like the Robert Wood Johnson Foundation, which has long been committed to funding substance abuse research and the study of public policies and programs that are most effective in decreasing teen substance abuse. In a recent paper posted online, Bond, Peck, and Scott (2004) provide a primer on the role that philanthropy in general, and various charitable foundations in particular, have played and can play in promoting the conduct and dissemination of evidence-based health-care research. They readily acknowledge that the funds involved will never match those available from public, governmental agencies. However, they note that Kenneth Shine, President of the Institute of Medicine, has commented that private organizations have a unique capacity to invest in research that is "risky" or politically unpopular (as research on teen drug abuse is often considered to be) and to augment and support further leverage of federal research dollars so that they are utilized to maximum effect.

The road ahead: policy as the missing link between research and practice

The aim of this book was to present some of the most interesting and important scientific advances in adolescent drug abuse treatment. We also wanted to highlight key, and in some cases unresolved, issues in the field. On many, or perhaps most, occasions, these issues have involved basic science, methodological, or treatment development topics. The issue highlighted in this final chapter is that policy and politics are topics and areas of work that are underrepresented in our specialty. The numerous advances and developments in the specialty are being translated into practice settings but as yet they have been insufficiently recognized or utilized in the relevant policy circles. This final chapter's basic premise is that policy work on behalf of the specialty can be the next big advance in the field. Many articles and conferences have been held that bemoan the research–practice gap. Adding the domain of policy to the research–practice framework transforms the current conceptual paradigm about this gap. It presents a new way of thinking about this issue and adds a concrete set of alternatives to narrow it and make research and practice interact more productively.

We end with the words of Professor Carol Weiss, a pioneer in the area of how science can be utilized to influence and make effective public policy. Weiss (1977) believed that research must be accessible to policy makers, to the network or web of people that are in the loop of policy making (generally more broad than one first imagines). Weiss noted that research and evidence is best understood as a contributor to a policy decision, but it is rarely the single source of motivation or justification. Evidence-based policy formation, a dynamic process in which decisions are informed by research, is part of a complex and rich web or network of people, institutions, historical precedent, and contemporary circumstances. Weiss' contextual, multidimensional view (1998) offers excellent counsel as we enter into the next phase of development in our complex and rapidly changing specialty.

Governments do not use research directly very often, but research helps by allowing people to reconsider issues; it helps them to think differently, to reconceptualize what the problem is and how prevalent it is, to discard some old assumptions, and to abandon old myths. It takes time and reconceptualization before research actually leads to a change in policy. In the meantime, many other things happen. So it is very hard to say that social science triggered a particular change. There had to be a lot of supporting and reinforcing conditions in place. A good example is the role of women in society. In the 1950s and 1960s, sociologists studied women in the professions and showed that women were not being treated equally. They were being held back: not being made partner in law firms and so on. Research uncovered all of these situations and the dynamics of the problem. However, it was not until the women's movement came along and mobilized support for change that something happened. Research alone did not lead to a change in policy. However, research and activism supported each other and resulted in change.

REFERENCES

Addiction Technology Transfer Center Network (2004). *The Change Book: A Blueprint for Technology Transfer*. Kansas City, KA: Addiction Technology Transfer Center of the Substance Abuse and Mental Health Services Administration. Retrieved October 29, 2004, from http://www.nattc.org/pdf/The_Change_Book_2nd_Edition.pdf.

Alcohol and Public Policy Group (2003). Summary and commentary on the WHO report, *Alcohol: No ordinary commodity. Addiction*, **98**, 1343–1367.

Anon. (1995), The policy implications. [An edited version of Ch. 10 of *Alcohol Policy and the Public Good.*] *Addiction*, 90, 173–203.

American Psychological Association (2004). *APA Fellows Testify on Adolescent Substance Abuse.* Retrieved October 29, 2004, from http://www.apa.org/ppo/issues/samhsahrg04.html.

Babor, T. F., Caetano, R., Casswell, S., *et al.* (2003). *Alcohol: No Ordinary Commodity – Research and Public Policy.* Oxford: Oxford University Press.

Belenko, S. & Dembo, R. (2003). Treating adolescent substance abuse problems in the juvenile drug court. *International Journal of Law and Psychiatry*, **26**, 87–110.

Bond, E. C., Peck, M. G., & Scott, M. (2004). *The Future of Philanthropic Support for Medical/Health Research.* Washington, DC: American Association for the Advancement of Science. Retrieved October 29, 2004, from http://www.aaas.org/spp/cstc/pne/pubs/fundscience/papers/bond.htm.

Brown, S. A. (2004). Measuring youth outcomes from alcohol and drug treatment. *Addiction*, **99**(Suppl. 2), S38–S46.

Bukstein, O. G. & Winters, K. (2004). Salient variables for treatment research of adolescent alcohol and other substance use disorders. *Addiction*, **99**(Suppl. 2), S23–S37.

Burniston, S., Dodd, M., Elliott, L., Orr, L., & Watson, L. (2002). *Drug Treatment Services for Young People: A Research Review.* Edinburgh: Effective Interventions Unit, Substance Misuse Division, Scottish Executive.

Catalano, R. F., Berglund, M. L., Ryan, J. A. M., Lonczak, H. S., & Hawkins, J. D. (2004). Positive youth development in the United States: research findings on evaluations of positive youth development programs. *Annals of the American Academy of Political and Social Science*, **591**, 98–124.

Clark, D. M. (2004). Developing new treatments: on the interplay between theories, experimental science and clinical innovation. *Behaviour Research and Therapy*, **42**, 1089–1104.

Clayton, R. R., Cattarello, A., Day, L. E., & Walden, K. P. (1991). Persuasive communication and drug abuse prevention: an evaluation of the DARE program. In L. Donohew, H. Sypher, & W. Bukosi (eds.), *Persuasive Communication and Drug Abuse Prevention* (pp. 195–313). Hillside, NJ: Lawrence Erlbaum.

Colby, S. M., Lee, C. S., Lewis-Esquerre, J., Esposito-Smythers, C., & Monti, P. M. (2004). Adolescent alcohol misuse: methodological issues for enhancing treatment research. *Addiction*, **99**(Suppl. 2), S47–S62.

CSAT (Center for Substance Abuse Treatment) (1999). *Treatment of Adolescents with Substance Abuse Problems.* [*Treatment Improvement Protocol Series*, No. 32.] Rockville, MD: Substance Abuse and Mental Health Services Administration.

Davies, H. T. O., Nutley, S, M., & Smith, P. C. (eds.) (2000). *What Works? Evidence-based Policy and Practice in Public Services.* Bristol: Policy Press.

DiClemente, R. J. (1998). Preventing sexually transmitted infections among adolescents: a clash of ideology and science. *Journal of the American Medical Association*, **279**, 1574–1575.

Drug Strategies (2003). *Treating Teens: A Guide to Adolescent Drug Problems.* Washington, DC: Drug Strategies.

Edwards, G. (1997). Alcohol policy and the public good. *Addiction*, **92**(Suppl. 1), S73–S79.

Edwards, G., Anderson, P., Babor, T. F., *et al.* (1994). *Alcohol Policy and the Public Good.* Oxford: Oxford University Press.

European Monitoring Centre for Drugs and Drug Addiction (2003). *2003 Annual Report on the Drug Situation in the EU and Norway: Some "Cautious Optimism" but Beware of Complacency, Warns Agency.* Retrieved June 21, 2004 from http://annualreport.emcdda. eu.int/download/mainreport-en.pdf.

Fals-Stewart, W., Birchler, G. R., & O'Farrell, T. J. (2005). Family therapy techniques. In F. Rodgers, D. S. Keller, & J. Morgenstern (eds.), *Treating Substance Abuse: Theory and Technique* (pp. 140–165). New York: Guilford Press.

Gregrich, R. J. (2003). A note to researchers: communicating science to policy makers and practitioners. *Journal of Substance Abuse Treatment*, **25**, 233–237.

Henderson, C. E., Dakof, G. A., Rowe, C. L., Greenbaum, P., & Liddle, H. A. (2004). Subtypes of treatment response among adolescent substance abusers: An application of general growth mixture modeling. In *Proceedings of the 2004 Annual Meeting of the College on Problems of Drug Dependence*, San Juan, Puerto Rico [poster].

Henggeler, S. W. (2001). Multisystemic therapy. *Residential Treatment for Children and Youth*, **18**, 75–85.

Henggeler, S. W., Climgempeel, W. G., Brondino, M. J., & Pickrel, S. G. (2002). Four-year follow-up of multisystemic therapy with substance-abusing and substance-dependent juvenile offenders. *Journal of the American Academy of Child and Adolescent Psychiatry*, **41**, 868–874.

Hogue, A., Liddle, H. A., Rowe, C., Turner, R. M., Dakof, G. A., & LaPann, K. (1998). Treatment adherence and differentiation in individual versus family therapy for adolescent substance abuse. *Journal of Counseling Psychology*, **45**, 104–114.

Hogwood, B. & Gunn, L. (1984). *Policy Analysis and the Real World.* Oxford: Oxford University Press.

Huey, S. J., Henggeler, S. W., Brondino, M. J., & Pickrel, S. G. (2000). Mechanisms of change in multisystemic therapy: reducing delinquent behavior through therapist adherence and improved family and peer functioning. *Journal of Consulting and Clinical Psychology*, **68**, 451–467.

Huey, S. J., Henggeler, R., Rowland, M. D., *et al.* (2004). Multisystemic therapy effects on attempted suicide by youths presenting psychiatric emergencies. *Journal of the American Academy of Child and Adolescent Psychiatry*, **43**, 183–190.

Institute of Medicine (1989). *Confronting AIDS: Directions for Public Health, Health Care, and Research.* Washington, DC: National Academy Press.

Jenkins, R. (2001). Making psychiatric epidemiology useful: the contribution of epidemiology to government policy. *Acta Psychiatrica Scandinavica*, **103**, 2–14.

Johnston, L. D., O'Malley, P. M., Bachman, J. G., & Schulenberg, J. E. (2003). *Monitoring the Future National Survey Results on Drug Use, 1975–2003*, Vol. 1: *Secondary School Students.* [Publication No. 04–5507] Bethesda, MD: National Institute on Drug Abuse.

Kazdin, A. E. (1994). Methodology, design, and evaluation in psychotherapy research. In S. L. Garfield & A. E. Bergin (eds.), *Handbook of Psychotherapy and Behavior Change* (pp. 19–71). Oxford: John Wiley.

Krausz, M. (2000). Addictive behaviour of adolescents and young adults. *European Addiction Research*, **6**, 161–162.

Liddle, H. A. (1999). Theory development in a family-based therapy for adolescent drug abuse. *Journal of Clinical Child Psychology*, **28**, 521–532.

——— (2004). Family-based therapies for adolescent alcohol and drug use: research contributions and future research needs. *Addiction*, **99**(Suppl. 2), S76–S92.

Liddle, H. A., Diamond, G. M., & Becker, D. (1997). Family therapy supervision. In C. Watkins (ed.), *Handbook of Psychotherapy Supervision* (pp. 400–418). New York: John Wiley.

Liddle, H. A., Rowe, C. L., Quille, T., *et al.* (2002). Transporting a research-developed drug abuse treatment into practice. *Journal of Substance Abuse Treatment*, **22**, 231–243.

Little Hoover Commission (2003). *For our Health and Safety: Joining Forces to Defeat Addiction.* [Report 169] Sacramento, CA: Little Hoover Commission.

McArdle, P., Weigersma, A., Gilvarry, E., *et al.* (2002). European adolescent substance abuse: the roles of family structure, function and gender. *Addiction*, **97**, 329–336.

MacIntyre, J. (1997). Understanding your state legislator. *American Academy of Child and Adolescent Psychiatry News*, **March/April**.

McKeganey, N., McIntosh, J., MacDonald, F., *et al.* (2003). *Preteens and Illegal Drug Use: Use, Offers, Exposure and Prevention.* Glasgow: Department of Health Policy Research Program.

NIDA (National Institute on Drug Abuse) (2002a). *Improving Behavioral Health Services and Treatment for Adolescent Drug Abuse.* [RFA DA-03-003] Retrieved October 29, 2004, from http://grants2.nih.gov/grants/guide/rfa-files/RFA-DA-03-003.html.

——— (2002b). *Guidance for Behavioral Treatment Providers: Research on Knowledge and Skill Enhancement.* [RFA DA-03-005] Retrieved May 15, 2004, from http://grants.nih.gov/grants/guide/rfa-files/RFA-DA-03-005.html.

——— (2002c). *National Criminal Justice Drug Abuse Treatment Services Research System.* [RFA DA-02-011] Retrieved May 15, 2004, from http://grants2.nih.gov/grants/guide/rfa-files/RFA-DA-02-011.html.

——— (2003). *Treatment of Adolescents with Alcohol Use Disorders.* [PA 03–088] Retrieved May 15, 2004, from http://grants2.nih.gov/grants/guide/pa-files/PA-03-088.html.

——— (2004a). *Criminal Justice Drug Abuse Treatment System (CJ–DATS).* Retrieved October 29, 2004, from http://www.cjdats.org/ka/ka-2.cfm?folder_id=157.

——— (2004b). *Clinical Trials Network.* Retrieved October 29, 2004, from http://www.drugabuse.gov/CTN/Index.htm.

NIH (National Institutes of Health) (2004a). *Health Disparities among Minorities and Underserved Women.* Retrieved October 29, 2004, from http://grants.nih.gov/grants/guide/pa-files/PA-04-153.html.

——— (2004b). *Consensus Conference on Violence Prevention Among Adolescents.* Retrieved October 29, 2004, from http://consensus.nih.gov/ta/023/preventviolenceintro.html.

Neilson, S. (2001). *Knowledge Utilization and Public Policy Processes: A Literature Review.* Retrieved October 29, 2004, from http://www.idrc.ca/evaluation/litreview_e.html.

Newcomb, M. D. & Bentler, P. M. (1989). Substance use and abuse among children and teenagers. *American Psychologist*, **44**, 242–248.

Nutley, S. M. (2003). Bridging the policy/research divide: Reflections and lessons from the UK. [Keynote paper] In *National Institute of Governance Conference, Facing the Future: Engaging Stakeholders and Citizens in Developing Public Policy*. Canberra, Australia.

Nutley, S., Walter, F., & Davies, H. (2002). *From Knowing to Doing: A Framework for Understanding the Evidence-into-practice Agenda*. St. Andrews, UK: Research Unit for Research Utilisation. Retrieved October 29, 2004 from http://www.st-andrews.ac.uk/~ruru/KnowDo%20paper.pdf.

Overseas Development Institute (2004). *Bridging the Gap between Research and Policy in Combating HIV/AIDS in Developing Countries*. Retrieved December 29, 2004 from http://www.odi.org.uk/RAPID/Meetings/BR&P_HIV-AIDS/Index.html.

Pawar, M. (2004). Social policy curricula for training social workers: towards a model. *Australian Social Work*, **57**, 3–18.

Plant, M. & Miller, P. (2001). Young people and alcohol: an international insight. *Alcohol and Alcoholism*, **36**, 513–515.

Rahdert, E. (1990). *The Problem Oriented Screening Instrument (POSIT)*. Rockville, MD: National Institute on Drug Abuse.

Rigter, H. (2004). Treating cannabis dependence in adolescents: a European initiative based on current insights. In *Proceedings of a Conference on Youth Cannabis Culture: Risks and Interventions*, Berlin, November.

Rowe, C. L. & Liddle, H. A. (2003). Substance abuse. *Journal of Marital and Family Therapy*, **29**, 97–120.

Rowe, C. L., Liddle, H. A., Caruso, J., & Dakof, G. A. (2004). Clinical variations of adolescent substance abuse: an empirically based typology. *Journal of Child and Adolescent Substance Abuse*, **14**, 19–40.

Robbins, M. S., Turner, C., Alexander, J. F., & Perez, G. (2003). Alliance and dropout in family therapy for adolescents with behavior problems: individual and systemic effects. *Journal of Family Psychology*, **17**, 534–544.

Robbins, M. S., Liddle, H. A., Turner, C., Kogan, S., & Alexander, J. (2005). Early stage parental and adolescent therapeutic alliance predicts early stage dropout and completion of multi-dimensional family therapy. *Journal of Family Psychology*, in press.

Ryder, D. (1996). The analysis of policy: understanding the process of policy development. *Addiction*, **91**, 1265–1270.

Schmidt, S. E., Liddle, H. A., & Dakof, G. A. (1996). Changes in parental practices and adolescent drug abuse during multi-dimensional family therapy. *Journal of Family Psychology*, **10**, 12–27.

Scottish Executive Effective Interventions Unit (2003). *A Guide to Working in Partnership: Employability Provision for Drug Users*. Edinburgh: Effective Interventions Unit.

Shatkin, J. P. & Belfer, M. L. (2004). The global absence of child and adolescent mental health policy. *Child and Adolescent Mental Health*, **9**, 104–108.

Shelef, K., Diamond, G. M., Diamond, G. S., & Liddle, H. A. (2005). Adolescent and parent alliance and treatment outcome in multidimensional family therapy. *Journal of Consulting and Clinical Psychology*, **73**, in press.

Shonkoff, J. P. (2000). Science, policy, and practice: three cultures in search of a shared mission. *Child Development*, **71**, 181–187.

Stevens, S. J. & Morral, A. R. (eds.) (2002). *Adolescent Substance Abuse Treatment in the United States: Exemplary Models from a National Evaluation Study*. Binghampton, NY: Haworth Press.

Teplin, L. A., Abram, K. M., McClelland, G. M., Dulcan, M. K., & Mericle, A. A. (2002). Psychiatric disorders in youth in juvenile detention. *Archives of General Psychiatry*, **59**, 1133–1143.

UK Home Office Drug Strategy Directorate (2002). *Updated Drug Strategy 2002*. London: Home Office Research.

Waldron, H. B. & Kaminer, Y. (2004). On the learning curve: the emerging evidence supporting cognitive–behavioral therapies for adolescent substance abuse. *Addiction*, **99**(Suppl. 2) S93–S105.

Walter, I., Nutley, S. M., & Davies, H. T. O. (2003). *Developing a Taxonomy of Interventions Used to Increase the Impact of Research*. St. Andrews, UK: Research Unit for Research Utilisation.

Weiss, C. (1977). Research for policy's sake: the enlightenment function of social research. *Policy Analysis*, **3**, 531–545.

(1998). *Evaluation Methods for Studying Programs and Policies*, 2nd edn. Upper Saddle River, NJ: Prentice Hall.

Whiteford, H. (2001). Can research influence mental health policy? *Australian and New Zealand Journal of Psychiatry*, **35**, 428–434.

Williams, J. (2005). Presentation. In *Proceedings of the 18th Annual Conference of the Florida Mental Health Institute; A System of Care for Children's Mental Health: Expanding the Research Base*, Tampa, FL.

Williams, R. J. & Chang, S. Y. (2000). A comprehensive and comparative review of adolescent substance abuse treatment outcome. *American Psychological Association*, **7**, 138–166.

Wyatt, A. (2002). Evidence-based policy making: the view from a centre. *Public Policy and Administration*, **17**, 12–28.

Young, K., Ashby, D., Boaz, A., & Grayson, L. (2002). Social science and the evidence-based policy movement. *Social Policy and Society*, **1**, 215–224.

Index

Page numbers in *italics* refer to figures. Page numbers in **bold** denote entries in tables.

LaVergne, TN USA
10 October 2010
200154LV00002BA/1/P